STEDMAN'S

MEDICAL
EQUIPMENT
WORDS

Edited by
Catherine S. Baxter, CMT
Department of Medical Records
M.D. Anderson Cancer Center
Houston, Texas

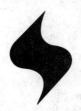

Stedman's

MEDICAL EQUIPMENT WORDS

STEDMANS

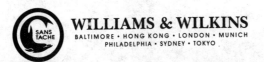

WILLIAMS & WILKINS
BALTIMORE · HONG KONG · LONDON · MUNICH
PHILADELPHIA · SYDNEY · TOKYO

Series Editor: Elizabeth Randolph
Editorial Consultant: Rhonda M. Kumm
Editor: Catherine S. Baxter, CMT
Production Manager: Cordelia Slaughter
Cover Design: Carla Frank

Copyright © 1993
Williams & Wilkins
428 East Preston Street
Baltimore, Maryland 21202, USA

Printed in the United States of America

Library of Congress Cataloging-in-Publication Data
Stedman's medical equipment words.
    p.   cm.
    Developed from the Stedman's medical dictionary, 25th ed. and supplemented by terminology found in the current medical literature.
    ISBN 0-683-07954-9
    1. Medical instruments and apparatus—Terminology.   2. Medical technology—Terminology.   I. Stedman, Thomas Lathrop, 1853–1938. Medical dictionary.   II. Title: Medical equipment words.
    [DNLM: 1. Equipment and Supplies—dictionaries.]
R123.S698   1992
DNLM/DLC
for Library of Congress   92-5510
                                        CIP
                93 94 95 96 97
      1 2 3 4 5 6 7 8 9 10

Preface

It all started with the Veress needle and an intense dedication to my profession as a medical transcriptionist. As most veteran MTs will recall, the Veress pneumoperitoneum needle had always been spelled "Verres." However, while I was doing some personal medical research during a bout of hepatitis of unknown origin, I began to notice that in texts written by those specializing in laparoscopic procedures Verres was most often spelled "Veress." My curiosity and impulsive desire to do it right kept me at the library that Saturday until the doors closed, but I was back on Sunday with yellow pad of paper in hand and lots of dimes for the copy machine. I leafed through text after text keeping a talley of Verres vs. Veress, and Veress was in the lead. Eventually, my search through bibliographies led me into the musty archives. My quest came to an end in a 1930's German medical journal which contained Dr. Veress' original article introducing his patented Veress pneumoperitoneum spring-action needle for instilling gas into the abdominal cavity.

I may as well have discovered a cache of gold!

Those same feelings of elation and satisfaction over a job well done I so vividly recall experiencing that Sunday afternoon in the archives, I have felt over and over again as I worked this past year with the supportive, talented wordsmiths from Williams & Wilkins.

Stedman's Medical Equipment Words brings to fruition my dream of providing medical transcriptionists and others in the allied healthcare arena an up-to-date, easy to use reference list of medical equipment used in hospitals, clinics, and doctors' offices. I have stacks of file cards with manufacturers' names, addresses, and 1-800 numbers that I amassed while researching my word columns for the local, state, and national members of the American Association for Medical Transcription. But, I never had the time or resources to put it all together. In stepped Williams & Wilkins, who has done what other publishers have often failed to do: listen to the professionals that comprise their market.

We have all faced this dilemma during our medical careers: How can we satisfy our insatiable appetite for spelling medical words correctly? I frequently describe medical transcriptionists to those outside the profession as artists—having a child-like curiosity, sometimes temperamental, always questing to know more, and never wanting to stop until the job is complete. I hope that the *Stedman's Medical Equipment Words* will satisfy that "need to know!"

Stedman's Medical Equipment Words was compiled primarily from manufacturers' catalogs, FDA lists, journals, and lists provided by specialists in a particular area. Every effort was made to search and research until the editors were reasonably certain of the correctness of a particular spelling; however, there are still those words that are on the continue-to-research list. Some were included and others were held out of this edition until they could be further verified. Oftentimes, we found that the original spelling in the native tongue of the inventor had been Americanized. The decision was made to use the original spelling with proper diacritical marks noted and to cite alternate forms of spelling when appropriate.

An editorial decision was made to follow the AAMT recommendation not to use an apostrophe "s" on the possessive form of an eponym unless it is truly difficult to say properly without using an apostrophe "s," as with "Joe's hoe." Also, we attempted to consistently use the modifying form of the word placed before a noun, as in "Schnidt tonsillar forceps" or "Rankin arterial forceps." However, when referring to a particular vessel, as in the "De-Bakey-Diethrich coronary artery forceps," "coronary artery" is considered a phrase modifying "forceps" and, thus, "artery" is left as a noun. I must admit that I drew the line at using some modifying forms, such as "mastoidal," simply because it just doesn't roll off the tongue easily nor does it look right. In most instances, the AAMT standards of style were abided by.

As a final note, I hope that this reference book will assist medical language specialists in all allied healthcare fields to do their re-

Contents

Acknowledgments

"Where can we find a single, comprehensive listing of generic, trade, and eponymic medical equipment names?", we asked when we embarked on this project. The answer, we soon realized, was "nowhere." Yet many people desperately wanted and needed this information.

Development of a high-quality, comprehensive medical equipment word reference is the result of many hours of investigation, research, keyboarding, reviewing, proofreading, and editing. This would not have been possible without the hard work, determination, and expertise of many individuals.

Editor Catherine S. Baxter, CMT, has accomplished an extraordinary feat in less than a year. Of course, her years of experience and superlative word research capabilities helped!

Susan D. Dooley, CMT, also spent many hours reviewing dozens of wordlists as we entered the editing phase of the project. Before this, Susan slogged through reams of FDA data and transformed them into clean, comprehensible wordlists. Other dogged members of this team were: Sandra Manzo; Suzanne L. Minnick, CMT; Donna M. Taylor, CMT; Laurie J. Spangler, CMT; Carolyn A. Cadigan, CMT; and Dorothy Vickers.

Special thanks for this tremendous effort go to Rhonda M. Kumm, RN, MSN, editorial consultant, and the members of the Williams & Wilkins MT Advisory Board, whose expertise, ideas, and words contribute to the overall quality of this and other Stedman's word books: LaVonne Alexis, CMT; Joan Bachman; Addie M. Garner; Suzanne Minnick, CMT; Susan Pierce, CMT, ART; Laurie J. Spangler, CMT; Harriet Stewart, CMT; and Dorothy Vickers.

It is important to recognize the many sources of information used to compile this book. Dozens of equipment manufacturers provided us with catalogs and product information. The FDA Center for Devices and Radiological Health, particularly its Division of Small Manufacturers Assistance and the Registration and Listing Branch, pointed us to public information that we could use as "raw material." Several professional and medical specialty organizations were extremely helpful in identifying the most frequently performed procedures nationwide.

Chief medical residents in several clinical specialties provided us with lists of commonly performed procedures and related instrument words they would typically dictate. Transcriptionists, such as those mentioned above, provided us with information about terms encountered in dictation. Also, several institutions obliged our requests for equipment word information: special thanks to Brigham and Women's Hospital, Cleveland Clinic, Gurnett Hospital, Johns Hopkins University Hospital, and Shady Grove Adventist Hospital.

Elizabeth B. Randolph
Reference Division
Williams & Wilkins

Explanatory Notes

It is with great pleasure that we introduce **Stedman's Medical Equipment Words**, the first medical word resource of its kind and one that many have long clamored for, especially medical transcriptionists. If you have ever been "stumped" by an equipment term, with nowhere to turn for verification, this is the reference for you. Now, **Stedman's Medical Equipment Words** can be used to validate both the spelling and accuracy of medical equipment, device, and instrument names in all of the major clinical specialties. This extraordinary compilation of over 75,000 entries, fully cross-indexed for quick access, was built from a base vocabulary of 38,000 medical equipment, device, and instrument terms. It includes generic, trade, AND eponymic names.

This extensive A-Z list was developed from a variety of sources, including physicians, transcriptionists, hospitals, professional associations, manufacturers, government agencies, and the current medical literature. **Stedman's Medical Equipment Words** covers equipment terminology in general and plastic surgery, OB/GYN, gastroenterology, orthopaedics, radiology, neurology and neurosurgery, cardiology, ophthalmology, urology, otorhinolaryngology, and dentistry.

Medical transcription is an art as well as a science. Both are needed to correctly interpret a physician's dictation, whose language is a product of education, training, and experience. This variety in medical language means that there are several acceptable ways to express certain terms. In addition, equipment terminology is one of the hardest areas due to the lack of standards and consistency.

Stedman's Medical Equipment Words provides a thoroughly researched, reviewed, and edited guide through an often murky and perplexing area of terminology. The user will find variant spellings and phrasings for many terms. This, in addition to complete cross-indexing, makes **Stedman's Medical Equipment Words** a valuable resource for determining the validity of equipment, instrument, and device names as they are encountered.

A special feature of this book is the APPENDICES section. The most commonly performed procedures—**and their corresponding instrumentation**—are listed at the back of the book.

Alphabetical Organization

Alphabetization of entries is **letter by letter** as spelled, ignoring punctuation, spaces, prefixed numbers, Greek letters, or other characters. For example:

> **Expander mammary implant material**
> **expanding reamer**
> **Expand-O-Graft cutter**
> **expansile dilator**

In subentries, the abbreviated singular form or the spelled-out plural form of the noun main entry word is ignored in alphabetization.

Format and Style

All main entries are in **boldface** to speed up location of a sought-after entry, to enhance distinction between main entries and subentries, and to relieve the textual density of the pages.

Irregular plurals and variant spellings are shown on the same line following the singular or preferred form of the word. For example:

> **speculum, pl. specula**
> **curette, curet**
> **Fyodorov, Federov, Fydorov, Fyoderov**
> **lacrimal, lachrymal**

Some variants are listed separately, indicating the preferred spelling where subentries are to be found:

> **erisophake** (var. of **erysiphake**)
> **erysiphake, erisophake**
> > Barraquer e.
> > Bell e.
> > Castroviejo e.
> > etc.

Wherever possible, abbreviations that appear in equipment terms are separately defined and cross-referenced. For example:

ACS
> Alcon Closure System
>> ACS Angioject
>> ACS angioplasty catheter

Alcon
> A. Closure system (ACS)
> A. cystitome

endoscopic
> e. retrograde
> cholangiopancreatography (ERCP)

ERCP
> endoscopic retrograde
> cholangiopancreatography
>> ERCP cannula
>> ERCP catheter

The use of the possessive form in medical language remains somewhat controversial, as there is often no absolute right or wrong. In equipment terminology, usage tipped the scales. Since equipment and instrument names **usually** are referred to and appear in the nonpossessive, we have used that form throughout this reference in the interest of being consistent.

Cross-indexing

The word list is in an index-like main entry-subentry format that contains two combined alphabetical listings:

(1) A noun main entry-subentry organization typical of the A-Z section of medical dictionaries like *Stedman's*:

amniotome	**hysteroscope**
Baylor a.	ACMI h.
Beacham a.	AMSCO h.
Glove-n-Gel a.	Baggish h.
	contact h.

(2) An adjective main entry-subentry organization, which lists words and phrases **as you hear them**. The main entries are the adjectives or descriptors in a multi-word term. The subentries are the nouns around which the terms are constructed and to which the adjectives or descriptors pertain:

corneal
    c. bur
    c. chisel
    c. curette
    c. dissector

Farabeuf
    F. bone clamp
    F. bone-holding forceps
    F. double-ended retractor
    F. forceps

This format provides the user with more than one way to locate and identify a multi-word term. For example:

esophagoscope
    Jesberg e.

Jesberg
    J. esophagoscope

probe
    Geldmacher tendon-
       passing p.

Geldmacher
    G. tendon-passing probe

It also allows the user to see together all terms that contain a particular descriptor as well as all types, kinds, or variations of a noun entity. For example:

Surgitek
    S. catheter
    S. double-J ureteral
       catheter
    S. double-J ureteral
       stent
    S. Flexi-Flate II penile
       implant
    S. graduated cysto-
       scope

tube
    Abbott t.
    Abbott-Rawson t.
    abdominal suction t.
    Adson aspirating t.
    Adson brain suction t.

medium
    m. chromic suture
    m. forceps
    Gastrovist contrast m.

References

Stedman's abbreviations, acronyms & symbols. Baltimore: Williams & Wilkins; 1992.

Stedman's medical dictionary, 25ed. Baltimore: Williams & Wilkins; 1990.

Szulec, Syllabus for the surgeon's secretary, 4ed. Grosse Pointe: Medical Arts; 1990.

Tessier, The surgical word book, 2ed. Philadelphia: W. B. Saunders; 1991.

Your Medical Word Resource Publisher

We strive to provide you with the most up-to-date and accurate word references available. Your use of this word book will prompt new editions, which will be published as often as justified by updates and revisions. We welcome your suggestions for improvements, changes, corrections, and additions—whatever will make this **Stedman's** product more useful to you. Please use the postpaid card at the back of this book and send your recommendations to the Reference Division at Williams & Wilkins.

A1-Askari needle holder
AA1 single-chamber pacemaker
Aagesen
    A. disposable rasp
    A. file
AAI pacemaker
AAIR pacemaker
AAT pacemaker
Abadie
    A. clamp
    A. enterostomy clamp
    A. self-retaining retractor
Abanda drape sheet
Abbey needle holder
Abbott
    A. scoop
    A. tube
Abbott-Mayfield forceps
Abbott-Rawson tube
ABCH curette
abdominal
    a. aortic counterpulsation
      device
    a. bandage
    a. belt
    a. brace
    a. left ventricular assist
      device (ALVAD)
    a. needle
    a. retractor
    a. ring retractor
    a. scissors
    a. scoop
    a. suction tube
    a. trocar
    a. vascular retractor
abduction
    a. finger splint
    a. pillow
    a. pillow cover splint
    a. splint
    a. thumb splint
Abel-Aesculap-Pratt tenaculum
Abeli corneal scissors
Abelson
    A. adenotome
    A. cannula
    A. cricothyrotomy cannula
    A. cricothyrotomy trocar

    A. curved cricothyrotomy
      cannula
Aberhart
    A. disposable urinal bag
    A. hemostatic bag
Abernaz strut forceps
Abiomed BVAD 5000
Ablaza
    A. aortic wall retractor
    A. clamp
    A. patent ductus clamp
    A. retractor
Ablaza-Blanco
    A.-B. cardiac valve retractor
    A.-B. retractor
Ablaza-Morse
    A.-M. approximator
    A.-M. rib approximator
abortion scoop
Abradabloc dermabrasion
  instrument
abrader
    a. bur
    cartilage a.
    Dingman otoplasty
      cartilage a.
    Haverhill dermal a.
    Howard corneal a.
    Lieberman a.
    Montague a.
Abraham
    A. cannula
    A. contact lens
    A. elevator
    A. iridectomy laser lens
    A. laryngeal cannula
    A. rectal curette
    A. tonsillar knife
    A. YAG laser lens
Abrams
    A. biopsy punch
    A. needle
    A. pleural biopsy punch
    A. pleural needle
Abrams-Lucas flap heart valve
Abramson
    A. catheter
    A. hook
    A. retractor
    A. sump drain

Abramson-Allis breast clamp
Abramson-Dedo microlaryngoscope
abscess forceps
abscission needle
Absolok
    A. endoscopic clip
      applicator
    A. forceps
absorbable
    a. dressing
    a. gauze
    a. surgical suture
    a. suture
absorbent gauze
absorber
    laser fume a.
accessory
    cystoscope a.
    a. instrument
    pneumatic drill a.
ACCO
    ACCO appliance
    ACCO cotton roll
    ACCO impression material
    ACCO orthodontic appliance
ACCOR dental matrix
accordion
    a. drain
    a. graft
    a. implant
Accu-Brush
Accucare TENS unit
Accucore II biopsy needle
Accufilm articulating film
Accufix pacemaker
Accuflex impression material
Accu-Flo
    A.-F. bur-hole button
    A.-F. bur-hole cover
    A.-F. button
    A.-F. connector
    A.-F. CSF reservoir
    A.-F. distal catheter
    A.-F. distal slit-valve
      catheter
    A.-F. dural film
    A.-F. dural substitute
    A.-F. infant end catheter
    A.-F. pressure valve
    A.-F. reservoir
    A.-F. spring catheter
    A.-F. spring distal slit
      catheter

    A.-F. U-channel stripping
      cannula
    A.-F. ventricular cannula
    A.-F. ventricular catheter
Accuflo ultrafiltration system
Accu-Gel impression material
Accu-Line
    A.-L. knee instrumentation
    A.-L. surgical marker
Acculith pacemaker
Accu-Mix
    A.-M. amalgamator
    A.-M. impression material
Accu-o-Matic TENS unit
Accura hydrocephalus shunt
Accurate Surgical and Scientific
    Instruments (ASSI)
Accu-Sorb
    A.-S. gauze sponge
    A.-S. laparotomy sponge
Accu-Temp cautery
Ace
    A. adherent bandage
    A. adherent dressing
    A. elastic dressing
    A. intramedullary femoral
      nail system
    A. longitudinal strips
      dressing
    A. pin
    A. rubber elastic dressing
    A. spica bandage
    A. wire tension assembly
    A. wrap
Ace-Fischer
    A.-F. external fixator
    A.-F. frame
Ace-Hesive dressing
Ace intramedullary (AIM)
acetabular
    a. angle guide
    a. component
    a. cup
    a. cup peg drill guide
    a. grater
    a. shell guide
    a. skid
achalasia dilator
acid
    polyglycolic a. (PGA)
Ackerman
    A. clip
    A. lingual bar

A. needle
A. overdenture retention
Acland
A. clamp
A. clamp approximator
A. clasp
A. clip
A. double clamp
A. double clamp
  approximator
A. microvascular clamp
A. microvascular clamp-
  applying forceps
A. needle
A. single clamp
Acland-Banis arteriotomy set
Acland-Bunke counterpressor
ACL drill
Aclec resin
AC lens
ACMI
ACMI Alcock catheter
ACMI antroscope
ACMI bag
ACMI biopsy loop electrode
ACMI Bunts catheter
ACMI catheter
ACMI cautery
ACMI coated Foley catheter
ACMI cystoscopic tip
ACMI cystourethroscope
ACMI duodenoscope
ACMI Emmett hemostatic
  catheter
ACMI endoscope
ACMI esophagoscope
ACMI examining
  gastroscope
ACMI fiberoptic
  esophagoscope
ACMI fiberoptic
  proctosigmoidoscope
ACMI flexible
  sigmoidoscope
ACMI forceps
ACMI gastroscope
ACMI hysteroscope
ACMI laparoscope
ACMI Marici bronchoscope
ACMI Martin endoscopy
  forceps
ACMI Martin forceps

ACMI microlens Foroblique
  telescope
ACMI microlens telescope
ACMI monopolar electrode
ACMI operating coloscope
ACMI Owens catheter
ACMI Pezzer drain
ACMI positive pressure
  catheter
ACMI proctoscope
ACMI resectoscope
ACMI retrograde electrode
ACMI severance catheter
ACMI telescope
ACMI Thackston catheter
ACMI ulcer-measuring
  device
ACMI ureteral catheter
ACMI Word Bartholin
  gland catheter
Acmistat catheter
Acmix Foley catheter
acorn cannula
acorn-shaped
a.-s. eye implant
a.-s. implant
acorn-tipped
a.-t. bougie
a.-t. catheter
acoustic otoscope
Acrad HS catheter
Acrotorque bur
acrylic
a. ball eye implant
a. bar
a. bar prosthesis
a. bite block
a. cap splint
a. conformer eye implant
Dentex a.
Durabase a.
Durabase soft rebase a.
Durahue a.
Duralay a.
Dura-Liner a.
a. eye implant
Flexacryl hard rebase a.
a. graft
a. implant material
a. lens
a. mold
a. resin dressing
Setacure denture repair a.

acrylic *(continued)*
  Splintline a.
  TAB a.
  TMJ a.
  Vita-Gel a.
ACS
  Alcon Closure System
  ACS Angioject
  ACS angioplasty catheter
  ACS balloon catheter
  ACS catheter
  ACS exchange guiding
    catheter
  ACS JI4 catheter
  ACS mini catheter
  ACS needle
  ACS percutaneous
    introducer
  ACS RX coronary dilatation
    catheter
  ACS SULP II balloon
Action Eyes
Activase
activated balloon expandable
  intravascular stent
activator
  Andresen a.
  Andresen-Haupl a.
  Bimler a.
  cutout a.
  Karwetsky U-bow a.
  Klammt elastic open a.
  Metzelder modification a.
  Nuva-Lite ultraviolet a.
  palate-free a.
  Pfeiffer-Grobety a.
  Schmuth modification a.
  Schwarz bow-type a.
  Schwarz modification a.
  Wunderer modification a.
active length needle
Activitrax
  A. pacemaker
  A. single-chamber responsive
    pacemaker
  A. variable-rate pacemaker
activity-sensing pacemaker
Acu-Brush brush
Acucise ureteral cutting cautery
Acufex
  A. alignment guide
  A. arthroscope
  A. basket

A. curved basket forceps
A. drill
A. femoral guide tip
A. guide
A. handle
A. rotary basket forceps
A. straight basket forceps
A. straight forceps
Acufex-Suretac implant
Acuflex intraocular lens implant
ACUTENS transcutaneous nerve
  stimulator
Acutrol suture
Adair
  A. adenotome
  A. breast clamp
  A. breast tenaculum
  A. breast tenaculum forceps
  A. breast tissue tenaculum
    forceps
  A. clamp
  A. forceps
  A. screw compressor
  A. tenaculum forceps
  A. tissue forceps
  A. tissue-holding forceps
  A. uterine forceps
  A. uterine tenaculum
    forceps
Adair-Allis
  A.-A. forceps
  A.-A. tissue forceps
Adam and Eve rib belt splint
Adams
  A. aspirator
  A. clasp
  A. kidney stone filter
  A. modification of Bethune
    tourniquet
  A. orthodontic clip
  A. retractor
  A. rib contractor
  A. saw
Adams-DeWeese
  A.-D. inferior vena caval
    clip
  A.-D. vena caval clip
  A.-D. vena caval serrated
    clip
Adamson retractor
adaptable class III mask headgear
adapter, adaptor
  Air-Lon a.

Alcock conical catheter a.
AMSCO Hall a.
ASC torque vise a.
Bard-Tuohy-Borst a.
B-D a.
Bernaco a.
Biolas laser a.
butterfly a.
cannula tubing a.
catheter a.
catheter tubing a.
chuck a.
Coherent laser a.
coil machine a.
Cooper laser a.
Cordis-Dow shunt a.
Curry hip nail counterbore
  with Lloyd a.
cystoscope-urethroscope a.
ear suction a.
electrode terminal a.
fiberoptic cable a.
Freestyle CAPD catheter a.
Greenberg Maxi-Vise a.
Hamm electrode terminal a.
House a.
House cutoff a.
House suction a.
House suction tube a.
Hudson a.
Jacobs chuck a.
Kaufman a.
King connector a.
KleenSpec otoscope a.
Luer a.
Luer lock a.
Luer suction cannula a.
manual dermatome a.
Mayfield skull clamp a.
Merrimack laser a.
metal a.
Morch swivel a.
Neuroguide suction-
  irrigation a.
Nickell cystoscope a.
resectoscope a.
rotating a.
Sanders ventilation a.
sheath with side-arm a.
side-arm a.
sleeve a.
Storz catheter a.
Storz fiberoptic cable a.

suction a.
T-a.
terminal electrode a.
tubing a.
Universal T-a.
venous Y-a.
ventilation a.
Venturi ventilation a.
Wullstein chuck a.
Xanar laser a.
adapter-stopcock
  arterial a.-s.
Adaptic
  A. gauze dressing
  A. II dental restorative
    material
  A. non-adherent dressing
adaptometer
adaptor (*var. of* adapter)
Ada scissors
Addix needle
A-Dec
  A.-D. amalgamator
  A.-D. handpiece
adenoid
  a. curette
  a. cutter
  a. forceps
  a. punch
adenotome
  Abelson a.
  Adair a.
  a. blade
  Box a.
  Box-DeJager a.
  Breitman a.
  Cullom-Mueller a.
  Daniel a.
  direct-vision a.
  guillotine a.
  Kelly a.
  Kelly direct vision a.
  LaForce a.
  LaForce-Grieshaber a.
  LaForce-Stevenson a.
  LaForce-Storz a.
  Mueller-LaForce a.
  Myles a.
  Myles guillotine a.
  reverse a.
  Shambaugh a.
  Shambaugh reverse a.
  Shulec a.

adenotome *(continued)*
Sluder a.
St. Clair-Thompson a.
Stevenson-LaForce a.
Storz-LaForce a.
Storz-LaForce-Stevenson a.
V. Mueller-LaForce a.
Aderer alloy
Ad-Hese-Away dressing
adhesive
a. absorbent dressing
a. bandage
Bond-Eze bond a.
Brimms Denturite
denture a.
Chewrite denture a.
Dentlock denture a.
a. drape
a. dressing
Endslip denture a.
Fasteeth denture a.
Firmdent denture a.
Fixodent denture a.
Klutch denture a.
MDS a.
Orahesive denture a.
Orthomite II a.
Perma-Grip denture a.
a. plastic drape
Plastodent dental
impression a.
Rigident denture a.
Secure denture a.
Silastic medical a.
silicone a.
a. silicone implant
Staze denture a.
Suxion denture a.
adjustable
a. breast implant
a. headrest
a. skull traction tongs
a. vaginal stent
Adjust-A-Flow colostomy irrigation kit
Adjusta-Rak
A.-R. hanger
Adkins strut
Adler
A. attic ear punch
A. bone forceps
A. forceps
A. punch forceps

A. tripronged lens error
loop
Adler-Kreutz forceps
Adler loop
adnexal forceps
adolescent vaginal speculum
adrenal medullary implant
Adson
A. aneurysm needle
A. arterial forceps
A. aspirating tube
A. bayonet dressing forceps
A. bipolar forceps
A. blunt dissecting hook
A. bone rongeur
A. brain clip
A. brain-exploring cannula
A. brain forceps
A. brain hook
A. brain retractor
A. brain suction tube
A. bur
A. cannula
A. cerebellar retractor
A. chisel
A. clamp
A. clip
A. clip-applying forceps
A. clip-introducing forceps
A. conductor
A. cranial rongeur
A. cranial rongeur forceps
A. dissecting hook
A. dissector
A. drainage cannula
A. dressing forceps
A. drill
A. drill guide
A. drill guide forceps
A. dural hook
A. dural knife
A. dural needle holder
A. dural protector
A. elevator
A. enlarging bur
A. exploring cannula
A. forceps
A. ganglion scissors
A. Gigli-saw guide
A. headrest
A. hemostat
A. hemostatic forceps
A. hypophyseal forceps

A. knot tier
A. knot tier hook
A. laminectomy chisel
A. microforceps
A. monopolar forceps
A. needle
A. needle holder
A. neurosurgical suction tube
A. perforating bur
A. periosteal elevator
A. pickup
A. retractor
A. rongeur
A. scalp clip
A. scalp clip-applying forceps
A. scalp hemostasis clip
A. scalp needle
A. scissors
A. sharp knife
A. speculum
A. spiral drill
A. splanchnic retractor
A. straight bipolar forceps
A. suction tube
A. suture needle
A. thumb forceps
A. tissue forceps
A. tooth forceps
A. twist drill
A. Vital tissue forceps
Adson-Beckman retractor
Adson-Biemer forceps
Adson-Brown
A.-B. clamp
A.-B. forceps
A.-B. tissue forceps
Adson-Callison
A.-C. forceps
A.-C. tissue forceps
Adson-Love periosteal elevator
Adson-Mixter
A.-M. forceps
A.-M. neursurgical forceps
Adson-Murphy
A.-M. needle
A.-M. trocar point needle
Adson-Rogers
A.-R. cranial bur
A.-R. perforating drill
Adsorba hemoperfusion cartridge

adult
a. laryngoscope
a. retractor set
a. retractor set ring
a. reverse-bevel laryngoscope
a. sigmoidoscope
Advanced Medical Systems fetal monitoring system
advancement
a. forceps
a. needle
Advent Flurofocon contact lens
adventitial bed
AE-60-I-2 implantable pronged unipolar electrode
AE-60-K-10 implantable unipolar endocardial electrode
AE-60-KB implantable unipolar endocardial electrode
AE-60-KS-10 implantable unipolar endocardial electrode
AE-85-I-2 implantable pronged unipolar electrode
AE-85-K-10 implantable unipolar endocardial electrode
AE-85-KB implantable unipolar endocardial electrode
AE-85-KS-10 implantable unipolar endocardial electrode
Aebli
A. corneal scissors
A. corneal section scissors
A. tenotomy scissors
Aebli-Manson scissors
AEC pacemaker
Aequitron pacemaker
Aero-flo tip catheter
Aeroflow syringe
aeroplane splint
Aeroplast dressing
AES Amplatz guide wire
Aesculap
A. drill
A. forceps
A. needle holder
A. traction bow
Aesculap-Pratt tenaculum
AFO
ankle-foot orthosis
AFO brace
AFP pacemaker
AF tube
Agarloid impression material

AG Bovie electrosurgical unit
AGC
    AGC Biomet total knee system
    AGC dual-pivot resection guide
    AGC knee program implant
    AGC Modular Tibial II component
    AGC porous anatomic femoral component
    AGC unicondylar knee component
Agee 4-pin fixation device
Aggressor meniscal blade
agility drill
Agnew
    A. canaliculus knife
    A. keratome
    A. needle
    A. splint
    A. tattooing needle
Agosteril dressing
agraffe clamp
Agrikola
    A. eye speculum
    A. lacrimal sac retractor
    A. retractor
    A. speculum
Agris rasp
AgX antimicrobial Foley catheter
Ahlm
Ahlquist-Durham
    A.-D. clip
    A.-D. embolism clamp
    A.-D. vena caval clip
AICD
    automatic implantable cardioverter-defibrillator
    AICD device
    AICD pacemaker
aid
    air-conduction hearing a.
    Argosy in-the-ear hearing a.
    Audibel ear a.
    Audicraft VIP-I hearing a.
    Audionics PB Max hearing a.
    Audiotone hearing a.
    Audivisette hearing a.
    Auriculina hearing a.
    Bansaton behind-the-ear hearing a.

    behind-the-ear hearing a.
    bone-conduction hearing a.
    Crystal Tone I in-the-ear hearing a.
    Dahlberg hearing a.
    Ear-Tronics hearing a.
    Euroton hearing a.
    eyeglass hearing a.
    Fonix hearing a.
    Giller hearing a.
    hearing a.
    in-the-ear hearing a.
    Jade Audio-Starr hearing a.
    Lion hearing a.
    Listening Glass hearing a.
    Magnatone hearing a.
    MasterCraft hearing a.
    Mecon-I hearing a.
    Metavox hearing a.
    Microson hearing a.
    Nuway in-the-ear hearing a.
    Omnitone hearing a.
    Ovation in-the-ear hearing a.
    Pacific Coast hearing a.
    Panasonic hearing a.
    postauricular hearing a.
    Prescriptor hearing a.
    Quantum hearing a.
    Rexton hearing a.
    Rionet hearing a.
    Servox hearing a.
    Star Optica hearing a.
    Tactaid I vibrotactile a.
    Unitron hearing a.
    Widex hearing a.
AID-B pacemaker
AIDS tray
    Alcon Instrument Delivery System tray
AIM
    Ace intramedullary
    AIM femoral nail system
aimer
    Puddu tibial a.
Aim retractor
Ainslie acrylic splint
Ainsworth
    A. arch
    A. punch
air
    a. aspirator needle
    a. bag

a. bed
a. cannula
a. compressor
a. cystotome
a. dermatome
a. drill
a. foam splint
a. inflatable vessel occluder
  clamp
a. injection cannula
a. pressure dressing
a. saw
a. splint
a. turbine
a. uterine displacer
air-boot
Jobst postoperative a.-b.
Aircast
A. air-stirrup leg brace
A. brace
A. fracture brace
A. pneumatic brace
air-conduction hearing aid
air-fluidized bed
airfoam splint
airgun retractor
Air-Lon
A.-L. adapter
A.-L. decannulation plug
A.-L. inhalation cannula
A.-L. inhalation catheter
A.-L. laryngectomy tube
A.-L. tracheal tube
A.-L. tracheal tube brush
airplane splint
Air Plus low-air-loss bed
Air-Shield-Vickers syringe tip
air-spaced electrode
air-stirrup ankle brace
airway
Beck mouth tube a.
Berman a.
Berman disposable a.
Berman intubating
  pharyngeal a.
binasal pharyngeal a.
Coburg-Connell a.
Connell a.
disposable a.
esophageal a.
Foerger a.
Guedel a.
Guedel rubber a.

Lumbard a.
major a.
nasal a.
Portex nasopharyngeal a.
rubber a.
Safar-S a.
AK-10 dialysis machine
Aker lens pusher
Akins valve re-do forceps
AL-1 catheter
Alabama
A. needle holder
A. University forceps
A. University utility forceps
Alabama-Green needle eye holder
alar
a. protector
a. retractor
alar-columellar implant
alarm
Bárány a.
Albany eye guard
Albarran
A. bridge
A. laser
A. laser cystoscope
A. lens
Albarran-Reverdin needle
Albee
A. bone graft
A. bone graft calipers
A. drill
A. orthopaedic table
A. osteotome
A. saw
Albert
A. slotted bronchoscope
A. Smith pessary
A. suture
Albert-Andrews laryngoscope
Albin-Bunegin pressure sensor
albumin-coated vascular graft
Alcatel pacemaker
Alcock
A. bag
A. bladder syringe
A. catheter
A. conical catheter adapter
A. hemostatic bag
A. hemostatic catheter
A. lithotrite
A. plug

Alcock *(continued)*
  A. return-flow hemostatic
    catheter
Alcock-Timberlake obturator
Alcon
  A. Closure System (ACS)
  A. cryoextractor
  A. cystitome
  A. indirect ophthalmoscope
  A. Instrument Delivery
    System tray (AIDS tray)
  A. intraocular lens
  A. ophthalmic knife
  A. phacoemulsifier
  A. sponge
  A. suture
Alcott catheter
aldehyde-tanned bovine graft
Alden retractor
Alden-Senturia specimen collector
Alderkreutz
  A. forceps
  A. tissue forceps
Aleman meniscotomy knife
Alesen tube
Alexander
  A. antrostomy punch
  A. approximator
  A. bone chisel
  A. bone gouge
  A. bone lever
  A. chisel
  A. costal periosteotome
  A. dressing forceps
  A. elevator
  A. gouge
  A. mastoid chisel
  A. mastoid gouge
  A. needle
  A. otoplasty knife
  A. perforating osteotome
  A. periosteotome
  A. raspatory
  A. retractor
  A. rib raspatory
  A. tonsillar needle
Alexander-Ballen orbital retractor
Alexander-Farabeuf
  A.-F. costal periosteotome
  A.-F. elevator
  A.-F. forceps
  A.-F. periosteotome
Alexander-Matson retractor

Alexander-Reiner ear syringe
Alexian
  A. Brothers overhead
    fracture frame
  A. Hospital model retractor
Alfonso eye speculum
Alfreck retractor
Alfred
  A. Becht temporary crown
  A. M. Large vena caval
    clamp
  A. snare
Algee impression material
Alger
  A. brush
  A. brush rust ring remover
Alginate impression material
Algitec impression material
aligner
  orthodontic a.
AL II guiding catheter
alimentation catheter
Alivium prosthesis cup
alkaline battery cautery
Alldress multilayered wound
  dressing
Allen
  A. anastomosis clamp
  A. applicator
  A. cecostomy trocar
  A. clamp
  A. eye implant
  A. eye introducer
  A. forceps
  A. implant
  A. intestinal anastomosis
    clamp
  A. intestinal anastomosis
    forceps
  A. intestinal clamp
  A. intestinal forceps
  A. orbital implant
  A. retractor
  A. root pliers
  A. sphere introducer
  A. Supramid implant
  A. uterine forceps
  A. wire threader
Allen-Barkan knife
Allen-Brailey intraocular lens
  implant
Allen-Brown prosthesis
Allen-Burian trabeculotome

Allen-Hanbury knife
Allen-headed screwdriver
Allen-Heffernan nasal speculum
Allen-Kocher clamp
Allen-Powell air turbine
Allen-Schiotz plunger retractor
  tonometer
Allen-Thorpe gonioscopic prism
Allen-type hex key
Allerdyce
  A. approximator
  A. dissector
  A. elevator
  A. elevator-dissector
Allergan
  A. Advent contact lens
  A. Medical Optics (AMO)
  A. Medical Optics lens
Allergan-Simcoe C-loop intraocular
  lens
Allevyn dressing
Allgower suture
alligator
  a. crimper forceps
  a. ear forceps
  a. forceps
  a. grasping forceps
  a. jaws forceps
  a. nasal forceps
  a. scissors
Allingham rectal speculum
all-in-the-bag intraocular lens
Allis
  A. catheter
  A. clamp
  A. delicate tissue forceps
  A. dissector
  A. dry dissector
  A. forceps
  A. intestinal forceps
  A. lung retractor
  A. Micro-Line pediatric
    forceps
  A. pediatric forceps
  A. periosteal elevator
  A. retractor
  A. thoracic forceps
  A. tissue clamp
  A. tissue forceps
  A. tissue-holding forceps
Allis-Abramson breast biopsy
  forceps

Allis-Adair
  A.-A. forceps
  A.-A. intestinal forceps
  A.-A. tissue forceps
Allis-Coakley
  A.-C. forceps
  A.-C. tonsillar forceps
  A.-C. tonsil-seizing forceps
Allis-Duval forceps
Allis-Ochsner
  A.-O. forceps
  A.-O. tissue forceps
  A.-O. tonsillar forceps
Allison
  A. clamp
  A. lung retractor
  A. lung spatula
  A. retractor
  A. suture
Allis-Willauer
  A.-W. forceps
  A.-W. tissue forceps
allogeneic lyophilized bone grafts
  implant material
alloy
  Aderer a.
  amalgam a.
  Arjalloy a.
  Ceradelta a.
  Ceramalloy a.
  Cerapall a.
  Cer-Mate a.
  Cer-On R a.
  CoCrMo a.
  Coltene a.
  Coronet a.
  Co-Span a.
  Degucast a.
  Degudent a.
  Densilay a.
  Dentsply a.
  E-G a.
  Everest a.
  Fulcast a.
  GFH a.
  GM a.
  Hammond a.
  Imperial a.
  Leff a.
  Lumi a.
  Phase-A-Caps a.
  Phasealloy a.
  Primallor a.

alloy *(continued)*
    Remanium a.
    Safco a.
    Shasta a.
    Sierra a.
    Stabilor a.
    Steldent a.
    Summar a.
    Summit a.
    Thriftcast a.
    Tivanium Ti-6A1-4V a.
    Ultracast a.
    UTK a.
    Vera bond a.
    Victory a.
    Wilgnath a.
    Wilkadium a.
    Wilkoro a.
    Wil-Tex a.
    Zimaloy cobalt-chromium-molybdenum a.

Allport
    A. bur
    A. eustachian bur
    A. gauze packer
    A. hook
    A. mastoid bayonet retractor
    A. mastoid retractor
    A. mastoid searcher
    A. mastoid sound
    A. retractor

Allport-Babcock
    A.-B. mastoid searcher
    A.-B. retractor

Allport-Gifford retractor
all-purpose
    a.-p. transilluminator
    a.-p. urethral catheter

Alm
    A. clip applier
    A. dilator
    A. microsurgery retractor
    A. minor surgery retractor
    A. retractor
    A. self-retaining retractor

Almeida forceps
Alnico Magneprobe magnet
aloe tape dressing
Alpar
    A. implant
    A. intraocular lens implant
alpha-chymotrypsin cannula

ALR cystoresectoscope
already-threaded suture
Alta
    A. cancellous screw
    A. channel bone plate
    A. cortical screw
    A. cross-locking screw
    A. distal fracture bone plate
    A. femoral intramedullary rod
    A. lag screw
    A. modular system
    A. proximal-angled bone plate
    A. supracondylar bone plate
    A. transverse screw

Altchek vaginal mold
Alter lip retractor
alternating suture
Altmann needle
Alukart hemoperfusion cartridge
Alumafoam nasal splint
aluminum
    a. band
    a. cortex retractor
    a. eye shield
    a. fence splint
    a. finger cot splint
    a. shell
    a. splint
    a. wire splint
    a. wire suture

aluminum-bronze wire suture
Aluwax impression wax
ALVAD
    abdominal left ventricular assist device

Alvarado Orthopedic Research (AOR)
Alvarado surgical knee holder
Alvarez-Rodriguez cardiac catheter
Alvis
    A. curette
    A. eye curette
    A. fixation forceps
    A. forceps
    A. foreign body curette
    A. foreign body spud
    A. spud

Alvis-Lancaster sclerotome
Alway groover

Alyea
  A. clamp
  A. vas clamp
amalgam
  a. alloy
  a. carrier
  a. carver
  a. condenser
  a. plugger
  a. scraper
amalgamator
  Accu-Mix a.
  A-Dec a.
  Bantex a.
  Capmix a.
  Dentomat a.
  McShirley a.
  Vari-Mix II a.
Amalgan plugger elevator
amber latex catheter
AMBI compression hip screw system
Ambler dilator
amblyoscope
  Major a.
  Orthoptic Therapy a.
Ambrose eye forceps
Ambu
  A. bag
  A. respirator
Ambu-E valve
Amcath catheter
AMC needle
Amdent ultrasonic scaler
AMD urinary sphincter
Amdur lid forceps
Amenabar
  A. capsular forceps
  A. lens loupe
  A. loop
  A. retractor
Amercal intraocular lens
Amercal-Shepard intraocular lens
American
  A. artificial larynx
  A. circle nephrostomy tube
  A. dilation system dilator
  A. endoscopy dilator
  A. endoscopy esophageal dilator
  A. Hanks uterine dilator
  A. Heyer-Schulte brain retractor

  A. Heyer-Schulte chin prosthesis
  A. Heyer-Schulte elastomer
  A. Heyer-Schulte-Hinderer malar prosthesis
  A. Heyer-Schulte mammary prosthesis
  A. Heyer-Schulte prosthesis
  A. Heyer-Schulte Radovan tissue expander prosthesis
  A. Heyer-Schulte rhinoplasty prosthesis
  A. Heyer-Schulte-Robertson suprapubic trocar
  A. Heyer-Schulte sphere
  A. Heyer-Schulte stent
  A. Heyer-Schulte suction tube
  A. Heyer-Schulte testicular prosthesis
  A. Heyer-Schulte T-tube
  A. Lapidus bed
  A. Medical Electronics, Inc. PinSite shield
  A. Medical Optics lens
  A. Medical Systems (AMS)
  A. Opitical Cardiocare pacemaker
  A. Optical coagulator
  A. Optical ophthalmometer
  A. Optic R-inhibited pacemaker
  A. Optics photocoagulator
  A. umbilical scissors
  A. vascular stapler
Amerson bone elevator
Ames ventriculoperitoneal shunt
Amico
  A. chisel
  A. drill
Amicon arteriovenous blood tubing set
aminotome
AML
  anatomic medullary locking
  AML total hip prosthesis
Amnihook amniotic membrane perforator
amnioscope
  Erosa a.
  Saling a.
amniotome
  Baylor a.

amniotome *(continued)*
    Beacham a.
    Glove-n-Gel a.
AMO
    Allergan Medical Optics
    AMO intraocular lens implant
    AMO laser
    AMO lens
    AMO phacoemulsification lens-folder forceps
    AMO refractometer
    AMO scleral implant
    AMO vitreous aspiration cutter
Amoena breast form
Amoils
    A. cryopencil
    A. iris retractor
    A. probe
    A. retractor
Amoils-Keeler cryo unit
Amplatz
    A. anchor system
    A. angiography needle
    A. aortography catheter
    A. cardiac catheter
    A. catheter
    A. coronary catheter
    A. dilator
    A. femoral catheter
    A. guide wire
    A. high-flow torque-control catheter
    A. needle
    A. renal dilator and sheath
    A. retinal snare
amplifier
    Cona-Tone office-use hearing a.
Amplitone-3
Ampoxen sling
amputating saw
amputation
    a. knife
    a. retractor
AMS
    American Medical Systems
    AMS 700CX Inflatable penile prosthesis
    AMS 700CXM inflatable penile prosthesis

AMS Malleable 600M penile prosthesis
AMS Malleable 800 urinary prosthesis
AMS penile prosthesis
AMS Sphincter 800 urinary prosthesis
AMS urethral stent
AMSCO
    AMSCO Hall adapter
    AMSCO head holder
    AMSCO hysteroscope
    AMSCO light
    AMSCO Orthairtome
Amsler
    A. aqueous transplant needle
    A. grid
    A. needle
Amsterdam
    A. biliary stent
    A. stent
Amtech-Killeen pacemaker
Amussat probe
anal
    a. dilator
    a. retractor
    a. speculum
analyzer
    Friedmann visual field a.
Anastasia bougie
anastigmatic aural magnifier
anastomosis
    a. apparatus
    a. clamp
    a. forceps
anastomotic button
Anatomic hip system
Anatomic/Intracone reamer
anatomic medullary locking (AML)
Ancap
    A. braided silk suture
    A. silk suture
Anchor
    A. all-nylon hand brush
    A. IIa osseointegrated titanium implant system
    A. needle holder
    A. plate
    A. sterilizer box
    A. surgical needle
    A. tapered spring-needle holder

anchor
- a. band
- Hall sacral a.
- Lemoine-Searcy a.
- Mitek a.
- a. needle holder
- Searcy fixation a.
- a. splint
- a. suture

anchoring suture
Ancrofil clasp wire
Andersen mercury-weighted tube
Anderson
- A. columellar prosthesis
- A. curette
- A. flexible suction tube
- A. nasal strut
- A. splint
- A. traction bow
- A. tractor

Anderson-Adson
- A.-A. retractor
- A.-A. scalp retractor
- A.-A. self-retaining retractor

Anderson-Neivert osteotome
Ando
- A. aortic clamp
- A. motor-driven probe

Andre hook
Andresen activator
Andresen-Haupl activator
Andrews
- A. applicator
- A. chisel
- A. comedo extractor
- A. cotton applicator
- A. forceps
- A. frame
- A. gouge
- A. infant laryngoscope
- A. laryngoscope
- A. mastiod gouge
- A. retractor
- A. rigid chest support holder
- A. tongue depressor
- A. tonsillar forceps
- A. tonsil-seizing forceps
- A. tracheal retractor

Andrews-Hartmann
- A.-H. forceps
- A.-H. rongeur
- A.-H. rongeur forceps

Andrews-Pynchon
- A.-P. aspirating tube
- A.-P. suction tube
- A.-P. tongue depressor

Andries stethoscope
Anel lacrimal probe
anesthesia
- a. block needle
- a. needle

Aneuroplast acrylic material
aneuroplastic
- Codman a.
- a. kit

aneurysm
- a. clamp
- a. clip
- a. clip-applier
- a. forceps
- a. neck dissector
- a. needle

Angelchik antireflux prosthesis
Angell
- A. curette
- A. gauze packer

Angell-James
- A.-J. angled dissector
- A.-J. dissector
- A.-J. hypophysectomy forceps
- A.-J. punch forceps
- A.-J. reverse-action hypophysectomy forceps

Angell-Shiley heart valve
Anger camera
Angestat hemostasis introducer
Angetear tear-away introducer
angiocatheter
- Deseret a.
- Mikro-tip a.

Angiocath PRN catheter
Angioflow high-flow catheter
angiogram
angiographic
- a. balloon occlusion catheter
- a. catheter
- a. tubing

angiography needle
Angioject
- ACS A.

Angio-Kit catheter
angiolaser
- pulsed a.

angiopigtail catheter

angioplasty
balloon a.
a. balloon catheter
Excimer laser coronary a.
(ELCA)
percutaneous transluminal
coronary a. (PTCA)
angioscope
Baxter a.
Masy a.
Mitsubishi a.
Olympus a.
Optiscope a.
angiotribe
Ferguson a.
a. forceps
Zweifel a.
Angiovist contrast material
angle
a. arch
a. band
a. drain
a. splint
a. suture
angled
a. ball-end electrode
a. balloon catheter
a. biter
a. clamp
a. clip
a. curette
a. DeBakey clamp
a. decompression retractor
a. forceps
a. guide wire
a. peripheral vascular clamp
a. pigtail catheter
a. probe
a. ring curette
a. scissors
a. stone forceps
a. suture-carrying forceps
a. vein retractor
Angle-Pezzer drain
Angle's appliance
angle-tip electrode
angle-tipped
a.-t. guide wire
a.-t. urethral catheter
angular
a. elevator
a. knife
a. needle

a. scissors
a.-tip electrode
angulated
a.-blade electrode
a. catheter
a. forceps
Angus-Esterline recorder
Anis
A. aspirating cannula
A. ball capsular polisher
A. ball reverse-curvature
capsular polisher
A. capsulotomy forceps
A. corneal forceps
A. corneal scissors
A. corneoscleral forceps
A. disk capsular polisher
A. forceps
A. intraocular lens forceps
A. microforceps
A. microsurgical tying
forceps
A. needle holder
A. straight corneal forceps
A. two flexible closed loops
intraocular lens
A. tying forceps
Anis-Barraquer needle holder
Ankeney
A. retractor
A. sternal retractor
ankle
a. hitch
a. orthosis (AO)
a. prosthesis
Smith total a.
a. traction kit
ankle-foot
a.-f. orthosis (AFO)
a.-f. orthotic splint
Ann Arbor
A. A. clamp
A. A. double towel clamp
A. A. phrenic retractor
A. A. retractor
anomaloscope
Nagel a.
anorectal dressing
anoscope
Bacon a.
Bensaude a.
Bodenheimer a.
Boehm a.

Brinkerhoff a.
Buie-Hirschman a.
Burnett a.
Disposo-Scope a.
Fansler a.
Fansler-Ives a.
fiberoptic a.
Goldbacher a.
Hirschman a.
Ives a.
Ives-Fansler a.
KleenSpec disposable a.
Muer a.
Munich-Crosstreet a.
Otis a.
Pratt a.
Proscope a.
Pruitt a.
rotating a.
rotating speculum a.
Sims a.
Sklar a.
Smith a.
speculum a.
Welch Allyn a.
anosigmoidoscope
Anprolene sterilizer
Anspach
    A. leg holder
    A. system
antegrade
    a. internal stent
    a. valvulotome
anterior
    a. acute flexion elbow
      splint
    a. bulbi camera
    a. capsule forceps
    a. cervical retractor set
    a. chamber cannula
    a. chamber gauge
    a. chamber intraocular lens
    a. chamber irrigating
      cannula
    a. chamber irrigator
    a. chamber maintainer
    a. chamber receiving needle
    a. chamber retaining wire
    a. commissure laryngoscope
    a. commissure laryngoscope
      blade
    a. commissure
      microlaryngoscope

a. crurotomy nipper
a. footplate pick
a. forceps
a. palatine suture
a. prostatic retractor
a. resection clamp
a. resection intestinal
    forceps
a. retractor
a. segment forceps
anterior-posterior
    a.-p. cutting block
    a.-p. cystoresectoscope
Anthony
    A. aspirating tube
    A. compressor
    A. elevator
    A. enucleation compressor
    A. gorget
    A. mastoid suction tube
    A. orbital enucleation
      compressor
    A. pillar retractor
    A. retractor
    A. suction tube
Anthony-Fisher
    A.-F. antral balloon
    A.-F. forceps
Anthron heparinized catheter
anticavitation drill
anticoagulator
    argon gas a.
antiembolism stockings
antifog tube
antirotation guide
antiseptic dressing
anti-siphon device
Antoni-Hook lumbar puncture
   cannula
antral
    a. balloon
    a. bur
    a. cannula
    a. chisel
    a. curette
    a. drain
    a. forceps
    a. gouge
    a. irrigator
    a. needle
    a. perforator
    a. punch
    a. rasp

antral *(continued)*
    a. retractor
    a. sinus cannula
    a. trocar
    a. trocar needle
    a. wash tube
antroscope
    ACMI a.
    Nagashima right-angle a.
    Reichert a.
antrum
antrum-exploring needle
Anustim electronic neuromuscular stimulator
Anzio catheter
A-O
    A-O minus cylinder phoroptors
    A-O plus cylinder phoroptors
AO
    ankle orthosis
    AO brace
    AO compression plate
    AO lens
AOA cervical immobilization brace
AO/ASIF orthopaedic implant
A-OK
    A-OK crescent knife
    A-OK ophthalmic knife
    A-OK phacoemulsification slit knife
AOO pacemaker
AOR
    Alvarado Orthopedic Research
    AOR check traction device
    AOR collateral ligament retractor
aortic
    a. aneurysm clamp
    a. aneurysm forceps
    a. arch cannula
    a. cannula
    a. cannula clamp
    a. catheter
    a. clamp
    a. cuff
    a. curette
    a. dilator
    a. forceps
    a. occluder
    a. occlusion clamp
    a. occlusion forceps
    a. perfusion cannula
    a. punch
    a. retractor
    a. retractor
    a. root perfusion needle
    a. sump tube
    a. valve brush
    a. valve retractor
    a. vent needle
    a. vent needle
aortogram
    a. catheter
    a. needle
aortographic catheter
aortography needle
A-P cutting block
Apexo elevator
Apex pin
Apfelbaum
    A. bipolar forceps
    A. cerebellar retractor
    A. forceps
    A. micromirror
APF Moore-type femoral stem
apicitis curette
apicoaortic
    a. conduit heart valve
    a. shunt heart valve
apicolysis retractor
apparatus
    anastomosis a.
    aspiration a.
    automatic systematic desensitization a.
    Bárány alarm a.
    Bárány noise a.
    Belzer a.
    Belzer for donor kidney a.
    biphase Morris fixation a.
    blow-by a.
    Brawley suction a.
    Buck extension a.
    Calandruccio compression a.
    cryosurgical a.
    Davidson pneumothorax a.
    Desault a.
    Deyerle a.
    Doppler a.
    electro-oculogram a.
    extension a.
    Fell-O'Dwyer a.
    fixation a.
    Frac-Sur a.

fracture-banding a.
Frigitronics nitrous oxide
  cryosurgery a.
Georgiade visor halo
  fixation a.
Gibson-Cooke sweat test a.
Golgi a.
Hodgen a.
Holman flushing a.
Howse-Coventry hip a.
ICLH a.
Jaquet a.
Killian a.
Killian suspension a.
Killian suspension
  gallows a.
Kirschner a.
Kirschner traction a.
Kroner a.
Küntscher traction a.
lacrimal a.
Lewy suspension a.
Light-Veley a.
Lynch suspension a.
Malgaigne a.
Marstock a.
McAtee a.
McKesson pneumothroax a.
Morwel silhouette suction a.
Nakayama anastomosis a.
Naugh os calcis a. tractor
Osteo-Stim a.
Parham-Martin fracture a.
Parham-Martin fracture-
  banding a.
Pearson flexed-knee a.
Plummer-Vinson a.
pneumothoracic a.
Potain a.
R&B portable
  pneumothorax a.
Reichert steriotaxic brain a.
Robinson artifical a.
Robinson artificial
  pneumothorax a.
Roger Anderson a.
Ruth-Hedwig
  pneumothorax a.
Sayre a.
Seldinger a.
Semm pneumoperitoneum a.
Singer portable a.

Singer portable
  pneumothorax a.
Stader extraoral a.
Stryker Constavac closed
  wound suction a.
suction a.
surgical exhaust a.
suspension a.
Swenko gastric-cooling a.
Tallerman a.
Taylor a.
Taylor spinal support a.
Tobold a.
Tobold laryngoscopic a.
Todd-Wells stereotaxic a.
traction a.
vacuum a.
Venturi a.
Volutrol a.
von Petz a.
von Petz suturing a.
Wagner a.
Waldenberg a.
Wangensteen a.
Watanabe a. for
  cystolithotripsy
Zander a.
Zavod aneroid
  pneumothorax a.
Zund-Burguet a.
appendage clamp
appendectomy retractor
appendiceal retractor
applamatic tonometer
applanation tonometer
appliance
    ACCO a.
    ACCO orthodontic a.
    Angle's a.
    arch bar facial fracture a.
    Balters a.
    Begg a.
    Bimler a.
    Bipro a.
    Bipro orthodontic a.
    Bradford fracture a.
    Brooks a.
    Buck fracture a.
    Case a.
    craniofacial a.
    craniofacial fracture a.
    Crozat a.
    Denholtz a.

appliance *(continued)*
Denholtz muscle anchorage a.
dental a.
dental arch bar facial fracture a.
Dewald halo spinal a.
double-band naval a.
Erich facial fracture a.
extraoral a.
Fairdale orthodontic a.
fixed a.
Frac-Sur a.
fracture a.
Fränkel a.
Gerster fracture a.
Goldthwait fracture a.
Graber a.
Hasund a.
Hawley a.
Hibbs fracture a.
ileostomy a.
Janes fracture a.
Jelenko facial fracture a.
Jewett fracture a.
Johnson twin-wire a.
Joseph septal clamp facial fracture a.
Joseph septal fracture a.
Karaya adhesive a.
Karaya ring ileostomy a.
Karaya seal ileostomy a.
Margolis a.
Marlen colostomy a.
microstomia prevention a. (MPA)
Mitek quick anchor a.
Nu-Comfort colostomy a.
orthodontic a.
ostomy a.
prosthetic a.
Remedy colostomy a.
Remedy ileostomy a.
removable a.
Roger Anderson a.
Schacht colostomy a.
Seep-Pruf ileostomy a.
"stick-and-carrot" a.
Stockfisch a.
Universal a.
Vasocillator fracture a.
Whip a.
Whitman fracture a.

Wilson fracture a.
Winter facial fracture a.
wire a.
W. W. Walker a.

applicator
Absolok endoscopic clip a.
Allen a.
Andrews a.
Andrews cotton a.
Bárány a.
Barth double-end a.
beta irradiation a.
beta therapy eye a.
Brown a.
Brown-Dean a.
Brown-Dean cotton a.
Buck a.
Buck ear a.
Buck nasal a.
Campbell-type Heyman fundus a.
Chaoul a.
Cohen suture a.
Copalite a.
cotton a.
Dean a.
ear a.
Ernst radium a.
Falope-ring a.
Farrell a.
Farrior a.
Farrior suction a.
a. forceps
Gass dye a.
Gifford corneal a.
Gorney rubber band a.
Grafco cotton tip a.
Holinger a.
Huzly a.
Ivan laryngeal a.
Ivan nasopharyngeal a.
Jackson laryngeal a.
Jobson-Horne cotton a.
Kevorkian-Younge uterine a.
Kyle a.
laryngeal a.
Lathbury a.
Lathbury cotton a.
Lejeune a.
Lejeune cotton a.
Ludwig middle ear a.
Mayfield clip a.
Milex Jel-Jector vaginal a.

minilaparotomy Falope-
ring a.
Montrose dressing a.
Playfair uterine caustic a.
Plummer-Vinson radium
esophageal a.
Pynchon a.
Ralks sinus a.
Roberts a.
Sawtell a.
Sawtell laryngeal a.
Stille laryngeal a.
Storz a.
strontium-90 ophthalmic
beta ray a.
Ter-Pogossian cervical
radium a.
Turnbull a.
Uckermann cotton a.
Uebe a.
University of Iowa
cotton a.
Wolf-Yoon a.
Yoon a.
Yoon-ring a.
applier
Alm clip a.
aneurysm clip-a.
Autoclip a.
automatic hemoclip a.
Auto Suture Clip-A-Matic
clip a.
bulldog clamp a.
clip a.
Endoclip a.
Gam-Mer clip a.
Hamby right-angle clip a.
Heifitz bayonet clip a.
Heifitz clip a.
hemostatic clip a.
Hulka clip a.
Kaufman hemostat clip a.
Kees clip a.
Kerr clip a.
Malis clip a.
Mayfield clip a.
McFadden Vari-Angle
clip a.
Mount-Olivecrona clip a.
Mt. Clemens Hospital
clip a.
pivot clip a.
Schwartz clip a.

Scoville clip a.
Scoville-Drew clip a.
Spetzler clip a.
Sugita jaws clip a.
surgical clip a.
surgical staple a.
vari-angle McFadden clip a.
Weck clip a.
Yasargil clip a.
Zmurkiewicz clip a.
applying forceps
Appolionio eye implant
Appolito suture
Appose
A. disposable skin stapler
A. skin stapler
apposition suture
approximation
a. forceps
a. suture
approximator
Ablaza-Morse a.
Ablaza-Morse rib a.
Acland clamp a.
Acland double clamp a.
Alexander a.
Allerdyce a.
Bailey rib a.
Biemer a.
Bruni-Wayne clamp a.
Brunswick-Mack a.
Bunke-Schulz clamp a.
clamp a.
double clamp a.
Henderson a.
Henderson clamp a.
hook a.
Ikuta clamp a.
Iwashi clamp a.
Kleinert-Kutz clamp a.
Lalonde tendon a.
Leksell sternal a.
Lemmon rib a.
Lemmon sternal a.
Link a.
micro-anastomosis a.
micro-anastomosis clip a.
Microspike a.
Nunez a.
Nunez sternal a.
Pilling-Wolock a.
Pilling-Wolvek sternal a.
pivot micro-anastomosis a.

approximator *(continued)*
>sternal a.
>Tamai clamp a.
>vari-angle temporary clip a.
>Wolvek a.
>Wolvek sternal a.

APR acetabular cup
apron
>Grafco x-ray a.

Aquaflex contact lens
Aquaflo dressing
Aquamatic dressing
Aquaphor gauze dressing
Aqua-Purator suction device
Aquasonic gel
AR-1 catheter
AR-2
>AR-2 diagnostic catheter
>AR-2 guiding catheter

arachnoid knife
arachnoid-shape
>a.-s. Beaver blade
>a.-s. blade

Arani
>A. catheter
>A. double-loop guiding catheter

Arans pulley passer
Arbuckle
>A. probe
>A. sinus probe

Arbuckle-Shea trocar
arch
>Ainsworth a.
>angle a.
>a. bar
>a. bar facial fracture appliance
>a. bars frame
>Bimler a.
>extramedullary alignment a.
>lingual a.
>a. rake retractor
>Simon expansion a.

Archer
>A. forceps
>A. splinter forceps

Archimedean drill
archwire
>Tru-Arch preformed a.

Arco
>A. atomic pacemaker

>A. lithium pacemaker
>A. pacemaker

arcuate
>a. skin stapler
>a. suture

ARD
>ARD bandage
>ARD dressing

Ardee denture liner
Arem-Madden retractor
Arenberg
>A. dural palpator elevator
>A. endolymphatic sac knife

Arenberg-Denver inner-ear valve implant
Aren retractor
Argen dental attachment
argon
>a. beam coagulator
>a. gas anticoagulator
>a. guide wire
>a. laser
>a. laser coagulator
>a. laser photocoagulator
>a. spring guide
>a. vessel dilator

argon-krypton laser
Argosy in-the-ear hearing aid
Argyle
>A. catheter
>A. endotracheal tube
>A. esophageal stethoscope
>A. lubricating jelly
>A. Medicut R catheter
>A. oxygen catheter
>A. Penrose tubing
>A. trocar

Argyle-Dennis tube
Argyll Robertson suture
Arion
>A. implant
>A. rod eye prosthesis

Arjalloy alloy
Arkan sharpening-stone needle
ARK-Juno refractor
Arlt
>A. fenestrated lens scoop
>A. lens loop
>A. lens loupe
>A. lens scoop
>A. suture

arm
>Budde halo flex a.

a. elevator sling
flexible a.
flexible retractor
  extension a.
Huang Universal flexible a.
Leyla flexible a.
pediatric retractor
  adjustable a.
a. retractor
retractor adjustable a.
a. and shoulder immobilizer
Wittmoser optical a.
armed bougie
Armstrong
  A. grommet ventilation tube
  A. ventilation tube
  A. "V" tube suction
    inserter
  A. V-Vent tube
Army
  A. bone gouge
Army-Navy retractor
Army-pattern
  A.-p. bone gouge
  A.-p. chisel
  A.-p. osteotome
Arndorfer esophageal motility probe
Arnold brace
Arnold-Bruening intracordal injection set
Arnott
  A. bed
  A. dilator
  A. one-piece all-PMMA
    intraocular lens
Aronson
  A. esophageal retractor
  A. lateral sternomastoid
    retractor
  A. medical esophageal
    retractor
  A. retractor
Aronson-Fletcher antrum cannula
Array ultrasound transducer
Arrow
  A. articulation paper
    forceps
  A. balloon wedge catheter
  A. multilumen catheter
  A. pneumothorax kit
  A. pulmonary artery
    catheter

  A. tube
  A. Twin Cath
  A. Twin Cath catheter
Arrow-Berman balloon catheter
Arrow-Clarke thoracentesis device
Arrow-Howes
  A.-H. catheter
  A.-H. multilumen catheter
arrow pin clasp
Arrowsmith
  A. electrode
  A. fixation forceps
Arrowsmith-Clerf pin-closing forceps
Arruga
  A. capsular forceps
  A. curved capsular forceps
  A. curved forceps
  A. encircling suture
  A. expressor
  A. extraction hook
  A. eye holder
  A. eye implant
  A. eye retractor
  A. eye speculum
  A. eye trephine
  A. globe retractor
  A. globe speculum
  A. implant
  A. lacrimal trephine
  A. lens expressor
  A. movable eye implant
  A. needle holder
  A. protector
  A. retractor
  A. surface electrode
  A. tip forceps
  A. trephine
Arruga-Gill forceps
Arruga-McCool
  A.-M. capsular forceps
  A.-M. forceps
Arruga-Moura-Brazil orbital implant
arterial
  a. adapter-stopcock
  a. blood needle
  a. cannula
  a. catheter
  a. clamp
  a. embolectomy catheter
  a. filter
  a. forceps

arterial *(continued)*
- a. graft prosthesis
- a. irrigation catheter
- a. line pressure bag
- a. needle
- a. oscillator endarterectomy instrument
- a. sheath
- a. silk suture

arteriography needle
arteriotomy scissors
arteriovenous (AV)
Arthrex arthroscope
Arthrofile orthopaedic rasp
Arthro-Flo powered irrigation system
Arthro Force
- A. F. basket cutting forceps
- A. F. hook scissors

Arthro-Lok
- A.-L. knife
- A.-L. system of Beaver blades

arthroplasty
- total articular replacement a. (TARA)

ArthroProbe
- SLT Contact A.

Arthroscan video system
arthroscope
- Acufex a.
- Arthrex a.
- Circon a.
- Codman a.
- Concept Intravision a.
- Downs a.
- Dyonics a.
- Dyonics needle scope a.
- Dyonics rod lens a.
- Eagle a.
- examining a.
- fiberoptic a.
- Flexiscope a.
- Hopkins a.
- LUMINA rod lens a.
- O'Connor operating a.
- Richard Wolf a.
- spinal a.
- standard a.
- Storz a.
- Storz examining a.
- Takagi a.
- Watanabe a.

arthroscopic
- a. ankle holder
- a. banana blade
- a. blade
- a. leg holder
- a. meniscus repair instrument set
- a. mini-meniscus blade
- a. surgical table

arthroscopy
- a. bur set
- a. knife

arthrotome
- Hall a.

Arthur splinter forceps
articular insert
articulated
- a. chin implant
- a. external fixator

articulating paper
articulation paper forceps
articulator
- Galetti a.
- Handy II a.
- KSK a.
- Oliair a.
- Olyco a.
- Olympia a.
- Steele a.

artificial
- a. eye
- a. joint implant
- a. pacemaker

Arti-holder tweezers
Artilk forceps
Artmann
- A. chisel
- A. disarticulation chisel
- A. elevator
- A. raspatory

Artus power system
Arzco
- A. electrode
- A. pacemaker

AS
- Auto Suture

Asahi
- A. blood plasma pump
- A. hollow fiber dialyzer
- A. Plasmaflo plasma separator
- A. pressure controller

ASC
   ASC Alpha balloon
   ASC Monorel catheter
   ASC RX perfusion balloon
    catheter
   ASC torque vise adapter
Asch
   A. clamp
   A. forceps
   A. nasal splint
   A. nasal-straightening
    forceps
   A. septal forceps
   A. septal straightener
   A. septum-straightening
    forceps
   A. uterine secretion scoop
ASE
  axilla, shoulder, elbow
   ASE bandage
aseptic saw
Asepto
   A. bulb syringe
   A. suction tube
Ash
   A. catheter
   A. dental forceps
   A. septum-straightening
    forceps
Ashbell hook
Ashby
   A. fluoroscopic forceps
   A. fluoroscopic foreign body
    forceps
   A. forceps
Ashhurst leg splint
Ashley
   A. breast prosthesis
   A. cleft palate elevator
   A. retractor
Ashworth-Blatt implant
ASIF
  Association for the Study of
   Internal Fixation
   ASIF plate
   ASIF screw pin
   ASIF twist drill
ASIS femoral head locator
**ASI uroplasty TCU dilatation
  catheter**
ASN
  automatic single-needle monitor
   ASN monitor

Asnis
   A. guided screw system
   A. pin
ASP
   ASP clip
   ASP clip staple
Aspen
   A. electrocautery
   A. laparoscopic electrode
aspheric
   a. lens
   a. lens implant
Aspiradeps dissector
aspirating
   a. cannula
   a. curette
   a. dissector
   a. needle
   a. syringe
   a. tube
aspiration
   a. apparatus
   a. biopsy needle
   a. cannula
   Laparostat with irrigation
    and a.
aspirator
   Adams a.
   Aspirette endocervical a.
   blue-tip a.
   bronchoscopic a.
   Broyles a.
   Cairtron ultrasonic a.
   a. cannula
   Carabelli a.
   Carmody a.
   Carmody electric a.
   cataract a.
   Cavitron a.
   Cavitron ultrasonic
    surgical a. (CUSA)
   clamp-on a.
   Clerf a.
   Cogsell tip a.
   Cook County Hospital a.
   DeLee meconium trap a.
   DeLee trap a.
   DeVilbiss Vacu-Aide a.
   Dia pump a.
   Dieulafoy a.
   Egnell uterine a.
   electric a.
   faucet a.

aspirator *(continued)*
Flex-O-Jet a.
Fritz a.
Frye a.
Frye portable a.
gallbladder a.
Gesco a.
Gomco a.
Gomco portable suction a.
Gomco suction a.
Gomco uterine a.
Gottschalk a.
Gottschalk middle ear a.
Gradwhol sternal bone
    marrow a.
Gynosampler endometrial a.
Hahnenkratt a.
Huzly a.
Hydrojette a.
Junior Tompkins portable a.
Kelman a.
Leasure a.
Lukens a.
meconium a.
middle ear a.
Monoject bone marrow a.
nasal a.
Nugent a.
Nugent soft cataract a.
Penberthy double-action a.
phacoemulsifer-a.
Pilling-Negus clamp-on a.
portable a.
portable suction a.
Potain a.
Printz a.
red-tip a.
Senoran a.
Sklar-Junion Tompkins a.
soft cataract a.
Sonop ultrasonic a.
Stedman a.
Stedman suction pump a.
suction a.
suction pump a.
Taylor a.
Thorek a.
Thorek gallbladder a.
Tompkins a.
Universal a.
uterine a.
Vabra a.
Vabra cervical a.
vacuum a.
Vent-O-Vac a.
Walker a.
yellow-tip a.
Aspirette endocervical aspirator
ASR
ASR blade
ASR scalpel
assembly
Ace wire tension a.
Dosick bellows a.
Feild retractable blade a.
proximal drill guide a.
ASSI
Accurate Surgical and Scientific
    Instruments
ASSI bipolar coagulating
    forceps
ASSI cranial blades
ASSI forceps
ASSI wire pass drill
**Association for the Study of
    Internal Fixation (ASIF)**
Aston face-lift scissors
Astra pacemaker
Astron
A. dental resin
A. dental wax
A. investment material
A. resin
A. teeth
Astropulse cuff
ASVIP pacemaker
asynchronous
a. mode pacemaker
a. pacemaker
a. ventricular VOO
    pacemaker
atelectatic band
Aten olecranon screw
Athens forceps
atherectomy device
atheroblation laser
AtheroCath spinning blade catheter
ATI forehead thermometer
Atkins
A. esophagoscopic telescope
A. nasal splint
A. tonsillar knife
Atkins-Cannard tracheotomy tube
Atkinson
A. keratome
A. needle

A. retrobulbar needle
A. sclerotome
Atkinson-Walker scissors
Atkins-Tucker
    A.-T. antiembolism stockings
    A.-T. laryngoscope
    A.-T. shadow-free
      laryngoscope
    A.-T. surgical shield
Atlanta hip brace
Atlanta-Scottish Rite brace
Atlantic ileostomy catheter
Atlas
    A. balloon dilatation
      catheter
    A. orthogonal percussion
      instrument
Atlas-Storz eye magnet
Atlee
    A. bronchus clamp
    A. clamp
    A. dilator
    A. uterine dilator
Atmolit suction unit
atomizer
    DeVilbiss a.
    Jackson laryngeal a.
    laryngeal a.
    Ono laryngobronchoscope a.
Atrac-II double-balloon catheter
Atrac multipurpose balloon
  catheter
Atra-Grip
    A.-G. clamp
Atraloc needle
atraumatic
    a. braided silk suture
    a. chromic suture
    a. clamp
    a. forceps
    a. grasper
    a. needle
    a. stomach clamp
    a. suture
    a. suture needle
    a. tissue forceps
    a. visceral forceps
Atraum with Clotstop drain
atrial
    a. cannula
    a. clamp
    a. cuff

a. electrode
a. pacemaker
a. retractor
a. septal retractor
a. synchronous pacemaker
a. synchronous ventricular-
  inhibited pacemaker
a. tracking pacemaker
a. triggered ventricular-
  inhibited pacemaker
Atricor
    A. Cordis pacemaker
    A. pacemaker
atrioseptostomy catheter
atrioventricular
    a. junctional pacemaker
    a. sequential demand
      pacemaker
    a. sequential pacemaker
attachment
    Argen dental a.
    cerebellar a.
    Distaflex dental a.
    Hader dental a.
    Hudson cerebellar a.
    Preci-Slot dental a.
    Stern dental a.
    Strauss dental a.
    Tach-EZ dental a.
Attenborough
    A. knee prosthesis
    A. total knee prosthesis
attic
    a. cannula
    a. dissector
    a. hook
Atwood
    A. crown and bridge
      remover
    A. loupe
    A. orthodontic cement
A-type dental implant
Audibel ear aid
Audicraft VIP-I hearing aid
audiometer
    AudioScope 3 a.
    Crib-O-Gram neonatal
      screening a.
Audionics PB Max hearing aid
AudioScope 3 audiometer
Audiotone hearing aid
Audisil silicone ear mold material

auditory
  a. canal dissector set
  a. trainer
Audivisette hearing aid
Aufranc
  A. arthroplasty gouge
  A. awl
  A. cobra retractor
  A. cup
  A. dissector
  A. femoral neck retractor
  A. finishing ball reamer
  A. finishing cup reamer
  A. hip retractor
  A. hook
  A. offset reamer
  A. periosteal elevator
  A. psoas retractor
  A. push retractor
  A. retractor
  A. trochanteric awl
Aufranc-Turner hip prosthesis
Aufricht
  A. glabellar rasp
  A. nasal rasp
  A. nasal retractor
  A. rasp
  A. retractor
  A. retractor-speculum
  A. scissors
  A. septal speculum
Aufricht-Lipsett nasal rasp
auger
  Hough footplate a.
  Hough stapedial footplate a.
  stapedial footplate a.
Augmen bone-grafting material
August automatic gauze packer
Augustine boat nail
Ault
  A. clamp
  A. intestinal clamp
  A. intestinal occlusion
    clamp
aural
  a. forceps
  a. magnifier
  a. speculum
Aureomycin
  A. gauze dressing
  A. suture

auricular
  a. appendage catheter
  a. appendage clamp
  a. appendage forceps
  a. clamp
Auriculina hearing aid
Aurora dual-chamber pacemaker
Aurovest investment material
Aus-Jena-Gullstrand lens loupe
Austin
  A. attic dissector
  A. awl
  A. chisel
  A. clip
  A. dental knife
  A. dental retractor
  A. dissection knife
  A. dissector
  A. duckbill elevator
  A. duckbill knife elevator
  A. elevator
  A. endolymph dispersment
    shunt
  A. excavator
  A. footplate elevator
  A. forceps
  A. gauge
  A. measuring guage
  A. middle ear instrument
  A. Moore curved
    endoprosthesis
  A. Moore head
  A. Moore hip prosthesis
  A. Moore inside-outside
    calipers
  A. Moore mortising chisel
  A. Moore-Murphy bone
    skid
  A. Moore outside calipers
  A. Moore pin
  A. Moore prosthesis
  A. Moore rasp
  A. Moore reamer
  A. Moore straight-stem
    endoprosthesis
  A. needle
  A. oval curette
  A. pick
  A. piston
  A. retractor
  A. right-angle elevator

A. sickle knife
A. strut calipers
Australian orthodontic wire
Auth knife
Autima
  A. II dual-chamber cardiac
    pacemaker
  A. II pacemaker
Auto-Band Steri-Drape
autoclave sterilizer
Autoclip
  A. applier
  Totco A.
autologous fat graft
automatic
  a. catheter
  a. cranial drill
  a. hemoclip applier
  a. implantable cardioverter-
    defibrillator (AICD)
  a. ratchet snare
  a. screwdriver
  a. single-needle monitor
    (ASN)
  a. skin retractor
  a. stapling device
  a. suction device
  a. systematic desensitization
    apparatus
  a. tourniquet
Automator
autopsy
  a. blade
  a. handle
Autoref keratometer
**Autostat ligating and hemostatic
clip**
Auto Suture (AS)
  AS clip
  AS Clip-A-Matic clip
    applier
  AS curette
  AS device
  AS endoscopic suction-
    irrigation device
  AS forceps
  AS GIA stapler
  AS Multifire Endo GIA 30
  AS stapler
  AS surgical mesh
  AS surgical stapler
  AS suture
autotome drill

Autraugrip
  A. forceps
  A. tissue forceps
Auvard
  A. clamp
  A. cranioclast
  A. speculum
  A. vaginal speculum
  A. weighted speculum
  A. weighted vaginal
    retractor
  A. weighted vaginal
    speculum
Auvard-Britetrac speculum
Auvard-Remine vaginal speculum
Auvard-Zweifel
  A.-Z. basiotribe
  A.-Z. forceps
AV
  arteriovenous
  AV fistula needle
  AV Gore-Tex graft
  AV junctional pacemaker
  AV sequential demand
    pacemaker
  AV synchronous pacemaker
Avalox skin clip
AVCO aortic balloon
Avenida dilator
Avenida-Torres dilator
Averett
  A. head and neck
    endoprosthesis
  A. total hip
Avitene
  A. collagen hemostat
AVIT unit
Avius sequential pacemaker
awl
  Aufranc a.
  Aufranc trochanteric a.
  Austin a.
  bone a.
  Carroll a.
  curved a.
  DePuy a.
  Kelsey-Fry bone a.
  Kirklin sternal a.
  Mustarde a.
  Obwegeser a.
  reamer a.
  rib brad a.
  Rochester a.

awl *(continued)*
    Rush pin reamer a.
    starter a.
    sternal perforating a.
    trochanteric a.
    Uniflex distal targeting a.
    Wangensteen a.
    Wilson a.
    Wilson right-angled a.
    Zuelzer a.
Axenfeld
    A. nerve loop
    A. suture
Axhausen needle holder
axial tractor
axilla, shoulder, elbow (ASE)
Axiom
    A. DG balloon angioplasty catheter
    A. drain
Axios pacemaker
axis-traction forceps
Ayers
    A. chalazion forceps
    A. forceps

Ayer stopcock
Ayre
    A. brush
    A. cervical spatula
    A. cone knife
    A. tube
Ayre-Scott cervical cone knife
Azar
    A. corneal scissors
    A. cystitome
    A. intraocular forceps
    A. intraocular lens
    A. iris retractor
    A. lens forceps
    A. lens-holding forceps
    A. lens hook
    A. lens-manipulating hook
    A. Mark II intraocular lens
    A. needle holder
    A. Tripod eye implant
    A. tying forceps
    A. utility forceps

B-12 dental curette
Babcock
- B. clamp
- B. empyema trocar
- B. forceps
- B. intestinal forceps
- B. jointed vein stripper
- B. lung-grasping forceps
- B. needle
- B. plate
- B. raspatory
- B. retractor
- B. stainless steel suture wire
- B. suture wire
- B. thoracic tissue forceps
- B. thoracic tissue-holding forceps
- B. tissue clamp
- B. tissue forceps
- B. Vital atraumatic forceps
- B. Vital intestinal forceps
- B. Vital tissue forceps
- B. wire
- B. wire suture

Babcock-Beasley forceps
Babinski percussion hammer
baby
- b. Adson brain retractor
- b. Adson forceps
- b. Allis forceps
- b. Balfour retractor
- b. Barraquer needle holder
- b. Bishop clamp
- b. Collin abdominal retractor
- b. Crile forceps
- b. Crile needle holder
- b. Crile-Wood needle holder
- b. dressing forceps
- b. hemostatic forceps
- b. Inge bone spreader
- b. Inge laminar spreader
- b. intestinal tissue forceps
- b. Kocher clamp
- b. Lane bone-holding forceps
- b. Lane forceps
- b. Metzenbaum scissors
- b. Mikulicz forceps

- b. Miller blade
- b. Miller laryngoscope
- b. Mixter forceps
- b. mosquito forceps
- b. Overholt forceps
- b. pylorus clamp
- b. retractor
- b. rib contractor
- b. Roux retractor
- b. Satinsky clamp
- b. Senn-Miller retractor
- b. spur crusher
- b. tissue forceps
- b. Weitlaner retractor
- b. Weitlaner self-retaining retractor

BABYbird respirator
bacitracin dressing
back-and-forth suture
backbiting forceps
back brace
Backhaus
- B. cervical knife
- B. clamp
- B. clip
- B. dilator
- B. forceps
- B. towel clamp
- B. towel forceps

Backhaus-Jones
- B.-J. clamp
- B.-J. towel clamp

Backhaus-Kocher
- B.-K. clamp
- B.-K. towel clamp

backing
- Hahnenkratt b.

back, leg and chest dynamometer
Backmann thyroid retractor
back-stop laser probe
Bacon
- B. anoscope
- B. cranial bone rongeur
- B. cranial forceps
- B. cranial retractor
- B. cranial rongeur
- B. cranial rongeur forceps
- B. forceps
- B. periosteal raspatory
- B. retractor

Bacon *(continued)*
    B. rongeur
    B. shears
Badgley
    B. laminectomy retractor
    B. plate
    B. retractor
Baer
    B. bone-cutting forceps
    B. forceps
bag
    Aberhart disposable
      urinal b.
    Aberhart hemostatic b.
    ACMI b.
    air b.
    Alcock b.
    Alcock hemostatic b.
    Ambu b.
    arterial line pressure b.
    Bard b.
    Bardex b.
    Bardex hemostatic b.
    Barnes b.
    bile b.
    Bomgart stomal b.
    bowel b.
    Brake hemostatic b.
    Brodney hemostatic b.
    Bunyan b.
    b. catheter
    Champetier de Ribes
      obstetrical b.
    Coloplast b.
    Coloplast colostomy b.
    colostomy b.
    coudé b.
    coudé hemostatic b.
    Curity leg b.
    Daimed leg b.
    Davol b.
    dialysate b.
    Douglas b.
    drainage b.
    Duval b.
    Dynacor leg b.
    Emmet hemostatic b.
    exudate disposal b.
    Foley b.
    Foley-Alcock b.
    Foley-Alcock hemostatic b.
    Foley hemostatic b.
    Frenta enteral feeding b.

    gauze tissue b.
    Grafco colostomy b.
    Grafco ileostomy b.
    Greck ileostomy b.
    Hagner b.
    Hagner hemostatic b.
    Hagner urethral b.
    Hemofreeze blood b.
    hemostatic b.
    Hendrickson b.
    Hendrickson hemostatic b.
    Heyer-Schulte disposal b.
    Heyer-Schulte Pour-Safe
      exudate b.
    Higgins b.
    Higgins hemostatic b.
    Hofmeister drainage b.
    Hollister b.
    Hollister colostomy b.
    Hollister drainage b.
    Hope b.
    hydrostatic b.
    ice b.
    ileostomy b.
    Incono b.
    intestinal b.
    intracervical b.
    Karaya seal ileostomy
      stomal b.
    Lahey b.
    Lapadis ileostomy b.
    Lapides collecting b.
    latex b.
    Lyster water b.
    Mac-Lee enema b.
    manual resuscitation b.
    Marlen ileostomy b.
    Marlen leg b.
    Marlen weightless b.
    micturition b.
    millinery b.
    3M limb isolation b.
    Mosher b.
    Nesbit hemostatic b.
    ostomy b.
    Owen hemostatic b.
    Paul condom b.
    Paul hemostatic b.
    Pearman transurethral
      hemostatic b.
    pear-shaped fluted b.
    pear-shaped fluted
      hemostatic b.

Peel Pak b.
Pennine leg b.
Perry b.
Perry ileostomy b.
Petersen b.
Petersen rectal b.
Pilcher b.
Pilcher hemostatic b.
Pilcher hemostatic
  suprapubic b.
Pilcher suprapubic
  hemostatic b.
Plummer b.
Plummer hydrostatic b.
pneumatic b.
Politzer b.
Politzer air b.
prostatectomy b.
rebreathing b.
replacement collection b.
Robinson b.
Rusch leg b.
Rutzen b.
SEMI leg b.
severance transurethral b.
severance transurethral
  hemostatic b.
Shea-Anthony b.
short-tip b.
short-tip hemostatic b.
sleeve b.
Sones hemostatic b.
stomal b.
suprapubic b.
suprapubic hemostatic b.
Sur-Fit colostomy b.
Sur-Fit urinary drainage b.
Surgi-Flo leg b.
Swenko b.
Tassett vaginal cup b.
Thackston retropubic b.
Thackston retropublic
  hemostatic b.
Travenol b.
Travenol heart b.
two-way b.
two-way hemostatic b.
vaginal b.
Van Hove b.
Voorhees b.
Whitmore b.
Wolf hemostatic b.
Bagby compression plate

bag-fixated intraocular lens
Baggish hysteroscope
Bagley-Wilmer
  B.-W. expressor
  B.-W. lens expressor
Bahama suture scissors
Bahnson
  B. aortic aneurysm clamp
  B. aortic cannula
  B. aortic clamp
  B. appendage clamp
  B. cannula
  B. clamp
  B. retractor
  B. sternal retractor
Bahnson-Brown forceps
Bailey
  B. aortic clamp
  B. aortic occlusion clamp
  B. aortic rongeur
  B. aortic valve-cutting
    forceps
  B. aortic valve rongeur
  B. baby rib contractor
  B. bur
  B. cannula
  B. catheter
  B. chalazion forceps
  B. clamp
  B. conductor
  B. conductor saw
  B. contractor
  B. dilator
  B. drill
  B. duckbill clamp
  B. forceps
  B. foreign body remover
  B. Gigli-saw guide
  B. guide
  B. lacrimal cannula
  B. leukotome
  B. punch
  B. rib approximator
  B. rib contractor
  B. rib spreader
  B. round knife
  B. saw conductor
  B. skull bur
  B. transthoracic catheter
Bailey-Cowley clamp
Bailey-Gibbon
  B.-G. contractor
  B.-G. rib contractor

Bailey-Glover-O'Neil
  commissurotomy knife
Bailey-Morse
  B.-M. clamp
  B.-M. mitral knife
Bailey-Williamson
  B.-W. forceps
  B.-W. obstetrical forceps
Bailliart
  B. ophthalmodynamometer
  B. tonometer
bail-lock brace
bailout catheter
Baim catheter
Bainbridge
  B. anastomosis clamp
  B. clamp
  B. forceps
  B. hemostatic forceps
  B. intestinal clamp
  B. intestinal forceps
  B. resection forceps
  B. thyroid forceps
  B. vessel clamp
Baird
  B. chalazion forceps
  B. forceps
Bakelite
  B. dental chisel
  B. mallet
  B. retractor
  B. spatula
Baker
  B. continuous flow capillary drain
  B. forceps
  B. jejunostomy tube
  B. tissue forceps
Bakes
  B. bile duct dilator
  B. common bile duct dilator
  B. common duct dilator
  B. dilator
  B. duct dilator
  B. gall duct dilator
  B. probe
Bakes-Pearce dilator
Bakst
  B. cardiac scissors
  B. valvulotome

balanced
  b. salt solution (BSS)
  b. traction device
Baldwin butterfly ventilation tube
Balectrode
  B. pacing catheter
  B. pacing probe
Balfour
  B. abdominal retractor
  B. baby retractor
  B. bladder blade
  B. blade
  B. center blade
  B. center-blade abdominal retractor
  B. center-blade retractor
  B. clamp
  B. detachable-blade abdominal retractor
  B. lateral blade
  B. malleable center-blade abdominal retractor
  B. pediatric abdominal retractor
  B. pediatric retractor
  B. retractor
  B. retractor with fenestrated blade
  B. self-retaining retractor
  B. wire side blade
Balkan
  B. bed
  B. femoral splint
  B. fracture frame
Ball
  B. coagulator
  B. dissector
  B. forceps
  B. reusable electrode
ball
  cotton b.
  b. electrode
  b. extractor
  b. joint block
  KBM cotton b.
  b. nerve hook
  roller b.
  b. tipped scissors
Ballade needle
Ballance mastoid spoon
Ballantine
  B. clamp
  B. forceps

B. hemilaminectomy
  retractor
B. hysterectomy forceps
B. uterine curette
Ballantine-Drew coagulator
Ballantine-Peterson
  B.-P. forceps
  B.-P. hysterectomy forceps
Ballen-Alexander
  B.-A. orbital retractor
  B.-A. retractor
ball-end elevator
Ballenger
  B. bur
  B. cartilage knife
  B. chisel
  B. curette
  B. electrode
  B. ethmoid curette
  B. follicle electrode
  B. forceps
  B. gouge
  B. hysterectomy forceps
  B. mastoid bur
  B. mucosal knife
  B. nasal knife
  B. periosteotome
  B. raspatory
  B. septal elevator
  B. septal knife
  B. sponge forceps
  B. sponge-holding forceps
  B. swivel knife
  B. tonsillar forceps
  B. tonsil-seizing forceps
Ballenger-Foerster forceps
Ballenger-Hajek
  B.-H. chisel
  B.-H. elevator
Ballenger-Lillie
  B.-L. bur
  B.-L. mastoid bur
Ballenger-Sluder
  B.-S. guillotine
  B.-S. tonsillectome
Ballobes gastric balloon
balloon
  ACS SULP II b.
  b. angioplasty
  Anthony-Fisher antral b.
  antral b.
  ASC Alpha b.
  AVCO aortic b.

Ballobes gastric b.
banana-shaped b.
Baxter Intrepid b.
Baylor b.
Baylor cervical b.
b. biliary catheter
Brighton b.
Brighton epistaxis b.
b. catheter
catheter b.
counterpulsation b.
Datascope b.
detachable silicone b. (DSB)
b. dilatation catheter
b. dilating catheter
b. embolectomy catheter
epistaxis b.
esophageal b.
b. expandable intravascular
  stent
b. flotation catheter
Fogarty b.
Fox b.
Fox postnasal b.
Garren-Edwards gastric b.
gastric b.
Gau gastric b.
Giesy ureteral dilatation b.
Grüntzig b.
Hartzler angioplasty b.
Honan b.
Honan single-use b.
Hunter-Sessions b.
hydrostatic b.
inflated b.
intra-aortic b. (IAB)
intragastric b.
intraocular b.
Katzin-Long b.
Kay b.
kissing b.
Kontron b.
Kontron intra-aortic b.
laser b.
Lo-Profile b.
LPS b.
Mansfield b.
mercury-containing b.
Microvasic Rigiflex b.
occlusive b.
Olbert b.
Percival gstric b.
Percor-Stat intra-aortic b.

balloon *(continued)*
postnasal b.
pulmonary b.
b. pump
b. pumping catheter
QuickFurl double-lumen b.
QuickFurl single-lumen b.
Rashkind b.
rectal b.
RediFurl double-lumen b.
RediFurl single-lumen b.
Reipe-Bard gastric b.
Rigiflex b.
Rushkin b.
scintigraphic b.
Sengstaken b.
Sengstaken-Blakemore b.
Sengstaken-Blakemore
  esophageal varices b.
Shea-Anthony b.
Simpson epistaxis b.
sinus b.
Slinky b.
stone retrieval b.
Taylor gastric b.
transluminal b.
Trefoil b. for percutaneous
  valvuloplasty
b. uterine elevator cannula
  (BUEC)
b. valvuloplasty catheter
b. wedge pressure catheter
Wilson-Cook gastric b.
balloon-centered argon laser
ballooning esophagoscope
balloon-tipped angiographic catheter
ball-peen splint
ball-tip coagulating electrode
ball-type retractor
Balmer tongue depressor
Balnetar implant
Balser hook plate
Balters appliance
Baltherm thermal dilution catheter
Baltimore nasal scissors
Bamby clamp
banana blade
banana-shaped balloon
band
adhesive b.
aluminum b.
anchor b.
angle b.

atelectatic b.
BB b.
belly b.
broad b.
broad adhesive b.
coffer b.
copper b.
Dentaform b.
elastic rubber b.
encircling b.
Falope-ring tubal
  occlusion b.
Flexi-Ty vessel b.
fracture b.
Fränkel head b.
Hahnenkratt matrix b.
Harris b.
His b.
hymenal b.
Johnson dental b.
Ladd b.
Lane b.
lateral b.
latex b.
latex O b.
Lukens orthodontic b.
Magill b.
Magill orthodontic b.
Marlex b.
Matas b.
Matas vessel b.
matrix b.
MB b.
Meckel b.
Mersilene b.
mesocolic b.
metal b.
MM b.
oligodonal b.
omental b.
omental adhevise b.
Ormco preformed b.
Orthoband traction b.
orthodontic b.
Parham b.
Parham-Martin b.
Parma b.
PD b.
PD copper b.
PD SS matrix b.
peritoneal b.
Q-b.
Ray-Tec b.

[Handwritten marginal annotations: Powerflex, Rocket, Slalom, Synergy, Trakstar, Uropas II (Vlach), TX-2000, Stack 40-S perfusion, Titan]

Remak b.
scleral b.
scultetus binder b.
Silastic b.
silicone elastomer b.
Simonart b.
snap b.
Storz b.
T-b.
table b.
tissue b.
Tofflemire matrix b.
tooth b.
T-type matrix b.
ventricular b.'s
vessel b.
Vistnes rubber band
   applier b.

bandage
abdominal b.
Ace adherent b.
Ace spica b.
adhesive b.
ARD b.
ASE b.
Band-Aid b.
Band-Aid adhesive b.
barrel b.
Barton b.
Bennell b.
binocular b.
Borsch b.
Buller b.
capeline b.
Cellamin b.
Cellamin resin plaster-of-
  Paris b.
Cellona b.
Cellona resin plaster-of-
  Paris b.
Champ elastic b.
circular b.
Coban b.
collodion-treated self-
  adhesive b.
Comperm tubular elastic b.
compression b.
cotton elastic b.
cotton-wool b.
Cover-Roll stretch b.
cravat b.
crepe b.
crucial b.

Curad plastic b.
demigauntlet b.
Desault b.
Dyna-Flex elastic b.
E-cotton b.
elastic b.
elastic adhesive b.
elastic foam b.
Elastikon b.
Elastomull b.
Elastomull elastic gauze b.
Elastoplast b.
Esmarch b.
eye b.
figure-of-eight b.
fixation b.
flat eye b.
Flexicon gauze b.
Flexilite conforming
  elastic b.
Flexilite gauze b.
FoaMTrac traction b.
four-tailed b.
Fractura Flex b.
Fractura Flex elastic b.
Fricke b.
Galen b.
Garretson b.
gauntlet b.
gauze b.
Gauztex b.
Genga b.
Gibney b.
Guibor Expo flat eye b.
Haftelast self-adhering b.
Hamilton b.
hammock b.
Heliodorus b.
Hermitex b.
Hippocrates b.
Hueter b.
Hydron Burn b.
Hypertie b.
immobilizing b.
immovable b.
Kerlix b.
Kiwisch b.
Kling b.
Kling gauze b.
Larrey b.
Lister b.
Maisonneuve b.
many-tailed b.

bandage *(continued)*
    Marlex b.
    Martin b.
    moleskin b.
    monocular b.
    Morton b.
    oblique b.
    Orthoflex elastic plaster b.
    Ortho-Trac adhesive skin
      traction b.
    Pearlcast polymer plaster b.
    perineal b.
    plano T-b.
    plaster b.
    plaster-of-Paris b.
    b. plaster shears
    POP b.
    pressure b.
    Priessnitz b.
    protective b.
    recurrent b.
    reverse b.
    reversed b.
    Ribble b.
    Richet b.
    Robert Jones b.
    roller b.
    rubber-reinforced b. (REB)
    Sayre b.
    scarf b.
    b. scissors
    scultetus b.
    Seutin b.
    b. shears
    Silesian b.
    sling-and-swathe b.
    Sof-Band bulky b.
    Sof-Kling b.
    Sof-Kling conforming b.
    spica b.
    spiral b.
    spiral reverse b.
    spray b.
    starch b.
    stockinette b.
    stockinette amputation b.
    Surgiflex b.
    suspensory b.
    T-b.
    Telfa 4 x 4 b.
    Theden b.
    Thermophore b.
    Thillaye b.

    triangular b.
    Tubigrip elastic support b.
    Tubiton tubular b.
    Tuffnell b.
    Velpeau b.
    Webril b.
    wet b.
    woven elastic b.
    Y-b.
BandageGuard half-leg guard
Band-Aid
    B.-A. adhesive bandage
    B.-A. bandage
    B.-A. dressing
Bandeloux bed
bandsaw
    microcut b.
    minicut b.
Bane
    B. forceps
    B. hook
    B. mastoid rongeur
    B. rongeur
    B. rongeur forceps
Bane-Hartmann rongeur
Bangerter
    B. angled iris spatula
    B. forceps
    B. muscle forceps
Bangs bougie
banjo
    b. curette
    b. splint
    b. tractor
Bankart
    B. rasp
    B. rectal retractor
    B. retractor
    B. shoulder retractor
Banks bone graft
Banner enucleation snare
Banno catheter
Bansaton behind-the-ear hearing
    aid
Bantam
    B. Bovie coagulator
    B. coagulator
    B. irrigation set
    B. wire cutter
    B. wire cutting scissors
Bantex amalgamator
bar
    Ackerman lingual b.

acrylic b.
arch b.
Bendick arch b.
Bendick dental arch b.
Bookwalter horizontal b.
Bookwalter horizontal
  flex b.
Bose b.
Buck extension b.
Burns prism b.
clasp b.
connector b.
cross b.
dental arch b.
b. drill
Erich arch b.
Erich arch malleable b.
Erich dental arch b.
Erich-Winter arch b.
Essig arch b.
facial fracture appliance
  dental arch b.
Fillauer b.
fixed arch b.
fracture b.
Gerster traction b.
Goldman b.
Goldthwait b.
Hahnenkratt lingual b.
hex b.
Instra-Rack count b.
intramedullary b.
Jelenko b.
Jelenko arch b.
Jewett b.
Joseph septal b.
Kazanjian b.
Kazanjian T-b.
Kennedy b.
labial b.
lingual b.
Livingston b.
Livingston intramedullary b.
lumbrical b.
major connector b.
mandibular arch b.
maxillary arch b.
minor connector b.
Niro arch b.'s
occlusal rest b.
palatal b.
Passavant b.
retainer arch b.

Roger Anderson fixation b.
Simonart b.
spreader b.
stabilizing b.
stall b.
strut b.
tarsal b.
Tommy b.
Tommy hip b.
traction b.
trapeze b.
b. T-tube
unilateral b.
unsegmented b.
valgus b.
Vistnes applier b.
Winter arch b.

Bárány
  B. alarm
  B. alarm apparatus
  B. applicator
  B. noise apparatus
  B. noise apparatus whistle
  B. speculum
Barbara needle
barbed
  b. broach
  b. myringotome
  b. plastic washer
  b. Richards staple
  b. staple
  b. stapler
Bard
  B. arterial cannula
  B. bag
  B. balloon-directed pacing
    catheter
  B. biopsy needle
  B. catheter
  B. clamp
  B. coil stent
  B. dilator
  B. electrode
  B. electrophysiology catheter
  B. evacuator
  B. graft
  B. guiding catheter
  B. helical catheter
  B. implant
  B. PTFE graft
  B. resectoscope
  B. soft double-pigtail stent
  B. sterilizer

Bard *(continued)*
   B. tip
   B. ureteroscopic cytology
    brush
   B. urethral dilator
   B. x-ray ureteral catheter
Bardam
   B. catheter
   B. red rubber catheter
Bardco catheter
Bardeleben bone-holding forceps
Bardex
   B. bag
   B. catheter
   B. drain
   B. Foley balloon catheter
   B. Foley catheter
   B. Foley return-flow
    rentention catheter
   B. hemostatic bag
   B. Lubricath Foley catheter
   B. stent
Bardex-Bellini drain
Bard-Hamm fulgurating electrode
Bardic
   B. cannula
   B. catheter
   B. curette
   B. cutdown catheter
   B. translucent catheter
   B. tube
   B. vein catheter
Bardic-Deseret Intracath catheter
Bard-Parker
   B.-P. autopsy blade
   B.-P. blade
   B.-P. dermatome
   B.-P. forceps
   B.-P. handle
   B.-P. knife
   B.-P. laboratory handle
   B.-P. scalpel
   B.-P. surgical blade
   B.-P. surgical handle
   B.-P. transfer forceps
Bard-Tuohy-Borst adapter
barium contrast material
Barkan
   B. forceps
   B. goniotomy knife
   B. illuminator
   B. implant
   B. infant lens

   B. iris forceps
   B. operating lens
   B. scissors
Barker
   B. calipers
   B. needle
   B. Vacu-tome
   B. Vacu-tome suction knife
Barker-Vacutome dermatome
Barlow forceps
Barnes
   B. bag
   B. cervical dilator
   B. common duct dilator
   B. compressor
   B. dilator
   B. internal decompression
    trocar
   B. intestinal decompression
    trocar
   B. spirometer
   B. suction tube
   B. vessel scissors
Barnes-Crile
   B.-C. forceps
   B.-C. hemostatic forceps
Barnes-Dormia stone basket
Barnes-Hill forceps
Barnes-Hind
   B.-H. contact lens cleaning
    and soaking solution
   B.-H. ophthalmic dressing
   B.-H. wetting solution
Barnes-Simpson
   B.-S. forceps
   B.-S. obstetrical forceps
Barnhill
   B. adenoid curette
   B. curette
Barnhill-Jones curette
Baron
   B. ear knife
   B. ear suction tube
   B. ear tube
   B. forceps
   B. intraocular lens
   B. knife
   B. retractor
   B. suction tube
   B. suction tube-cleaning
    wire
Baron-Frazier suction tube

Barr
B. anal speculum
B. bolt
B. bolt nail
B. crypt hook
B. fistular hook
B. fistular probe
B. pin
B. probe
B. rectal crypt hook
  retractor
B. rectal hook
B. rectal probe
B. rectal retractor
B. rectal speculum
B. retractor
B. self-retaining retractor
Barraquer
B. baby needle holder
B. blade
B. bladebreaker
B. brush
B. cannula
B. ciliary forceps
B. conjunctival forceps
B. corneal dissector
B. corneal knife
B. corneal section scissors
B. corneal trephine
B. corneal utility forceps
B. curved holder
B. cyclodialysis spatula
B. erysiphake
B. eye needle holder
B. eye shield
B. eye speculum
B. fixation forceps
B. forceps
B. implant
B. iris scissors
B. iris spatula
B. irrigator
B. J-loops intraocular lens
B. lens
B. lid retractor
B. mosquito forceps
B. needle
B. needle holder
B. sable brush
B. sable eye brush
B. silk suture
B. solid speculum

B. speculum
B. suture
B. suture forceps
B. tonometer
B. vitreous strand scissors
B. wire guide
B. wire speculum
Barraquer-Colibri eye speculum
Barraquer-DeWecker iris scissors
Barraquer-Douvas eye speculum
Barraquer-Floyd speculum
Barraquer-Karakashian scissors
Barraquer-Katzin forceps
Barraquer-Troutman
  B.-T. corneal forceps
  B.-T. forceps
  B.-T. needle holder
Barraquer-Vogt needle
**Barraquer-von Mandach clot
  forceps**
Barraya
  B. forceps
  B. tissue forceps
barrel
  b. bandage
  b. cutting bur
  b. dressing
  b. knot suture
Barrett
  B. appendix inverter
  B. flange lens manipulator
  B. forceps
  B. hebosteotomy needle
  B. hydrogel intraocular lens
  B. intestinal forceps
  B. irrigating lens
  manipulator
  B. lens forceps
  B. needle
  B. placental forceps
  B. tenacular forceps
  B. tenaculum
  B. uterine knife
  B. uterine tenaculum
  B. uterine tenaculum
  forceps
Barrett-Adson
  B.-A. cerebellum retractor
  B.-A. retractor
Barrett-Allen
  B.-A. forceps
  B.-A. placental forceps

Barrett-Allen *(continued)*
  B.-A. uterine-elevating
    forceps
  B.-A. uterine forceps
Barrett-Murphy
  B.-M. forceps
  B.-M. intestinal forceps
Barrie-Jones
  B.-J. angled crocodile
    forceps
  B.-J. forceps
barrier
  Interceed absorbable
    adhesion b.
  Interceed adhesion b.
  sterile field b.
Barrier drape
Barron
  B. alligator forceps
  B. hemorrhoidal ligator
  B. ligator
  B. retractor
  B. seizing alligator
    hemorrhoidal forceps
Barr-Shuford speculum
Barsky
  B. cleft palate raspatory
  B. elevator
  B. forceps
  B. nasal osteotome
  B. nasal rasp
  B. nasal retractor
  B. nasal scissors
  B. retractor
Barth
  B. curette
  B. double-end applicator
  B. mastoid curette
Bartholdson-Stenstrom rasp
Bartholin gland catheter
Bartkiewicz two-sided drain
Bartlett fascial stripper
Bartley
  B. anastomosis clamp
  B. partial-occlusion clamp
Barton
  B. bandage
  B. blade
  B. double hook
  B. dressing
  B. forceps
  B. obstetrical forceps
  B. skull traction tongs

  B. suction
  B. traction device
  B. traction handle
  B. wrench
Barton-Cone
  B.-C. tongs
  B.-C. traction tractor
Baruch circumcision scissors
Baschui pigtail catheter
base
  fixation b.
  Getz rubber b.
  Lok-Mesh bonding b.
baseball
  b. finger splint
  b. suture
Basek chisel
basilar suture
Basile hip screw
basin
  urological soaking b.
basiotribe
  Auvard-Zweifel b.
  Tarnier b.
Basis breast pump
Basix pacemaker
basket
  Acufex b.
  Barnes-Dormia stone b.
  biliary stone b.
  Browne stone b.
  Councill b.
  Councill stone b.
  disposable stone b.
  Dormia b.
  Dormia biliary stone b.
  Dormia gallstone b.
  Dormia stone b.
  Dormia ureteral b.
  Dormia ureteral stone b.
  Ellik kidney stone b.
  Ellik stone b.
  endotriptor stone-crushing b.
  Ferguson b.
  Ferguson stone b.
  b. forceps
  gallstone b.
  Glassman b.
  Hobbs stone b.
  Howard b.
  Howard stone b.
  instrument b.
  Johns Hopkins stone b.

Johnson b.
Johnson stone b.
Johnson ureteral b.
Johnson ureteral stone b.
Levant stone dislodger b.
Medi-Tech stone b.
Mill-Rose spiral stone b.
Mill-Rose stone b.
Mitchell b.
Mitchell stone b.
parrot-beak b.
Pfister-Schwartz stone b.
Pfister stone b.
b. retriever
Robinson stone b.
rotary b.
Rutner stone b.
Schutte b.
Segura-Dretler stone b.
Segura stone b.
spincterotomy b.
sterilizing b.
stone b.
stone-holding b.
stone retrieval b.
ultrasonic cleaner b.
ultrasonic cleaner with
  folding handles
  instrument b.
ultrasonic cleaner with rigid
  handles instrument b.
ureteral stone b.
Vantec stone b.
VPI stone b.
Wilson-Cook stone b.
basket-cutting forceps
basket-punch forceps
basket-type crushing forceps
Basswood splint
bastard suture
Bastow raspatory
bat
    Mexican b.
Batchelor plate
Bateman
    B. finger prosthesis
    B. UPF II bipolar system
bath
    sitz b.
Bath respirator
Batson-Carmody elevator

battery pack
    rechargeable nerve
      stimulator b.p.
battery-powdered endoscope
bat-wing catheter
Baudelocque pelvimeter
Bauer
    B. dissecting forceps
    B. forceps
    B. hernia belt
    B. kidney pedicle clamp
    B. sponge forceps
Bauer-Black suture
Baum
    B. needle holder
    B. tonsillar needle holder
Baumberger forceps
Baumgarten wire twister
Baumgartner
    B. forceps
    B. holder
    B. needle holder
    B. punch
Baum-Hecht
    B.-H. forceps
    B.-H. tarsorrhaphy forceps
Baum-Metzenbaum
    B.-M. needle holder
    B.-M. sternal needle holder
Baumrucker
    B. clamp irrigator
    B. electrode
    B. incontinence clamp
    B. post-TUR irrigation
      clamp
    B. resectoscope
    B. urinary incontinence
      clamp
Baumrucker-DeBakey clamp
Bausch
    B. articulation paper forceps
    B. and Lomb Duoloupe
      lens loupe
Bausch-Lomb Thorpe slit lamp
Bavarian splint
Baxter
    B. angioplasty catheter
    B. angioscope
    B. dilatation catheter
    B. disposable blade
    B. Intrepid balloon
    B. surgical clipper
Baxter-V. Mueller catheter

Bay external fixator
Bayless neurosurgical head holder
Baylor
    B. adjustable cross splint
    B. amniotome
    B. balloon
    B. cervical balloon
    B. intracardiac sump tube
    B. metatarsal splint
    B. pelvic traction belt
    B. sump tube
Baynton dressing
bayonet
    b. bipolar electrosurgical forceps
    b. bipolar forceps
    b. clip
    b. curette
    b. forceps
    b. knife
    Lucae b.
    b. molar forceps
    b. needle holder
    b. scissors
    b. separator
    b. transsphenoidal mirror
bayonet-shaped
    b.-s. needle holder
    b.-s. scissors
bayonet-tip electrode
BB band
B-B graft
BCC
    Bushey compression clamp
B-D
    B-D adapter
    B-D bone marrow biopsy needle
    B-D butterfly swab dressing
    B-D needle
    B-D spinal needle
beach
    b. bum rocker-bottom cast sandle shoe
    b. chair positioner
Beacham amniotome
Bead
    B. ethmoidal forceps
    B. forceps
bead
    b. bed
beaded
    b. cerclage wire

    b. guide wire
    b. hip pin
    b. pin wrench
beaded-tip scissors
beaked
    b. cowhorn forceps
    b. sheath
Beall
    B. bulldog clamp
    B. circumflex artery scissors
    B. disk heart valve
    B. heart valve
    B. scissors
Beall-Feldman-Cooley sump tube
Beall-Morris ascending aortic clamp
beam
    Omni b.
bean forceps
Bear
    B. adult-volume ventilator
    B. Cub infant ventilator
    B. respirator
    B. ventilator
Beard
    B. cystitome
    B. eye speculum
    B. lid knife
Beardsley
    B. aortic dilator
    B. cecostomy trocar
    B. clamp
    B. dilator
    B. empyema tube
    B. esophageal retractor
    B. forceps
    B. intestinal clamp
bearing
    radial b.
    ulnar b.
bearing-seating forceps
Beasley-Babcock
    B.-B. forceps
    B.-B. tissue forceps
Beath
    B. needle
    B. pin
Beatty
    B. pillar retractor
    B. tongue depressor
Beaulieu camera
Beaupre
    B. ciliary forceps

B. epilation forceps
B. forceps
Beaver
 B. Arthro-Lok blade
 B. bent blade
 B. blade
 B. cataract blade
 B. cataract cryoextractor
 B. cataract knife blade
 B. curette
 B. DeBakey blade
 B. discission blade
 B. discission knife blade
 B. disposable cryoextractor
 B. dissector
 B. ear knife
 B. electrode
 B. eye blade
 B. eyesurgery blade
 B. goniotomy needle knife
 B. keratome
 B. keratome blade
 B. lamellar blade
 B. limbus blade
 B. Lundsgaard blade
 B. microblade
 B. microsharps blade
 B. Mini-blade
 B. myringotomy blade
 B. Okamura blade
 B. phacokeratome blade
 B. retractor
 B. rhinoplasty blade
 B. ring cutter
 B. scleral Lundsgaard blade
 B. tail-tip electrode
 B. tonsillar knife
 B. tosillectomy blade
 B. variblade blade
Beaver-Ziegler needle blade
Bechert
 B. capsular polisher
 B. forceps
 B. intraocular lens cannula
 B. intraocular lens implant
 B. IOL cannula
 B. lens
 B. nucleus rotator
 B. one-piece all-PMMA
  intraocular lens
 B. rotator
 B. spatula

Bechert-Hoffer nucleus rotator
Bechert-Kratz
 B.-K. cannulated nucleus
  retractor
 B.-K. nucleus rotator
Bechert-McPherson
 B.-M. angled tying forceps
 B.-M. tying forceps
Bechert-Sinskey needle holder
Bechtol
 B. implant
 B. system prosthesis
Beck
 B. abdominal scoop
 B. aortic clamp
 B. clamp
 B. forceps
 B. gastrostomy
 B. loupe
 B. miniature aortic clamp
 B. mouth tube airway
 B. pericardial raspatory
 B. pliers
 B. tonsillar knife
 B. twisted wire loop
 B. twisted wire snare loop
 B. vascular clamp
 B. vessel clamp
Becker
 B. gonioscopic prism
 B. probe
 B. retractor
 B. scissors
 B. screwdriver
 B. septal scissors
 B. skull trephine
 B. spatulated corneal
  section scissors
Becker-Joseph saw
Becker-Park speculum
Beckman
 B. adenoid curette
 B. goiter retractor
 B. nasal scissors
 B. nasal speculum
 B. probe
 B. retractor
 B. self-retaining retractor
 B. Silastic bulb
 B. speculum
 B. stomach electrode
 B. thyroid retractor

Beckman-Adson
  B.-A. laminectomy retractor
  B.-A. retractor
Beckman-Colver nasal speculum
Beckman-Eaton
  B.-E. laminectomy retractor
  B.-E. retractor
Beckman-Weitlaner
  B.-W. laminectomy retractor
  B.-W. retractor
Beck-Mueller tonsillectome
Beck-Potts
  B.-P. aortic and pulmonic
    clamp
  B.-P. clamp
Beck-Satinsky clamp
Beck-Schenck
  B.-S. tonsillar snare
  B.-S. tonsillectome
  B.-S. tonsillectome loop
Beck-Storz tonsillar snare
Béclard suture
Becton-Dickinson
  B.-D. guide wire
  B.-D. Teflon-sheathed needle
bed
  adventitial b.
  air b.
  air-fluidized b.
  Air Plus low-air-loss b.
  American Lapidus b.
  Arnott b.
  Balkan b.
  Bandeloux b.
  bead b.
  Biomet b.
  capillary b.
  carotid arterial b.
  CircOlectric b.
  Clinicare b.
  Clinitron b.
  Clinitron air-fluidized b.
  electric b.
  ether b.
  Fisher b.
  Flexicair b.
  Flexicair low-air-loss b.
  Foster b.
  fracture b.
  gallbladder b.
  Gatch b.
  head of b.
  hepatic b.

  Hough b.
  hydrostatic b.
  hyperbaric b.
  IC b.
  KinAir b.
  Klondike b.
  Lapidus b.
  liver b.
  Medicus b.
  Mediscus low-air-loss b.
  monitored b.
  nail b.
  portal vascular b.
  pulmonary b.
  Roto Kinetic b.
  Roto-Rest b.
  Sanders b.
  sawdust b.
  scleral b.
  Skytron air-fluidized b.
  tissue b.
  ulcer b.
  vascular b.
  venouscapacitance b.
  water b.
Bedrossian eye speculum
Beebe
  B. forceps
  B. hemostatic forceps
  B. lens loupe
  B. wire-cutting forceps
  B. wire scissors
Beekhuis-Supramid mentoplasty
  augmentation implant
Beer
  B. cataract knife
  B. ciliary forceps
  B. forceps
Beeson
  B. cast spreader
  B. plaster cast spreader
Beeth needle
Begg appliance
B.E. glass abdominal retractor
Behen ear forceps
behind-the-ear (BTE)
  b.-t.-e. hearing aid
Behrend
  B. cystic duct forceps
  B. periosteal elevator
Beird eye catheter
Belcher clamp

Belin
- B. double-ended needle holder
- B. needle holder

Bell
- B. circumcision clamp
- B. clamp
- B. erysiphake
- B. suture

Bellavar medical support stockings
Bellfield wire retractor
bellied bougie
Bellman retractor
Bellocq
- B. cannula
- B. sound
- B. tube

Bellow CO2 cryoextractor
Bellows cryoextractor extractor
Bellucci
- B. alligator scissors
- B. cannula
- B. curette
- B. ear forceps
- B. elevator
- B. forceps
- B. hook
- B. knife
- B. lancet knife
- B. middle ear instrument
- B. pick
- B. scissors
- B. suction tube
- B. tube

Belluci-Wullstein retractor
belly band
Bel-O-Pak suction tube
Belos compression pin
Belscope
- B. blade
- B. laryngoscope

belt
- abdominal b.
- Bauer hernia b.
- Baylor pelvic traction b.
- Billi Button abdominal b.
- Black hernia b.
- Conco abdominal b.
- Dover abdominal b.
- Grafco pelvic traction b.
- Grotena abdominal b.
- Grotena lumbar b.
- Hackett sacral b.
- pelvic b.
- pelvic traction b.
- Posey b.
- Pro-Comelastic abdominal b.
- Reed cast b.
- traction b.
- Universal pelvic traction b.

Belz
- B. lacrimal rongeur
- B. lacrimal sac rongeur

Belzer
- B. apparatus
- B. for donor kidney apparatus

Benaron
- B. forceps
- B. scalp-rotating forceps

Benda finger vise
bender
- plate b.
- rod b.

Bendick
- B. arch bar
- B. dental arch bar

bending pliers
Bendixen-Kirschner traction bow
Benedict
- B. gastroscope
- B. operating gastroscope

Beneventi
- B. retractor
- B. self-retaining retractor

Beneys tonsillar compressor
Bengash needle
Benger
- B. probe
- B. probe hook

Bengolea
- B. arterial forceps
- B. forceps

Béniqué
- B. catheter
- B. catheter guide
- B. dilator
- B. sound

Benjamin
- B. binocular slimline laryngoscope
- B. pediatric laryngoscope

Benjamin-Havas fiberoptic light clip

Bennell
  B. bandage
  B. forceps
Bennett
  B. bone elevator
  B. bone lever
  B. bone retractor
  B. ciliary forceps
  B. common duct dilator
  B. elevator
  B. epilation forceps
  B. foreign body spud
  B. pressure-cycled ventilator
  B. raspatory
  B. respirator
  B. retractor
  B. tibial retractor
  B. ventilator
Bensaude anoscope
Benson
  B. baby pyloric separator
  B. pyloric clamp
  B. pylorus spreader
  B. wire
bent
  b. blade
  b. blade plate
  b. needle
Bentley button
Bentson
  B. exchange straight guide wire
  B. guide wire
benzoin scrub soap
Berbecker
  B. needle
  B. pliers
Berci-Schore choledochoscope-nephroscope
Berci-Ward
  B.-W. laryngonasopharyngoscope
  B.-W. laryngopharyngoscope
Berens
  B. bident electrode
  B. calipers
  B. capsular forceps
  B. clamp
  B. common duct scoop
  B. compressor
  B. conical eye implant
  B. corneal transplant forceps
  B. corneal transplant scissors
  B. corneoscleral punch
  B. dilator
  B. enucleation compressor
  B. esophageal retractor
  B. expressor
  B. eye implant
  B. eye retractor
  B. eye speculum
  B. forceps
  B. graft
  B. implant
  B. iridocapsulotomy scissors
  B. iris knife
  B. keratome
  B. lens expressor
  B. lens loupe
  B. lens scoop
  B. lid everter
  B. lid retractor
  B. mastectomy retractor
  B. mastectomy skin flap retractor
  B. muscle clamp
  B. muscle clamp forceps
  B. muscle forceps
  B. muscle recession forceps
  B. orbital compressor
  B. orbital implant
  B. punctum dilator
  B. pyramidal eye implant
  B. recession forceps
  B. retractor
  B. scleral hook
  B. sclerotomy knife
  B. skin flap retractor
  B. sphere eye implant
  B. sterilizing case
  B. thyroid retractor
Berens-Rosa
  B.-R. eye implant
Berens-Tolman
  B.-T. indicator
  B.-T. ocular hypertension indicator
Bergen retractor
Berger
  B. biopsy forceps
  B. forceps
  B. loupe
  B. spur crusher
Bergeret-Reverdin needle

Bergeron pillar forceps
Berges-Reverdin needle
Berget lens loupe
Bergh ciliary forceps
Berghmann-Foerster sponge forceps
Bergman
- B. forceps
- B. mallet
- B. plaster saw
- B. plaster scissors
- B. scalpel
- B. tissue forceps
- B. tracheal retractor
- B. wound retractor

Bergstrom-Stille muscle cannula
Berke
- B. ciliary forceps
- B. clamp
- B. double-end lid everter
- B. forceps
- B. ptosis clamp
- B. ptosis forceps

Berke-Jaeger lid plate
Berkeley
- B. cannula
- B. clamp
- B. forceps
- B. Medevices, Inc. syringe tip
- B. retractor

Berkeley-Bonney
- B.-B. retractor
- B.-B. self-retaining abdominal retractor
- B.-B. vaginal clamp

Berlin curette
Berlind-Auvard
- B.-A. retractor
- B.-A. speculum
- B.-A. vaginal speculum

Berliner
- B. neurological hammer
- B. percussion hammer

Berman
- B. airway
- B. angiographic catheter
- B. aortic clamp
- B. cardiac catheter
- B. catheter
- B. clamp
- B. disposable airway
- B. intubating pharyngeal airway

- B. locator
- B. magnet
- B. vascular clamp

Bermen-Werner probe
Berna
- B. infant abdominal retractor
- B. retractor

Bernaco adapter
Bernard uterine forceps
Bernay
- B. gauze packer
- B. retractor
- B. tracheal retractor

Berndt hip ruler
Berne
- B. forceps
- B. nasal forceps
- B. nasal rasp

Bernell
- B. grid
- B. tangent screen

Bernhard
- B. clamp
- B. towel forceps

Bernstein
- B. catheter
- B. gastroscope
- B. nasal retractor
- B. retractor

Berry
- B. clamp
- B. forceps
- B. needle holder
- B. pile clamp
- B. rib raspatory
- B. rotating inlet
- B. uterine-elevating forceps

Berry-Lambert periosteal elevator
Bertillon calipers
Bertrandi suture
Best
- B. clamp
- B. colon clamp
- B. common duct stone forceps
- B. direct forward-vision telescope
- B. forceps
- B. gallstone forceps
- B. intestinal clamp
- B. right-angle colon clamp

Best *(continued)*
  B. stone forceps
  B. telescope
beta
  b. irradiation applicator
  b. therapy eye applicator
Betacel-Biotronik pacemaker
Betadine
  B. gel
  B. scrub soap
Bethea sheet holder
Bethune
  B. clamp
  B. elevator
  B. lung tourniquet
  B. nerve hook
  B. periosteal elevator
  B. phrenic retractor
  B. retractor
  B. rib shears
Bethune-Coryllos rib shears
Bettman empyema tube
Bettman-Forvash thoracotome
Bettman-Noyes forceps
Bevan
  B. forceps
  B. gallbladder forceps
  B. hemostatic forceps
beveled chisel
bevel-point Rush pin
Bever surgical blade
Beyer
  B. atticus punch
  B. bone rongeur
  B. endaural rongeur
  B. forceps
  B. needle
  B. paracentesis needle
  B. pigtail probe
  B. rongeur
  B. rongeur forceps
Beyer-Lempert rongeur
bezel
  Miller injector b.
B. F. Wehmer cephalometer
B-H
  B-H forceps
  B-H irrigating cannula
biangled hook
BIAS
  BIAS slaphammer
  BIAS total hip system
bias-cut stockinette dressing

BICAP
  Bipolar Circumactive Probe
  BICAP cautery
  BICAP probe
Bicek
  B. retractor
  B. vaginal retractor
Biceps bipolar coagulator
Bicer-val mitral heart valve
Bickle microsurgical knife
Bicol collagen sponge
biconvex intraocular lens
bicoudé catheter
bicycle ergometry
bident retractor
Biegelseisen needle
Bielawski heart clamp
Biemer
  B. approximator
  B. vessel clip
biepharoplasty clip
Bierman needle
Biestek thyroid retractor
Bietti eye implant
bifid
  b. gallbladder retractor
  b. retractor
bifocal
  b. demand pacemaker
  b. eye implant
  b. lens
bifurcated
  b. drain extension
  b. retractor
  b. seamless prosthesis
  b. vascular graft
Bigelow
  B. calvarium clamp
  B. clamp
  B. evacuator
  B. forceps
  B. lithotrite
  B. suture
Biggs
  B. mammaplasty retractor
  B. retractor
bike brace
BiLAP bipolar cautery unit
bile bag
biliary
  b. balloon catheter
  b. balloon dilator
  b. balloon probe

b. catheter
b. dilator catheter
b. duct dilator
b. endoprosthesis
b. retractor
b. stent
b. stone basket
Bill
B. traction handle
B. traction handle forceps
Billeau
B. curette
B. ear curette
B. ear hook
B. ear loop
B. loop
Billeau-House ear loop
Billi Button abdominal belt
Billroth
B. curette
B. forceps
B. retractor
B. tube
B. tumor forceps
B. uterine tumor forceps
Billroth-Stille retractor
Bilos pin extractor
bilumen mammary implant
Bi-Metric
Bi-M. Interlok femoral prosthesis
Bi-M. PMMA centering sleeve
Bi-M. porous primary femoral prosthesis
Bi-M. tapered reamer with Zimmer-Hudson shank
Bimler
B. activator
B. appliance
B. arch
binangled chisel
binasal pharyngeal airway
binder
Texal-Muller chest b.
Binder submalar implant
Binkhorst
B. collar stud intraocular lens
B. eye implant
B. hooked cannula
B. implant
B. intraocular lens

B. irrigating cannula
B. lens forceps
B. lens implant
B. mustache lens intraocular lens
B. two modified J-loops intraocular lens
Binner
B. diaphanoscope
B. head lamp
binocular
b. bandage
b. dressing
b. eye dressing
b. indirect ophthalmoscope with SPF
b. loupe
b. shield
Bio-Absorbable staple
Biobrane
B. dressing
B. wound dressing
bioceramic implant material
Bioclad with pegs reinforced acetabular prosthesis
Bioclusive
B. drape
B. dressing
B. transparent dressing
Biocon impedance plethysmography cardiac output monitor
Biodrape dressing
biofeedback
b. device
b. electroencephalograph
b. electromyometer
b. galvanic skin response device
biofil
Trio-Temp X b.
Bio-Fit total hip system
Biofix
B. absorbable fixation system
B. fixation rod
Bioglass prosthesis
biograft
Dardik b.
Meadox Dardik b.
Bio-Groove
B.-G. femoral prosthesis
B.-G. hip
B.-G. stem

51

Biolas laser adapter
Biolite ventilation tube
Bio-Medicus percutaneous cannula set
Bio-Med MVP-10 pediatric ventilator
Biomer microsuturing instrument
Biomet
    B. bed
    B. Bi-Polar component
    B. fracture brace
    B. hip
    B. plug
biometry probe
biomicroscope
Bio-Modular
    B.-M. humeral rasp
    B.-M. shoulder component
Bio-Moore
    B.-M. II instrumentation
    B.-M. II provisional neck spacer
    B.-M. II stem impactor
    B.-M. rasp
Bionicare stimulator
Bionic ear prosthesis
Bionit vascular graft
Biopac gingival retraction cord
Biophysic Medical laser
Bio-Plug
    B.-P. canal plug
    B.-P. component
    B.-P. provisional
BioPolyMeric
    B. femoropopliteal bypass graft
    B. vascular graft
Bioport collection and transportation system
bioprosthesis
    Carpentier-Edwards b.
Bioprosthesis heart valve
biopsy
    b. cannula
    b. curette
    b. forceps
    b. forceps handle
    b. forceps shaft
    b. kit
    b. loop electrode
    b. needle

    b. punch
    b. punch forceps
    b. specimen forceps
    b. suction curette
    b. telescope
bioptic telescope
bioptome
    King cardiac b.
Biosearch
    B. anal biofeedback device
    B. catheter
    B. jejunostomy kit
    B. needle
Bio-sentry telemetry
Biospal hemodialyzer
Biostil
    B. blood transfusion set
BioTac biopsy cannula
biotelemetry system
biothesiometer
Biotronik demand pacemaker
biparietal suture
biphase Morris fixation apparatus
biplane sector probe
bipolar
    b. catheter
    b. catheter electrode
    b. cautery
    b. coagulating forceps
    b. coagulation-suction forceps
    b. coagulator
    b. coaptation forceps
    b. connection cord
    b. cutting forceps
    b. depth electrode
    b. electrocautery
    b. electrode
    b. eye forceps
    b. forceps
    b. hemostasis probe
    b. irrigating forceps
    b. irrigating stylet
    b. Medtronic pacemaker
    b. myocardial electrode
    b. needle
    b. pacemaker
    b. pacing catheter
    b. pacing electrode catheter
    b. probe
    b. suction forceps

b. temporary pacemaker
catheter
b. transsphenoidal forceps
Bipolar Circumactive Probe
(BICAP)
Bipro
B. appliance
B. orthodontic appliance
Bipulse micro stimulator
Bircher
B. bone-holding clamp
B. cartilage clamp
B. hyfrecator
Bircher-Ganske
B.-G. forceps
B.-G. meniscal forceps
Birch trocar
Bird
B. Mark 8 respirator
B. modified vacuum
extractor
B. pressure-cycled ventilator
B. vacuum extractor
bird's
b. nest filter
b. nest IVC filter
Bireks dissecting forceps
Birkett
B. forceps
B. hemostatic forceps
Birtcher
B. cautery
B. coagulator
B. electrode
B. electrosurgical needle
B. hyfrecator electrosurgical
unit
B. hyfrecatur coagulator
Bishop
B. antral perforator
B. bone clamp
B. chisel
B. gouge
B. mastoid chisel
B. mastoid gouge
B. oscillatory bone saw
B. tendon tucker
B. tendon tucker forceps
B. tissue forceps
Bishop-Black tendon tucker
Bishop-DeWitt tendon tucker

Bishop-Harman
B.-H. anterior chamber
cannula
B.-H. anterior chamber
irrigating cannula
B.-H. anterior chamber
irrigator
B.-H. cannula
B.-H. dressing
B.-H. dressing forceps
B.-H. eye dressing forceps
B.-H. forceps
B.-H. foreign body forceps
B.-H. iris forceps
B.-H. irrigating cannula
B.-H. mules
B.-H. spud
B.-H. tissue forceps
Bishop-Peter tendon tucker
bistoury
b. blade
Converse b.
Converse button-end b.
Jackson tracheal b.
Jackson tracheotomic b.
b. knife
straight b.
tracheal b.
tracheotomic b.
bit
drill b.
b. drill
femoral drill b.
bite
b. block
Leivers formed-type b.
Leivers swivel-type b.
b. protector
b. stick
Bitefork face bowe
biter
angled b.
suction b.
biterminal electrode
Bite wafer denture bite wax
biting
b. forceps
b. rongeur
BIVAD centrifugal left and right
ventricular assist device
bivalved
b. anal speculum
b. cannula

53

bivalved *(continued)*
    b. retractor
    b. speculum
biventricular assist device (BVAD)
Bivona tracheostomy tube
Bizzarri-Guiffrida laryngoscope
Bjerrum screen
Björk
    B. diathermy forceps
    B. drill
    B. prosthesis
    B. rib drill
Björk-Shiley
    B.-S. heart valve
    B.-S. heart valve holder
    B.-S. heart valve sizer
Björk-Stille diathermy forceps
Black
    B. clamp
    B. hernia belt
    B. meatal clamp
    B. retractor
black
    b. braided suture
    b. silk suture
    b. suture
    b. twisted suture
Blackburn
    B. skull traction tractor
    B. trephine
Black-Decker needle
Blackmon needle
Black-Wylie
    B.-W. dilator
    B.-W. obstetric dilator
bladder
    b. blade
    b. catheter
    b. dilator
    b. evacuator
    b. flap
    b. forceps
    b. irrigation control clamp
    b. pacemaker
    b. retractor
    b. sound
    b. specimen forceps
    b. specimen forceps shaft
  blade
    adenotome b.
    Aggressor meniscal b.
    anterior commissure
      laryngoscope b.

arachnoid-shape b.
arachnoid-shape Beaver b.
Arthro-Lok system of
  Beaver b.'s
arthroscopic b.
arthroscopic banana b.
arthroscopic mini-
  meniscus b.
ASR b.
ASSI cranial b.'s
autopsy b.
baby Miller b.
Balfour b.
Balfour bladder b.
Balfour center b.
Balfour lateral b.
Balfour retractor with
  fenestrated b.'s
Balfour wire side b.
banana b.
#15 Bard-Parker b.
Bard-Parker b.
Bard-Parker autopsy b.
Bard-Parker surgical b.
Barraquer b.
Barton b.
Baxter disposable b.
Beaver b.
Beaver Arthro-Lok b.
Beaver bent b.
Beaver cataract b.
Beaver cataract knife b.
Beaver DeBakey b.
Beaver discission b.
Beaver discission knife b.
Beaver eye b.
Beaver eyesurgery b.
Beaver keratome b.
Beaver lamellar b.
Beaver limbus b.
Beaver Lundsgaard b.
Beaver microsharps b.
Beaver Mini-b.
Beaver myringotomy b.
Beaver Okamura b.
Beaver phacokeratome b.
Beaver rhinoplasty b.
Beaver scleral
  Lundsgaard b.
Beaver tosillectomy b.
Beaver variblade b.
Beaver-Ziegler needle b.
Belscope b.

bent b.
Bever surgical b.
bistoury b.
bladder b.
Blount bent b.
Blount V-b.
bone saw b.
Bookwalter-Balfour
  retractor b.
Bookwalter-Gelpi point
  retractor b.
Bookwalter-Harrington
  retractor b.
Bookwalter-Kelly retractor b.
Bookwalter rectal b.
Bookwalter retractor b.
Bookwalter vaginal
  Deaver b.
Bookwalter vaginal
  lateral b.
Bookwalter vaginal
  posterior b.
breakable b.
Brown dermatome b.
capsulotomy b.
carbolized knife b.
carbon steel b.
Castroviejo b.
Castroviejo slimline b.
cataract b.
center b.
cervical b.
cervical biopsy b.
chisel b.
chondroplastic b.
chondroplastic Beaver b.
circular b.
Cloward b.
Cloward retractor b.
Cloward single-tooth
  retractor b.
Collin radiopaque sternal b.
Concept disposable intra-
  articular b.
conization instrument b.
Converse retractor b.
Cooley-Pontius b.
Cooley-Pontius sternal b.
copper b.
Cottle nasal knife b.
Cottle Universal nasal saw
  replacement b.
crescentic b.

Crile b.
Crockard curved retractor b.
Crockard retractor b.
Crockard small-tongue
  retractor b.
Curdy b.
curved b.
curved meniscotome b.
cutting hemostatic
  tonsillectome b.
Davis b.
Davis-Crowe tongue b.
Davis b. with groove
Dean b.
Deaver b.
DeBakey b.
deep spreader b.
Denis Browne abdominal
  retractor b.
Denis Browne-Hendren
  pediatric retractor b.
Denis Browne malleable
  copper retractor b.
Denis Browne mastoid
  pediatric retractor b.
Denis Browne mastoid
  retractor b.
Denis Browne pediatric
  abdominal retractor b.
Denis Browne pediatric
  retractor hook b.
Denis Browne retractor
  hook b.
dermatome b.
diamond b.
Dingman mouth gag tongue
  depressor b.
discission b.
Dixon b.
Dixon center b.
double-angled b.
ear b.
ear surgery b.
ear surgery Beaver b.
b. electrode
electrodermatome sterile b.
Emir razor b.
English MacIntosh fiberoptic
  laryngoscope b.
Epstein b.
Epstein hemilaminectomy b.
expandable b.
eye b.

blade *(continued)*
eyeknife b.
eye surgery b.
Feather carbon breakable b.
Finochietto laminectomy
retractor b.
Flagg stainless steel
laryngoscope b.
Fleming conization
instrument b.
folding b.
Gigli-saw b.
Gill b.
Goulian b.
Grieshaber b.
Guedel b.
Guedel laryngoscope b.
Hammond b.
Hammond winged
retractor b.
b. handle
Hebra b.
hemilaminectomy b.
Hendren b.
Hendren pediatric
retractor b.
Henley retractor center b.
Henley retractor set
center b.
Henley retractor side b.
Hibbs b.
Hibbs retractor b.
Hibbs spinal retractor b.
Hopp b.
Hopp anterior commissure
laryngoscope b.
Hopp laryngoscope b.
Horgan b.
Horgan center b.
House b.
House detachable b.
House knife b.
House ophthalmic b.
infant urethrotome b.
instrument set for angled b.
Katena b.
keratome b.
Kjelland b.
Knapp b.
knife b.
LaForce adenotome b.
lamellar b.
laminectomy b.

Lange b.
laryngoscope b.
laryngoscope folding b.
Leivers b.
Lemmon b.
Lundsgaard b.
M-b.
MacIntosh b.
MacIntosh fiberoptic
laryngoscope b.
MacIntosh stainless steel
laryngoscope b.
Magrina-Bookwalter vaginal
Deaver b.
Magrina-Bookwalter vaginal
lateral b.
Magrina-Bookwalter vaginal
posterior b.
malleable b.
Martin b.
M Beaver b.
McIntosh laryngoscope b.
McIvor mouth gag
tongue b.
McPherson-Wheeler b.
meniscectomy b.
Meyerding laminectomy b.
Meyerding retractor b.
Micro-Sharp b.
microvitreoretinal b.
Miller fiberoptic
laryngoscope b.
Miller stainless steel
laryngoscope b.
Millin side b.
Millin solid malleable
center b.
Morse b.
mouth gag tongue b.
mouth gag tongue
depressor b.
Mueller tongue b.
Mullins b.
Murphy-Balfour center b.
MVR b.
Myocure b.
myringotomy ear b.
myringotomy knife b.
myringotomy knife
ophthalmic b.
nasal knife b.
nasal saw b.
notchplasty b.

Nounton b.
nubular b.
ocutome vitreous b.
ophthalmic b.
Organdi b.
Padgett b.
Padgett dermatome b.
Park b.
Parker-Bard b.
Paufique b.
pediatric abdominal
  retractor b.
pediatric Hendren
  retractor b.
pediatric hook retractor b.
pediatric mastoid
  retractor b.
Personna b.
Personna surgical b.
b. plate
b. plate fixation device
razor b.
Reese dermatome b.
b. retractor
retractor b.
retractor abdominal b.
retractor center b.
retractor hook b.
retractor malleable
  copper b.
retractor mastoid b.
retractor side b.
retrograde b.
retrograde Beaver b.
retrograde meniscal b.
Rew-Wyly b.
ring b.
ring retractor b.
ring tongue b.
rosette b.
Rusch laryngoscope b.
Satterlee bone saw b.
b. scalpel
scimitar b.
sclerotome b.
Scoville b.
Scoville retractor b.
Scoville retractor hook with
  cross b.
self-retaining retractor b.
semilunar-tip b.
serrated b.
Sharpoint V-lance b.

shoulder b.
sickle-shaped b.
sickle-shaped Bever b.
side b.
side-cutting b.
slimline b.
slit b.
Sofield retractor b.
solid-center malleable b.
spear b.
special b.
spinal retractor b.
stainless steel b.
sterile electrodermatome b.
sternal b.
sternal retractor b.
Storz b.
Storz disposable b.
straight b.
Stryker b.
surgical b.
surgical saw b.
Swann-Morton b.
Swann-Morton surgical b.
Swiss b.
Taylor b.
Taylor laminectomy b.
Taylor retractor b.
Taylor spinal retractor b.
throw-away manual
  dermatome b.
tongue b.
tongue retractor b.
Tooke b.
Torpin vectis b.
trephine b.
Troutman b.
Tucker-Luikart b.
Turner-Warwick b.
Universal nasal saw b.
urethrotome b.
Vascutech circular b.
vectis b.
V. Mueller b.
V. Mueller ear b.
V. Mueller mini b.
V. Mueller myringotomy
  ear b.
Weck-Prep b.
Weinberg b.
Welch Allyn laryngoscope b.
Wheeler b.
winged retractor b.

blade *(continued)*
wire side b.
Wisconsin laryngoscope b.
Wisconsin stainless steel
laryngoscope b.
wood tongue b.
Zalkind-Balfour b.
Ziegler b.
Zimmer Gigli-saw b.'s
bladebreaker
Barraquer b.
Castroviejo b.
Castroviejo minirazor b.
Castroviejo razor b.
Castroviejo-style mini b.
b. holder
I-tech-Castroviejo b.
Jarit b.
minirazor b.
razor b.
Swiss b.
Troutman b.
Blade-Wilde ear forceps
Blair
B. chisel
B. cleft palate clamp
B. cleft palate elevator
B. cleft palate knife
B. elevator
B. four-prong retractor
B. Gigli-saw guide
B. head drape
B. modification of Gellhorn
pessary
B. nasal chisel
B. palate hook
B. retractor
B. serrefine
B. silicone drain
Blair-Brown
B.-B. graft
B.-B. implant
B.-B. needle
B.-B. needle holder
B.-B. retractor
B.-B. skin graft knife
B.-B. vacuum retractor
Blake
B. curette
B. drain
B. dressing forceps
B. ear forceps
B. embolus forceps

B. forceps
B. gallstone forceps
B. gingivectomy knife
B. silicone drain
B. uterine curette
Blakemore
B. esophageal tube
B. nasogastric tube
Blakemore-Sengstaken tube
Blakesley
B. ethmoidal forceps
B. forceps
B. lacrimal trephine
B. laminectomy rongeur
B. retractor
B. septal bone forceps
B. septal compression
forceps
B. septal forceps
B. tongue depressor
B. uvular retractor
Blakesley-Wilde
B.-W. ear forceps
B.-W. nasal forceps
Blalock
B. clamp
B. forceps
B. pulmonary artery clamp
B. pulmonary clamp
B. pulmonary stenosis
clamp
B. stenosis clamp
B. suture
Blalock-Kleinert forceps
Blalock-Niedner
B.-N. clamp
B.-N. pulmonary stenosis
clamp
B.-N. pulmonic clamp
Blanchard
B. clamp
B. cryptotome
B. forceps
B. hemorrhoidal forceps
B. pile clamp
Blanco
B. retractor
B. scissors
B. valve spreader
Bland
B. cervical traction forceps
B. perineal retractor

B. vulsellum
B. vulsellum forceps
blank
  implant b.
blanket suture
Blasucci
  B. catheter
  B. clamp
  B. curved-tip ureteral
    catheter
  B. pigtail ureteral catheter
  B. ureteral catheter
Blauth knee prosthesis
Blaydes
  B. angled-lens forceps
  B. corneal forceps
  B. forceps
  B. lens-holding forceps
Bledsoe
  B. brace
  B. cast brace
  B. knee brace
  B. leg brace
Blenderm surgical tape dressing
blepharostat
  b. clamp
  McNeil-Goldman b.
  b. ring
  Schachar b.
BlisterFilm dressing
block
  acrylic bite b.
  b. anesthesia needle
  anterior-posterior cutting b.
  A-P cutting b.
  ball joint b.
  bite b.
  Brightbill corneal cutting b.
  calipers b.
  cutting b.
  4-in-1 cutting b.
  cutting Delrin b.
  cutting Teflon b.
  ENT bite b.
  ESI bite b.
  Guilford-Wright cutting b.
  House cutting b.
  House-Delrin cutting b.
  House Teflon cutting b.
  Jackson bite b.
  Neumann calipers b.
  New Orleans corneal
    cutting b.

Oxyguard mouth b.
Shepard calipers b.
Shepard-Kramer calipers b.
Southern Eye Bank corneal
  cutting b.
Speed-E-Rim denture bite b.
Stahl calipers b.
Tanne corneal cutting b.
tibial augmentation b.
  (TAB)
tibial cutting b.
Wright-Guilford cutting b.
blocker
  hook b.
  Wallach cryosurgical pain b.
Block-Potts intestinal forceps
Block right coronary guiding
  catheter
Blohmka
  B. tonsillar forceps
  B. tonsillar hemostat
Blom-Singer esophagoscope
blood
  b. perfusion monitor (BPM)
  b. pressure cuff
  b. warmer cuff
blood-flow probe
bloodless circumcision clamp
Bloodwell
  B. forceps
  B. tissue forceps
  B. vascular forceps
  B. vascular tissue forceps
Bloodwell-Brown forceps
Bloomberg lens forceps
Blount
  B. bent blade
  B. bone retractor
  B. brace
  B. double-prong retractor
  B. epiphyseal staple
  B. fracture staple
  B. hip retractor
  B. knee retractor
  B. nylon mallet
  B. plate
  B. retractor
  B. scoliosis osteotome
  B. single-prong retractor
  B. staples
  B. V-blade
Blount-Schmidt-Milwaukee brace

blow-by
    b.-b. apparatus
    b.-b. ventilator
blower
    DeVilbiss powder b.
    powder b.
    Rica powder b.
    SMIC powder b.
blue
    b. cotton suture
    b. ring pessary
    b. sponge dressing
    b. twisted cotton suture
blue-black monofilament suture
Blue Max
    B. M. cannula
    B. M. triple-lumen catheter
blue-tip aspirator
Blum
    B. arterial scissors
    B. forceps
Blumenthal
    B. bone rongeur
    B. intraocular lens
    B. rongeur
    B. uterine dressing forceps
blunt
    b. dissecting hook
    b. dissector
    b. elevator
    b. hook
    b. iris hook
    b. needle
    b. palpator
    b. probe
    b. rake retractor
    b. retractor
    b. trocar
blunt-point needle
blunt-tip probe
board
    cartilage cutting b.
    cutting b.
    Fisher tape b.
    Gabarro b.
    Gibson-Ross b.
    graft b.
    pivoting surgical arm b.
    b. splint
    tape b.
boardlike retractor
Boari button
boat nail

Bobath snare
bobbin-type laryngectomy button
Boberg-Ans
    B.-A. implant
    B.-A. intraocular lens
Boberg lens
Bock
    B. knee prosthesis
    B. knife
Bodenham
    B. dermabrasion cylinder
    B. saw
    B. surgical saw
Bodenham-Blair skin graft knife
Bodenham-Humby skin graft knife
Bodenheimer
    B. anoscope
    B. rectal speculum
    B. speculum
Bodian
    B. discission knife
    B. lacrimal pigtail probe
    B. minilacrimal probe
    B. pigtail probe
Bodnar knee retractor
body
    Cloward lumbar retractor b.
    Crockard transoral
      retractor b.
    b. jacket
    b. positioner
Boebinger tongue depressor
Boehler (*var. of* Böhler)
Boehm
    B. anoscope
    B. drop syringe
    B. proctoscope
    B. sigmoidoscope
Boer craniotomy forceps
Boerma obstetrical forceps
Boettcher
    B. antral trocar
    B. arterial forceps
    B. forceps
    B. hemostat
    B. pulmonary artery clamp
    B. pulmonary artery forceps
    B. scissors
    B. tonsillar artery forceps
    B. tonsillar forceps
    B. tonsillar hook
    B. tonsillar scissors
Boettcher-Farlow snare

Boettcher-Jennings mouth gag
Boettcher-Schmidt
    B.-S. antral trocar
    B.-S. forceps
Bogle rongeur
Bograb Universal offset ossicular
  prosthesis
Böhler, Boehler
    B. clamp
    B. extension bow
    B. hip nail
    B. os calcis clamp
    B. pin
    B. plaster cast breaker
    B. reducing fracture frame
    B. rongeur
    B. tongs
    B. traction bow
    B. tractor
    B. wire splint
Böhler-Braun
    B.-B. leg sling
    B.-B. splint
Böhler-Braun fracture frame
Böhler-Knowles hip pin
Böhler-Steinmann
    B.-S. pin
    B.-S. pin holder
Bohlman pin
Bohm dropper sponge
Boies
    B. cutting forceps
    B. cutting forceps tip
    B. forceps
    B. nasal elevator
    B. nasal fracture elevator
Boies-Lombard mastoid rongeur
Boiler septal trephine
Boilo retinoscope
bold
    short b.
Boldrey brace
Bolex
    B. camera
    B. cinecamera
    B. gastrocamera
Boley
    B. dental gouge
    B. retractor
bolster
    retention suture b.
    b. suture
    tie-over b.

bolt
    Barr b.
    Camino ventricular b.
    cannulated b.
    DePuy b.
    Fenton b.
    Fenton tibial b.
    Herzenberg b.
    hexhead b.
    Hubbard b.
    Hubbard-Nylok b.
    Norman tibial b.
    Nylok b.
    Recon proximal drill
      guide b.
    Richmond b.
    solid hex b.   *I bolts*
    tibial b.
    transfixion b.
    Webb b.
    Webb stove b.
    Wilson b.
    wire fixation b.
    Zimmer b.
    Zimmer tibial b.
Bolton forceps
bolus dressing
Bomgart stomal bag
Bonaccolto
    B. capsule fragment forceps
    B. eye implant
    B. forceps
    B. jeweler's forceps
    B. magnet
    B. monoplex orbital implant
      material
    B. new cup jaws forceps
    B. utility forceps
    B. utility pickup forceps
Bonaccolto-Flieringa scleral ring
Bonchek-Shiley cardiac jacket
Bond
    B. arm splint
    B. forceps
    B. placental forceps
Bond-Eze bond adhesive
bone
    b. abduction instrument
    b. awl
    b. biopsy trephine set
    b. bur
    b. calipers
    cancellous b.

bone *(continued)*
- b. cement
- b. chisel
- b. clamp
- b. crusher
- b. curette
- b. drill
- b. drill set
- b. elevator
- b. extension clamp
- b. file
- b. fixation wire
- b. forceps standard set
- b. gouge
- b. guide
- b. hand drill
- b. hook
- b. implant material
- b. lever
- b. mallet
- b. marrow biopsy needle
- b. plate
- b. plating set
- b. plug
- b. prosthesis
- b. rasp
- b. reamer
- b. retractor
- b. rongeur
- b. saw
- b. saw blade
- b. scalpel
- b. screw
- b. screw depth gauge
- b. skid
- b. wax
- b. wax dressing
- b. wax suture

bone-biting forceps
bone-conduction hearing aid
bone-cutting
- b.-c. double-action forceps
- b.-c. forceps
- b.-c. rongeur

Bone-Dri femoral surgical wick
bone elevator
bone-graft holder
bone-holding
- b.-h. clamp
- b.-h. forceps

bone-measuring calipers
bone-splitting forceps
Bonfiglio bone graft

Bongort urinary diversion pouch
Bonn
- B. European suturing forceps
- B. forceps
- B. iris forceps
- B. iris hook
- B. iris scissors
- B. microhook
- B. micro-iris hook
- B. peripheral iridectomy forceps
- B. suturing forceps

Bonnano catheter
Bonney
- B. cervical dilator
- B. clamp
- B. clip
- B. curved needle
- B. forceps
- B. insufflator
- B. needle
- B. retrograde inflator
- B. suture
- B. suture needle
- B. tissue forceps
- B. uterine tube

Bonta mastectomy knife
bony suture
Bookwalter
- B. horizontal bar
- B. horizontal flex bar
- B. rectal blade
- B. rectal kit
- B. retractor
- B. retractor blade
- B. retractor ring
- B. round ring
- B. segmented ring
- B. small incision kit
- B. vaginal Deaver blade
- B. vaginal lateral blade
- B. vaginal posterior blade
- B. vaginal retractor ring

Bookwalter-Balfour
- B.-B. retractor
- B.-B. retractor blade

Bookwalter-Gelpi point retractor blade
Bookwalter-Harrington
- B.-H. retractor
- B.-H. retractor blade

Bookwalter-Kelly
B.-K. retractor
B.-K. retractor blade
Bookwalter-Magrina vaginal retractor
boomerang
b. bladder needle
b. needle
b. needle holder
Booster clip
boot brace
Boplant graft
Borchard
B. Gigli-saw guide
B. wire threader
Bores
B. corneal fixation forceps
B. forceps
B. incision spreader
B. U-shaped forceps
Borge
B. bile duct clamp
B. catheter
B. clamp
Boros esophagoscope
Borsch
B. bandage
B. dressing
Borst side-arm introducer set
Bortone shears
Bortz clamp
Bose
B. bar
B. retractor
B. tracheostomy hook
Bosher commissurotomy knife
Bosker TMI mandibular fixation device
boss
spica cast b.
Bossi
B. cervical dilator
B. dilator
Bostick staple
Boston
B. bivalve brace
B. brace
B. gauze sponge
B. Lying-In cervical forceps
B. Lying-In cervical-grasping forceps
B. stethoscope

Bosworth
B. coracoclavicular screw
B. crown drill
B. drill
B. headband
B. Joseph nasal saw
B. nasal snare
B. nasal wire speculum
B. nerve root retractor
B. osteotomy spline
B. retractor
B. saw
B. spline plate
B. temporary crown
B. tongue depressor
bottle
Ohio safety trap overflow b.
Botvin
B. forceps
B. iris forceps
B. vulsellum forceps
Boucheron
B. ear speculum
B. speculum
Bouchut laryngeal tube
bougie
acorn-tipped b.
Anastasia b.
armed b.
Bangs b.
bellied b.
b. à boule
Buerger dilating b.
bulbous b.
Chevalier Jackson b.
conic b.
cylindrical b.
dilatable b.
dilating b.
b. dilator
Dittel dilating b.
Dittel urethral b.
Dourmashkin tunneled b.
ear b.
elastic b.
elbowed b.
esophageal mercury-filled b.
esophageal tapered mercury-filled b.
eustachian b.
filiform b.
Fort urethral b.

bougie *(continued)*
Friedman-Otis b.
Friedman-Otis b. à boule
fusiform b.
Gabriel Tucker b.
Garceau b.
Gruber b.
b. guide
Guyon dilating b.
Guyon exploratory b.
Harold Hayes eustachian b.
Holinger-Hurst b.
Holinger infant b.
Hurst mercury-filled
  esophageal b.
Jackson b.
Jackson filiform b.
Jackson radiopaque b.
Jackson tracheal b.
Klebanoff b.
LeFort filiform b.
Maloney tapered b.
Maloney tapered mercury-
  filled esophageal b.
mercury-filled esophageal b.
Miller b.
olive-tipped b.
Otis b.
Otis b. à boule
Phillips urethral whip b.
Plummer modified b.
Ravich b.
retrograde b.
rosary b.
Royalt-Street b.
Rusch b.
Ruschelit urethral b.
spiral-tipped b.
Szuler eustachian b.
Trousseau esophageal b.
Tucker retrograde b.
Urbantschitsch eustachian b.
b. urethrotome
Wales rectal b.
Waltham-Street b.
wax b.
whalebone filiform b.
whip b.
Whistler b.
yellow-eyed dilating b.
Bourassa catheter

Bourns
B. infant respirator
B. infant ventilator
Bourns-Bear ventilator
Boutin optic
boutonniere splint
Bovie
B. cautery
B. cautery holder
clinic B.
B. coagulating forceps
B. coagulator
B. conization electrode
B. electrocautery
B. electrode
B. electrosurgical unit
B. holder
liquid conductor B.
B. liquid conductor
B. needle
Ritter B.
B. suction device
underwater B.
bovied
Bovino scleral-spreading forceps
Bovin-Stille vaginal speculum
Bovin vaginal speculum
bow
Aesculap traction b.
Anderson traction b.
Bendixen-Kirschner
  traction b.
Böhler extension b.
Böhler traction b.
Crego-McCarroll traction b.
extension b.
Granberry finger traction b.
Hare lip traction b.
Keys-Kirschner traction b.
Kirschner extension b.
Kirschner wire traction b.
lip traction b.
Logan lip traction b.
Pease-Thomson traction b.
Peterson skeletal traction b.
Schwarz traction b.
Steinmann extension b.
traction b.
Bow & Arrow cannulated drill
  guide
bowe
Bitefork face b.
Hanau face b.

bowel
    b. bag
    b. retractor
Bowen
    B. chisel
    B. gooseneck chisel
    B. gouge
    B. osteotome
    B. periosteal elevator
    B. suction loose body
      forceps
    B. suture drill
Bowen-Grover meniscotome
Bowers cannula
Bowlby arm splint
Bowls septal gouge
Bowman
    B. cataract needle
    B. dilator
    B. eye needle
    B. eye speculum
    B. iris needle
    B. lacrimal dilator
    B. lacrimal probe
    B. needle
    B. needle stop
    B. probe
    B. strabismus scissors
Box
    B. adenotome
    B. osteotome
box
    Anchor sterilizer b.
    sterilizer b.
Box-DeJager adenotome
box-joint forceps
Boxwood mallet
Boyce holder
Boyd
    B. bone graft
    B. dissecting scissors
    B. retractor
    B. scissors
    B. tonsillar scissors
Boyd-Stille tonsillar scissors
Boyes
    B. clamp
    B. muscle clamp
Boyes-Goodfellow
    B.-G. hook
    B.-G. hook retractor
Boyle-Davis mouth gag
Boyle-Rosin clip

Boynton needle holder
Boys-Allis
    B.-A. forceps
    B.-A. tissue forceps
    B.-A. tissue-holding forceps
Bozeman
    B. catheter
    B. clamp
    B. curette
    B. dilator
    B. dressing forceps
    B. forceps
    B. LR dressing forceps
    B. LR packing forceps
    B. LR uterine-dressing
      forceps
    B. needle holder
    B. packing forceps
    B. scissors
    B. speculum
    B. suture
    B. uterine-dressing forceps
    B. uterine forceps
    B. uterine-packing forceps
Bozeman-Douglas dressing forceps
Bozeman-Finochietto needle holder
Bozeman-Fritsch catheter
Bozeman-Wertheim needle holder
BPM
    blood perfusion monitor
bra
    Circumpress compression b.
    Woods Surgitek b.
Braasch
    B. bladder specimen forceps
    B. bladder specimen forceps
      shaft
    B. bulb catheter
    B. bulb ureteral catheter
    B. catheter
    B. direct catheterization
      cystoscope
    B. forceps
    B. ureteral catheter
    B. ureteral dilator
Braasch-Kaplan direct vision
    cystoscope
Braastad
    B. costal arch retractor
    B. retractor
brace
    abdominal b.
    AFO b.

brace *(continued)*
Aircast b.
Aircast air-stirrup leg b.
Aircast fracture b.
Aircast pneumatic b.
air-stirrup ankle b.
AO b.
AOA cervical
  immobilization b.
Arnold b.
Atlanta hip b.
Atlanta-Scottish Rite b.
back b.
bail-lock b.
bike b.
Biomet fracture b.
Bledsoe b.
Bledsoe cast b.
Bledsoe knee b.
Bledsoe leg b.
Blount b.
Blount-Schmidt-Milwaukee b.
Boldrey b.
boot b.
Boston b.
Boston bivalve b.
Buck knee b.
cage-back b.
Callender b.
Camp b.
Can-Am b.
canvas b.
Capener b.
CASH b.
cast b.
cervical b.
cervical collar b.
chair-back b.
Cincinnati ACL b.
clam-shell b.
collar b.
Cook walking b.
Count'R-Force arch b.
CTI b.
Cunningham b.
DePuy fracture b.
derotation b.
DonJoy knee b.
double Becker ankle b.
drop-foot b.
Duncan shoulder b.
elastic-hinge knee b.
49er knee b.

Fisher b.
flexor hinge hand splint b.
Florida b.
Forrester b.
Forrester cervical collar b.
four-point cervical b.
functional fracture b.
Futuro wrist b.
gaiter b.
Galveston metacarpal b.
Gauvain b.
Gillette b.
Goldthwait b.
Guilford b.
hand b.
head b.
Hessing b.
high-Knight b.
Hilgenreiner b.
Hudson b.
Hudson-Jones knee cage b.
hyperextension b.
InCare b.
ischial b.
ischial weightbearing b.
ischial weightbearing leg b.
Jewett b.
Jewett hyperextension b.
Jones b.
Joseph nasal b.
King b.
King cervical b.
Klenzak b.
Kling cervical b.
Knight b.
KSO b.
Kuhlman b.
Kuhlman cervical b.
Küntscher-Hudson b.
Kydex b.
LeCocq b.
leg b.
Lenox Hill b.
Lenox Hill knee b.
Lenox Hill Spectralite
  knee b.
Lerman hinge b.
Lofstrand b.
long-leg b.
Lorenz b.
LSU reciprocation-gait
  orthosis b.
Lyman-Smith b.

Lyman-Smith toe drop b.
Maliniac nasal b.
McDavid knee b.
McKee b.
McLight PCL b.
MD b.
Medical Design b.
Metcalf spring drop b.
Miami fracture b.
Milwaukee b.
Milwaukee scoliosis b.
Multi-Lock knee b.
Murphy b.
nonweightbearing b.
Northville b.
Omni knee b.
Opiela b.
Oppenheim b.
Orthomedics b.
Ortho-Mold spinal b.
Orthoplast fracture b.
Palumbo dynamic
  patellar b.
Palumbo knee b.
Patten Bottom Perthes b.
Phelps b.
Power Play knee b.
PPG-AFO b.
PPG-TLSO b.
PTB b.
Raney flexion jacket b.
ratchet-type b.
Rolyan b.
Rolyan tibial fracture b.
Samiento b.
Schanz b.
Schanz collar b.
scoliosis b.
Scottish Rite b.
seton hip b.
short-leg b.
shoulder b.
shoulder subluxation
  inhibitor b.
Smedberg b.
snap-lock b.
SOMI b.
SSI b.
Stille b.
stirrup b.
Swede-O b.
Taylor b.
Taylor back b.

Taylor-Knight b.
Taylor spine b.
Teufel b.
Teufel cervical b.
Thomas b.
Thomas cervical collar b.
Thomas walking b.
thoracolumbar standing
  orthosis b. (TLSO brace)
TLSO b.
toedrop b.
Tomasini b.
Tracker knee b.
Trinkle b.
UBC b.
UCLA functional long-leg b.
University of British
  Columbia b.
Verlow b.
Von Lackum transection
  shift jacket b.
walking b.
Warm Springs b.
weightbearing b.
Wilke b.
Wilke boot b.
Williams b.
b. with burs
Wright Universal b.
brachial coronary catheter
Bracken
  B. anterior chamber cannula
  B. cannula
  B. fixation forceps
  B. forceps
  B. iris forceps
  B. irrigating cannula
  B. scleral fixation forceps
  B. tissue-grasping forceps
Bracken-Forkas corneal forceps
bracket
  Lee b.
  Lee-Fischer plastic b.
  Ormco wire b.
  orthodontic b.
bracketed splint
Brackett
  B. dental probe
  B. probe
bradawl
Braden flushing reservoir
Bradford
  B. enucleation neurotome

Bradford *(continued)*
- B. forceps
- B. fracture appliance
- B. fracture frame
- B. thyroid forceps
- B. thyroid traction forceps
- B. thyroid traction vulsellum forceps

Bradshaw-O'Neill
- B.-O. aortic clamp
- B.-O. clamp

Brady balanced suspension splint
Bragg-Paul respirator
Brahler ultrasonic dental scaler
braided
- b. Ethibond suture
- b. Mersilene suture
- b. Nurolone suture
- b. nylon suture
- b. polyamide suture
- b. silk suture
- b. suture
- b. wire suture

brain
- b. biopsy cannula
- b. biopsy needle
- b. cannula
- b. clip
- b. clip carrier
- b. depressor
- b. dressing forceps
- b. forceps
- b. probe
- b. retractor
- b. scissors
- b. silicone-coated retractor
- b. spatula
- b. spatula forceps
- b. tissue forceps
- b. tumor forceps

brain-exploring cannula
Braithwaite
- B. clip remover
- B. forceps
- B. nasal chisel
- B. skin graft knife

Brake hemostatic bag
Brand
- B. forceps
- B. passing forceps
- B. shunt-introducing forceps
- B. tendon forceps
- B. tendon-holding forceps
- B. tendon passer
- B. tendon-pulling forceps
- B. tendon stripper
- B. tendon-tunneling forceps

Branemark osseointegration implant
Bransford-Lewis
- B.-L. dilator
- B.-L. ureteral dilator

Brant aluminum splint
Brantley-Turner
- B.-T. retractor
- B.-T. vaginal retractor

Branula cannula
brassiere
- Foerster surgical support b.

brassiere-type dressing
brass mallet
Brauer chisel
Braun
- B. cranioclast
- B. decapitation hook
- B. episiotomy scissors
- B. forceps
- B. frame
- B. graft
- B. implant
- B. ligature carrier
- B. needle
- B. obstetrical hook
- B. speculum
- B. tenaculum
- B. tenaculum forceps
- B. uterine depressor
- B. uterine tenaculum
- B. uterine tenaculum forceps
- B. vaginal depressor

Braun-Schroeder single-tooth tenaculum
Braun-Stadler
- B.-S. episiotomy scissors
- B.-S. scissors
- B.-S. sternal shears

Braunstein fixed calipers
Braunwald
- B. heart valve
- B. valve

Braun-Wangensteen graft
Braun-Yasargil right-angle clip
Brawley
- B. nasal suction tube
- B. retractor
- B. scleral wound retractor

B. sinus rasp
B. suction apparatus
Brawner
B. eye implant
B. orbital implant
breakable blade
breakaway splice
breaker
Böhler plaster cast b.
cast b.
Jarit-Mason cast b.
Jarit-Mason pediatric cast b.
Wölfe-Böhler cast b.
break knife valvulotome
breast
b. calipers
b. form
b. implant
b. localization needle
b. reduction pattern
b. tenaculum
b. tenaculum forceps
Brecht feeder
Breck
B. pin
B. pin cutter
Breen
B. retractor
bregmatomastoid suture
Breinin suction cup
Breisky
B. vaginal retractor
B. vaginal speculum
Breisky-Navratil
B.-N. speculum
B.-N. vaginal speculum
Breisky-Stille speculum
Breitman adenotome
Brenman camera
Brenner
B. carotid bypass shunt
B. forceps
B. rectal probe
brephoplastic graft
Bresgen
B. cannula
B. catheter
B. frontal sinus probe
B. probe
B. sinus probe
Brett bone graft
Brewer vaginal speculum

Brewster
B. phrenic retractor
B. retractor
Bridge
B. clamp
B. deep-surgery forceps
B. forceps
B. hemostatic forceps
B. intestinal forceps
B. telescope
bridge
Albarran b.
Burns converting b.
catheter deflecting b.
double b.
one-horn b.
pediatric b.
retention suture b.
Short b.
single b.
three-way b.
Wappler b.
bridle suture
Briesky pelvimeter
Briggs
B. laryngoscope
B. retractor
B. transilluminator
Brigham
B. brain tumor forceps
B. dressing forceps
B. forceps
B. thumb tissue forceps
B. tissue forceps
Brightbill corneal cutting block
Brighton
B. balloon
B. epistaxis balloon
Brilliant
B. Dentin resin
B. light-cured resin
Brimfield
B. cannulated blade holder
B. cannulated grasping hook
B. magnetic retriever
Brimms
B. denture reliner
B. Denturite denture adhesive
B. Quik-Fix denture repair kit

Brinkerhoff
  B. anoscope
  B. rectal speculum
Brinker hygienic tissue retractor
Bristow
  B. elevator
  B. lever
  B. periosteal elevator
Bristow-Bankart
  B.-B. humeral retractor
  B.-B. soft tissue retractor
Britetrac
  B. fiberoptic instrument
  B. illuminator
  B. speculum
Brittain
  B. chisel
  B. twin pattern chisel
Britt argon laser
broach
  barbed b.
  Charley b.
  crescent b.
  endodontic b.
  b. extractor
  femoral b.
  Firtel b.
  glenoid fin b.
  intramedullary b.
  metacarpal b.
  metatarsal stem b.
  Monaco b.
  orthopaedic b.
  phalangeal b.
  root canal b.
  starter b.
  Swanson intramedullary b.
  tibial b.
broad
  b. adhesive band
  b. band
broadbill hemostat with push fork
broad-blade forceps
Brock
  B. auricular clamp
  B. biopsy forceps
  B. cardiac dilator
  B. clamp
  B. dilator
  B. infundibular punch
  B. mitral valve knife
  B. probe

  B. pulmonary valve knife
  B. valvulotome
Brockenbrough
  B. catheter
  B. curved needle
  B. curved-tip occluder
  B. mapping catheter
  B. modified bipolar catheter
  B. needle
  B. transseptal catheter
  B. transseptal needle
Brockington pile clamp
Brodi director
Brodie
  B. fistular probe
  B. probe
Brodmerkel colon decompression set
Brodney
  B. cannula
  B. catheter
  B. clamp
  B. hemostatic bag
  B. urethrographic cannula
  B. urethrographic clamp
Broggi-Kelman dipstick gauge
Bromley uterine curette
Brompton Hospital retractor
bronchial
  b. biopsy forceps
  b. brush biopsy set
  b. catheter
  b. dilator
  b. forceps
  b. suture
  b. tube
bronchial-grasping forceps
bronchocele
  b. sound
  b. sound raspatory
bronchodilator
bronchofiberscope
  Pentax b.
bronchography set
bronchoscope
  ACMI Marici b.
  Albert slotted b.
  Broyles b.
  Broyles-Negus b.
  Bruening b.
  Chevalier Jackson b.
  Davis b.
  Doesel-Huzly b.

double-channel irrigating b.
Dumon-Harrell b.
Emerson b.
fiberoptic b.
flexible b.
Foregger b.
Foroblique b.
Haslinger b.
Holinger b.
Holinger infant b.
Holinger-Jackson b.
Holinger ventilating
  fiberoptic b.
hook-on b.
infant b.
Jackson costophrenic b.
Jackson full-lumen b.
Jackson standard b.
Jackson staple b.
Jesberg b.
Jesberg infant b.
Kernan-Jackson
  coagluating b.
Marici b.
Michelson infant b.
Moersch b.
Negus b.
Negus-Broyles b.
Olympus fiberoptic b.
Overholt-Jackson b.
Pentax b.
Pilling b.
Riecker respiration b.
Safar ventilation b.
SFB-I right-angled b.
Sharpshay laser b.
Tucker b.
Waterman folding b.
Xaner laser b.
Yankauer b.
bronchoscopic
  b. aspirator
  b. biopsy forceps
  b. brush
  b. cleaner
  b. face shield
  b. forceps
  b. oval-cup biopsy forceps
  b. probe
  b. rotation forceps
  b. rule
  b. spectacles
  b. sponge

  b. sponge carrier
  b. telescope
bronchoscopy disposable suction tube
bronchospirometric catheter
bronchus forceps
bronchus-grasping forceps
Bronner clamp
Bronson
  B. magnet
  B. speculum
  B. ultrasonoscope
Bronson-Magnion magnet
Bronson-Ray
  B.-R. curette
  B.-R. pituitary curette
Bronson-Turner foreign body locator
Bronson-Turtz
  B.-T. iris retractor
  B.-T. speculum
bronze
  b. suture
  b. wire suture
Brooker-Wills nail
Brooks
  B. adenoidal punch
  B. appliance
  B. gallbladder scissors
  B. punch
Brophy
  B. bistoury knife
  B. cleft palate knife
  B. dressing forceps
  B. forceps
  B. gum
  B. mouth gag
  B. needle
  B. periosteal elevator
  B. periosteotome
  B. retractor
  B. scissors
  B. tenaculum
  B. tenaculum retractor
  B. tissue forceps
  B. tooth elevator
Brophy-Deschamps needle
Broviac
  B. atrial catheter
  B. catheter
  B. hyperalimentation catheter

Brown
  B. air dermatome
  B. applicator
  B. cannula
  B. chisel
  B. clamp
  B. cleft palate knife
  B. cleft palate needle
  B. dermatome
  B. dermatome blade
  B. dissecting scissors
  B. ear speculum
  B. electrodermatome
  B. forceps
  B. hook
  B. lip clamp
  B. mallet
  B. nasal splint
  B. needle
  B. needle holder
  B. periosteotome
  B. rasp
  B. retractor
  B. saw
  B. scissors
  B. side-grasping forceps
  B. side-grasping tissue
    forceps
  B. sphenoid cannula
  B. staphylorrhaphy needle
  B. thoracic forceps
  B. tissue forceps
  B. tonsillar snare
  B. tonsillectome
  B. tooth elevator
  B. uvula retractor
Brown-Adson
  B.-A. forceps
  B.-A. tissue forceps
Brown-Bahnson
  B.-B. bayonet forceps
  B.-B. forceps
Brown-Blair
  B.-B. dermatome
  B.-B. skin graft knife
Brown-Buerger
  B.-B. cystoscope
  B.-B. dilator
  B.-B. forceps
Brown-Burr modified Gillies retractor
Brown-Davis mouth gag

Brown-Dean
  B.-D. applicator
  B.-D. cotton applicator
Brown-Dohlman
  B.-D. corneal implant
  B.-D. eye implant
Browne
  B. splint
  B. stone basket
Brown-Fillebrown-Whitehead mouth gag
Brown-Joseph saw
Brown-McHardy
  B.-M. air-filled pneumatic dilator
  B.-M. dilator
  B.-M. pneumatic dilator
Brown-Pusey corneal trephine
Brown-Roberts-Wells
  B.-R.-W. headrest
  B.-R.-W. stereotactic system
Brown-Sanders fascial needle
Brown-Sharp gauge suture
Brown-Swan forceps
Brown-Whitehead mouth gag
brow tape
Broyle retrograde cystoscope
Broyles
  B. anterior commissure laryngoscope
  B. aspirator
  B. bronchoscope
  B. dilator
  B. esophageal dilator
  B. esophagoscope
  B. esophagoscope tube
  B. forceps
  B. laryngoscope
  B. nasopharyngoscope
  B. optical forceps
  B. optical laryngoscope
  B. telescope
  B. wasp-waist laryngoscope
Broyles-Negus bronchoscope
Bruch mastoid retractor
Bruecke tube
Brueckmann lead hand
Bruel-Kjaer transvaginal ultrasound probe
Bruening
  B. aural magnifier
  B. biting tip
  B. bronchoscope

B. cannula
B. chisel
B. cup biting punch
B. cutting-tip forceps
B. ear snare
B. electroscope
B. esophagoscope
B. esophagoscopy forceps handle
B. ethmoid exenteration forceps
B. forceps
B. forceps stylet
B. intracordal injection set
B. Japanese anastigmatic aural magnifier
B. nasal-cutting septal forceps
B. nasal snare
B. otoscope
B. otoscope set
B. pneumatic otoscope
B. pressure syringe
B. punch
B. retractor
B. septal forceps
B. speculum
B. tongue depressor
B. tonsillar snare
Bruening-Arnold intracordal injection set
Bruening-Citelli
B.-C. forceps
B.-C. rongeur
Bruening-Storz
B.-S. anastigmatic aural magnifier
B.-S. diagnostic head
Bruening-Work diagnostic head
Brughleman needle
Brun
B. bone curette
B. chisel
B. curette
B. ear curette
B. guarded chisel
B. mastoid curette
B. plaster shears
Bruner vaginal speculum
Brunetti chisel
Bruni counterpressor
Brunings esophagoscope
Bruni-Wayne clamp approximator

Brunner
B. chisel
B. colon clamp
B. dissector
B. forceps
B. goiter dissector
B. intestinal clamp
B. intestinal forceps
B. ligature needle
B. needle
B. probe
B. raspatory
B. retractor
B. rib shears
B. sigmoid anastomosis forceps
B. tissue forceps
Bruns
B. plaster scissors
B. plaster shears
B. sterlizing rack
Brunschwig
B. arterial forceps
B. forceps
B. retractor
B. visceral forceps
B. visceral retractor
Brunswick-Mack
B.-M. approximator
B.-M. bur
B.-M. chisel
B.-M. rotating drill
Brunswick serrefine
Brunton otoscope
brush
Acu-Brush b.
Air-Lon tracheal tube b.
Alger b.
Anchor all-nylon hand b.
aortic valve b.
Ayre b.
Bard ureteroscopic cytology b.
Barraquer b.
Barraquer sable b.
Barraquer sable eye b.
b. biopsy kit
bronchoscopic b.
bur b.
contour instrument cleaning b.
Contrangle dermabrasion b.
Cox cytology b.

brush *(continued)*
 cytological b.
 denture b.
 Diaflex cytology b.
 Edwards-Carpentier aortic
  valve b.
 endotracheal tube b.
 Geenen biliary cytology b.
 Gill biopsy b.
 Glassman b.
 Grafco tracheal tube b.
 Haidinger b.
 hand nylon scrub b.
 hand scrub b.
 Hobbs sheath b.
 intramedullary b.
 Kurtin planing
  dermabrasion b.
 Kurtin wire b.
 manual dermatome b.
 Marten hair eye b.
 Mill-Rose cytology b.
 nylon hand scrub b.
 nylon scrub b.
 ophthalmic sable b.
 polishing b.
 polypropylene hand b.
 protected bronchoscopic b.
 rectal snare stem b.
 Rusch cleaning b.
 sable b.
 scrub b.
 Sklar b.
 soft scrub b.
 stomach b.
 Storz cleaning b.
 tracheal tube b.
 Wagner laryngeal b.
 Wilson-Cook cytology b.
Bruus scoop
Bryant
 B. mitral hook
 B. nasal forceps
 B. tractor
Brymill probe
Brysmill cryosurgical probe
B&S gauge suture
BSS
 balanced salt solution
BTE
 behind-the-ear
BTF-37 arterial blood filter
BTM hip system

BT 77 turbine
bubble
 gastric b.
 Guibor Expo eye b.
Buchbinder catheter
Buchholz acetabular cup
Buchwald tongue depressor
Buck
 B. applicator
 B. bone curette
 B. convoluted traction unit
 B. curette
 B. ear applicator
 B. ear curette
 B. ear knife
 B. ear probe
 B. earring curette
 B. extension apparatus
 B. extension bar
 B. extension frame
 B. extension splint
 B. extension tractor
 B. femoral cement restrictor
 B. femoral cement restrictor
  inserter
 B. foreign body forceps
 B. fracture appliance
 B. hammer
 B. knee brace
 B. mastoid curette
 B. myringotome
 B. myringotomy knife
 B. nasal applicator
 B. neurological hammer
 B. percussion hammer
 B. probe
 B. traction
 B. traction device
 B. traction splint
 B. Universal convoluted
  traction unit
bucket handle tear set
Buck-Gramcko bone lever
Buckholz prosthesis
Buck-House curette
Buckingham mirror
Buckstein colonic insufflator
Buckston suture
Bucy
 B. cordotomy knife
 B. retractor
 B. spinal cord retractor
 B. suction tube

Bucy-Frazier
  B.-F. cannula
  B.-F. coagulating suction
    cannula
  B.-F. coagulating-suction
    cannula
  B.-F. coagulating suction
    cannula connection cord
  B.-F. coagulating suction
    cannula obturator
  B.-F. monopolar cautery
    cord
  B.-F. suction tube
Bud bur
Budde
  B. halo blade kit
  B. halo flex arm
  B. halo flex arm minivise
  B. halo hinged ring
  B. halo neurosurgical
    retractor
  B. halo patty tray
  B. halo sterilizing case
  B. halo wrench
BUEC
  balloon uterine elevator cannula
Buelan empyema trocar
Buerger
  B. dilating bougie
  B. needle
  B. prostatic needle
  B. punch
  B. snare
Buerger-McCarthy
  B.-M. bladder forceps
  B.-M. forceps
  B.-M. scissors
Buerhenne catheter
Buettner-Parel cutter
Buffalo
  B. dental cement
  B. dental sterilizer
  B. ultrasonic scaler
Buford Word Bartholin gland
  catheter
Bugbee
  B. electrode
  B. fulgurating electrode
Buie
  B. biopsy forceps
  B. cannula
  B. clamp
  B. electrode

  B. fistula probe
  B. forceps
  B. fulgurating electrode
  B. pile clamp
  B. probe
  B. ractal scissors
  B. rectal clamp
  B. rectal forceps
  B. rectal suction tube
  B. retractor
  B. sigmoidoscope
  B. sigmoidoscope dilating
    window
  B. sigmoidoscope light
    carrier
  B. sigmoidoscope
    replacement lamp
  B. specimen forceps
  B. suction tube
  B. tube
Buie-Hirschman
  B.-H. anoscope
  B.-H. clamp
  B.-H. pile clamp
Buie-Smith
  B.-S. anal retractor
  B.-S. rectal speculum
  B.-S. retractor
build-up eye implant
Bülau trocar
bulb
  Beckman Silastic b.
  b. catheter
  dilating b.
  lamp b.
  nystagmus b.
  b. retractor
  Selrodo b.
  b. suture
  b. syringe
  b. ureteral catheter
bulb-operated nebulizer
bulbous
  b. bougie
  b. catheter
bulbous-tip ear syringe
bulky
  b. compressive dressing
  b. dressing
  b. pressure dressing
bulldog
  b. clamp
  b. clamp applier

bulldog *(continued)*
    b. clamp-applying forceps
    b. forceps
    b. scissors
Buller
    B. bandage
    B. eye shield
bullet
    b. forceps
    b. probe
    b.-shaped tip stapler
    b. tip catheter
    tri-point b.
Bulnes-Sanchez retractor
Bumgardner dental holder
Bumm
    B. curette
    B. placental curette
    B. uterine curette
Bumpus
    B. forceps
    B. specimen forceps
bunching suture
Buncke quartz needle
Bunge
    B. curette
    B. evisceration spoon
    B. exenteration spoon
    B. scissors
    B. ureteral meatotome
Bunim
    B. forceps
    B. urethral forceps
bunion dissector
Bunke
    B. clamp
Bunker
    B. forceps
    B. implant
    B. modification of Jackson
      laryngeal forceps
Bunke-Schulz clamp approximator
Bunnell
    B. bone drill
    B. dissecting probe
    B. dressing
    B. drill
    B. forwarding probe
    B. hand drill
    B. knuckle bender splint
    B. needle
    B. outrigger splint
    B. probe

    B. suture
    B. tendon needle
    B. tendon passer
    B. tendon stripper
Bunnell-Howard arthrodesis clamp
Bunnell-Littler dressing
Bunt
    B. catheter
    B. forceps holder
    B. instrument holder
    B. tendon stripper
Bunyan bag
bur, burr
    abrader b.
    Acrotorque b.
    Adson b.
    Adson enlarging b.
    Adson perforating b.
    Adson-Rogers cranial b.
    Allport b.
    Allport eustachian b.
    antral b.
    Bailey b.
    Bailey skull b.
    Ballenger b.
    Ballenger-Lillie b.
    Ballenger-Lillie mastoid b.
    Ballenger mastoid b.
    barrel cutting b.
    bone b.
    brace with b.'s
    Brunswick-Mack b.
    b. brush
    Bud b.
    Burwell b.
    Burwell corneal b.
    Caparosa b.
    Caparosa cutting b.
    carbide b.
    carbide mastoid b.
    cataract b.
    Cavanaugh b.
    Cavanaugh-Israel b.
    Cavanaugh sphenoid b.
    choanal b.
    Concept Ophtho-b.
    Cone b.
    conical b.
    corneal b.
    cranial b.
    Cross corneal b.
    crosscut b.
    crosscut fissure b.

curetting b.
Cushing b.
Cushing cranial b.
cutting b.
Davidson b.
Densco b.
dental b.
D'Errico b.
D'Errico enlarging b.
D'Errico perforating b.
Dialom b.
diamond b.
diamond barrel b.
diamond-dust b.
Doyen b.
b. drill
Dyonics b.
electric b.
electrically-driven b.
enlarging b.
eustachian b.
Farrior b.
fenestration b.
Ferris Smith-Halle b.
Ferris Smith-Halle sinus b.
FG diamond b.
Fisch cutting b.
fissure b.
Frey-Freer b.
Gam-Mer b.
Guilford-Wright b.
Hall b.
Halle b.
Halle bone b.
Hall mastoid b.
Hannahan b.
high-speed b.
high-speed steel b.
b. hole cover
Hough-Wullstein crurotomy
  saw b.
House b.
House-Wullstein
  perforating b.
Hudson b.
Hudson brace with b.
Hudson conical b.
Hudson cranial b.
Hu-Friedy dental b.
inverted cone b.
Jordan b.
Jordan-Day b.
Jordan-Day cutting b.

Jordan-Day fenestration b.
Jordan-Day polishing b.
Jordan perforating b.
Kopetzky b.
Kopetzky sinus b.
Le Blond R diamond
  dental b.
Lee diamond b.
Lempert b.
Lempert diamond-dust
  polishing b.
Lempert fenestration b.
Light-Veley b.
Lindeman b.
Marin b.
Martin b.
mastoid b.
mastoid bone b.
McKenzie b.
McKenzie enlarging b.
Micro-Aire b.
M b. (M-1, M-2, etc.)
Mueller b.
neurosurgical b.
orthopaedic b.
Osteon b.
oval cutting b.
Paton b.
Patton b.
pear-shaped b.
perforating b.
polishing b.
primary trimming b.
Red Witch b.
rhinoplasty diamond b.
Rosen b.
round b.
round cutting b.
round diamond b.
Sachs b.
Sachs skull b.
Scheer-Wullstein cutting b.
Shea b.
side-cutting b.
sinus b.
skull b.
slotting b.
Somerset b.
sphenoidal b.
spherical b.
Storz corneal b.
straight shank b.
Stryker b.

bur *(continued)*
    Stumer perforating b.
    Surgair b.
    Surgitome b.
    Thomas b.
    Turbo-Jet dental b.
    vulcanite b.
    Wachsberger b.
    Wilkerson b.
    Wilkerson choanal b.
    wire pass b.
    Wullstein b.
    Wullstein diamond b.
    Wullstein high-speed b.
    Yazujian b.
    Yazujian cataract b.
    Zimmer b.

Burch
    B. biopsy forceps
    B. calipers
    B. eye calipers
    B. fixation pick
    B. forceps
    B. hook
    B. ophthalmic pick
    B. tendon tucker

Burch-Greenwood tendon tucker

Burdick
    B. cautery
    B. microwave diathermy
      electrosurgical unit
    B. short-wave diathermy
      electrosurgical unit

Buretrol device

Burford
    B. clamp
    B. coarctation forceps
    B. forceps
    B. retractor
    B. rib retractor
    B. rib spreader
    B. spreader

Burford-Finochietto
    B.-F. infant rib spreader
    B.-F. retractor
    B.-F. rib retractor
    B.-F. rib spreader

Burford-Lebsche sternal knife
Burgess Vibro-Graver
Burge vagotometer
bur-hole button
buried suture
Burlisher clamp

Burnett
    B. anoscope
    B. Pap smear kit
    B. Sani-Spec disposable
      speculum

Burnham
    B. bandage scissors
    B. biopsy forceps
    B. forceps
    B. scissors

burnisher
    Nordent b.
    SMIC b.

Burns
    B. bone forceps
    B. bridge telescope
    B. chisel
    B. converting bridge
    B. forceps
    B. guarded chisel
    B. prism bar
    B. telescope

burr *(var. of* bur)
bur-saw
burst pacemaker

Burton
    B. laryngoscope
    B. osteotome

Burwell
    B. bur
    B. corneal bur

Busch umbilical cord scissors
Bushey compression clamp (BCC)
bushing
    patellar planer b.
    reamer b.
    Uniflex drill b.
    Uniflex guide b.

Bush intervertebral curette
Butcher saw
Butler
    B. bayonet forceps
    B. dental retractor
    B. pillar retractor
    B. Red-Cote plaque
      disclosant
    B. retractor
    B. stimulator
    B. tonsillar suction tube

Butte dissector
Butterfield cystoscope
butterfly
    b. adapter

b. clip
b. drain
b. dressing
b. IV needle
b. needle
b. winged infusion set
button
Accu-Flo b.
Accu-Flo bur-hole b.
anastomotic b.
Bentley b.
Boari b.
bobbin-type laryngectomy b.
bur-hole b.
Chlumsky b.
collar b.
Converse fracture b.
Converse fracture-wiring b.
Davy surgical b.
Drummond b.
b. electrode
Emesay suture b.
fixation b.
gastrostomy b.
Graether collar b.
Helsper laryngectomy b.
Jaboulay b.
Kazanjian b.
Kazanjian tooth b.
Kistner b.
Lardennois b.
Lee lingual b.
b. lip lens manipulator
Moore b.
Moore tracheostomy b.
Murphy b.
Murphy-Johnson
  anastomosis b.
Norris b.
Panje b.
Panje voice b.
patellar b.
peritoneal b.

polyethylene collar b.
polypropylene b.
Reuter b.
Reuter bobbin collar b.
Sheehy b.
Sheehy collar b.
Silastic suture b.
Smithwick buttonhook b.
Smithwick silk
  buttonhook b.
stoma b.
b. suture
suture b.
Teflon b.
Teflon collar b.
Todd b.
Todd bur hole b.
tracheostomy b.
Villard b.
voice b.
button-end knife
buttonhook (*See also* hook)
Graether collar b.
b. nerve retractor
b. retractor
buttress
b. plate
Teflon pledget suture b.
Buttress thread screw
Buxton
B. clamp
B. uterine clamp
Buyes air-vent suction tube
BV100 needle
BV-2 needle
BVAD
biventricular assist device
B-W graft
Byars mandibular prosthesis
Bycroft-Brunswick thyroid retractor
Byford retractor
bypass
Byrel pacemaker

C

cable
    coaxial c.
    fiberoptic c.
    c. graft
    Sullivan variable stiffness c.
    c. wire suture
Cabot
    C. leg splint
    C. Medical Corporation
       diagnostic laparoscope
    C. Medical Corporation
       operating laparoscope
    C. Medical Corporation
       videoscope
    C. nephroscope
Cadogan-Hough footpedal suction
    control
caesarian (var. of cesarean)
Caffinière prosthesis
cage-back brace
Cairns
    C. clamp
    C. dissection forceps
    C. forceps
    C. hemostatic forceps
    C. retractor
    C. rongeur
    C. scalp retractor
Cairns-Dandy hemostasis forceps
Cairtron ultrasonic aspirator
Cal-20 central dialysate
    preparation unit
Calandruccio
    C. compression apparatus
    C. triangular compression
       device
calcar
    c. planer
    c. reamer
    c. replacement stem
    c. trimmer
    c. trimmer with Zimmer-
       Hudson shank
calcified tissue scissors
Calcipulpe cavity liner
Calcitite bone graft
calcium sodium alginate wound
    dressing

Calcutript
    Karl Storz C.
    C. by Karl Storz
Caldwell guide
Calgiswab dressing
Calhoun-Hagerless needle
Calhoun-Merz needle
Calhoun needle
calibrated
    c. clubfoot splint
    c. depth gauge
    c. grasping tube
    c. pin
    c. probe
    c. V-Lok cuff
calibrator
    Fogarty c.
    screw depth c.
Calibri forceps
caliceal cup
calipers
    Albee bone graft c.
    Austin Moore inside-
       outside c.
    Austin Moore outside c.
    Austin strut c.
    Barker c.
    Berens c.
    Bertillon c.
    c. block
    bone c.
    bone-measuring c.
    Braunstein fixed c.
    breast c.
    Burch c.
    Burch eye c.
    Castroviejo c.
    Castroviejo eye c.
    Castroviejo marking c.
    Castroviejo-Schacher
       angled c.
    Cone c.
    Cone ice tong c.
    Cottle c.
    ECG c.
    EKG c.
    electric c.
    eye c.
    Fat-O-Meter skinfold c.
    Green c.

calipers *(continued)*
Green eye c.
Harpenden skinfold c.
House c.
House strut c.
ice-tong c.
Jameson c.
Jameson eye c.
John Green c.
Ladd c.
Lange skinfold c.
Machemer c.
McGaw skinfold c.
Mendez degree c.
middle ear c.
ophthalmic c.
Osher internal c.
Paparella c.
Paparella rasp c.
Ruddy stapes c.
ruler c.
skinfold c.
Stahl c.
Storz c.
strut c.
Thorpe c.
tibial c.
tonsillar c.
Townley c.
Townley femur c.
Townley inside-outside
femur c.
Vernier c.
V. Mueller ruler c.
x-ray c.
Cali-Press graft press
Callaghan suture
Callahan
C. flange
C. forceps
C. lacrimal rongeur
C. lens loupe
C. modification speculum
C. retractor
C. scleral fixation forceps
Callahan forceps
Callender
C. brace
C. clip
Callison-Adson
C.-A. tissue
C.-A. tissue forceps

Calman
C. carotid clamp
C. ring clamp
Calnan-Nicole finger prosthesis
calomel electrode
Calot jacket
Caltagirone
C. chisel
C. skin graft knife
calvarium clamp
Calve cannula
cam blade-tipped catheter
Cambridge jelly electrode
**Cameco syringe pistol aspiration
device**
camera
Anger c.
anterior bulbi c.
Beaulieu c.
Bolex c.
Brenman c.
Circon c.
Circon video c.
Docustar fundal c.
DyoCam arthroscopic
video c.
endo-c.
EndoVideo-Five
endoscopic c.
Endo zoom lens c.
Fujica c.
fundal c.
fundus-retinal c.
gamma c.
Garcia-Ibanez M picture c.
Garcia-Ibanez super 8 c.
House-Urban Pentax c.
House-Urban-Stille c.
Icarex 25 Med mirror
reflex lens c.
Keeler c.
Kowa c.
Kowa angiographic c.
Kowa fundus c.
Kowa hand c.
Kowa Optimed c.
Kowa retinal c.
Leicaflex c.
Lester A. Dine c.
Medx c.
Mirrorreflex c.
Nikon c.
Nikon fundus c.

Olympus c.
Olympus OM-1
  endoscopic c.
Olympus operating c.
ophthalmoscope c.
Pentax Spotmatic c.
Polaroid c.
Polaroid CB-100 c.
Polavision Land c. for
  endoscopy
Reichert c.
Robot Starr II c.
Scheimpflug c.
Schepens binocular
  indirect c.
scintillation c.
Storz c.
Storz endo c.
Stryker c.
Stryker chip c.
Syn-optics c.
Topcon c.
Topcon SL-45 c.
Urban microsurgery closed-
  circuit color TV c.
video c.
Zeiss c.
Zeiss operating c.
Zeiss-Scheimpflug c.
camera-processor
Neuroguide c.-p.
Cameron
C. cautery
C. gastroscope
C. omni-angle gastroscope
C. periosteal elevator
Cameron-Haight
C.-H. elevator
C.-H. periosteal elevator
Cameron-Miller electrode
Cam guided trephine
Camino
C. catheter
C. ventricular bolt
camouflage prosthesis
Campbell
C. airplane splint
C. arthroplasty gouge
C. catheter
C. forceps
C. graft
C. infant catheter

C. lacrimal sac retractor
C. laminectomy rongeur
C. ligature-carrier forceps
C. miniature sound
C. miniature urethral sound
C. needle
C. nerve rongeur
C. nerve root retractor
C. osteotome
C. periosteal elevator
C. retractor
C. self-retaining retractor
C. slit lamp
C. suprapubic cannula
C. suprapubic retractor
C. suprapubic trocar
C. traction splint
C. ureteral catheter
C. ureteral catheter forceps
C. ureteral forceps
C. ureterotome
C. urethral catheter
C. urethral catheter forceps
C. ventricular needle
Campbell-Boyd tourniquet
Campbell-French sound
Campbell-type Heyman fundus
  applicator
Camp brace
Canadian
C. chest retractor
C. hip prosthesis
Canad meniscal knife
Canakis
C. beaded hip pin
C. wrench
canal
c. chisel
c. knife
c. reamer
canaliculus
c. dilator
c. knife
c. probe
canalicural scissors
Can-Am brace
cancellous
c. bone
c. bone screw
c. pin
c. screw
candle vaginal cesium implant

Cane
    C. bone-holding forceps
    C. forceps
Canfield tonsillar knife
cannister
    coil c.
    Evacupack disposable
     suction c.
Cannon
    C. Bio-Flek nasal splint
    C. endarterectomy loop
    C.-type stripper
Cannon-Rochester lamina elevator
Cannu-Flex guide wire
cannula
    Abelson c.
    Abelson cricothyrotomy c.
    Abelson curved
     cricothyrotomy c.
    Abraham c.
    Abraham laryngeal c.
    Accu-Flo U-channel
     stripping c.
    Accu-Flo ventricular c.
    acorn c.
    Adson c.
    Adson brain-exploring c.
    Adson drainage c.
    Adson exploring c.
    air c.
    air injection c.
    Air-Lon inhalation c.
    alpha-chymotrypsin c.
    Anis aspirating c.
    anterior chamber c.
    anterior chamber
     irrigating c.
    Antoni-Hook lumbar
     puncture c.
    antral c.
    antral sinus c.
    aortic c.
    aortic arch c.
    aortic perfusion c.
    Aronson-Fletcher antrum c.
    arterial c.
    aspirating c.
    aspiration c.
    aspirator c.
    atrial c.
    attic c.
    Bahnson c.
    Bahnson aortic c.

    Bailey c.
    Bailey lacrimal c.
    balloon uterine elevator c.
     (BUEC)
    Bard arterial c.
    Bardic c.
    Barraquer c.
    Bechert intraocular lens c.
    Bechert IOL c.
    Bellocq c.
    Bellucci c.
    Bergstrom-Stille muscle c.
    Berkeley c.
    B-H irrigating c.
    Binkhorst hooked c.
    Binkhorst irrigating c.
    biopsy c.
    BioTac biopsy c.
    Bishop-Harman c.
    Bishop-Harman anterior
     chamber c.
    Bishop-Harman anterior
     chamber irrigating c.
    Bishop-Harman irrigating c.
    bivalved c.
    Blue Max c.
    Bowers c.
    Bracken c.
    Bracken anterior chamber c.
    Bracken irrigating c.
    brain c.
    brain biopsy c.
    brain-exploring c.
    Branula c.
    Bresgen c.
    Brodney c.
    Brodney urethrographic c.
    Brown c.
    Brown sphenoid c.
    Bruening c.
    Bucy-Frazier c.
    Bucy-Frazier coagulating-
     suction c.
    Bucy-Frazier coagulating
     suction c.
    Buie c.
    Calve c.
    Campbell suprapubic c.
    Cantlie c.
    Carabelli c.
    Carabelli mirror c.
    cardiovascular c.
    Casselberry c.

Casselberry sphenoid c.
Castaneda c.
Castroviejo c.
Castroviejo cyclodialysis c.
cataract-aspirating c.
caval c.
Charlton c.
Chilcott c.
Chilcott venoclysis c.
Christmas-tree c.
Churchill cardiac suction c.
Clagett c.
Clagett S-c.
c. clamp
clysis c.
coagulating-suction c.
Coakley c.
Coakley frontal sinus c.
coaxial c.
Cobe small vessel c.
Codman c.
Cohen c.
Cohen-Eder c.
Cohen-Eder uterine c.
Cohen intrauterine c.
Cohen tubal insufflation c.
Colt c.
Concept c.
Concorde suction c.
Cone c.
cone biopsy c.
Cone-Bucy c.
Cone cerebral c.
Continental c.
Cooper c.
Cooper
  chemopallidectomy c.
Cooper double-lumen c.
Cope needle introducer c.
coronary c.
coronary artery c.
coronary perfusion c.
cortex-aspirating c.
c. cradle
c. cradle holder
cricothyrotomy c.
curved c.
curved cricothyrotomy c.
cyclodialysis c.
dacryocystorhinostomy c.
Day c.
Day attic c.
De La Vega c.

Delima ethmoid c.
Devonshire-Mack c.
DeWecker c.
DeWecker syringe c.
Digiflex c.
disposable cystotome c.
DLP aortic root c.
Dohrmann-Rubin c.
Dorsey c.
Dorsey ventricular c.
double c.
double-lumen c.
Dougherty anterior
  chamber c.
Douglas c.
Dow Corning c.
Drews c.
Drews irrigating c.
Duke c.
Dulaney antral c.
duodenoscope c.
Dupuis c.
ear c.
egress c.
Eichen c.
Eichen irrigating c.
Elecath ECMO c.
Elsberg c.
Elsberg brain-exploring c.
Elsberg ventricular c.
ERCP c.
Eriksson muscle c.
esophagoscopic c.
exploring c.
fallopian c.
Fasanella c.
Fasanella lacrimal c.
Fazio-Montgomery c.
Fein c.
femoral artery c.
femoral perfusion c.
Fink cul-de-sac c.
Fischer c.
Fischer silicone
  ventricular c.
Fish c.
Fisher c.
Fisher ventricular c.
Fish infusion c.
flattened irrigating c.
Fletcher-Pierce c.
Flexicath silicone
  subclavian c.

cannula *(continued)*
Flourotip c.
Floyd loop c.
Fluoro Tip ERCP c.
flute c.
Ford Hospital ventricular c.
Franklin-Silverman c.
Franklin-Silverman biopsy c.
Frazier c.
Frazier brain-exploring c.
Frazier exploring c.
Frazier suction c.
Frazier ventricular c.
Freeman Blue-Max c.
Freeman positioning c.
frontal sinus c.
Futch c.
Futch antral c.
gallbladder c.
Gans c.
Gans cyclodialysis c.
Gans eye c.
Gass c.
Gass cataract-aspirating c.
Gass retinal detachment c.
Gass vitreous-aspirating c.
Gill double irrigating-
  aspirating c.
Gill irrigating-aspirating c.
Gill sinus c.
Gill-Welsh c.
Gill-Welsh aspirating c.
Gill-Welsh double c.
Gill-Welsh double-barreled
  irrigating-aspirating c.
Gill-Welsh irrigating c.
Gill-Welsh irrigating-
  aspirating c.
Gill-Welsh olive-tip c.
Girard c.
Girard irrigating c.
Goldstein c.
Goldstein anterior
  chamber c.
Goldstein anterior chamber-
  irrigating c.
Goldstein irrigating c.
Goldstein lacrimal c.
Goodfellow c.
Goodfellow frontal sinus c.
Gott c.
Grafco c.
Gram c.

gravity infusion c.
Gregg c.
Grizzard c.
Grizzard subretinal c.
Gromley-Russell c.
Grüntzig femoral
  stiffening c.
c. guard
guiding c.
Hahn c.
Hajek c.
Harvard c.
Hasson c.
Hasson balloon uterine
  elevator c.
Hasson-Eder laparoscope c.
Haverfield c.
Haverfield brain c.
Havlicek c.
Havlicek spiral c.
Haynes c.
Haynes brain c.
Healon injection c.
Hendon venoclysis c.
Hepacon c.
Heyer-Schulte-Fischer
  ventricular c.
high-flow c.
high-flow coaxial c.
Hirschman hooked c.
Hoen c.
Hoen ventricular c.
Hoffer forward-cutting
  knife c.
c. holder
c. holder tray
Holinger c.
hollow c.
Holman-Mathieu c.
Holman-Mathieu
  salpingography c.
Hudgins c.
Hudgins salpingography c.
Hudson All-Clear nasal c.
Hulka c.
Hulka uterine c.
Hulten-Stille c.
HUMI c.
Hunt-Reich secondary c.
Huse c.
Hyde "frog" irrigating c.
iliac-femoral c.
Illouz c.

Illouz suction c.
inflow c.
infusion c.
Ingals c.
Ingals antral c.
Ingals flexible silver c.
Ingals rectal injection c.
ingress/egress c.
inhalation c.
injection c.
inlet c.
inner c.
inner coaxial irrigating c.
c. instrument cleaner
intra-arterial c.
intracardiac c.
intraocular c.
intraocular lens c.
intrauterine c.
IPAS flexible c.
irrigating c.
irrigating and aspirating
  coaxial c.
I-tech c.
Jarcho c.
Jarcho self-retaining
  uterine c.
Jarcho uterine c.
Jarit air injection c.
Jarit lacrimal c.
Jensen-Thomas irrigating-
  aspirating c.
J-shaped I&A c.
Judd c.
Kahn c.
Kahn trigger c.
Kahn uterine c.
Kahn uterine trigger c.
Kanavel c.
Kanavel brain-exploring c.
Kanavel exploring c.
Kara cataract-aspirating c.
Katzenstein rectal c.
Keisler lacrimal c.
Kelman c.
Kelman cyclodialysis c.
Kesilar c.
Keyes-Ultzmann-Luer c.
Kidde uterine c.
Killian c.
Killian antral c.
Killian-Eichen c.
Killian nasal c.

Kleegman c.
Knolle c.
Knolle anterior chamber
  irrigating c.
Knolle-Pearce c.
Knolls irrigating c.
Kos c.
Kos attic c.
Krause c.
Krause nasal snare c.
Kreutzmann c.
lacrimal c.
Lamb c.
Landolt c.
laparoscopic c.
large antral c.
large-bore c.
laryngeal c.
lens c.
Lewicky threaded
  infusion c.
Lichtwicz antral c.
Lifemed c.
ligature c.
Lillie c.
Lillie attic c.
Lindeman c.
Lindeman self-retaining
  uterine vacuum c.
Littell c.
Litwak c.
Look coaxial flexible
  disposable c.
Look single-use c.
Luer tracheal c.
Lukens c.
lumen c.
Luongo c.
Luongo sphenoid
  irrigating c.
LV apex c.
Malette-Spencer coronary c.
Malström-Westman c.
Mandelbaum c.
maxillary sinus c.
Mayo c.
Mayo coronary perfusion c.
Mayo-Ochsner c.
Mayo-Ochsner suction
  trocar c.
McCaskey sphenoid c.
McGoon c.
McIntyre c.

cannula *(continued)*

McIntyre angled c.
McIntyre anterior
  chamber c.
McIntyre-Binkhorst
  irrigating c.
McIntyre coaxial c.
McIntyre lacrimal c.
McIntyre staight anterior
  chamber c.
mediastinal c.
Medicut c.
Medi-Tech flexible
  stiffening c.
Menghini c.
Mercedes tip c.
metal c.
metallic-tip c.
middle ear suction c.
mirror c.
Moncrieff c.
Moncrieff anterior
  chamber c.
Moncrieff anterior chamber
  irrigating c.
monitoring c.
Montgomery tracheal c.
Morris c.
Morwel c.
Müller coronary perfusion c.
MVS c.
Myerson-Moncrieff c.
Myles c.
Myles sinus c.
Myles sinus antral c.
nasal c.
nasal snare c.
Neal c.
Neal fallopian c.
Neubauer c.
Neubauer lancet c.
New York Eye and Ear c.
nucleus c.
nucleus delivery c.
O'Gawa irrigating c.
O'Gawa two-way
  aspirating c.
O'Gawa two-way cataract-
  aspirating c.
O'Gawa two-way irrigating
  and aspirating c.
Osher air bubble removal c.
Osher lens vacuuming c.

outer coaxial irrigating c.
outflow c.
outlet c.
pacifico c.
Packo pars plana c.
Padgett-Concorde suction c.
Padgett shark-mouth c.
Park irrigating c.
Paterson c.
Paterson laryngeal c.
Patton c.
Pearce coaxial c.
Peczon I & A c.
Pereyra c.
Pereyra ligature c.
perfusion c.
Pierce c.
Pierce attic c.
plastic c.
polyethylene c.
Polystan perfusion c.
portal c.
Portex c.
Portex nylon c.
Portnoy ventricular c.
Post washing c.
Pritchard c.
Pye c.
Pynchon c.
Randolph c.
Randolph cyclodialysis c.
Ranfac c.
rectal injection c.
Reipen c.
return-flow c.
Rica tracheostomy c.
Rigg c.
Riordan flexible silver c.
Robb c.
Robb antral c.
Rockey c.
Rockey mediastinal c.
Rockey tracheal c.
Rohrschneider c.
Rolf-Jackson c.
Roper c.
Roper alpha-chymotrypsin c.
Rowsey c.
Rowsey fixation c.
Rubin c.
Rubin fallopian tube c.
Rycroft c.
S-c.

Sachs c.
Sachs brain-exploring c.
saphenous vein c.
Sarns c.
Sarns aortic arch c.
Sarns two-stage c.
Sarns venous drainage c.
Scheie c.
Scheie anterior chamber c.
Scheie cataract-aspirating c.
Scott c.
Scott attic c.
Scott rubber ventricular c.
Scott ventricular c.
Seletz c.
Seletz ventricular c.
self-retaining infusion c.
Semm c.
Semm uterine c.
Semm vacuum c.
Sewall c.
Sewall antral c.
Shahinian lacrimal c.
Sheets c.
Sheets irrigating vectis c.
Shepard c.
Shepard incision
  irrigating c.
Shepard radial keratotomy
  irrigating c.
side-port c.
sidewall infusion c.
Silastic c.
Silastic coronary artery c.
silicone c.
silicone oil c.
c. silicone support cradle
silicone tip c.
Silver c.
Silver curved c.
Silverman-Boeker c.
Simcoe cortex c.
Simcoe double c.
Simcoe double-barreled c.
Simcoe nucleus delivery c.
Simcoe reverse aperture c.
Simcoe reverse irrigating-
  aspirating c.
Sims c.
sinoscopy c.
sinus c.
sinus antral c.
sinus-irrigating c.

Skillern c.
Skillern sphenoidal c.
Smcoe I&A c.
SMI c.
Soresi c.
Southey c.
Spencer c.
sphenoidal c.
Spielberg sinus c.
Spizziri-Simcoe c.
stable access c. (SAC)
Stangel fallopian tube c.
Storz needle c.
straight lacrimal c.
Strauss c.
subclavian c.
subretinal fluid c.
suction c.
suprapubic c.
surgical c.
Sylva irrigating c.
Teflon c.
Teflon ERCP c.
Tenner c.
Tenner eye c.
Tenner lacrimal c.
Thomas irrigating-
  aspirating c.
three-hole aspiration c.
Thurmond nucleus-
  irrigating c.
Thurmond two-way air
  bubble removal c.
Tibbs arterial c.
Topper c.
Torchia c.
Torchia aspirating c.
Torchia nucleus c.
tracheal c.
tracheostomy c.
tracheotomy c.
transseptal c.
Tremble sphenoid c.
Trendelenburg c.
trigeminus c.
trigger c.
Troutman c.
Troutman alpha-
  chymotrypsin c.
tubal insufflation c.
c. tubing adapter
Tulevech lacrimal c.
Turnbull c.

cannula *(continued)*
two-stage Sarns c.
two-way cataract
aspirating c.
Uldall subclavian
hemodialysis c.
Universal c.
urethral instillation c.
urethrographic c.
U-shaped c.
uterine self-retaining c.
uterine trigger c.
uterine vacuum c.
Vabra c.
vacuum intrauterine c.
vacuum uterine c. (VUC)
Van Alyea c.
Van Alyea antral c.
Van Alyea frontal sinus c.
Van Alyea sphenoid c.
Vance prostatic aspiration c.
Van Osdel irrigating c.
vein graft c.
Veirs c.
vena caval c.
Venflon c.
venoclysis c.
venous c.
ventricular c.
Veress c.
Veress laparoscopic c.
Veress peritoneum c.
Viking c.
Viscoflow angled c.
Visitec c.
Visitec anterior chamber c.
Vitalcor cardioplegia
infusion c.
Von Eichen c.
Von Eichen antral c.
washout c.
Webb c.
Webster infusion c.
Weil c.
Weil lacrimal c.
Weiner c.
Weisman c.
Wells c.
Wells Johnson c.
Welsh c.
West c.
West lacrimal c.
wire-wound c.

Wolf c.
Wolf drainage c.
Wolf return-flow c.
Yankauer middle meatus c.
Zinn endoilluminiation
infusion c.
Zylik c.
cannular scissors
cannulated
c. bolt
c. bronchoscopic forceps
c. cortical step drill
c. drill
c. forceps
c. four-flute reamer
c. nail
c. obturator
c. reamer
c. screw
c. wire threader
cannulation catheter
Canon automatic keratometer
Cantlie cannula
Cantor
C. intestinal tube
C. tube
canvas brace
cap
Cloward drill guard c.
Lehnhardt Universal c.
c. splint
Zimmer tibial nail c.
Caparosa
C. bur
C. cutting bur
C. wire crimper
CAPD
continuous ambulatory
peritoneal dialysis
capeline bandage
Capener
C. brace
C. nail
C. nail plate
Capes clamp
capillary
c. bed
c. flow dialyzer
CAPIS
CAPIS bone plate system
CAPIS compression plate
CAPIS individual plate
CAPIS kit

CAPIS reconstruction plate
CAPIS screw
CAPIS screw assortment
   tray
CAPIS screwdriver
CAPIS sterilizing tray
capitonnage suture
Caplan
   C. angular scissors
   C. dorsal scissors
   C. nasal scissors
   C. scissors
Capmix amalgamator
Capner gouge
caps
   Supramid quarter globe c.
Capsitome cystitome
capsular
   c. forceps
   c. scraper
   c. scrubber
   c. style lens
capsule
   c. applier system
   c. coupeur
   Crosby-Kugler biopsy c.
   Crosby-Kugler pediatric c.
   dental c.
   c. fragment forceps
   c. knife
   NK dental c.
   Saf-T-Fit amalgamator c.
   Watson intestinal biopsy c.
capsule-grasping forceps
Capsulform lens
capsulorrhexis forceps
capsulotome
   Darling c.
capsulotomy
   c. blade
   c. forceps
   c. scissors
caput forceps
Carabelli
   C. aspirator
   C. cancer cell collector
   C. cannula
   C. endobronchial tube
   C. irrigator
   C. lumen finder
   C. mirror cannula
Carapace face shield
Carass ventilator

Carb-Bite
   C.-B. needle holder
   C.-B. tissue forceps
Carb-Edge scissors
carbide
   c. bur
   c. mastoid bur
carbide-jaw forceps
carbolized knife blade
Carbomedics cardiac valve
   prosthesis
carbon
   c. dioxide (CO_2) laser
      scalpel
   c. dioxide laser
   c. fiber half ring
   c. steel blade
CARD
   cardiac automatic resuscitative
   device
Cardak percutaneous catheter
   introducer
Cardens retractor
cardiac
   c. automatic resuscitative
      device (CARD)
   c. catheter
   c. dilator
   c. infant catheter
   c. monitor
   c. pacemaker
   c. probe
   c. valve dilator
Cardillo retractor
cardinal suture
cardiodilator
cardioesophageal junction dilator
cardiograph
   Minnesota impedance c.
Cardio-Grip
   C.-G. anastomosis clamp
   C.-G. aortic aneurysm
      clamp
   C.-G. aortic clamp
   C.-G. bronchus clamp
   C.-G. iliac forceps
   C.-G. ligature carrier
   C.-G. multipurpose clamp
   C.-G. pediatric clamp
   C.-G. renal artery clamp
   C.-G. tangential occulusion
      clamp

Cardio-Grip *(continued)*
    C.-G. tissue forceps
    C.-G. vascular clamp
Cardiomarker catheter
Cardiomemo device
Cardiometrics cardiotomy reservoir
Cardio-Pace Medical Durapulse pacemaker
cardioplegic needle
cardioscope
    Carlens Universal c.
cardiospasm dilator
Cardiotach fetal monitor
cardiotomy reservoir
cardiovascular
    c. anastomotic clamp
    c. bulldog clamp
    c. cannula
    c. clamp
    c. forceps
    c. implant
    c. needle holder
    c. Prolene suture
    c. retractor
    c. scissors
    c. stylet
    c. suture
    c. tissue forceps
cardioverter-defibrillator
    automatic implantable c.-d. (AICD)
Cardona
    C. corneal prosthesis forceps
    C. corneal trephine
    C. focalizing fundus lens
    C. focalizing goniolens
    C. forceps
    C. keratoprosthesis prosthesis
    C. threading lens forceps
Carey-Coons soft stent
Cargile suture
Carl
    C. P. Jones traction splint
    C. Zeiss myringotomy tube
Carlens
    C. bronchospirometric catheter
    C. catheter
    C. curette
    C. forceps
    C. mediastinoscope
    C. needle

    C. tracheotomy retractor
    C. tube
    C. Universal cardioscope
Carlens-Stille tracheal retractor
Carmack
    C. curette
    C. ear curette
Carmalt
    C. arterial forceps
    C. clamp
    C. forceps
    C. hemostatic forceps
    C. hysterectomy forceps
    C. splinter forceps
    C. thoracic forceps
Carman rectal tube
Carmel clamp
Carmody
    C. aspirator
    C. drill
    C. electric aspirator
    C. forceps
    C. perforator drill
    C. thumb tissue forceps
    C. tissue forceps
Carmody-Batson elevator
Carmody-Brophy forceps
Caroline finger retractor
Carolon life support antiembolism stockings
carotid
    c. angiogram needle
    c. arterial bed
    c. artery bypass clamp
    c. artery clamp
    c. artery forceps
    c. clamp
carpal
    c. lunate implant
    c. scaphoid screw
Carpenter
    C. dissector
    C. tonsillar knife
Carpentier
    C. ring
    C. ring heart valve
    C. stent
Carpentier-Edwards
    C.-E. bioprosthesis
    C.-E. heart valve
    C.-E. xenograft
Carpule needle

Carrel
   C. clamp
   C. hemostatic forceps
   C. mosquito forceps
   C. suture
   C. tube
Carrel-Girard screw
carrier
   amalgam c.
   brain clip c.
   Braun ligature c.
   bronchoscopic sponge c.
   Buie sigmoidoscope light c.
   Cardio-Grip ligature c.
   clamp c.
   Cooley ligature c.
   cotton c.
   DeBakey ligature c.
   DeBakey-Semb ligature c.
   deep ligature c.
   Deschamps c.
   Deschamps ligature c.
   ear snare wire c.
   Favaloro ligature c.
   Favaloro-Semb ligature c.
   fiberoptic light c.
   Finochietto clamp c.
   Fitzwater ligature c.
   foil c.
   Fragen c.
   gauze pad c.
   goiter ligature c.
   Jackson sponge c.
   Kilner suture c.
   Krause nasal snare wire c.
   Kwapis ligature c.
   Lahey c.
   Lahey ligature c.
   laryngeal sponge c.
   ligature c.
   light c.
   London College foil c.
   Macey tendon c.
   Madden ligature c.
   Mayo c.
   Mayo goiter ligature c.
   Mija ligature c.
   nasal snare wire c.
   proctological cotton c.
   Raz double-prong ligature c.
   Rica cotton c.
   sigmoidoscope light c.
   sponge c.

   Storz cotton c.
   suture c.
   Tauber ligature c.
   tendon c.
   tube c.
   Wangensteen c.
   Wangensteen deep
      ligature c.
   Wangensteen ligature c.
   Yasargil ligature c.
   Young ligature c.
Carrington wound gel
Carrion penile prosthesis
Carrion-Small penile implant
Carr lobectomy tourniquet
Carroll
   C. aluminum mallet
   C. awl
   C. bone-holding forceps
   C. bone hook
   C. finger goniometer
   C. forearm tendon stripper
   C. hook curette
   C. needle
   C. offset hand retractor
   C. osteotome
   C. periosteal elevator
   C. retractor
   C. rongeur
   C. self-retaining spring
      retractor
   C. skin hook
   C. tendon passer
   C. tendon-passing forceps
   C. tendon-pulling forceps
   C. tendon retriever
Carroll-Adson
   C.-A. dural forceps
   C.-A. forceps
Carroll-Bennett finger retractor
Carroll-Bunnell drill
Carroll-Legg
   C.-L. osteotome
   C.-L. periosteal elevator
Carroll-Smith-Petersen osteotome
Carson
   C. catheter
   C. model catheter
Cartella eye shield
Carter
   C. clamp
   C. curette
   C. eye sphere introducer

Carter *(continued)*
    C. intranasal splint
    C. mitral valve retractor
    C. retractor
    C. septal knife
    C. septal speculum
    C. sphere introducer
    C. submucous curette
    C. submucous elevator
Carter-Glassman
    C.-G. clamp
    C.-G. resection clamp
cartilage
    c. abrader
    c. chisel
    c. clamp
    c. crusher
    c. cutting board
    c. elastic pullover kneecap
      splint
    c. forceps
    c. guide
    c. implant
    c. knife
    c. scissors
cartilage-holding forceps
Carti-Loid syringe
Cartmill feeding tube kit
cartridge
    Adsorba hemoperfusion c.
    Alukart hemoperfusion c.
    Diakart hemoperfusion c.
    Hemocal hemoperfusion c.
    Hemokart hemoperfusion c.
Cartwright
    C. heart prosthesis
    C. implant
caruncle
    c. clamp
    c. forceps
carver
    amalgam c.
    Cooley wax c.
    dental wax c.
    Frahm c.
    G-C wax c.
    modelling c.
    Nordent c.
    SMIC c.
Carver dental wax
Carvex
case
    Berens sterilizing c.

    Budde halo sterilizing c.
    Cloward PLIF c.
    Codman dilator c.
    Contique contact lens c.
    Cooley neonatal set c.
    Mazzariello-Caprini stone
      forceps sterilizing c.
Case appliance
CA 125 serum tumor marker
Casey pelvic clamp
CASH brace
Caspar
    C. alligator forceps
    C. forceps
    C. hook
    C. retractor
    C. rongeur
    C. speculum
Casselberry
    C. cannula
    C. sphenoid cannula
    C. sphenoid tube
cassette cup collecting device
Cassidy-Brophy
    C.-B. dressing forceps
    C.-B. forceps
cast
    c. brace
    c. breaker
    c. lingual splint
    c. padding
    c. spreader
CastAlert device
Castallo
    C. eyelid retractor
    C. eye speculum
    C. lid retractor
    C. retractor
Castanares
    C. face-lift scissors
Castaneda
    C. anastomosis clamp
    C. cannula
    C. clamp
    C. forceps
    C. IMM vascular clamp
    C. infant sternal retractor
    C. kit
    C. multipurpose clamp
    C. partial occlusion clamp
    C. retractor
    C. suture tag forceps

C. vascular clamp
C. vascular forceps
Castaneda-Mixter
C.-M. clamp
C.-M. forceps
C.-M. thoracic clamp
Castelli-Paparella colar button tube
Castens
C. ascites trocar
C. hydrocele trocar
Castex rigid dressing
Casteyer prostatic punch
CastGuard guard
Castillo catheter
casting wax sheet
Castle
C. Daystar surgical
television system
C. surgical light
Castmate plaster bandage dressing
**cast-molded PMMA intraocular
lens**
Castorit investment material
Castro-Martinez keratome
Castroviejo
C. acrylic implant
C. adjustable retractor
C. angled keratome
C. anterior synechia scissors
C. bay forceps
C. blade
C. bladebreaker
C. blade holder
C. calipers
C. cannula
C. capsular forceps
C. clamp
C. compressor
C. corneal dissector
C. corneal scissors
C. corneal section scissors
C. corneal trephine
C. corneoscleral forceps
C. corneoscleral punch
C. corneoscleral suture
forceps
C. cross-action capsule
forceps
C. cyclodialysis cannula
C. cyclodialysis spatula
C. dermatome
C. dilator
C. dissector

C. double-end dilator
C. double-end lacrimal
dilator
C. double-end spatula
C. electrode
C. electromucotome
C. enucleation snare
C. erysiphake
C. eye calipers
C. eye implant
C. eye needle holder
C. eye speculum
C. fixation forceps
C. forceps
C. implant
C. improved trephine
C. iris scissors
C. keratome
C. keratoplasty scissors
C. lacrimal dilator
C. lip clamp
C. marking calipers
C. microcorneal scissors
C. minicorneal scissors
C. minirazor bladebreaker
C. mosquito lid clamp
C. needle
C. needle holder
C. ophthalmic knife
C. oscillating razor
C. razor
C. razor bladebreaker
C. razor holder
C. retractor
C. scissors
C. scleral marker
C. sclerotome
C. slimline blade
C. spatula
C. spoon
C. surface electrode
C. suture forceps
C. synechia spatula
C. tenotomy scissors
C. transplant forceps
C. transplant-grafting forceps
C. transplant trephine
C. trephine
C. tying forceps
Castroviejo-Arruga
C.-A. capsular forceps
C.-A. forceps
Castroviejo-Barraquer needle holder

Castroviejo-Colibri
 C.-C. corneal forceps
 C.-C. forceps
Castroviejo-Furness corneal-holding forceps
Castroviejo-Kalt eye needle holder
Castroviejo-McPherson keratectomy scissors
Castroviejo-Schacher angled calipers
Castroviejo-Simpson forceps
Castroviejo-Steinhauser mucotome
Castroviejo-style mini bladebreaker
Castroviejo-Troutman
 C.-T. eye needle holder
 C.-T. needle holder
 C.-T. scissors
Castroviejo-Vannas
 C.-V. capsulotomy scissors
 C.-V. scissors
Castroviejo-Wheeler discission knife
Catalano
 C. capsular forceps
 C. corneoscleral forceps
 C. dilator
 C. forceps
 C. intubation set
 C. muscle hook
 C. needle holder
 C. tying forceps
cataract
 c. aspirator
 c. blade
 c. bur
 c. knife
 c. needle
 c. probe
 c. rotoextractor extractor
 c. scissors
 c. spoon
cataract-aspirating
 c.-a. cannula
 c.-a. needle
Catford visual acuity test
catgut
 c. needle
 Rica surgical c.
 SMIC surgical c.
 c. suture (CGS, CS)
Cathcart orthocentric hip prosthesis
cathematic catheter

catheter
 Abramson c.
 Accu-Flo distal c.
 Accu-Flo distal slit-valve c.
 Accu-Flo infant end c.
 Accu-Flo spring c.
 Accu-Flo spring distal slit c.
 Accu-Flo ventricular c.
 ACMI c.
 ACMI Alcock c.
 ACMI Bunts c.
 ACMI coated Foley c.
 ACMI Emmett hemostatic c.
 ACMI Owens c.
 ACMI positive pressure c.
 ACMI severance c.
 Acmistat c.
 ACMI Thackston c.
 ACMI ureteral c.
 ACMI Word Bartholin gland c.
 Acmix Foley c.
 acorn-tipped c.
 Acrad HS c.
 ACS c.
 ACS angioplasty c.
 ACS balloon c.
 ACS exchange guiding c.
 ACS JI4 c.
 ACS mini c.
 ACS RX coronary dilatation c.
 c. adapter
 c. adaptor
 Aero-flo tip c.
 AgX antimicrobial Foley c.
 Air-Lon inhalation c.
 AL-1 c.
 Alcock c.
 Alcock hemostatic c.
 Alcock return-flow hemostatic c.
 Alcott c.
 AL II guiding c.
 alimentation c.
 Allis c.
 all-purpose urethral c.
 Alvarez-Rodriguez cardiac c.
 amber latex c.
 Amcath c.
 Amplatz c.

Amplatz aortography c.
Amplatz cardiac c.
Amplatz coronary c.
Amplatz femoral c.
Amplatz high-flow torque-
  control c.
Angiocath PRN c.
Angioflow high-flow c.
angiographic c.
angiographic balloon
  occlusion c.
Angio-Kit c.
angiopigtail c.
angioplasty balloon c.
angled balloon c.
angled pigtail c.
angle-tipped urethral c.
angulated c.
Anthron heparinized c.
Anzio c.
aortic c.
aortogram c.
aortographic c.
AR-1 c.
Arani c.
Arani double-loop guiding c.
AR-2 diagnostic c.
AR-2 guiding c.
Argyle c.
Argyle Medicut R c.
Argyle oxygen c.
Arrow balloon wedge c.
Arrow-Berman balloon c.
Arrow-Howes c.
Arrow-Howes multilumen c.
Arrow multilumen c.
Arrow pulmonary artery c.
Arrow Twin Cath c.
arterial c.
arterial embolectomy c.
arterial irrigation c.
ASC Monorel c.
ASC RX perfusion
  balloon c.
Ash c.
ASI uroplasty TCU
  dilatation c.
AtheroCath spinning
  blade c.
Atlantic ileostomy c.
Atlas balloon dilatation c.
Atrac-II double-balloon c.

Atrac multipurpose
  balloon c.
atrioseptostomy c.
auricular appendage c.
automatic c.
Axiom DG balloon
  angioplasty c.
bag c.
Bailey c.
Bailey transthoracic c.
bailout c.
Baim c.
Balectrode pacing c.
balloon c.
c. balloon
balloon biliary c.
balloon dilatation c.
balloon dilating c.
balloon embolectomy c.
balloon flotation c.
balloon pumping c.
balloon-tipped
  angiographic c.
balloon valvuloplasty c.
balloon wedge pressure c.
Baltherm thermal dilution c.
Banno c.
Bard c.
Bardam c.
Bardam red rubber c.
Bard balloon-directed
  pacing c.
Bardco c.
Bard electrophysiology c.
Bardex c.
Bardex Foley c.
Bardex Foley balloon c.
Bardex Foley return-flow
  rentention c.
Bardex Lubricath Foley c.
Bard guiding c.
Bard helical c.
Bardic c.
Bardic cutdown c.
Bardic-Deseret Intracath c.
Bardic translucent c.
Bardic vein c.
Bard x-ray ureteral c.
Bartholin gland c.
Baschui pigtail c.
bat-wing c.
Baxter angioplasty c.
Baxter dilatation c.

catheter *(continued)*
Baxter-V. Mueller c.
Beird eye c.
Béniqué c.
Berman c.
Berman angiographic c.
Berman cardiac c.
Bernstein c.
bicoudé c.
biliary c.
biliary balloon c.
biliary dilator c.
Biosearch c.
bipolar c.
bipolar pacing c.
bipolar pacing electrode c.
bipolar temporary
  pacemaker c.
bladder c.
Blasucci c.
Blasucci curved-tip
  ureteral c.
Blasucci pigtail ureteral c.
Blasucci ureteral c.
Block right coronary
  guiding c.
Blue Max triple-lumen c.
Bonnano c.
Borge c.
Bourassa c.
Bozeman c.
Bozeman-Fritsch c.
Braasch c.
Braasch bulb c.
Braasch bulb ureteral c.
Braasch ureteral c.
brachial coronary c.
Bresgen c.
Brockenbrough c.
Brockenbrough mapping c.
Brockenbrough modified
  bipolar c.
Brockenbrough transseptal c.
Brodney c.
bronchial c.
bronchospirometric c.
Broviac c.
Broviac atrial c.
Broviac hyperalimentation c.
Buchbinder c.
Buerhenne c.
Buford Word Bartholin
  gland c.

bulb c.
bulbous c.
bulb ureteral c.
bullet tip c.
Bunt c.
cam blade-tipped c.
Camino c.
Campbell c.
Campbell infant c.
Campbell ureteral c.
Campbell urethral c.
cannulation c.
cardiac c.
cardiac infant c.
Cardiomarker c.
Carlens c.
Carlens
  bronchospirometric c.
Carson c.
Carson model c.
Castillo c.
cathematic c.
Cathlon IV c.
caval c.
cecostomy c.
central c.
central venous c.
central venous pressure c.
  (CVP)
cephalad c.
cerebral c.
Chaffin c.
Chaffin tube c.
Chemo-Port c.
cholangiography c.
chorionic villus sampling c.
Clark expanding mesh c.
Clark helix c.
Clark rotating cutter c.
cloverleaf c.
coaxial c.
Cobe-Tenckhoff peritoneal
  dialysis c.
cobra c.
cobra-shaped c.
Codman-Holter c.
coil-tipped c.
colon motility c.
Comfort Cath c.
Comfort Cath II c.
condom c.
conductance c.
cone tip c.

Cholangiocath

conformation of right
   heart c.
conical c.
conical-tip c.
Constantine c.
Constantine flexible
   metal c.
ConstaVac c.
continuous irrigation c.
Cook c.
Cook arterial c.
Cook pigtail c.
Cook TPN c.
Cordis c.
Cordis guiding c.
Cordis Lumelec c.
Cordis pigtail c.
Corlon c.
coronary c.
coronary dilatation c.
coronary guiding c.
coronary perfusion c.
coronary sinus
   thermodilution c.
Cotton graduated dilation c.
coudé c.
coudé assist c.
coudé suction c.
coudé-tip c.
coudé-tip demeure c.
coudé urethral c.
Councill c.
Councill retention c.
Cournand c.
Cournand quadpolar c.
Coxeter c.
Coxeter prostatic c.
CPV c.
Critikon c.
Critikon balloon temporary
   pacing c.
Critikon balloon
   thermodilution c.
Critikon balloon-tipped end-
   hole c.
Critikon balloon wedge
   pressure c.
Critikon Berman
   angiographic balloon c.
cryoablation c.
CUI 1 drain or c.
Cummings c.
Cummings four-wing c.

Cummings four-wing
   Malecot retention c.
Cummings nephrostomy c.
Cummings-Pezzer c.
Cummings-Pezzer head c.
Curl Cath c.
curved c.
cutdown c.
CVIS intravascular US
   imaging c.
CVP c.
CVS c.
Cynosar c.
Dacron c.
Dakin c.
Datascope intra-aortic
   balloon pump c.
Davis c.
Davol c.
Davol rubber c.
Dearor model c.
decompression c.
decompressive enteroclysis c.
c. deflecting bridge
DeKock two-way
   bronchial c.
DeLee c.
DeLee infant c.
DeLee suction c.
DeLee tracheal c.
à demeure c.
Deseret c.
Deseret flow-directed
   thermodilution c.
Desilets c.
Devonshire c.
Devonshire-Mack c.
DeWeese caval c.
Diaflex ureteral dilatation c.
diagnostic c.
dialysis c.
dilating c.
dilating pressure balloon c.
dilation c.
dilation balloon c.
dilator c.
disposable c.
distal slit valve c.
DLP cardioplegic c.
Doppler c.
Doppler coronary c.
Dormia stone basket c.

catheter *(continued)*

Dorrost brachial internal
mammary guiding c.
Dotter caged-balloon c.
Dotter coaxial c.
double-current c.
double-J-stent c.
double-lumen c. (DLC)
double-lumen balloon stone
extractor c.
double-lumen Broviac c.
double-lumen Hickman c.
double-lumen Hickman-
Broviac c.
double-lumen Silastic c.
Dover c.
Dow Corning c.
Dow Corning ileal pouch c.
drainage c.
Drew-Smythe c.
Ducor angiographic c.
Ducor balloon c.
Ducor cardiac c.
DVI Simpson AtheroCath c.
Dynacor Foley c.
Dynacor suction c.
Easy c.
echo transponder
electrode c.
Edslab c.
Edslab cholangiography c.
Edwards c.
Edwards diagnostic c.
Eichelter-Schenk vena
caval c.
eight-lumen esophageal
manometry c.
eight-lumen manometry c.
elbowed c.
Elecath c.
Elecath thermodilution c.
electrode c.
electrohemostasis c.
El Gamal coronary
bypass c.
El Gamal guiding c.
embolectomy c.
Encapsulon epidural c.
en chemise c.
end-hole c.
end-hole pigtail c.
endoscopic retrograde
cholangiopancreatography c.

endotracheal c.
Enhanced Torque 8F
guiding c.
Entract dilation and
occlusion c.
Eppendorfer c.
Eppendorfer cardiac c.
ERCP c.
Erythroflex c.
esophageal balloon c.
esophageal manometry c.
esophageal motility
perfused c.
esophagoscopic c.
eustachian c.
Evermed c.
Express PTCA c.
external c.
extrusion balloon c.
6-eye c.
fallopian c.
FAST balloon c.
FAST right heart
cardiovascular c.
faucial c.
faucial eustachian c.
female c.
femoral guiding c.
fenestrated c.
fiberoptic oximeter c.
filiform c.
filiform-tipped c.
Finesse guiding c.
Finesse large-lumen
guiding c.
flat-blade-tipped c.
flexible c.
flexible metal c.
Flextip c.
floating c.
flotation c.
flow-directed c.
flow-directed balloon
cardiovascular c.
flow-directed balloon-
tipped c.
flow-directed
thermodilution c.
flow-oximetry c.
fluid-filled c.
Fogarty c.
Fogarty arterial
embolectomy c.

Fogarty arterial irrigation c.
Fogarty balloon c.
Fogarty balloon biliary c.
Fogarty-Chin c.
Fogarty-Chin extrusion
  balloon c.
Fogarty-Chin peripheral
  dilatation c.
Fogarty dilation c.
Fogarty embolus c.
Fogarty gallstone c.
Fogarty irrigation c.
Fogarty occlusion c.
Fogarty venous irrigation c.
Fogarty venous
  thrombectomy c.
Folatex c.
Foley c.
Foley acorn-bulb c.
Foley-Alcock c.
Foley-Alcock bag c.
Foley balloon c.
Foley cone-tip c.
Foltz c.
Foltz-Overton cardiac c.
c. forceps
Formex barium c.
four-eye c.
four-wing c.
four-wing Malecot
  retention c.
Freedom external c.
Frekatheter vena caval c.
French c.
French angiographic c.
5-French angiographic c.
French curve out-of-plane c.
French Foley c.
French in-plane guiding c.
French JR4 Schneider c.
French MBIH c.
French mushroom-tip c.
French red-rubber
  Robinson c.
French Robinson c.
French SAL c.
French Silastic Foley c.
5-French stiff c.
French tripolar His c.
Friend c.
Friend-Hebert c.
Fritsch c.
Furness c.

Gambro c.
Ganz-Edwards coronary
  infusion c.
Garceau c.
Garceau ureteral c.
gastroenterostomy c.
Geenen graduated
  dilation c.
Gensini c.
Gensini Teflon c.
Gentle-Flo suction c.
Gesco c.
Gibbon c.
Gibbon urethral c.
Gilbert c.   *Goetz*
Gilbert balloon c.
Gilbert pediatric c.
Gilbert pediatric balloon c.
Gilbert plug sealing c.
Gilbert-type Bardex Foley c.
Goodale-Lubin c.
Goodale-Lubin cardiac c.
Gore-Tex c.
Gore-Tex peritoneal c.
Gorlin c.
Gorlin pacing c.
Gould PentaCath 5-lumen
  thermodilution c.
Gouley c.
Gouley whalebone
  filiform c.
Goutz c.
graduated c.
graduated-size c.
Grigor fiber light guide c.
Grollman c.
Grollman pigtail c.
Groshong c.
Groshong double-lumen c.
Groshong dual-lumen c.
Grüntzig c.
Grüntzig c.
Grüntzig arterial balloon c.
Grüntzig balloon c.
Grüntzig balloon
  angiography c.
Grüntzig D dilating c.
Grüntzig D-G dilating c.
Grüntzig Dilaca c.
Grüntzig 20-30 dilating c.
Grüntzig G dilating c.
Grüntzig S dilating c.
Grüntzig steerable c.

catheter *(continued)*
  guide c.
  c. guide
  c. guide holder
  c. guide wire
  guiding c.
  Guyon ureteral c.
  H-1 c.
  Hagner c.
  Hagner bag c.
  Hakim c.
  Hakko Dwellcath c.
  Hamilton-Steward c.
  Hanafee c.
  Hancock coronary
    perfusion c.
  Hancock embolectomy c.
  Hancock fiberoptic c.
  Hancock hydrogen
    detection c.
  Hancock luminal
    electrophysiologic
    recording c.
  Hancock thermodilution c.
  Hancock wedge-pressure c.
  Harris c.
  Harris uterine injector c.
  Hartmann c.
  Hartmann eustachian c.
  Hartzler c.
  Hartzler ACS coronary
    dilation c.
  Hartzler ACX balloon c.
  Hartzler balloon c.
  Hartzler dilatation c.
  Hartzler Micro c.
  Hartzler Micro II c.
  Hartzler Micro XT c.
  Hartzler Ultra-Lo-Profile c.
  Hatch c.
  headhunter c.
  headhunter visceral
    angiography c.
  helical c.
  helical PTCA dilatation c.
  hemostatic c.
  Hepacon c.
  heparin-coated c.
  hexapolar c.
  Heyer-Schulte c.
  Heyer-Schulte-Portnoy c.
  Heyer-Schulte-Pudenz
    cardiac c.

  H-H open-end
    alimentation c.
  Hickman c.
  Hickman-Broviac c.
  Hickman indwelling c.
  Hickman indwelling right
    atrial c.
  Hidalgo c.
  Hieshima coaxial c.
  Higgins c.
  high-fidelity c.
  high-flow c.
  His c.
  Hi-Torque floppy guide c.
  Hobbs medical dilatation
    balloon c.
  Hohn c.
  c. holder
  Hollister c.
  Hollister external c.
  Hollister self-adhesive c.
  Holter c.
  Holter distal atrial c.
  Holter distal peritoneal c.
  Holter-Hausner c.
  Holter lumboperitoneal c.
  Holter ventricular c.
  Holt self-retaining c.
  Hopkins Percuflex
    drainage c.
  hot-tipped c.
  Hryntschak c.
  HUI c.
  Huibregtse-Katon ERCP c.
  Hunter-Sessions vena cava-
    occluding balloon c.
  Hurwitt c.
  Hyams c.
  Hyams double-lumen c.
  HydraCross TLC PTCA c.
  hydrostatic balloon c.
  hyperalimentation c.
  hysterosalpingography c.
  IAB c.
  ICP c.
  ileal reservoir c.
  Imperson c.
  Impra peritoneal c.
  indwelling c.
  infant c.
  infant female c.
  infant male c.
  inflatable c.

inflatable Foley bag c.
Infusaid c.
infusion c.
Ingram c.
Inoue balloon c.
Intact c.
intercostal c.
internal mammary artery c.
interventional c.
Intimax biliary c.
Intimax cholangiography c.
Intimax occlusion c.
Intimax vascular c.
intra-aortic balloon c.
intra-arterial
  chemotherapy c.
intracardiac c.
Intracath c.
intracoronary guiding c.
intracoronary perfusion c.
intracranial pressure c.
Intran disposable
  intrauterine pressure
  measurement c.
Intrasil c.
intrauterine c.
intrauterine insemination c.
  (IUI)
intrauterine pressure c.
intravenous c.
intravenous pacing c.
intraventricular pressure
  monitoring c.
Intrepid balloon c.
Intrepid percutaneous
  transluminal coronary
  angioplasty c.
Intrepid PTCA c.
c. introducer
introducer c.
irrigating c.
irrigation c.
Itard c.
Itard eustachian c.
IV c.
Jackson-Pratt c.
Jaeger-Whiteley c.
James lumbar peritoneal c.
Javid c.
JB c.
JB-1 c.
Jehle coronary perfusion c.
Jelco c.

Jelm c.
Jelm two-way c.
Jinotti dual-purpose c.
JL-4 c.
JL-5 c.
Jo-Kath c.
Josephson c.
Josephson quadpolar c.
Jostra c.
JR-4 c.
JR-5 c.
Judkins c.
Judkins coronary c.
Judkins guiding c.
Judkins-4 guiding c.
Judkins left coronary c.
Judkins right coronary c.
Judkins torque-control c.
Judkins USCI c.
J-Vac c.
Kaminsky c.
Karmen c.
Katon c.
Katzen balloon c.
Kaufman c.
KDF-2.3 intrauterine
  insemination c.
Kearns bag c.
Kensey atherectomy c.
kidney internal splint c.
kidney internal stent c.
Kifa c.
Kifa green, grey, red,
  yellow c.
Kimball c.
King c.
King guiding c.
King multipurpose c.
King multipurpose coronary
  graft c.
kink-resistant c.
kink-resistant peritoneal c.
Kish urethral c.
KISS c.
Lahey c.
Lane c.
Lane rectal c.
Lapides c.
LAP-13 Ranfac
  cholangiographic c.
large-bore c.
large-lumen c.
laser c.

catheter *(continued)*
latex c.
lavaging c.
Ledor pigtail c.
LeFort c.
LeFort male c.
LeFort urethral c.
left ventricular clamp c.
Lehman c.
Lehman aortographic c.
Lehman pancreatic
  manometry c.
Lehman ventriculography c.
LeRoy c.
LeVeen c.
Levin tube c.
Lifecath c.
Lillehei-Warden c.
Lincoff c.
Lincoff design of Storz
  scleral buckling balloon c.
Lloyd c.
Lloyd bronchial c.
Lloyd double c.
Lloyd esophagoscopic c.
lobster-tail c.
Lofric disposable urethral c.
Longdwel c.
Longdwel Teflon c.
Lo-Profile balloon c.
Lo-Profile II balloon c.
Lo-Profile steerable
  dilatation c.
LPS c.
Lucae eustachian c.
Lumaguide infusion c.
lumbar peritoneal c.
lumbar subarachnoid c.
Lumelec c.
Magill endotracheal c.
Maglinte c.
Mahurkar c.
Mahurkar dual-lumen
  dialysis c.
Mahurkar dual-lumen
  femoral c.
male c.
Malecot c.
Malecot nephrostomy c.
Malecot self-retaining
  urethral c.
Malecot Silastic c.
Malecot suprapubic c.

Malecot suprapubic
  cystostomy c.
Malecot urethral c.
Malecot 2-wing c.
Malecot 4-wing c.
Mallinckrodt c.
Mallinckrodt angiographic c.
Maloney c.
Mandelbaum c.
Mani c.
Mani cerebral c.
manometer-tipped c.
Mansfield balloon c.
Mansfield balloon
  dilatation c.
Mansfield dilatation
  balloon c.
Marlin thoracic c.
Maryfield introducer c.
mastoid c.
Max Force biliary balloon
  dilatation c.
McCarthy c.
McCaskey c.
McCaskey antral c.
McGood coronary
  perfusion c.
McGoon coronary
  perfusion c.
McIntosh double-lumen c.
McIntosh hemodialysis c.
McIver c.
McIver nephrostomy c.
Meadox Surgimed c.
Med-Co flexible c.
Medena continent
  ileostomy c.
mediastinal c.
Medicut c.
Medina c.
Medina ileostomy c.
MediPort-DL double-
  lumen c.
Medi-Tech c.
Medi-Tech arterial
  dilatation c.
Medi-Tech balloon c.
Medi-Tech Mansfield
  dilating c.
Medi-Tech steerable c.
Medrad c.
Medrad angiographic c.
Medtronic balloon c.

Mentor coudé c.
Mentor Foley c.
Mentor Tele-Cath ileal
  conduit sampling c.
Mentor-Urosan external c.
Mercier c.
metal c.
metal ball-tip c.
Metaport c.
Metras c.
Metras bronchial c.
Mewissen infusion c.
Micro-Guide c.
micro-invasive c.
micromanometer-tip c.
Micross c.
Micross dilatation c.
midstream aortogram c.
Mikaelsson c.
Millar micromonometer c.
Millar pigtail
  angiographic c.
Miller-Abbott c.
Mills operative peripheral
  angioplasty c.
Mini-Profile dilatation c.
Minispace IUI c.
Mitsubishi angioscopic c.
Mixtner c.
Monorail angioplasty c.
Morris c.
Morris thoracic c.
MP-A-1 c.
MP-A-2 c.
MPF c.
MPR drain c.
Mueller c.
Mullins c.
Mullins transseptal c.
multielectrode impedance c.
multilumen c.
Multi-Med triple-lumen
  infusion c.
multipolar impedance c.
multipurpose c.
Multistim electrode c.
mushroom c.
Mylar c.
Namic c.
nasal c.
nasobiliary c.
nasotrachael c.
NBIH c.

Neal c.
c. needle
needle tip c.
Nélation urethralc.
Nélaton c.
Neoplex c.
nephrostomy c.
Neplaton c.
Nestor guiding c.   *Niogra c.*
Neuroguide Visicath
  viewing c.
Nichols-Jehle coronary
  multihead c.
NIH c.
NIH left ventriculography c.
Nir Lat male external c.
Norfolk aspiration c.
Norton flow-directed Swan-
  Ganz thermodilution c.
Nova thermodilution c.
Novoste c.
Nutricath c.
Nycore c.
Nycore angiography c.
occlusion c.
Odman-Ledin c.
Olbert balloon c.
Olbert balloon dilatation c.
olivary c.
olive-tipped c.
Omni c.
Omniflex balloon c.
Opaca-Garcea ureteral c.
Opticath oximeter c.
Optiscope c.
ORC-B Ranfac
  cholangiographic c.
c.-over-needle
Owatusi double c.
Owen c.
Owen Lo-Profile dilation c.
oximetric c.
oximetry c.
pacemaker c.
Paceport c.
pacifico c.
pacing c.
Paparella c.
Park blade septostomy c.
Pathfinder c.
PDT guiding c.
pediatric c.
pediatric balloon c.

catheter *(continued)*
  pediatric Foley c.
  pediatric pigtail c.
  Pedicat c.
  peel-away c.
  peel-off c.
  pennate suction c.
  Pennine Nélaton c.
  PE Plus II balloon
    dilatation c.
  PE Plus II peripheral
    balloon c.
  Percor-DL c.
  Percor dual-lumen intra-
    aortic balloon c.
  Percor intra-aortic
    balloon c.
  Percor-Stat-DL c.
  percutaneous c.
  percutaneous transhepatic
    pigtail c.
  percutaneous transheptatic
    biliary drainage c.
  percutaneous transluminal
    coronary angioplasty c.
  perfusion c.
  peripheral atherectomy c.
  peripheral long-line c.
  peripherally inserted
    central c. (PICC)
  peritoneal c.
  peritoneal dialysis c.
  peritoneal reflux control c.
  Perma-Cath c.
  permanent silicone c.
  Per-Q-Cath percutaneously
    inserted central venous c.
  Perry c.
  Perry-Foley c.
  Perry pediatric Foley
    latex c.
  Per-Stat-DL c.
  pervenous c.
  Pezzer c.
  Pezzer mushroom-tipped c.
  Pezzer self-retaining c.
  Pezzer self-retaining
    urethral c.
  Pezzer suprapubic
    cystostomy c.
  Pharmaseal c.
  Pharmaseal disposable c.
  Pharmex disposable c.

  Phillips c.
  Phillips urethral c.
  Phillips urologic c.
  PIBC c.
  Picolino monorail c.
  pigtail c.
  Pilcher c.
  Pilcher bag c.
  Pilotip c.
  Pinkerton c.
  plastic c.
  plastic Tiemann c.
  Pleurovac chest c.
  c. plug
  pneumatic balloon c.
  Polaris c.
  polyethylene c.
  Polysil-Foley c.
  Polystan c.
  Polystan venous return c.
  polyvinyl c.
  Port-A-Cath implantable c.
  portal c.
  Portex chorionic villus
    sampling c.
  Portex-Gibbon c.
  Portnoy c.
  Portnoy ventricular c.
  Porto-Vac c.
  Positrol c.
  Positrol II Bernstein c.
  Positrol USCI c.
  Pousson pigtail c.
  preformed c.
  preformed Cordis c.
  preshaped c.
  Priestly c.
  probe c.
  probing c.
  Procath electrophysiology c.
  Profile Plus c.
  Profile Plus balloon
    dilatation c.
  Profile Plus dilatation c.
  Proflex dilatation c.
  Pro-Flo c.
  prostatic c.
  Pruitt irrigation c.
  Pruitt occlusion c.
  PTBD c.
  PTCA c.
  Pudenz barium cardiac c.
  Pudenz cardiac c.

Pudenz-Heyer vascular c.
Pudenz infant cardiac c.
Pudenz peritoneal c.
Pudenz ventricular c.
pulmonary arterial c.
pulmonary flotation c.
pulmonary triple-lumen c.
pusher c.
Putnam evacuator c.
quadpolar W/Damato
  curve c.
Quadra-Flo infusion c.
quadripolar c.
Quanticor c.
Quinton c.
Quinton biopsy c.
Quinton Mahurkar double-
  lumen c.
Quinton Mahurkar dual-
  lumen peritoneal c.
Quinton Q-Port c.
Raaf c.
Raaf Cath vascular c.
Raaf double-lumen c.
Raaf dual-lumen c.
radial arterial c.
Radiofocus Glidewire
  angiography c.
radiopaque c.
railway c.
Raimondi c.
Raimondi peritoneal c.
Raimondi ventricular c.
Ramirez winged c.
Ranfac cholangiographic c.
rapid exchange balloon c.
Rashkind c.
Rashkind balloon c.
Rashkind septostomy
  balloon c.
rat-tail c.
RC1 c.
RC2 c.
recessed balloon
  septostomy c.
rectal c.
Reddick cystic duct
  cholangiogram c.
RediFurl c.
red Robinson c.
red rubber c.
Reif c.
Reif design c.

Rentrop c.
Rentrop infusion c.
Replogle c.
retention c.
retroperfusion c.
return-flow c.
return-flow hemostatic c.
return-flow retention c.
Revivac c.
Reynolds infusion c.
RF balloon c.
Rica eustachian c.
right-angle chest c.
right coronary c.
Ring c.
Ring biliary drainage c.
Ring-McLean c.
Robinson c.
Robinson urethral c.
Rockey-Thompson c.
Rodriguez c.
Rodriguez-Alvarez c.
Rolnel c.
Rosch c.
Ross c.
Rothene c.
round-tip c.
Royal Flush angiographic
  flush c.
rubber c.
rubber-shod c.
Rumel c.
Rusch c.
Rusch bronchial c.
Rusch coudé c.
Ruschelit c.
Rusch external c.
Rusch-Foley c.
Rusch nephrostomy c.
Rutner c.
Rutner nephrostomy
  balloon c.
Rutner wedge c.
Safe-T-Coat heparin-coated
  thermodilution c.
Saratoga sump c.
Schneider c.
Schneider-Shiley c.
Schneider-Shiley dilatation c.
Schoonmaker c.
Schoonmaker femoral c.
Schoonmaker
  multipurpose c.

catheter *(continued)*
    Schrotter c.
    Schwarten balloon-
      dilatation c.
    Science-Med balloon c.
    Sci-Med angioplasty c.
    Sci-Med guiding c.
    Sci-Med skinny c.
    scleral buckling c.
    Scoop transtracheal c.
    Seidel c.
    Seldinger c.
    Seldinger cardiac c.
    Selective-HI c.
    Seletz c.
    self-retaining c.
    Sellheim uterine c.
    semirigid c.
    Semm uterine c.
    Semm vacuum c.
    sensing c.
    septostomy balloon c.
    Shadow-Stripe c.
    shaver c.
    Sheldon c.
    shellac-covered c.
    shepherd's hook c.
    Shiley c.
    Shiley guiding c.
    Shiley-Ionescu c.
    Shiley irrigation c.
    Shiley JL-4 guiding c.
    Shiley MultiPro c.
    Shiley soft-tip guiding c.
    SHJR4s c.
    Shulitz c.
    side-hole c.
    side-hole Judkins right,
      curved 4, short c.
    side-hole pigtail c.
    sidewinder c.
    sidewinder percutaneous
      intra-aortic balloon c.
    Silastic c.
    Silastic elastomer
      infusion c.
    Silastic ileal reservoir c.
    Silastic mushroom c.
    Silcath subclavian c.
    silicone elastomer c.
    silicone elastomer
      infusion c.

silicone rubber Dacron-
  cuffed c.
Silicore c.
Silitek c.
silk-and-wax c.
Simmons c.
Simplus c.
Simplus dilatation c.
Simpson atherectomy c.
Simpson AtheroCath c.
Simpson coronary
  AtheroCath c.
Simpson-Robert c.
Simpson-Robert ACS
  dilatation c.
Simpson suction c.
Simpson Ultra Lo-Profile
  balloon c.
single-lumen c.
single-lumen balloon stone
  extractor c.
single-lumen infusion c.
single-stage c.
six-eye c.
Skene c.
Skinny balloon c.
Slinky balloon c.
Slinky PTCA c.
smart position-sensing c.
SMIC eustachian c.
Soehendra Universal c.
soft c.
SOF-T guiding c.
Softip c.
Softip arteriography c.
Softip diagnostic c.
Softouch Cobra 1 c.
Softouch Cobra 2 c.
Softouch guiding c.
Softouch Headhunter 1 c.
Softouch Multipurpose
  B2 c.
Softouch Simmons 1 c.
Softouch Simmons 2 c.
Softouch spinal
  angiography c.
solid-state esophageal
  manometry c.
solid-tip c.
Sones c.
Sones Cardio-Marker c.
Sones coronary c.
Sones Hi-Flow c.

Sones Positrol c.
Sones vent c.
Spectraprobe-PLS laser
  angioplasty c.
Spetzler c.
Spetzler subarachnoid c.
c. spigot
spiral-tipped c.
split-sheath c.
Squire c.
Stack perfusion c.
Stack perfusion coronary
  dilatation c.
Stamey c.
Stamey ureteral c.
standard 6-lumen
  perfused c.
Stanford end-hole pigtail c.
St. Bartholomew barium c.
steerable c.
Stertzer c.
Stertzer brachial guiding c.
stimulating c.
Stitt c.
stone basket outer c.
Storz c.
Storz bronchial c.
Storz-DeKock two-way
  bronchial c.
Storz scleral buckling
  balloon c.
straight c.
straight flush
  percutaneous c.
Stress Cath c.
Stretzer bent-tip USCI c.
Stringer tracheal c.
Stripseal c.
styletted c.
styletted tracheobronchial c.
subclavian c.
subclavian dialysis c.
suction c.
Suggs c.
Sugita c.
SULP II c.
sump c.
sump pump c.
Supercath intravenous c.
suprapubic c.
Sureflow c.
Surgitek c.
Surgitek double-J ureteral c.

Swan-Ganz c.
Swan-Ganz balloon type c.
Swan-Ganz guide-wire
  TD c.
Swan-Ganz pulmonary
  artery c.
Swan-Ganz
  thermodilution c.
Switzerland dilatation c.
TAC atherectomy c.
tapered c.
taper tip c.
Tauber c.
Tauber male
  urethrographic c.
Teflon c.
Teflon needle c.
Teflon-tipped c.
temporary pacing c.
Tenckhoff c.
Tenckhoff peritoneal c.
Tenckhoff renal dialysis c.
Tennis Racquet c.
Tennis Racquet
  angiographic c.
Terumo Surflo
  intravenous c.
Texas c.
thermal dilution c. (TDC)
thermistor c.
thermodilution c.
thermodilution balloon c.
thermodilution pacing c.
thermodilution Swan-
  Ganz c.
Thompson c.
Thompson bronchial c.
thoracic c.
three-way c.
three-way Foley c.
three-way irrigating c.
thrombectomy c.
Thruflex PTCA balloon c.
Tiemann c.
Tiemann coudé c.
Tiemann Foley c.
Tiemann Neoflex c.
Timberlake c.
tip-deflecting c.
c. tip occluder
TLC Baxter balloon c.
Tolantins bone marrow
  infusion c.

catheter *(continued)*
Tomac c.
Tomac Nélaton c.
toposcopic c.
Torcon c.
Torcon angiographic c.
Torktherm torque control c.
torque-control balloon c.
Touchless c.
TPN c.
tracheal c.
transducer-tipped c.
transluminal angioplasty c.
transluminal extraction c.
transluminal extraction-
  endarterectomy c. (TEC)
transseptal c.
transthoracic c.
transvenous pacemaker c.
Trattner c.
Trattner urethrographic c.
triple-lumen c.
triple-lumen biliary
  manometry c.
triple-lumen central c.
triple-lumen manometric c.
triple thermistor coronary
  sinus c.
tripolar c.
tripolar W/Damato curve c.
Trocath peritoneal
  dialysis c.
Troeltsch eustachian c.
T-tube c.
c. tubing adapter
Tuohy c.
twist drill c.
two-way c.
Tygon c.
Ultramer c.
umbilical c.
umbilical artery c. (UAC)
umbilical vein c.
Unicath all-purpose c.
UNI shunt c.
Universal drainage c.
Uresil biliary c.
Uresil embolectomy-
  thrombectomy c.
Uresil irrigation c.
Uresil occlusion balloon c.
ureteral c.
ureteral dilatation c.

ureteral occlusion c.
urethral c.
urethrographic c.
Uridome c.
Uridrop c.
urinary c.
Urocare Foley c.
Urocath external c.
urological c.
Uro-San Plus external c.
USCI c.
USCI Bard c.
USCI Finesse guiding c.
USCI guiding c.
USCI Mini-Profile balloon
  dilatation c.
USCI Positrol coronary c.
Vabra c.
Vacurette c.
vacuum aspiration c.
valvuloplasty balloon c.
Van Aman pigtail c.
Vance-Kish urethral
  illuminated c.
Vance percutaneous Malecot
  nephrostomy c.
van Sonnenberg c.
van Sonnenberg sump c.
Van Tassel angled pigtail c.
Van Tassel pigtail c.
Vantec occlusion balloon c.
Vantec ureteral balloon
  dilatation c.
Variflex c.
Vas-Cath Opti-Plast
  peripheral angioplasty c.
Vas-Cath peritoneal
  dialysis c.
vascular c.
vascular access c.
venous c.
venous irrigation c.
venous thrombectomy c.
venting c.
ventricular c.
ventriculography c.
Versaflex steerable c.
vertebrated c.
Virden c.
Virden rectal c.
Visicath viewing c.
Vitalcor c.
Vitalcor venous c.

Vitalcor venous return c.
Vitax female c.
Vivonex jejunostomy c.
V. Mueller c.
V. Mueller embolectomy c.
Von Andel c.
Von Andel biliary
  dilation c.
Vygon Nutricath S c.
Walther c.
Walther female c.
Walther female dilator c.
wash c.
washing c.
Watanabe c.
water-infusion esophageal
  manometry c.
wave guide c.
3-way c.
3-way Foley c.
3-way irrigating c.
Weber c.
Weber rectal c.
Weber winged c.
Webster coronary sinus c.
wedge c.
wedge balloon c.
Wedge Cook c.
wedge pressure balloon c.
Western external urinary c.
whalebone filiform c.
whistle-tip c.
whistle-tip Foley c.
whistle-tip ureteral c.
Wholey-Edwards c.
Wick c.
Williams c.
Williams L-R guiding c.
Wilson-Cook c.
Wilton-Webster coronary
  sinus c.
Winer c.
winged c.
Winston SD c.
wire stylet c.
Wishard c.
Wishard tip c.
Wishard tip ureteral c.
Witzel enterostomy c.
Wolf c.
Wolf nephrostomy c.
Wolf nephrostomy bag c.
Woodruff c.

Woodruff
  ureteropyelographic c.
Word c.
woven c.
woven-silk c.
Wurd c.
XL-11 Ranfac percutaneous
  cholangiographic c.
Yankauer c.
Yankauer eustachian c.
Y-trough c.
Zavod c.
Zavod bronchospirometry c.
Zimmon c.
Zucker c.
Zucker cardiac c.
Zucker multipurpose
  bipolar c.
Zurich dilatation c.
catheter-introducing forceps
catheterizing Foroblique telescope
Cath-Lok catheter locking device
Cathlon IV catheter
Catlin amputing knife
cat's paw retractor
Cattell
  C. forked-type T- tube
  C. gallbladder tube
caudal needle
caulking gun
Cault punch
Causse piston
cautery
  Accu-Temp c.
  ACMI c.
  Acucise ureteral cutting c.
  alkaline battery c.
  BICAP c.
  bipolar c.
  Birtcher c.
  Bovie c.
  Burdick c.
  Cameron c.
  c. clamp
  Codman-Mentor wet-field c.
  cold (carbon dioxide) c.
  Concept c.
  Corrigan c.
  cutting c.
  Davis-Bovie c.
  Downes c.
  electrocautery c.
  c. electrode

cautery *(continued)*
- eraser c.
- eraser-tip c.
- Geiger c.
- Goodhill c.
- Hildreth c.
- Hildreth ocular c.
- Hildreth rechargable c.
- Khosia c.
- c. knife electrode
- Magielski coagulation c.
- Mueller alkaline battery c.
- Mueller Currentrol c.
- National c.
- needlepoint c.
- ocular c.
- Op-Temp c.
- Paquelin c.
- pencil c.
- pencil-tip c.
- phacoemulsification c.
- Prince eye c.
- Rommel-Hildreth c.
- Scheie ophthalmic c.
- Schepens eye c.
- c. snare
- Souttar c.
- Statham c.
- stepped-down c.
- suction c.
- unipolar c.
- Wadsworth-Todd c.
- Wadsworth-Todd eye c.
- Walker c.
- Wappler c.
- Wappler cold c.
- Wepsic fiberoptic c.
- wet-field c.
- Wills Hospital eye c.
- Ziegler c.

Linvatec (handwritten annotation)

caval
- c. cannula
- c. catheter
- c. occlusion clamp

Cavanaugh
- C. bur
- C. sphenoid bur

Cavanaugh-Israel bur
Cavanaugh-Wells tonsillar forceps
Cav-Clean cavity degreaser
Cave
- C. cartilage knife
- C. knee retractor

- C. retractor
- C. scaphoid gouge
- C. scaphoid spatula

Cavi-Jet dental prophylaxis device
Cavit
Cavitec cavity liner
Cavitron
- C. aspirator
- C. dissector
- C. I&A handpiece
- C. machine
- C. phacoemulsifier
- C. scalpel
- C. ultrasonic surgical aspirator (CUSA)

Cavitron-Kelman phacoemulsification machine
Cavoline cavity liner
Cawood nasal splint
Caylor scissors
C-block
CCK femoral stem provisional guide
CCS endocardial pacing lead
C-Dak dialyzer
CDH Precoat Plus hip prosthesis
CE-2 cryostat
Cebotome drill
Cecar electrode
Cecil dressing
cecostomy
- c. catheter
- c. retractor

Cedar anesthesia face rest
Celestin
- C. endoesophageal prosthesis
- C. endoesophageal tube
- C. graduated dilator
- C. graft material
- C. implant
- C. tube

celiac clamp
Cellamin
- C. bandage
- C. resin plaster-of-Paris bandage

Cellona
- C. bandage
- C. resin plaster-of-Paris bandage

cellophane dressing
celltrifuge device

celluloid
c. implant
c. implant material
c. linen suture
c. suture
cellulose
Oxycel oxidized c.
Celluron dental roll
cement
Atwood orthodontic c.
bone c.
Buck femoral c. restrictor
Buffalo dental c.
Ceramco dental c.
Ceramcore dental c.
Ceramlin dental c.
Ceramsave dental c.
Compacement dental c.
Conclude dental c.
dental c.
dermatome c.
Diaket root canal c.
Durelon dental c.
Eastman dental c.
c. eater
c. eater drill
Epoxylite dental resin c.
Fuji dental c.
Gembase dental c.
Gemcem dental c.
Gemcore dental c.
Howmedica c.
low-viscosity bone c.
Mynol endodontic c.
Neutrocim dental c.
Nobetec dental c.
Nogenol dental c.
orthodontic c.
Palacos c.
Palacos bone c.
Palacos radiopaque bone c.
Petralit dental c.
c. restrictor
Roth dental c.
Selfast dental c.
Shofu dental c.
c. spatula
Super-Dent orthodontic c.
Surgical Simplex P bone c.
Tempbond dental c.
Temrex dental c.
Zimmer bone c.
Centaur trial cup

center blade
centering drill
centimeter subtraction ruler
central
c. catheter
c. patient station (CPS)
c. terminal electrode
c. venous catheter
c. venous pressure catheter
(CVP)
centralizer
Integral distal c.
Centrax
C. bipolar component
C. bipolar endoprosthesis
C. endoprosthesis
Centrix PDQ ligator
Centry
C. 2 cps dialysis unit
C. 2 dialysis control unit
Century birthing chair
cephalad catheter
cephalic blade forceps
cephalometer
B. F. Wehmer c.
GX c.
Plasticeph c.
cephalotribe
Tarnier c.
Ceradelta alloy
Ceramalloy alloy
Ceramco
C. dental cement
C. porcelain kit
Ceramcore dental cement
ceramic ossicular prosthesis
Ceramlin dental cement
Ceramsave dental cement
Cerapall alloy
Ceravital incus replacement
prosthesis
cerclage wire
cerebellar
c. attachment
c. electrode
c. retractor
cerebral
c. angiography needle
c. angiography puncture
needle
c. catheter
c. retractor
cerebrospinal fluid (CSF)

Cer-Mate alloy
Cer-On R alloy
Cerva crane halter
Cervex-Brush
    C.-B. cervical cell collector
    C.-B. cervical cell sampler
    Unimar C.-B.
cervical
    c. accessory set
    c. biopsy blade
    c. biopsy curette
    c. biopsy forceps
    c. biopsy punch forceps
    c. blade
    c. brace
    c. collar brace
    c. cone knife
    c. conization electrode
    c. curette
    c. dilator
    c. disk retractor
    c. drill
    c. forceps
    c. grasping forceps
    c. hemostatic forceps
    c. mallet
    c. needle
    c. pillow
    c. punch
    c. punch forceps
    c. retractor
    c. suture
    c. suture needle
    c. traction forceps
    c. traction kit
    c. vulsellum
cervix
cesarean, caesarian
    c. forceps
CFI
    contour-facilitating instrument
CFV wrist component
CGI-1 contact lens
CGS
    catgut suture
Chadwick scissors
Chaffin
    C. catheter
    C. tube catheter
Chaffin-Pratt
    C.-P. bedside suction tube
    C.-P. drain

    C.-P. percolator hanger holder
chain
    c. saw
    c. suture
chair
    Century birthing c.
    OB/GYN c.
chair-back brace
chalazion
    c. clamp
    c. curette
    c. retractor
Chalnot valvulotome
Chamberlain-Fries atraumatic retractor
Chamberlain tongue depressor
Chamberlen
    C. forceps
    C. obstetrical forceps
Chambers
    C. doughnut pessary
    C. intrauterine cup
    C. intrauterine pessary
chamfer
    c. guide
    c. jig
Chamley
    C. bone clamp
    C. clamp
Chamois swab
Champ elastic bandage
Champetier de Ribes obstetrical bag
Championnière
    C. bone drill
    C. forceps
Champion suture
Chandler
    C. bone elevator
    C. elevator
    C. felt collar splint
    C. forceps
    C. iris forceps
    C. laminectomy retractor
    C. mallet
    C. retractor
    C. spinal-perforating forceps
    C. V-pacing probe
Chang bone-cutting forceps
channel retractor
Chaoul applicator

Chaput
    C. forceps
    C. tissue forceps
Chardack
    C. Medtronic pacemaker
    C. pacemaker
Chardack-Greatbatch pacemaker
Charest
    C. head fracture frame
    C. head frame
Charles
    C. fluted needle
    C. intraocular lens
    C. irrigating contact lens
    C. irrigating lens
    C. needle
    C. vacuuming needle
Charleston antral needle
Charley broach
Charlton
    C. antral needle
    C. antral trocar
    C. cannula
    C. needle
Charnley
    C. acetabular cup prosthesis
    C. acetabular scraper
    C. arthrodesis clamp
    C. bone clamp
    C. brace handle
    C. cement restrictor
    C. centering drill
    C. compressor
    C. cup
    C. cup-trimming scissors
    C. double-ended bone
      curette
    C. drain tube
    C. drill
    C. femoral condyle drill
    C. femoral lever
    C. femoral prosthesis pusher
    C. forceps
    C. gouge
    C. knee retractor
    C. pilot drill
    C. pin clamp
    C. reamer
    C. retractor
    C. saw
    C. socket-size gauge
    C. suction drain
    C. suture forceps

    C. total hip prosthesis
    C. trochanter file
    C. trochanter wire
Charnley-Mueller hip prosthesis
Charnley-Riches arterial forceps
Charnow notched ruler
Charriere
    C. amputation saw
    C. aseptic metacarpal saw
    C. bone saw
    C. saw
Chaston eye pad
Chatfield-Girdleston splint
Chatzidakis implant
Chauffen-Pratt tube
Chaussier tube
Chavantes-Zamorano
  neuroendoscope
Chavasse squint hook
Chayes handpiece
Cheanvechai-Favaloro retractor
Cheatle sterilizing forceps
cheek retractor
cheiroscope
Chelsea-Eaton
    C.-E. anal speculum
    C.-E. rectal speculum
chemonucleolysis table
Chemo-Port catheter
Chermel
    C. bone chisel
    C. bone gouge
    C. osteotome
Cherney suture
Chernov tracheostomy hook
Cheron
    C. dressing forceps
    C. forceps
    C. uterine dressing forceps
Cherry
    C. brain probe
    C. drill
    C. forceps
    C. laminectomy self-
      retaining retractor
    C. osteotome
    C. probe
    C. retractor
    C. screw extractor
    C. Secto dissector
    C. S-shaped brain retractor
    C. S-shape scissors

Cherry *(continued)*
    C. traction tongs
    C. traction tractor
Cherry-Adson forceps
Cherry-Austin drill
Cherry-Kerrison
    C.-K. forceps
    C.-K. laminectomy rongeur
    C.-K. laminectomy rongeur
      forceps
    C.-K. rongeur forceps
cherry sponge
Cheshire
    C. electrosurgical pencil
    C. suture removal set
Cheshire-Poole-Yankauer suction
  instrument
chessboard implant
chest
    c. dressing
    c. tube stripper
Chester
    C. forceps
    C. sponge forceps
Chevalier
    C. Jackson bougie
    C. Jackson
      bronchoesophagoscopy
      forceps
    C. Jackson bronchoscope
    C. Jackson esophagoscope
    C. Jackson forceps
    C. Jackson gastroscope
    C. Jackson laryngeal
      speculum
    C. Jackson laryngoscope
    C. Jackson scissors
Chewrite denture adhesive
Cheyne
    C. dissector
    C. dry dissector
    C. periosteal elevator
    C. retractor
Chiba
    C. biopsy needle
    C. eye needle
    C. needle
    C. transhepatic
      cholangiography needle
Chicco breast pump
Chick
    C. sterile dressing

    C. surgical light
    C. surgical table
chicken-bill rongeur forceps
Chid baby breast pump
Chilcott
    C. cannula
    C. venoclysis cannula
Child
    C. clip-applying forceps
    C. forceps
    C. intestinal forceps
child
    c. esophagoscope
    c. rectal dilator
Children's Hospital
    C. H. brain spatula
    C. H. clip
    C. H. dressing forceps
    C. H. forceps
    C. H. hand drill
    C. H. intestinal forceps
    C. H. mallet
    C. H. pediatric retractor
    C. H. retractor
    C. H. scalp clip
    C. H. screwdriver
Childs Cardio-cuff
Childs-Phillips
    C.-P. forceps
    C.-P. intestinal plication
      needle
    C.-P. needle
Chimani pharyngeal forceps
Chinese
    C. fingerstraps traction
      device
    C. twisted silk suture
chin implant
C-2 hip system
chiropractic adjusting instrument
chisel
    Adson c.
    Adson laminectomy c.
    Alexander c.
    Alexander bone c.
    Alexander mastoid c.
    Amico c.
    Andrews c.
    antral c.
    Army-pattern c.
    Artmann c.
    Artmann disarticulation c.
    Austin c.

Austin Moore mortising c.
Bakelite dental c.
Ballenger c.
Ballenger-Hajek c.
Basek c.
beveled c.
binangled c.
Bishop c.
Bishop mastoid c.
c. blade
Blair c.
Blair nasal c.
bone c.
Bowen c.
Bowen gooseneck c.
Braithwaite nasal c.
Brauer c.
Brittain c.
Brittain twin pattern c.
Brown c.
Bruening c.
Brun c.
Brunetti c.
Brun guarded c.
Brunner c.
Brunswick-Mack c.
Burns c.
Burns guarded c.
Caltagirone c.
canal c.
cartilage c.
Chermel bone c.
Cinelli c.
Cinelli-McIndoe c.
Clawicz c.
Clevedent-Gardner c.
Clevedent-Wakefield c.
Cloward c.
Cloward-Harman c.
Cloward puka c.
Cloward spinal fusion c.
Cobb c.
Compere c.
Compere bone c.
Converse c.
Converse guarded c.
Converse nasal c.
Cooley c.
corneal c.
costotome c.
Cottle c.
Cottle antral c.
Cottle crossbar c.

Cottle crossbar fishtail c.
Cottle curved c.
Cottle fishtail c.
Cottle nasal c.
Councilman c.
Crane c.
Crane bone c.
crossbar c.
crossbar fishtail c.
crurotomy c.
curved c.
Dautrey c.
Derlacki c.
Derlacki-Shambaugh c.
D'Errico laminar c.
D'Errico laminectomy c.
disarticulation c.
dissecting c.
double-guarded c.
Duray-Read c.
Duray-Wood c.
Dworacek-Farrior canal c.
Ecker-Roopenian c.
Eicher c.
Eicher tri-fin c.
c. elevator
endaural surgery c.
ethmoidal c.
Farrior-Derlacki c.
Farrior-Dworacek canal c.
Faulkner c.
Faulkner antral c.
Faulkner-Browne c.
Faulkner trocar c.
fishtail c.
Fomon c.
Fomon nasal c.
footplate c.
fracture c.
Freer c.
Freer bone c.
Freer lacrimal c.
Freer nasal c.
Freer submucous c.
French c.
frontal sinus c.
Gardner c.
Gardner bone c.
Gauje curved c.
Goldman c.
Goldman guarded c.
gooseneck c.
guarded c.

Epker

chisel *(continued)*
Hajek c.
Hajek septal c.
Halle c.
Hatch c.
Heermann c.
Henderson c.
Henderson bone c.
Hibbs c.
Hibbs bone c.
Hoke c.
hollow c.
Holmes c.
Hough c.
House c.
House-Derlacki c.
House footplate c.
Jenkins c.
J.E. Sheehan c.
Jordan-Hermann c.
Joseph c.
Katsch c.
Keyes c.
Keyes bone-splitting c.
Keyes splitting c.
Kezerian c.
Killian c.
Killian-Claus c.
Killian frontal sinus c.
Killian-Reinhard c.
Kilner c.
Kilner retrograde c.
Kos c.
Kreischer c.
Kreischer bone c.
lacrimal c.
Lambotte c.
Lambotte bone c.
Lambotte splitting c.
laminectomy c.
Lebsche c.
Lebsche sternal c.
Lever-Mini c.
Lexer c.
Lucas c.
MacAusland c.
Magielski c.
Magielski stapes c.
Mannerfelt c.
manual surgical c.
mastoid c.
McIndoe c.
McIndoe nasal c.

Metzenbaum c.
Meyerding c.
middle ear c.
Moberg c.
Moore c.
Moore hollow c.
Moore prosthesis-mortising c.
mortising c.
Murphy c.
nasal c.
Neivert c.
Nordent c.
Nordent bone c.
Nordent-Ochsenbein periodontic c.
Obwegeser splitting c.
orthopaedic c.
Partsch c.
Partsch bone c.
Passow c.
peapod c.
Pearson c.
Peck c.
pick c.
puka c.
Read c.
Rica mastoid c.
Richards c.
Richards-Hibbs c.
Rish c.
Roberts c.
Roberts hip dissecting c.
Rollet c.
Rubin nasal c.
Schuknecht c.
septal c.
Sewall c.
Sewall ethmoidal c.
Shambaugh-Derlacki c.
Sheehan c.
Sheehan nasal c.
Sheehy-House c.
Silver c.
Simmons c.
sinus c.
Skoog nasal c.
small bone c.
SMIC bone c.
SMIC mastoid c.
SMIC sternal c.
Smillie c.
Smillie cartilage c.

Smith-Petersen c.
spinal fusion c.
splitting c.
stapes c.
Stille c.
Stille bone c.
Stille-pattern bone c.
submucous c.
Swedish-pattern c.
Swiderski nasal c.
tri-fin c.
Troutman c.
Troutman mastoid c.
twin-pattern c.
U.S. Army c.
U.S. Army bone c.
Virchow c.
vulcanite c.
Walsh c.
Walsh footplate c.
Ward nasal c.
West c.
West bone c.
West lacrimal c.
West lacrimal sac c.
West nasal c.
White c.
White bone c.
Wilmer c.
Wilmer wedge c.
Worth c.
Chitten-Hill retractor
Chix cleaner
chloramine catgut suture
Chlumsky button
choanal bur
cholangiocatheter
cholangiography
c. catheter
c. clamp
cholangiopancreatography
endoscopic retrograde c.
(ERCP)
choledochocystonephrofiberscope
Pentax c.
choledochoscope
choledochoscope-nephroscope
Berci-Schore c.-n.
Storz c.-n.
chondroplastic
c. Beaver blade
c. blade

chondrotome
Stryker c.
chorda tympani pusher
chorionic
c. villus sampling (CVS)
c. villus sampling catheter
chorionscope
Chorus pacemaker
Choyce
C. eye implant
C. forceps
C. implant
C. intraocular eye implant
C. intraocular lens
C. intraocular lens forceps
C. lens
C. lens forceps
C. lens-inserting forceps
C. Mark intraocular lens
C. MK II keratoprosthesis
prosthesis
Choyce-Mark eye implant
Choyce-Tennant lens
Christie gallbladder retractor
Christmas-tree cannula
Christopher-Stille forceps
Chromaser dermatology laser
chromated catgut suture
chrome probe with eye
chromic
c. blue dyed suture
c. catgut mattress suture
c. catgut suture
c. collagen suture
c. gut suture
c. suture
chromicized catgut suture
chronaximeter
Chronicure protein hydrolysate
powder
Chronocor IV external pacemaker
Chronos pacemaker
chronowave
Chrys surgical CO_2 laser
CHS supracondylar bone plate
Chubb tonsillar forceps
chuck
c. adapter
c. drill
Gam-Mer c.
Jacobs snap-lock c.
pin c.
T-handle Zimmer c.

chuck *(continued)*
Trinkle c.
Wozniak Sur-Lok c.
Church
C. pediatric scissors
C. scissors
Churchill
C. cardiac suction cannula
C. sucker
Chux incontinent dressing
Cibis
C. electrode
C. needle
C. ski needle
Cibis-Vaiser muscle retractor
Cicherelli
C. bone rongeur
C. forceps
C. rongeur
C. rongeur forceps
Cidex solution
CIF needle
cigarette drain
cigar handle basket punch
Cikloid dressing
Cilacalcin double-chambered syringe
Cilco
C. intraocular lens
C. laser
C. lens forceps
C. MonoFlex PMMA lens
C. ophthalmic endoscope
C. Optiflex intraocular lens
C. posterior chamber intraocular lens
C. viscoelastic
ciliary forceps
cilia suture forceps
cilium pacemaker
Cincinnati ACL brace
cineangiogram
cinecamera
Bolex c.
House-Urban microsurgery c.
House-Urban UEM-100 c.
cinegastrocamera
Cinelli
C. chisel
C. elevator
C. osteotome
C. periosteal elevator

Cinelli-Fomon scissors
Cinelli-McIndoe chisel
Cintor knee prosthesis
circle knife
CircOlectric bed
Circon
C. arthroscope
C. camera
C. leg holder
C. video camera
Circon-ACMI
C.-A. diagnostic laparoscope
C.-A. electrohydraulic lithotriptor probe
circuit
Tygon tubing c.
circular
c. bandage
c. blade
c. cup bronchoscopic biopsy forceps
c. intraluminal stapler
c. mechanical stapler
c. stapler
c. stapling device
c. suture
circumcision
c. clamp
c. instrument
circumcisional
c. shield
c. suture
circumflex
c. artery scissors
c. scissors
Circumpress
C. chin strap
C. compression bra
C. face-lift dressing
C. gynecomastia vest
CISA dissector
Citelli
C. forceps
C. laminectomy punch
C. punch
C. rongeur
C. rongeur forceps
C. sphenoid rongeur
Citelli-Bruening ear forceps
Citelli-Meltzer atticus punch
Civiale forceps
Clagett
C. cannula

C. needle
C. S-cannula
Clairborne clamp
clamp
  Abadie c.
  Abadie enterostomy c.
  Ablaza c.
  Ablaza patent ductus c.
  Abramson-Allis breast c.
  Acland c.
  Acland double c.
  Acland microvascular c.
  Acland single c.
  Adair c.
  Adair breast c.
  Adson c.
  Adson-Brown c.
  agraffe c.
  Ahlquist-Durham
   embolism c.
  Alfred M. Large vena
   caval c.
  Allen c.
  Allen anastomosis c.
  Allen intestinal c.
  Allen intestinal
   anastomosis c.
  Allen-Kocher c.
  Allis c.
  Allison c.
  Allis tissue c.
  Alyea c.
  Alyea vas c.
  anastomosis c.
  Ando aortic c.
  aneurysm c.
  angled c.
  angled DeBakey c.
  angled peripheral vascular c.
  Ann Arbor c.
  Ann Arbor double towel c.
  anterior resection c.
  aortic c.
  aortic aneurysm c.
  aortic cannula c.
  aortic occlusion c.
  appendage c.
  c. approximator
  arterial c.
  Asch c.
  Atlee c.
  Atlee bronchus c.
  Atra-Grip c.

atraumatic c.
atraumatic stomach c.
atrial c.
Ault c.
Ault intestinal c.
Ault intestinal occlusion c.
auricular c.
auricular appendage c.
Auvard c.
Babcock c.
Babcock tissue c.
baby Bishop c.
baby Kocher c.
baby pylorus c.
baby Satinsky c.
Backhaus c.
Backhaus-Jones c.
Backhaus-Jones towel c.
Backhaus-Kocher c.
Backhaus-Kocher towel c.
Backhaus towel c.
Bahnson c.
Bahnson aortic c.
Bahnson aortic aneurysm c.
Bahnson appendage c.
Bailey c.
Bailey aortic c.
Bailey aortic occlusion c.
Bailey-Cowley c.
Bailey duckbill c.
Bailey-Morse c.
Bainbridge c.
Bainbridge anastomosis c.
Bainbridge intestinal c.
Bainbridge vessel c.
Balfour c.
Ballantine c.
Bamby c.
Bard c.
Bartley anastomosis c.
Bartley partial-occlusion c.
Bauer kidney pedicle c.
Baumrucker-DeBakey c.
Baumrucker incontinence c.
Baumrucker post-TUR
 irrigation c.
Baumrucker urinary
 incontinence c.
Beall bulldog c.
Beall-Morris ascending
 aortic c.
Beardsley c.
Beardsley intestinal c.

clamp *(continued)*
Beck c.
Beck aortic c.
Beck miniature aortic c.
Beck-Potts c.
Beck-Potts aortic and
  pulmonic c.
Beck-Satinsky c.
Beck vascular c.
Beck vessel c.
Belcher c.
Bell c.
Bell circumcision c.
Benson pyloric c.
Berens c.
Berens muscle c.
Berke c.
Berkeley c.
Berkeley-Bonney vaginal c.
Berke ptosis c.
Berman c.
Berman aortic c.
Berman vascular c.
Bernhard c.
Berry c.
Berry pile c.
Best c.
Best colon c.
Best intestinal c.
Best right-angle colon c.
Bethune c.
Bielawski heart c.
Bigelow c.
Bigelow calvarium c.
Bircher bone-holding c.
Bircher cartilage c.
Bishop bone c.
Black c.
Black meatal c.
bladder irrigation control c.
3-bladed c.
Blair cleft palate c.
Blalock c.
Blalock-Niedner c.
Blalock-Niedner pulmonary
  stenosis c.
Blalock-Niedner pulmonic c.
Blalock pulmonary c.
Blalock pulmonary artery c.
Blalock pulmonary
  stenosis c.
Blalock stenosis c.
Blanchard c.

Blanchard pile c.
Blasucci c.
blepharostat c.
bloodless circumcision c.
Boettcher pulmonary
  artery c.
Böhler c.
Böhler os calcis c.
bone c.
bone extension c.
bone-holding c.
Bonney c.
Borge c.
Borge bile duct c.
Bortz c.
Boyes c.
Boyes muscle c.
Bozeman c.
Bradshaw-O'Neill c.
Bradshaw-O'Neill aortic c.
Bridge c.
Brock c.
Brock auricular c.
Brockington pile c.
Brodney c.
Brodney urethrographic c.
Bronner c.
Brown c.
Brown lip c.
Brunner colon c.
Brunner intestinal c.
Buie c.
Buie-Hirschman c.
Buie-Hirschman pile c.
Buie pile c.
Buie rectal c.
bulldog c.
Bunke c.
Bunnell-Howard
  arthrodesis c.
Burford c.
Burlisher c.
Bushey compression c.
  (BCC)
Buxton c.
Buxton uterine c.
C-c.
Cairns c.
Calman carotid c.
Calman ring c.
calvarium c.
cannula c.
Capes c.

Cardio-Grip anastomosis c.
Cardio-Grip aortic c.
Cardio-Grip aortic
  aneurysm c.
Cardio-Grip bronchus c.
Cardio-Grip multipurpose c.
Cardio-Grip pediatric c.
Cardio-Grip renal artery c.
Cardio-Grip tangential
  occulusion c.
Cardio-Grip vascular c.
cardiovascular c.
cardiovascular
  anastomotic c.
cardiovascular bulldog c.
Carmalt c.
Carmel c.
carotid c.
carotid artery c.
carotid artery bypass c.
Carrel c.
c. carrier
Carter c.
Carter-Glassman c.
Carter-Glassman resection c.
cartilage c.
caruncle c.
Casey pelvic c.
Castaneda c.
Castaneda anastomosis c.
Castaneda IMM vascular c.
Castaneda-Mixter c.
Castaneda-Mixter thoracic c.
Castaneda multipurpose c.
Castaneda partial
  occlusion c.
Castaneda vascular c.
Castroviejo c.
Castroviejo lip c.
Castroviejo mosquito lid c.
cautery c.
caval occlusion c.
celiac c.
chalazion c.
Chamley c.
Chamley bone c.
Charnley arthrodesis c.
Charnley bone c.
Charnley pin c.
cholangiography c.
circumcision c.
Clairborne c.
c. clip

closing intestinal c.
cloth-shod c.
coarctation c.
Codman c.
Codman cartilage c.
Codman towel c.
Collier thoracic c.
Collin c.
Collin umbilical c.
colon c.
colostomy c.
columellar c.
Conger perineal
  urethrostomy c.
contour block c.
Cooley c.
Cooley acutely-curved c.
Cooley anastomosis c.
Cooley aortic c.
Cooley aortic aneurysm c.
Cooley aortic cannula c.
Cooley-Baumgarten aortic c.
Cooley-Beck c.
Cooley-Beck vessel c.
Cooley bronchus c.
Cooley bulldog c.
Cooley cardiovascular c.
Cooley carotid c.
Cooley caval occlusion c.
Cooley coarctation c.
Cooley cross-action
  bulldog c.
Cooley curved c.
Cooley curved
  cardiovascular c.
Cooley-Derra c.
Cooley-Derra anastomosis c.
Cooley double-angled c.
Cooley graft c.
Cooley iliac c.
Cooley multipurpose c.
Cooley multipurpose
  angled c.
Cooley multipurpose
  curved c.
Cooley neonatal c.
Cooley neonatal vascular c.
Cooley partial-occlusion c.
Cooley patent ductus c.
Cooley pediatric c.
Cooley pediatric vascular c.
Cooley peripheral
  vascular c.

clamp *(continued)*
Cooley renal c.
Cooley renal artery c.
Cooley-Satinsky c.
Cooley-Satinsky
  multipurpose c.
Cooley subclavian c.
Cooley tangential
  pediatric c.
Cooley vascular c.
Cooley vena caval c.
Cooley vena caval
  catheter c.
Cope c.
Cope crushing c.
Cope-DeMartel c.
Cope modification of a
  Martel intestinal c.
cordotomy c.
Cottle c.
Cottle columella c.
cotton-roll-rubber-dam c.
Crafoord c.
Crafoord aortic c.
Crafoord auricular c.
Crafoord coarctation c.
Crafoord-Sellor auricular c.
Crawford auricular c.
Crenshaw caruncle c.
Crile c.
Crile appendiceal c.
Crile appendix c.
Crile crushing c.
Crile-Crutchfield c.
Crile-type c.
Cross c.
cross-action c.
cross-action bulldog c.
Cruickshank c.
Cruickshank entropion c.
crush c.
crushing c.
Crutchfield c.
Crutchfield carotid artery c.
Cunningham c.
Cunningham incontinence c.
curved c.
curved-8 c.
curved cardiovascular c.
curved Mayo c.
curved peripheral
  vascular c.
Cushing c.

cystic duct catheter c.
Dacron graft c.
Daems c.
Daems bronchial c.
D'Allesandro c.
Dandy c.
Daniel c.
Daniel colostomy c.
Davidson c.
Davidson muscle c.
Davidson pulmonary
  vessel c.
Davidson vessel c.
Davila atrial c.
Davis c.
Davis aneurysm c.
Davis aortic aneurysm c.
Dean MacDonald c.
Dean MacDonald gastric
  resection c.
Deaver c.
DeBakey c.
DeBakey angled
  multipurpose c.
DeBakey aortic c.
DeBakey aortic aneurysm c.
DeBakey aortic exclusion c.
DeBakey arterial c.
DeBakey-Bahnson c.
DeBakey-Bahnson curved c.
DeBakey-Bahnson
  vascular c.
DeBakey-Bainbridge c.
DeBakey-Bainbridge
  vascular c.
DeBakey-Beck c.
DeBakey bulldog c.
DeBakey coarctation c.
DeBakey-Crafoord
  vascular c.
DeBakey cross-action
  bulldog c.
DeBakey curved c.
DeBakey curved peripheral
  vascular c.
DeBakey-Derra
  anastomosis c.
DeBakey-Harken c.
DeBakey-Harken
  aurricular c.
DeBakey-Howard c.
DeBakey-Howard aortic
  aneurysm c.

DeBakey-Kay c.
DeBakey-Kay aortic c.
DeBakey-McQuigg-Mixter
  bronchial c.
DeBakey miniature
  multipurpose c.
DeBakey multipurpose c.
DeBakey patent ductus c.
DeBakey pediatric c.
DeBakey peripheral
  vascular c.
DeBakey right-angled
  multipurpose c.
DeBakey ring-handled c.
DeBakey ring-handled
  bulldog c.
DeBakey-Satinsky vena
  caval c.
DeBakey-Semb c.
DeBakey-Semb ligature
  carrier c.
DeBakey sidewinder
  aortic c.
DeBakey S-shaped
  peripheral vascular c.
DeBakey tangential c.
DeBakey tangential
  occlusion c.
DeBakey vascular c.
DeCourcy c.
DeCourcy goiter c.
DeMartel c.
DeMartel vascular c.
DeMartel-Wolfson c.
DeMartel-Wolfson
  anastomosis c.
DeMartel-Wolfson colon c.
DeMartel-Wolfson
  intestinal c.
DeMartel-Wolfson intestinal
  anastomotic c.
DeMartel-Wolfson intestinal-
  closing c.
DeMartel-Wolfson intestinal-
  holding c.
DeMartel-Wolfson
  stomach c.
Demel wire c.
Demos tibial artery c.
Dennis c.
Dennis anastomotic c.
Dennis intestinal c.
Derra c.

Derra anastomosis c.
Derra aortic c.
Derra vena caval c.
Derra vestibular c.
Desmarres c.
Desmarres lid c.
Devonshire-Mack c.
DeWeese c.
DeWeese vena caval c.
Dick bronchus c.
Dick pressure c.
Dieffenbach c.
Dieffenbach bulldog c.
Diethrich c.
Diethrich aortic c.
Diethrich bulldog c.
Diethrich graft c.
Diethrich microcoronary
  bulldog c.
Diethrich shunt c.
Dingman c.
Dingman cartilage c.
disposable muscle biopsy c.
dissecting c.
distraction c.
Dixon-Thomas-Smith c.
Dixon-Thomas-Smith
  colonic c.
Dixon-Thomas-Smith
  intestinal c.
Dobbie-Trout c.
Dobbie-Trout bulldog c.
Doctor Collins c.
Doctor Collins fracture c.
Doctor Long c.
Dogliotti-Gugliel mini c.
Dolphin cord c.
Donald c.
double c.
double-angled c.
double Softjaw c.
double Softjaw handleless c.
double towel c.
Downing c.
Doyen c.
Doyen intestinal c.
Doyen towel c.
drape c.
dreamer c.
duckbill c.
ductus c.
duodenal c.
Duval lung c.

clamp *(continued)*
  Earle c.
  Earle hemorrhoidal c.
  Earle pile c.
  Eastman c.
  Eastman intestinal c.
  Edebohls c.
  Edebohls kidney c.
  Edna towel c.
  Edwards c.
  Edwards double c.
  Edwards double Softjaw c.
  Edwards double Softjaw
    handleless c.
  Edwards handleless c.
  Edwards single c.
  Edwards single Softjaw c.
  Edwards single Softjaw
    handleless c.
  Edwards spring c.
  Efteklar c.
  Ehrhardt lid c.
  Einsenstein c.
  Eisenstein c.
  English c.
  English-pattern c.
  enterostomy c.
  entropion c.
  Erhardt c.
  Erhardt lid c.
  Ericksson-Stille carotid c.
  Ewald-Hudson c.
  Ewing lid c.
  exclusion c.
  extension c.
  extension bone c.
  Falk c.
  Falk vaginal cuff c.
  Farabeuf bone c.
  Farabeuf-Lambotte c.
  Farabeuf-Lambotte bone c.
  Farabeuf-Lambotte bone-
    holding c.
  Fauer peritoneal c.
  Favaloro c.
  Favaloro proximal
    anastomosis c.
  Favorite c.
  feather c.
  Fehland c.
  Fehland intestinal c.
  Fehland right-angled
    colon c.

  femoral c.
  Ferguson bone c.
  ferrule c.
  fine-tooth c.
  Finochietto c.
  Finochietto arterial c.
  Finochietto bronchus c.
  Fitzgerald aortic
    aneurysm c.
  flexible aortic c.
  flexible retractor pressure c.
  flexible retractor sliding c.
  flexible vascular c.
  flow-regulator c.
  Fogarty c.
  Fogarty-Chin c.
  Fogarty Hydragrip c.
  folding approximating c.
  c. forceps
  Ford c.
  Forrester c.
  Foss c.
  Foss anterior resection c.
  Foss cardiovascular c.
  Foss intestinal c.
  Frahur c.
  Frahur cartilage c.
  Frazier-Adson c.
  Frazier-Adson osteoplastic c.
  Frazier-Adson osteoplastic
    flap c.
  Frazier-Sachs c.
  Freeman c.
  Friedrich c.
  Friedrich-Petz c.
  full-curved c.
  Furness c.
  Furness anastomosis c.
  Furness-Clute c.
  Furness-Clute anastomosis c.
  Furness-Clute duodenal c.
  Furness-McClure-Hinton c.
  gallbladder ring c.
  Gam-Mer aneurysm c.
  Gam-Mer occlusion c.
  Gandy c.
  Gant c.
  Garcia aortic c.
  Garcia classic aortic c.
  Gardner skull c.
  Garland c.
  Garland hysterectomy c.
  Gaskell c.

gastric c.
gastroenterostomy c.
gastrointestinal c.
gate c.
Gavin-Miller c.
Gemini c.
Gerald c.
Gerbode patent ductus c.
Gerster bone c.
GI c.
gingival c.
Glass liver-holding c.
Glassman c.
Glassman-Allis c.
Glassman anterior
  resection c.
Glassman
  gastroenterostomy c.
Glassman gastrointestinal c.
Glassman intestinal c.
Glassman liver-holding c.
Glassman noncrushing c.
Glassman noncrushing
  anterior resection c.
Glassman noncrushing
  gastroenterostomy c.
Glassman noncrushing
  gastrointestinal c.
Glover c.
Glover auricular c.
Glover auricular-
  appendage c.
Glover bulldog c.
Glover coarctation c.
Glover curved c.
Glover-DeBakey c.
Glover patent ductus c.
Glover spoon c.
Glover spoon
  anastomosis c.
Glover spoon-shaped c.
Glover-Stille c.
Glover-type bulldog c.
Glover vascular c.
goiter c.
Goldblatt c.
Gomco-Bell c.
Gomco bloodless
  circumcision c.
Gomco circumcision c.
Gomco umbilical cord c.
Goodhill tonsillar
  hemostat c.

Goodwin c.
Goodwin bone c.
Grafco incontinence c.
Grafco umbilical cord c.
graft c.
Grant c.
Grant abdominal aortic
  aneurysm c.
Grant aortic aneurysm c.
grasping c.
Gray c.
Green c.
Green bulldog c.
Green lid c.
Green suction tube-
  holding c.
Gregory c.
Gregory baby profunda c.
Gregory bulldog c.
Gregory carotid bulldog c.
Gregory external c.
Gregory stay suture c.
Gregory vascular
  miniature c.
Gross c.
Gross coarctation c.
Gross coarctation
  occlusion c.
Gross occluding c.
Grover c.
Grover Atra-grip c.
Grover auricular
  appendage c.
Gusberg hysterectomy c.
Gussenbauer c.
gut c.
Gutgeman c.
Gutgeman auricular
  appendage c.
Guyon c.
Guyon kidney c.
Guyon-Péan c.
Guyon-Péan vessel c.
Guyon vessel c.
Haberer intestinal c.
half-curved c.
Halsted c.
handleless c.
Harken c.
Harken auricular c.
Harrah lung c.
Harrington c.
Harrington-Carmalt c.

clamp *(continued)*
Harrington hook c.
Harrington-Mixter c.
Harrington-Mixter
   thoracic c.
Hartmann c.
Harvey Stone c.
Hausmann vascular c.
Haverhill c.
Haverhill-Mack c.
Hayes c.
Hayes anterior resection c.
Hayes anterior resection
   intestinal c.
Hayes colon c.
Hayes intestinal c.
Heaney c.
Heifitz cerebral aneurysm c.
Heitz-Boyer c.
hemoclip c.
hemorrhoidal c.
hemostatic c.
hemostatic thoracic c.
Hendren c.
Hendren cardiovascular c.
Hendren ductus c.
Hendren megaureter c.
Hendren ureteral c.
Henley subclavian artery c.
Henley vascular c.
Herbert Adams c.
Herbert Adams
   coarctation c.
Herff c.
Heritiz c.
Herrick c.
Herrick kidney c.
Herrick kidney pedicle c.
Herrick pedicle c.
Hesseltine c.
Hesseltine umbilical cord c.
Heyer-Schulte c.
Heyer-Schulte biopsy c.
Heyer-Schulte muscle
   biopsy c.
Heyer-Schulte Rayport
   muscle biopsy c.
Hibbs c.
Hirschman c.
Hirschman pile c.
Hirsch mucosal c.
Hoffmann c.
Hoffmann ligament c.

Hoff towel c.
Hohmann c.
Holcombe gastric
   tourniquet c.
c. holder
Hollister c.
Holter pump c.
Hopener c.
Hopkins c.
Hopkins aortic c.
Hopkins aortic occlusion c.
Hopkins hysterectomy c.
Howard-DeBakey aortic
   aneurysm c.
Hudson c.
Hufnagel c.
Hufnagel aortic c.
Hufnagel ascending aortic c.
Hufnagel valve-holding c.
Hugh Young pedicle c.
Hume c.
Hume aortic c.
Humphries c.
Humphries aortic c.
Humphries aortic
   aneurysm c.
Humphries reverse-curve
   aortic c.
Hunt c.
Hunt colostomy c.
Hunter-Satinsky c.
Hurson flexible pressure c.
Hurson flexible sliding c.
Hurwitz c.
Hurwitz esophageal c.
Hurwitz intestinal c.
Hyams c.
Hyams meatus c.
Hydragrip c.
hysterectomy c.
iliac c.
Iliff c.
incontinence c.
infant vascular c.
c. insert
intestinal c.
intestinal anastomosis c.
intestinal occlusion c.
intestinal resection c.
intestinal ring c.
Jackson c.
Jackson bone-extension c.
Jackson bone-holding c.

Jacob c.
Jacobs c.
Jacobson c.
Jacobson bulldog c.
Jacobson microbulldog c.
Jacobson modified vessel c.
Jacobson-Potts c.
Jacobson-Potts vessel c.
Jacobson vessel c.
Jahnke anastomosis c.
Jahnke-Cook-Seeley c.
Jako c.
Jameson muscle c.
Janko c.
Jansen c.
Jarit anterior resection c.
Jarit cartilage c.
Jarit intestinal c.
Jarit meniscal c.
Jarit small bone-holding c.
Jarvis c.
Jarvis pile c.
Javid c.
Javid bypass c.
Javid carotid c.
Javid carotid artery c.
Javid carotid artery
  bypass c.
Jesberg c.
Jesberg laryngectomy c.
Johns Hopkins c.
Johns Hopkins bulldog c.
Johns Hopkins
  coarctation c.
Johns Hopkins modified
  Potts c.
Johnston c.
Jones c.
Jones thoracic c.
Jones towel c.
Joseph c.
Joseph septal c.
Judd c.
Judd-Allis c.
Juevenelle c.
Julian-Damian c.
Julian-Fildes c.
Kane c.
Kane obstetrical c.
Kane umbilical c.
Kane umbilical cord c.
Kantor c.
Kantor circumcision c.

Kantrowitz c.
Kantrowitz hemostatic c.
Kantrowitz thoracic c.
Kapp c.
Kapp-Beck c.
Kapp-Beck bronchial c.
Kapp-Beck coarctation c.
Kapp-Beck colon c.
Kapp-Beck-Thomson c.
Kapp micro-arterial c.
Karamar-Mailatt
  tarsorrhaphy c.
Kartchner carotid c.
Kartchner carotid artery c.
Kaufman c.
Kaufman kidney c.
Kay c.
Kay aortic c.
Kay aortic anastomosis c.
Kay-Lambert c.
Kelly c.
Kelly hose c.
Kelsey c.
Kelsey pile c.
Kern c.
Kern bone c.
Kern bone-holding c.
Kersting colostomy c.
K-Gar c.
K-Gar umbilical c.
Khodadad c.
kidney c.
kidney pedicle c.
Kiefer c.
Kindt c.
Kindt arterial c.
Kindt carotid c.
Kindt carotid artery c.
Kinsella-Buie c.
Kinsella-Buie lung c.
Kitner c.
Kleinert-Kutz c.
Kleinschmidt
  appendectomy c.
Klevas c.
Klinikum-Berlin tubing c.
Klute c.
Knutsson penile c.
Knutsson urethrography c.
Kocher c.
Kocher intestinal c.
Kolodny c.

clamp *(continued)*

Krosnick vesicourethral suspension c.
Kutzmann c.
Ladd c.
Ladd lid c.
Lahey c.
Lahey bronchus c.
Lahey thoracic c.
Lambert aortic c.
Lambert-Kay c.
Lambert-Kay aortic c.
Lambert-Kay vascular c.
Lambert-Lowman c.
Lambert-Lowman bone c.
Lambotte bone-holding c.
Lamis patellar c.
Lane c.
Lane bone-holding c.
Lane gastroenterostomy c.
Lane intestinal c.
Lane towel c.
Large c.
Large vena caval c. (Alfred M. Large)
laryngectomy c.
Leahey c.
Lee bronchial c.
Lee microvascular c.
Lee right-angle c.
Lees c.
Lees right-angle c.
Lees vascular c.
Lees wedge resection c.
Leland-Jones c.
Leland-Jones peripheral vascular c.
Leland-Jones vascular c.
Lem-Blay c.
Lem-Blay circumcision c.
Lewin c.
Lewin bone c.
Lewin bone-holding c.
lid c.
Liddle c.
Liddle aortic c.
Life-Lok c.
ligament c.
Lillie rectus tendon c.
Lin c.
Lindner anastomosis c.
Linnartz c.
Linnartz intestinal c.
Linnartz stomach c.
Linton c.
Linton tourniquet c.
lion-jaw c.
lip c.
Litwak c.
liver-holding c.
Lloyd-Davis c.
Locke bone c.
locking c.
Lockwood c.
Longmire-Storm c.
Lorna nonperforating towel c.
lower occlusive c.
Lowman c.
Lowman bone c.
Lowman bone-holding c.
Lowman-Gerster bone c.
Lowman-Hoglund c.
Lulu c.
lung c.
lung exclusion c.
MacDonald c.
MacDonald gastric c.
Madden c.
Madden intestinal c.
Maingot c.
Malgaigne c.
Malis hinge c.
Marcuse tube c.
marginal c.
Martel c.
Martel intestinal c.
Martin c.
Martin cartilage c.
Martin muscle c.
Mason c.
Mason vascular c.
Masters intestinal c.
Masterson c.
Masterson curved c.
Masterson pelvic c.
Masterson straight c.
Masters-Schwartz intesstinal c.
Masters-Schwartz liver c.
Mastin c.
Mastin muscle c.
Mattox aortic c.
Mayfield aneurysm c.
Mayfield skull c.
May kidney c.

Mayo c.
Mayo-Guyon c.
Mayo-Guyon kidney c.
Mayo-Guyon vessel c.
Mayo kidney c.
Mayo-Lovelace c.
Mayo-Lovelace spur
 crushing c.
Mayo-Robson c.
Mayo-Robson intestinal c.
Mayo vessel c.
McCleery-Miller c.
McCleery-Miller intestinal c.
McCleery-Miller intestinal
 anastomosis c.
McCullough hysterectomy c.
McDonald c.
McGuire c.
McKenzie c.
McLean c.
McNealey-Glassman c.
McNealey-Glassman-
 Mixter c.
McQuigg c.
McQuigg right-angle c.
meatal c.
Meeker c.
Meeker gallstone c.
megaureter c.
meniscal c.
metal c.
metallic c.
Michel c.
Michel aortic c.
micro-arterial c.
microbulldog c.
micro cross-action
 bulldog c.
microvascular c.
Mikulicz c.
Mikulicz peritoneal c.
Mikulicz-Radecki c.
Miles c.
Miles rectal c.
Millin c.
miniature bulldog c.
miniature multipurpose c.
mini-Ullrich bone c.
Mitchel-Adam c.
Mitchel-Adam
 multipurpose c.
Mitchel aortotomy c.
Mixter c.

Mixter ligature-carrier c.
Mixter right-angle c.
Mixter thoracic c.
Mogen circumcision c.
Mohr c.
Mohr pinchcock c.
Moorehead c.
Moorehead lid c.
Moreno c.
Moreno gastroenterostomy c.
Morris aortic c.
mosquito c.
mosquito lid c.
mouse-tooth c.
Moynihan c.
Moynihan towel c.
Mueller c.
Mueller aortic c.
Mueller bronchial c.
Mueller pediatric c.
Mueller vena caval c.
Muir c.
Muir cautery c.
Muir rectal cautery c.
Mulligan anastomosis c.
multipurpose c.
multipurpose angled c.
multipurpose curved c.
muscle c.
muscle biopsy c.
mush c.
Myles c.
Myles hemorrhoidal c.
myocardial c.
Nakayama c.
neonatal vascular c.
nephrostomy c.
Nichol c.
Nichols aortic c.
Nicola c.
Nicola tendon c.
Niedner c.
Niedner anastomosis c.
Niedner pulmonic c.
noncrushing c.
noncrushing anterior
 resection c.
noncrushing bowel c.
noncrushing
 gastroenterostomy c.
noncrushing
 gastrointestinal c.
noncrushing intestinal c.

clamp *(continued)*
- noncrushing liver-holding c.
- noncrushing vascular c.
- nonperforating towel c.
- Noon AV fistular c.
- Nunez c.
- Nunez aortic c.
- Nunez auricular c.
- Nussbaum intestinal c.
- occluding c.
- occlusion c.
- occlusion multipurpose c.
- Ochsner c.
- Ochsner aortic c.
- Ochsner arterial c.
- Ochsner thoracic c.
- Ockerblad c.
- Ockerblad kidney c.
- Ockerblad vessel c.
- O'Connor c.
- O'Connor lid c.
- O'Hanlon gastrointestinal c.
- O'Hanlon intestinal c.
- Olivecrona aneurysm c.
- Omed bulldog vascular c.
- O'Neill c.
- O'Neill cardiac c.
- O'Neill double-curved c.
- O'Shaughnessy c.
- ossicle-holding c.
- osteoplastic flap c.
- padded c.
- parametrium c.
- Parham-Martin c.
- Parham-Martin bone c.
- Parham-Martin bone-holding c.
- Parker c.
- Parker-Kerr c.
- Parker-Kerr intestinal c.
- Parsonnet aortic c.
- partial occlusion c.
- Partipilo c.
- patellar c.
- patellar cement c.
- patent ductus c.
- Payr c.
- Payr gastrointestinal c.
- Payr intestinal c.
- Payr pylorus c.
- Payr resection c.
- Payr stomach c.
- Péan c.
- Péan hemostatic c.
- Péan hysterectomy c.
- Péan intestinal c.
- Péan vessel c.
- pediatric c.
- pediatric bulldog c.
- pedicle c.
- Peers c.
- Peers towel c.
- pelvic c.
- Pemberton c.
- Pemberton sigmoid c.
- Pemberton sigmoid anastomosis c.
- Pemberton spur-crushing c.
- penile c.
- penis c.
- Pennington c.
- Percy c.
- pericortical c.
- peripheral vascular c.
- peritoneal c.
- perticortical c.
- Phaneuf c.
- phantom c.
- Phillips c.
- Phillips rectal c.
- pile c.
- Pilling c.
- Pilling micro-anastomosis c.
- Pilling pediatric c.
- pinchcock c.
- placental c.
- Plastibell c.
- Plastibell circumcision c.
- Pomeranz aortic c.
- Poppen c.
- Poppen aortic c.
- Poppen-Blalock c.
- Poppen-Blalock carotid c.
- Poppen-Blalock carotid artery c.
- Poppen-Blalock-Salibi c.
- Poppen-Blalock-Salibi carotid c.
- post-TUR c.
- post-TUR irrigation c.
- post-TUR irrigation control c.
- Potts c.
- Potts aortic c.
- Potts cardiovascular c.
- Potts coarctation c.

Potts divisional c.
Potts ductus c.
Potts-Niedner c.
Potts-Niedner aortic c.
Potts patent ductus c.
Potts pulmonic c.
Potts-Satinsky c.
Potts-Smith aortic c.
Potts-Smith aortic
 occlusion c.
Potts-Smith pulmonic c.
Poutasse c.
Poutasse renal artery c.
Presbyterian Hospital c.
Presbyterian Hospital
 occluding c.
Presbyterian Hospital T-c.
Presbyterian Hospital
 tube c.
Presbyterian Hospital
 tubing c.
Preshaw c.
Price muscle c.
Price muscle biopsy c.
Price-Thomas c.
Price-Thomas bronchial c.
Price-Thomas bronchus c.
Prince c.
Pringle c.
Providence Hospital c.
ptosis c.
Pudenz-Heyer c.
pulmonary arterial c.
pulmonary embolism c.
pulmonary vessel c.
pulmonic c.
pulmonic stenosis c.
pylorus c.
Ralks c.
Ralks thoracic c.
Ramstedt c.
Ranieri c.
Rankin c.
Rankin anastomosis c.
Rankin intestinal c.
Rankin intestinal
 anastomosis c.
Rankin stomach c.
Ranzewski c.
Ranzewski intestinal c.
ratchet c.
Ravich c.
Rayport muscle c.

Rayport muscle biopsy c.
reamer c.
rectal c.
Redo intestinal c.
Reich-Nechtow c.
Reich-Nechtow arterial c.
Reinhoff swan neck c.
renal c.
renal artery c.
renal pedicle c.
resection c.
Reul aortic c.
reverse-curve c.
Reynolds c.
Reynolds dissecting c.
Reynolds resection c.
Reynolds vascular c.
Rhinelander c.
Rica c.
Rica arterial c.
Rica micro-arterial c.
Rica stem c.
Rica vessel c.
Richards c.
Richards bone c.
Rienhoff c.
Rienhoff arterial c.
right-angle c.
right-angle colon c.
ring c.
ring-handled bulldog c.
ring-jawed holding c.
R-N c.
Rochester c.
Rochester hook c.
Rochester-Kocher c.
Rochester-Péan c.
Rochester sigmoid c.
Rockey c.
Rockey vascular c.
Roe aortic c.
Roe aortic tourniquet c.
Roeder c.
Roeder towel c.
Roosevelt c.
Roosevelt
 gastroenterostomy c.
Roosevelt gastrointestinal c.
Roosevelt intestinal c.
rubber dam c.
rubber shod c.
Rubin c.
Rubin bronchial c.

clamp *(continued)*
Rubio wire-holding c.
Rubovits c.
Ruel aortic c.
Rumel c.
Rumel myocardial c.
Rumel rubber c.
Rumel thoracic c.
Rush c.
Rush bone c.
Salibi carotid artery c.
Santulli c.
Sarnoff c.
Sarnoff aortic c.
Sarot c.
Sarot arterial c.
Sarot bronchial c.
Satinsky c.
Satinsky anastomosis c.
Satinsky aortic c.
Satinsky pediatric c.
Satinsky vascular c.
Satinsky vena caval c.
Schaedel towel c.
Schlein c.
Schlesinger c.
Schmidt c.
Schnidt c.
Schoemaker intestinal c.
Schumacher aortic c.
Schutz c.
Schwartz c.
Schwartz arterial
  aneurysm c.
Schwartz bulldog c.
Schwartz intracranial c.
Schwartz temporary
  intracranial artery c.
Schwartz vascular c.
Scoville-Lewis c.
screw occlusive c.
Scudder c.
Scudder intestinal c.
Scudder stomach c.
Sehrt c.
Seidel bone-holding c.
Sellor c.
Selman c.
Selverstone c.
Selverstone carotid c.
Selverstone carotid artery c.
Semb bone-holding c.
Semb bronchus c.

Senning c.
Senning bulldog c.
Senning featherweight
  bulldog c.
Senning-Stille c.
septal c.
serrefine c.
c. set
Sheehy ossicle-holding c.
Sheldon c.
Shoemaker intestinal c.
shutoff c.
side-biting c.
sidewinder aortic c.
Siegler-Hellman c.
sigmoid c.
sigmoid anastomosis c.
Silber c.
Silber microvascular c.
Silber vasovasostomy c.
Sims-Maier c.
single c.
single Softjaw c.
single Softjaw handleless c.
Singley c.
Singley intestinal c.
Siniscal eyelid c.
skull c.
Slocum meniscal c.
SMIC intestinal c.
Smith c.
Smith bone c.
Smith cordotomy c.
Smith marginal c.
Smithwick c.
Smithwick anastomotic c.
Softjaw c.
Softjaw handleless c.
Somers c.
Somers uterine c.
Southwick c.
sponge c.
spoon c.
spoon anastomosis c.
spur-crushing c.
S-shaped peripheral
  vascular c.
stainless steel c.
Stallard head c.
Stanton c.
Stanton cautery c.
Stayce adjustable c.
Stay-Rite c.

Stemp c.
stenosis c.
Stepita c.
Stepita meatal c.
Stetten intestinal c.
Stevenson c.
Stille c.
Stille-Crawford
  coarctation c.
Stille kidney c.
Stille vessel c.
Stimson pedicle c.
Stiwer towel c.
St. Mark c.
Stockman c.
Stockman meatal c.
Stockman penile c.
stomach c.
Stone c.
Stone-Holcombe c.
Stone-Holcombe
  anastomosis c.
Stone-Holcombe intestinal c.
Stone intestinal c.
Stone intestinal
  anastomosis c.
Stone stomach c.
Stony splenorenal shunt c.
Storey c.
Storz meatal c.
straight c.
straight Crile c.
Stratte c.
Stratte kidney c.
Strauss c.
Strauss meatal c.
Strauss penile c.
Strauss-Valentine penis c.
Strelinger colon c.
Strelinger right-angle c.
Strelinger right-angle
  colon c.
St. Vincent tube c.
Subramanian c.
Subramanian aortic c.
Subramanian classic
  miniature aortic c.
Subramanian miniature
  aortic c.
Subramanian sidewinder
  aortic c.
Sugarbaker retrocolic c.
Sumner c.

surgical c.
Surgi-Med c.
Swan c.
Swan aortic c.
swan-neck c.
Swenson ring-jawed c.
Swenson ring-jawed
  holding c.
Swiss bulldog c.
Sztehlo c.
Sztehlo umbilical c.
T c.
tangential c.
tangential occlusion c.
tangential pediatric c.
Tatum c.
Tatum meatal c.
Taufic cholangiography c.
Tehl c.
temporalis transfer c.
tension c.
Textor vasectomy c.
Thoma c.
Thommy lid c.
Thompson c.
Thompson carotid c.
Thompson carotid artery c.
Thompson carotid
  vascular c.
Thomson lung c.
thoracic c.
Thorlakson lower
  occlusive c.
Thorlakson upper
  occlusive c.
three-bladed c.
tissue occlusion c.
tonsillar c.
towel c.
Trendelenburg-Crafoord c.
Trendelenburg-Crafoord
  coarctation c.
trochanter-holding c.
truncus c.
Trusler c.
Trusler infant vascular c.
tube-occluding c.
tubing c.
Tucker appendix c.
turkey-claw c.
Tydings tonsillar c.
Tyrrell c.
Ullrich tubing c.

clamp *(continued)*
   umbilical c.
   umbilical cord c.
   umbiliclamp c.
   Universal wire c.
   upper occlusive c.
   ureteral c.
   urethrographic c.
   urethrographic cannula c.
   urinary incontinence c.
   uterine c.
   vaginal cuff c.
   Valdoni c.
   Vanderbilt c.
   Vanderbilt University
     vessel c.
   Vanderbilt vessel c.
   Varco dissecting c.
   Varco gallbladder c.
   vas c.
   Vasconcelos-Barretto c.
   Vascuclamp minibulldog
     vessel c.
   Vascuclamp vascular c.
   vascular c.
   vascular graft c.
   vasovasostomy c.
   Veidenheimer c.
   Veidenheimer resection c.
   vena caval c.
   Verbrugge c.
   Verbrugge bone c.
   Verse-Webster c.
   vessel c.
   vessel-occluding c.
   vessel peripheral c.
   vestibular c.
   Virtus splinter c.
   V. Mueller aortic c.
   V. Mueller auricular
     appendage c.
   V. Mueller bulldog c.
   V. Mueller cross-action
     bulldog c.
   V. Mueller vena caval c.
   voltage c.
   von Petz c.
   von Petz intestinal c.
   von Petz stomach c.
   Vorse occluding c.
   Vorse tube-occluding c.
   Vorse-Webster c.

   Vorse-Webster tube-
     occluding c.
   Wadsworth lid c.
   Walther c.
   Walther-Crenshaw c.
   Walther-Crenshaw meatal c.
   Walther kidney pedicle c.
   Walther pedicle c.
   Walton c.
   Walton meniscal c.
   Wangensteen c.
   Wangensteen anastomosis c.
   Wangensteen gastric-crushing
     anastomotic c.
   Wangensteen patent
     ductus c.
   Warthen c.
   Warthen spur-crushing c.
   Watts c.
   Watts locking c.
   W. Dean McDonald
     gastric c.
   Weaver c.
   Weaver chalazion c.
   Weber aortic c.
   Weck c.
   Weck-Edna nonperforating
     towel c.
   wedge resection c.
   Weldon miniature
     bulldog c.
   Wells c.
   Wells pedicle c.
   Wertheim c.
   Wertheim-Cullen c.
   Wertheim-Cullen kidney
     pedicle c.
   Wertheim-Cullen pedicle c.
   Wertheim kidney pedicle c.
   Wertheim pedicle c.
   Wertheim-Reverdin c.
   Wertheim-Reverdin
     pedicle c.
   Wester c.
   Wester meniscal c.
   West Shur cartilage c.
   Whitver c.
   Whitver penile c.
   Wikstrom gallbladder c.
   Wikstrom-Stilgust c.
   Willett c.
   Williams c.
   Wilman c.

Wilson c.
Winkelmann circumcision c.
wire-tightening c.
Wirthlin splenorenal c.
Wirthlin splenorenal
  shunt c.
Wister c.
Wister vascular c.
Wolfson c.
Wolfson intestinal c.
Wolfson spur-crushing c.
Wood bulldog c.
Wylie c.
Wylie carotid artery c.
Wylie hypogastric c.
Wylie "J" c.
Wylie lumbar bulldog c.
X-c.
Yasargil c.
Yasargil carotid c.
Yellen c.
Yellen circumcision c.
Young c.
Young renal pedicle c.
Zachary-Cope c.
Zachary-Cope-DeMartel c.
Zachary-Cope-DeMartel
  colon c.
Zachary-Cope-DeMartel
  triple-colon c.
Ziegler-Furness c.
Zimmer c.
Zimmer cartilage c.
Zipser c.
Zipser meatal c.
Zipser penile c.
Zutt c.
Zweifel appendectomy c.
Zweifel pressure c.
clamp-on
  c.-o. aspirator
  c.-o. telescope
clam-shell brace
Clar head light
Clark
  C. capsule fragment forceps
  C. common duct dilator
  C. dilator
  C. expanding mesh catheter
  C. eye speculum
  C. forceps
  C. helix catheter

C. hemoperfusion system
C. rotating cutter catheter
C. vein stripper
Clarke-Reich ligator
Clark-Guyton forceps
Clark-Verhoeff
  C.-V. capsular forceps
  C.-V. forceps
clasp
  Acland c.
  Adams c.
  arrow pin c.
  c. bar
  Damon c.
  Duyzings c.
  eyelet c.
  Hahnenkratt dental c.
  preformed c.
  Sumpter c. spring-lock
Classix pacemaker
Classon pediatric scissors
Clas von Eichen needle
Claussen fragment stabilizer
clavate
  c. clove-hitch suture
  c. suture
Clawicz chisel
claw retractor
Clayman
  C. corneal forceps
  C. forceps
  C. guide
  C. intraocular guide
  C. iris hook
  C. lens
  C. lens forceps
  C. lens-holding forceps
  C. lens implant
  C. lens-inserting forceps
  C. lid retractor
  C. spatula
  C. suturing forceps
Clayman-Kelman
  C.-K. intraocular lens
    forceps
Clayman-Knolle
  C.-K. irrigating lens loop
  C.-K. lens loupe
Clayman-McPherson tying forceps
Clayman-Troutman corneal scissors
Clayman-Vannas scissors
Clayman-Westcott scissors

Clayton
> C. laminectomy shears
> C. osteotome

cleaner
> bronchoscopic c.
> cannula instrument c.
> Chix c.
> instrument c.
> Opti-Zyme enzymatic c.
> Soflens enzymatic contact lens c.
> Sofnet c.
> Surgikos c.
> ultrasonic denture c.
> Weck instrument c.
> Weck-Kare kit instrument c.
> Weck-Kleen instrument c.
> Wec-Wash instrument c.

cleanser
> Sklar sinus c.

CLEARPLAN Easy Ovulation Predictor

ClearSite wound dressing

Clearview hCG one-step pregnancy test

Cleasby iris spatula

cleaver
> fiber c.

cleft
> c. palate elevator
> c. palate forceps
> c. palate needle
> c. palate raspatory
> c. palate sharp hook

Clemetson uterine forceps

Clemons
> C. Tube-Tainer suction tube

Clerf
> C. aspirator
> C. cancer cell collector
> C. dilator
> C. forceps
> C. laryngeal saw
> C. laryngectomy tube
> C. laryngoscope

Clerf-Arrowsmith safety pin closer

Clev-Dent excavator

Clevedan positive pressure respirator

Clevedent
> C. forceps
> C. retractor

Clevedent-Gardner chisel

Clevedent-Lucas curette

Clevedent-Wakefield chisel

Cleveland bone-cutting forceps

Clevis dressing

clicker

C-line bipolar coagulator

clinic
> c. Bovie
> c. exolever elevator

Clinicare bed

Cliniguard

Cliniset infusion set

Clinitemp fever detector

Clinitron
> C. air-fluidized bed
> C. bed

clip
> Ackerman c.
> Acland c.
> Adams-DeWeese inferior vena caval c.
> Adams-DeWeese vena caval c.
> Adams-DeWeese vena caval serrated c.
> Adams orthodontic c.
> Adson c.
> Adson brain c.
> Adson scalp c.
> Adson scalp hemostasis c.
> Ahlquist-Durham c.
> Ahlquist-Durham vena caval c.
> aneurysm c.
> angled c.
> c. applier (*See* applier)
> c.-applying forceps
> ASP c.
> Austin c.
> Autostat ligating and hemostatic c.
> Auto Suture c.
> Avalox skin c.
> Backhaus c.
> bayonet c.
> Benjamin-Havas fiberoptic light c.
> Biemer vessel c.
> biepharoplasty c.
> Bonney c.
> Booster c.
> Boyle-Rosin c.
> brain c.

Braun-Yasargil right-angle c.
butterfly c.
Callender c.
Children's Hospital c.
Children's Hospital scalp c.
clamp c.
Codman c.
cranial aneurysm c.
curved c.
Cushing c.
Cushing-McKenzie c.
Dandy c.
DeWeese-Hunter c.
Drake c.
Drake aneurysm c.
Drew c.
Duane U-c.
Edslab jaw spring c.
Edwards c.
Edwards parallel-jaw
  spring c.
Elgiloy-Heifitz aneurysm c.
encircling c.
endo-GIA surgical c.
Ethicon c.
Feldstein blepharoplasty c.
fenestrated c.
fenestrated Drake c.
Filshie c.
c. forceps
Friedman c.
Friedman tantalum c.
gate c.
Guilford-Wright c.
Guilford-Wright suction
  tube c.
c. gun
c. gun tray kit
Heath c.
Hegenbarth c.
Hegenbarth-Adams c.
Heifitz c.
Heifitz aneurysm c.
hemostasis c.
hemostasis scalp c.
hemostasis silver c.
hemostatic c.
Herff c.
Horizon surgical ligating
  and marking c.
House neurovascular c.
Hoxworth c.
Hulka c.

Hylinks c.
implantable c.
implanted malleable c.
inferior vena caval c.
Ingraham-Fowler cranium c.
Ingraham-Fowler tantalum c.
Ingraham-Fowler tantalum
  cranium c.
Instra-Rack separator c.
jaw spring c.
Kapp c.
Keer aneurysm c.
Kerr c.
Khodadad c.
Kifa c.
Koln c.
LDS c.
lens c.
LeRoy c.
LeRoy disposable scalp c.
LeRoy infant scalp c.
LeRoy-Raney scalp c.
LeRoy scalp c.
Liga surgical c.
magazine c.
Mayfield c.
Mayfield CIS-RE
  aneurysm c.
Mayfield-Kees c.
McDermott c.
McFadden c.
McFadden aneurysm c.
McFadden Vari-Angle
  aneurysm c.
McKenzie c.
McKenzie brain c.
McKenzie hemostasis c.
McKenzie silver c.
McKenzie silver brain c.
McKenzie V-c.
metal c.
Michel c.
Michel scalp c.
Michel skin c.
Michel suture c.
Michel-Wachtenfeldt c.
Michel wound c.
micro-anastomosis c.
microbulldog c.
microclamp c.
Miles c.
Miles skin c.
Miles Teflon c.

clip *(continued)*
Miles vena caval c.
Moren-Moretz vena caval c.
Moretz c.
Morse towel c.
Mortson c.
Mortson V-shaped c.
Moynihan c.
Olivecrona c.
Olivecrona silver c.
partial occlusion inferior
 vena caval c.
Paterson long-shank brain c.
Penfield c.
Penfield silver c.
Phynox c.
Phynox cobalt alloy c.
pivot aneurysm c.
Pool Pfeiffer self-locking c.
Raney c.
Raney scalp c.
Raney scalp hemostasis c.
Raney spring steel c.
Raney stainless steel
 scalp c.
c. remover
retractor c.
Rica cross-action towel c.
Rica silver c.
Rica suture c.
scalp c.
scalp hemostasis c.
Scanlan aneurysm c.
Schaedel c.
Schepens c.
Schepens tantalum c.
Schulec silver c.
Schutz c.
Schwartz c.
Schwartz temporary c.
Schwasser brain c.
Schwasser microclip c.
Scoville c.
Scoville-Lewis c.
Scoville-Lewis aneurysm c.
Secu c.
Selman c.
Seraphim c.
Serature c.
Serature spur c.
silver c.
skin c.
Smith c.

Smith aneurysm c.
Smithwick c.
Smithwick silver c.
Sofield retractor c.
spring c.
Stichs wound c.
straight c.
suction tube c.
Sugar c.
Sugar aneurysm c.
Sugita c.
Sugita aneurysm c.
Sundt c.
Sundt encircling c.
Sundt-Kees c.
Sundt-Kees aneurysm c.
Sundt-Kees booster c.
Sundt-Kees Slim-Line
 aneurysm c.
Surgiclip c.
Surgidev iris c.
suture c.
Takaro c.
tantalum c.
tantalum hemostasis c.
Teflon c.
temporary c.
temporary vascular c.
temporary vessel c.
Tomac c.
Totco c.
towel c.
triangular encompassing c.
U-c.
umbilical c.
Uni-Shunt abdominal slip c.
Uni-Shunt anchoring c.
Uni-Shunt cranial
 anchoring c.
Uni-Shunt right-angle c.
V-c.
vari-angle c.
vari-angle temporary
 vessel c.
vascular c.
vena caval c.
vessel c.
Vitallium c.
von Petz c.
Wachtenfeldt c.
Wachtenfeldt butterfly c.
Wachtenfeldt suture c.
Wachtenfeldt wound c.

Weck c.
window c.
wing c.
wound c.
Yasargil c.
Zmurkiewicz brain c.
clip-applier
Sundt aneurysm c.-a.
Yasargil aneurysm c.-a.
clip-applying
c.-a. aneurysm forceps
c.-a. forceps
clip-introducing forceps
clipper
Baxter surgical c.
clip-removing
c.-r. forceps
c.-r. scissors
C-loop intraocular lens
Cloquet needle
closed
c. drain
c. hook
c. iris forceps
c. nail
c. suction drain
c. suction tube
c. water-seal suction tube
closed-loop intraocular lens
close encounter nut
closer
Clerf-Arrowsmith safety
pin c.
c. forceps
safety pin c.
closing
c. forceps
c. intestinal clamp
closure
retainer c.
clot forceps
clothesline drain
cloth-shod clamp
clovehitch suture
clove-hitch suture
cloverleaf
c. catheter
c. nail
c. pin
c. pin extractor
c. rod
Cloward
C. anterior fusion kit

C. blade
C. blade retractor
C. bone graft impactor
C. bone punch
C. brain retractor
C. cautery hook
C. cervical drill
C. cervical drill guard
C. cervical drill tip
C. cervical retractor
C. cervical retractor set
C. chisel
C. cross-bar handle
C. curette
C. depth gauge
C. dowel ejector
C. dowel handle
C. dowel impactor
C. drill
C. drill guard cap
C. drill shaft
C. dural hook
C. dural retractor
C. elevator
C. guard guide
C. guide
C. hammer
C. intervertebral disk
rongeur
C. intervertebral punch
C. laminectomy rongeur
C. lumbar retractor body
C. L-W gauge
C. nerve root retractor
C. osteotome
C. periosteal elevator
C. pituitary rongeur
C. PLIF case
C. PLIF II kit
C. posterior lumbar
interbody fusion kit
C. puka chisel
C. retractor
C. retractor blade
C. rongeur
C. self-retaining retractor
C. single-tooth retractor
blade
C. spanner gauge
C. spanner wrench
C. spinal fusion chisel
C. spinal fusion osteotome
C. spreader

Cloward *(continued)*
    C. square punch
    C. stitch suture
    C. tissue retractor
    C. vertebral spreader
Cloward-Cone ring curette
Cloward-Cushing vein retractor
Cloward-Dowel
    C.-D. cutter
    C.-D. punch
Cloward-English
    C.-E. punch
    C.-E. rongeur
Cloward-Harman chisel
Cloward-Harper
    C.-H. cervical punch
    C.-H. laminectomy rongeur
    C.-H. rongeur
Cloward-Hoen
    C.-H. laminectomy retractor
    C.-H. retractor
Cloward-type rongeur
Clyman endometrial curette
clysis cannula
CMI vacuum delivery system
coagulating
    c. electrode
    c. forceps
    c. suction cannula
      connection cord
    c. suction cannula obturator
coagulating-suction
    c.-s. cannula
    c.-s. forceps
coagulation
    c. forceps
    c. probe
    c. suction tube
coagulation-aspirator tube
coagulator
    American Optical c.
    argon beam c.
    argon laser c.
    Ball c.
    Ballantine-Drew c.
    Bantam c.
    Bantam Bovie c.
    Biceps bipolar c.
    bipolar c.
    Birtcher c.
    Birtcher hyfrecatur c.
    Bovie c.
    C-line bipolar c.

    Codman-Mentor wet-field c.
    Codman & Shurtleff neo-
      coagulator c.
    Coherent argon laser c.
    cold c.
    Concept bipolar c.
    Cut-Blot c.
    electricator c.
    Fabry c.
    Gam-Mer bipolar c.
    Hildreth c.
    hyfrecator c.
    Jarit bipolar c.
    Karl Storz c.
    Kirwan bipolar c.
    Magielski c.
    Malis c.
    Malis bipolar c.
    Malis CMC-II PC
      bipolar c.
    Mentor wet-field c.
    Mentor wet-field cordless c.
    Mira c.
    National c.
    Polar-Mate bipolar c.
    Poppen c.
    Poppen electrosurgical c.
    Resnick button bipolar c.
    Riddle c.
    Ritter c.
    Ritter-Bantam Bovie c.
    Scanlan bipolar c.
    Storz c.
    Storz microsurgical
      bipolar c.
    suction-c.
    Tekno c.
    Ultroid c.
    wet-field c.
    xenon c.
    xenon arc c.
    Zeiss c.
Coakley
    C. antral curette
    C. antral trocar
    C. cannula
    C. curette
    C. ethmoid curette
    C. forceps
    C. frontal sinus cannula
    C. nasal curette
    C. nasal probe
    C. nasal speculum

C. probe
C. sinus curette
C. suture
C. tonsillar forceps
C. wash tube
Coakley-Allis
C.-A. forceps
C.-A. tonsillar forceps
coaptation
c. forceps
c. plate
c. splint
c. suture
coarctation
c. clamp
c. forceps
c. hook
coated
c. polyester suture
c. suture
c. Vicryl suture
coating
porous c.
Teflon c.
Co-Axa light
coaxial
c. cable
c. cannula
c. catheter
c. irrigating-aspirating nylon
connector
**cobalt chrome modular head
component**
Coban
C. bandage
C. elastic dressing
Cobaugh eye forceps
Cobb
C. bone curette
C. chisel
C. curette
C. elevator
C. gouge
C. periosteal elevator
C. retractor
C. spinal curette
C. spinal elevator
C. spinal gouge
C. spinal instrument
C. sterilizing rack
Cobbett skin graft knife
cobbler's suture
Cobb-Ragde needle

Cobb-style bone curette
Cobe
C. AV fistular needle
C. AV shunt
C. cardiotomy reservoir
C. small vessel cannula
**Cobe-Tenckhoff peritoneal dialysis
catheter**
cobra
c. catheter
c. retractor
cobra-shaped catheter
Coburg-Connell airway
Coburn
C. anterior chamber
intraocular lens implant
C. haptic
C. intraocular lens
C. lens
C. Mark IX eye implant
C. Optical Industries-Feaster
intraocular lens
Coburn-Storz intraocular lens
cochlear implant
cock
stop c.
Cocke large flap retractor
cock-up
c.-u. arm splint
c.-u. splint
c.-u. wrist support
cocoon
c. dressing
c. thread suture
CoCrMo alloy
Codivilla graft
cod liver oil-soaked strips dressing
Codman
C. aneuroplastic
C. arthroscope
C. Bicol sponge
C. bone gouge
C. cannula
C. cartilage clamp
C. cervical rongeur
C. clamp
C. clip
C. cranioblade
C. cranioclast
C. cranioplastic
C. dilator case
C. disposable ICP kit

Codman *(continued)*
   C. disposable ICP Luer
      lock
   C. disposable perforator
   C. disposable vein stripper
   C. drill
   C. external drainage system
   C. external drainage
      ventricular set
   C. fallopian tube forceps
   C. gouge
   C. guide
   C.-Holter catheter
   C. ICP monitoring line
   C. IMA kit
   C. intracranial pressure
      monitor
   C. laminectomy rongeur
   C. lens loupe
   C. lumbar external drain
   C. magnifying loupe
   C. marker
   C. micro-impactor
   C. osteotome
   C. ovary forceps
   C. & Shurtleff neo-
      coagulator coagulator
   C. skull perforator guard
   C. spanner
   C. sternal saw
   C. surgical patty
   C. surgical strip
   C. towel clamp
   C. vein stripper
   C. wire cutter
   C. wire pass drill
Codman-Kerrison
   C.-K. laminectomy rongeur
   C.-K. rongeur
Codman-Leksell
   C.-L. laminectomy rongeur
   C.-L. rongeur
Codman-Mentor
   C.-M. wet-field cautery
   C.-M. wet-field coagulator
Codman-Schlesinger
   C.-S. cervical laminectomy
      rongeur
   C.-S. rongeur
Codman-Shurtleff
   C.-S. cranial drill
   C.-S. surgical instrument
      tray

Codman's Rhoton dissector
Cody
   C. magnetic probe
   C. sacculotomy tack
   C. tack
Coe
   C. impression material
   C. investment material
   C. orthodontic resin
Coe-Comfort tissue conditioner
Coe-Pak
   C.-P. periodontal dressing
   C.-P. periodontal paste
Coe-Rect denture reliner
Coe-Soft denture reliner
coffer band
Coffin plate
Cofield total shoulder system
Cogan-Boberg-Ans
   C.-B.-A. lens
   C.-B.-A. lens implant
Cogsell tip aspirator
Cohan
   C. corneal forceps
   C. corneal utility forceps
   C. needle holder
Cohan-Vannas iris scissors
Cohan-Westcott scissors
Cohen
   C. cannula
   C. elevator
   C. intrauterine cannula
   C. nasal-dressing forceps
   C. retractor
   C. sinus rasp
   C. suture applicator
   C. tubal insufflation
      cannula
Cohen-Eder
   C.-E. cannula
   C.-E. uterine cannula
Coherent
   C. argon laser
   C. argon laser coagulator
   C. argon laser
      photocoagulator
   C. laser adapter
   C. radiation argon laser
   C. system of CO_2 surgical
      laser
cohesive dressing
COH hip abduction splint
Cohney scissors

coil
    c. cannister
    c. machine adapter
    c. vascular stent
coiled spiral pusher wire
coil-tipped catheter
Colapinto transjugular biopsy set
CO₂ laser
Colclough
    C. laminectomy rongeur
    C. Love-Kerrison
      laminectomy rongeur
    C. rongeur
cold
    c. (carbon dioxide) cautery
    c. coagulator
    c. coning knife
    c. cup biopsy forceps
    c. cup forceps
    c. knife
    c. rolled rod
    c. soak solution
Coldite transilluminator
Coldlite-Graves speculum
Coldlite speculum
Cole
    C. duodenal retractor
    C. hyperextension fracture
      frame
    C. polyethylene vein
      stripper
    C. retractor
Coleman retractor
Colibri
    C. corneal forceps
    C. corneal utility forceps
    C. eye forceps
    C. forceps
    C. mules
Colibri-Pierce forceps
Colibri-Storz
    C.-S. corneal forceps
    C.-S. forceps
collagen
    c. implant
    c. shield
    c. suture
collar
    c. brace
    c. button
    c. button iris retractor
    c. button tube
    cone c.

    c. dressing
    implant c.
    Peterson cervical c.
    Philadelphia c.
    c. scissors
collarless stem
collector
    Alden-Senturia specimen c.
    Carabelli cancer cell c.
    Cervex-Brush cervical cell c.
    Clerf cancer cell c.
    Cuputi sputum c.
    Davidson c.
    Herchenson esophageal
      cytology c.
    Lukens c.
    Moffat-Robinson bone
      pate c.
    Pilling c.
    Senturia-Alden specimen c.
    stool c.
    Ware cancer cell c.
College
    C. forceps
    C. pliers
Collen-Pozzi tenaculum
Coller
    C. arterial forceps
    C. forceps
    C. hemostatic forceps
Colles
    C. external fixation frame
    C. needle holder
    C. snare
    C. splint
collet
    tibial c.
Colley
    C. tissue forceps
    C. traction forceps
Collier
    C. forceps
    C. hemostatic forceps
    C. needle holder
    C. thoracic clamp
Collier-Crile
    C.-C. forceps
    C.-C. hemostatic forceps
Collier-DeBakey
    C.-D. forceps
    C.-D. hemostat
    C.-D. hemostatic forceps
Collier-Martin hook

Collin
- C. abdominal retractor
- C. clamp
- C. dissector
- C. dressing forceps
- C. forceps
- C. intestinal forceps
- C. lung-grasping forceps
- C. mucous forceps
- C. osteoclast
- C. ovarian forceps
- C. pelvimeter
- C. pleural dissector
- C. radiopaque sternal blade
- C. raspatory
- C. shears
- C. sternal self-retaining retractor
- C. tissue forceps
- C. tongue forceps
- C. tongue-seizing forceps
- C. umbilical clamp
- C. uterine curette
- C. uterine-elevating forceps
- C. vaginal speculum

Collin-Duval
- C.-D. forceps
- C.-D. intestinal forceps

Collin-Duval-Crile intestinal forceps

Collings
- C. electrode
- C. fulguration electrode
- C. knife
- C. knife electrode

Collin-Hartmann retractor
Collin-Pozzi uterine forceps
Collins dynamometer
Collins-Mayo mastoid retractor
Collis
- C. anterior cervical retractor
- C. anterior cervical retractor set
- C. anterior lumbar accessory set
- C. cervical TDR accessory set
- C. forceps
- C. lumbar TDR accessory set
- C. microforceps
- C. microscissors
- C. micro-utility forceps
- C. mouth gag
- C. posterior lumbar retractor
- C. posterior lumbar retractor set
- C. Universal laminectomy set

Collis-Maumenee corneal forceps
Collison
- C. body drill
- C. cannulated hand drill
- C. drill
- C. screw
- C. screwdriver
- C. tap drill

Collis-Taylor retractor
collodion dressing
collodion-treated self-adhesive bandage
Collostat sponge
Collyer pelvimeter
colon
- c. clamp
- c. motility catheter

Colon-A-Sun colonic irrigation
Colonial retractor
colonic insufflator
colonofiberscope
- Pentax FC c.

colonoscope
- Olympus c.
- Pentax c.

Coloplast
- C. bag
- C. colostomy bag
- C. dressing

colorant
color vision test
coloscope
- ACMI operating c.

colostomy
- c. bag
- c. clamp
- c. rod

Coloviras-Rummel thoracic forceps
colposcope
- Cryomedics c.
- Frigitronics c.
- Jena c.
- Zeiss c.

colpostat
- Hejnosz radium c.
- Homiak radium c.

Landon c.
Regaud radium c.
Colt cannula
Coltene
C. alloy
C. Brilliant-Lux
C. direct inlay system
C. impression material
C. Magicap
Coltex impression material
Colton empyema tube
Colts cutting needle
columellar
c. clamp
c. implant
Colver
C. dissector
C. examining hook
C. forceps
C. needle
C. retractor
C. retractor hook
C. tonsillar dissector
C. tonsillar forceps
C. tonsillar knife
C. tonsillar needle
C. tonsillar pillar-grasping
forceps
C. tonsillar retractor
C. tonsil-seizing forceps
Colver-Coakley
C.-C. forceps
C.-C. tonsillar forceps
Colver-Dawson tongue depressor
comb
Cottle periosteal c.
periosteal c.
combilan electrosurgical unit
combination gel and inflatable
mammary prosthesis
combined wire guide bone elevator
comedo extractor
comeoscleral suture
Comfeel Ulcus occlusive dressing
Comfort
C. Cath catheter
C. Cath II catheter
Command PS pacemaker
commissure laryngoscope
committed mode pacemaker
common
c. bile duct dilator
c. duct dilator

c. duct-holding forceps
c. duct probe
c. duct scoop
c. duct stone forceps
c. duct stone scoop
c. McPherson forceps
CO_2mmO_2n sensor transcutaneous
gas electrode
Compacement dental cement
Compafill MH dental restorative
material
Compalay dental restorative
material
Compamolar dental restorative
material
Compass CT stereotaxic adaptation
system
Compere
C. bone chisel
C. chisel
C. fixation wire
C. threaded pin
Comperm tubular elastic bandage
complete traction unit
component
acetabular c.
AGC Modular Tibial II c.
AGC porous anatomic
femoral c.
AGC unicondylar knee c.
Biomet Bi-Polar c.
Bio-Modular shoulder c.
Bio-Plug c.
Centrax bipolar c.
CFV wrist c.
cobalt chrome modular
head c.
Deyerle c.
Duracon knee c.
Harris-Galante porous
acetabular c.
HGP II acetabular c.
Interlok primary femoral c.
Ionguard titanium modular
head c.
Judet impactor for
acetabular c.
Kirschner Universal self-
centering captive-head
bipolar c.
Kudo elbow c.
Mallory-Head Interlok
primary femoral c.

component *(continued)*
> OEC Dual-Op barrel/plate c.
> Omnifit HA femoral c.
> Opti-Fix femoral c.
> PCA hip c.
> PFC c.
> Precision Osteolock c.
> Press-Fit c. (PFC)
> Press-Fit condylar c.
> Pugh barrel c.
> Rothman Institute porous femoral c.
> supracondylar barrel/plate c.
> trial c.
> Universal radial c.
> Vitallium mesh c.

composite
> DRS c.
> Phaseafill dental c.
> c. spring elastic splint

compound
> c. curved rasp
> Dermatex c.
> c. dressing
> Finite dental glazing c.
> c. suture

compressible acrylic intraocular lens

compression
> c. bandage
> c. device
> c. dressing
> c. earrings
> c. forceps
> c. hook
> c. instrumentation

compression-molded PMMA intraocular lens

compressor
> Adair screw c.
> air c.
> Anthony c.
> Anthony enucleation c.
> Anthony orbital enucleation c.
> Barnes c.
> Beneys tonsillar c.
> Berens c.
> Berens enucleation c.
> Berens orbital c.
> Castroviejo c.
> Charnley c.

> Conn aortic c.
> continuous air c.
> Deschamps c.
> DeVilbiss Pulmo-Aide nebulizer with portable air c.
> enucleation c.
> orbital enucleation c.
> Riahl coronary c.
> screw c.
> Sehrt c.
> shot c.
> tonsillar c.
> tubing c.

Comprol dressing

computer
> Digitrace home c.
> thermodilution cardiac output c.

Comtesse medical support stockings

Comyns-Berkeley retractor

Cona-Tone office-use hearing amplifier

concave
> c. gouge
> c. obturator
> c. sheath

concentrate
> ERI-Lyte hemodialysis c.
> hemodialysis c.
> Sorbtrate dialysate c.

concentric needle electrode

Concept
> C. ACL/PCL graft passer
> C. arthroscopic knife
> C. arthroscopy power system
> C. arthroscopy rasp
> C. beachchair shoulder positioning system
> C. bipolar coagulator
> C. bone tunnel plug
> C. cannula
> C. cautery
> C. C-reamer
> C. curette
> C. dermatome
> C. digit trap
> C. disposable intra-articular blade
> C. Intravision arthroscope
> C. mesh grafter dermatome

C. Multi-Liner lining needle
C. nerve stimulator
C. Ophtho-bur
C. Ophtho-bur corneal rust ring remover
C. 2-pin passer
C. Precise ACL guide system
C. PuddleVac floor suction device
C. rotator cuff repair system
C. self-compressing cannulated screw system
C. shaver
C. Sterling arthroscopy blade system
C. suturing needle
C. Traction Tower
C. video imaging system
C. zone-specific cannula system
conchotome
Hartmann nasal c.
Henke-Stille c.
Olivecrona c.
Stille c.
Struyken c.
Watson-Williams c.
Weil-Blakesley c.
Conclude dental cement
Conco abdominal belt
Concorde
C. disposable skin stapler
C. suction cannula
condenser
amalgam c.
Nordent amalgam c.
conditioner
Coe-Comfort tissue c.
condom catheter
conductance catheter
conductive
c. device
c. V-Lok cuff
conductor
Adson c.
Bailey c.
Bailey saw c.
Bovie liquid c.
Davis c.
Kanavel c.

Martel c.
Souttar esophageal c.
Xomed Audiant bone c.
condyle
femoral c.
Cone
C. bone punch
C. bur
C. calipers
C. cannula
C. cerebral cannula
C. curette
C. forceps
C. guide
C. ice tong calipers
C. laminectomy retractor
C. nasal curette
C. needle
C. retractor
C. ring curette
C. scalp retractor
C. self-retaining retractor
C. skull punch
C. suction biopsy curette
C. suction tube
C. ventricular needle
C. wire-twisting forceps
cone
c. biopsy cannula
c. biopsy needle
c. collar
McIntyre truncated c.
shielded open-end c.
c. tip catheter
Cone-Bucy
C.-B. cannula
C.-B. suction cannula set
C.-B. suction tube
conformation of right heart catheter
conformer
Fox c.
Conger perineal urethrostomy clamp
conical
c. bur
c. catheter
c. eye implant
c. implant
c. inserter tip
c. probe
c. tip

conical-tip
    c.-t. catheter
    c.-t. electrode
conic bougie
conization
    c. electrode
    c. instrument
    c. instrument blade
conjunctival
    c. fixation forceps
    c. forceps
    c. scissors
Conley
    C. mandibular prosthesis
    C. pin
    C. tracheal stent
Conn
    C. aortic compressor
    C. pneumatic tourniquet
    C. Universal tourniquet
connecting tubing
connection cord
connector
    Accu-Flo c.
    c. bar
    coaxial irrigating-aspirating nylon c.
    Crockard retractor blade c.
    Denver c.
    drain-to-wall suction c.
    c. forceps
    Holter c.
    intracardiac sucker c.
    Luer c.
    Luer lock c.
    McIntyre nylon cannula c.
    neurosurgical c.
    pedicle c.
    Pudenz c.'s
    Universal c.
    venous Y c.
    c. with lock washer
Connell
    C. airway
    C. inverting suture
    C. suture
Conrad-Crosby
    C.-C. bone marrow biopsy needle
    C.-C. needle
Conray contrast material

Constantine
    C. catheter
    C. flexible metal catheter
ConstaVac catheter
constrained
    c. hinge knee prosthesis
    c. nonhinged knee prosthesis
contact
    c. hysteroscope
    c. lens
    c. shell implant
Contact Laser
    C. L. bullet probe
    C. L. chisel probe
    C. L. conical probe
    C. L. convex probe
    C. L. flat probe
    C. L. interstitial probe
    C. L. round probe
    C. L. scalpel
container
    dilution c.
    sterilizing and storage c.
Continental
    C. cannula
    C. needle
continuous
    c. air compressor
    c. ambulatory peritoneal dialysis (CAPD)
    c. catgut suture
    c. circular inverting suture
    c. cuticular suture
    c. interlocking suture
    c. inverting suture
    c. irrigation catheter
    c. key-pattern suture
    c. Lembert suture
    c. locked suture
    c. mattress suture
    c. over-and-over suture
    c. passive motion (CPM)
    c. passive motion device
    c. running locked suture
    c. running suture
    c. silk suture
    c. suction tube
    c. suture
    c. U-shaped suture
continuously perfused probe
Contique contact lens case
contiunous hemostatic suture

contour
  c. block clamp
  c. defect molding kit
  c. instrument cleaning brush
  c. retractor
  c. scalp retractor
contoured washer
contour-facilitating instrument
  (CFI)
contractor
  Adams rib c.
  baby rib c.
  Bailey c.
  Bailey baby rib c.
  Bailey-Gibbon c.
  Bailey-Gibbon rib c.
  Bailey rib c.
  Cooley rib c.
  Crafoord c.
  Effenberger c.
  Finochietto-Burford rib c.
  Finochietto infant rib c.
  Graham rib c.
  Lemmon c.
  Medicon c.
  rib c.
  Rienhoff-Finochietto rib c.
  Scanlan-Crafoord c.
  Sellor c.
  Sellor rib c.
  Stille-Bailey-Senning rib c.
  surgical c.
  Waterman rib c.
Contrangle dermabrasion brush
control
  Cadogan-Hough footpedal
    suction c.
  Hough-Cadogan footpedal
    suction c.
controlled drain
controller
  Asahi pressure c.
Control-Release
control-release needle
Contura medicated dressing
Convatec urostomy pouch
conventional
  c. needle
  c. reform eye implant
  c. shell-type eye implant
Converse
  C. alar elevator
  C. alar retractor

  C. bistoury
  C. blade retractor
  C. button-end bistoury
  C. chisel
  C. curette
  C. double-end curette
  C. double-ended retractor
  C. fracture button
  C. fracture-wiring button
  C. guarded chisel
  C. hinged skin hook
  C. hook
  C. knife
  C. nasal chisel
  C. nasal knife
  C. nasal retractor
  C. nasal root rongeur
  C. nasal saw
  C. nasal speculum
  C. needle holder
  C. osteotome
  C. periosteal elevator
  C. rasp
  C. retractor
  C. retractor blade
  C. saw
  C. scissors
  C. skin hook
  C. splint
  C. sweeper curette
Converse-Lange rongeur
Converse-MacKenty
  C.-M. elevator
  C.-M. periosteal elevator
Converse-Wilmer conjunctival
  scissors
convertible
  c. fin
  c. telescope
Convertors surgical drape
convex
  c. obturator
  c. rasp
  c. sheath
convexoconcave heart valve
Conway
  C. eye retractor
  C. lid retractor
  C. lid speculum
Conzett goniometer
Cook
  C. arterial catheter
  C. catheter

Cook *(continued)*
C. County Hospital aspirator
C. County tracheal suction tube
C. endoscopic curved needle driver
C. eye infection speculum
C. eye speculum
C. filter
C. flexible biopsy forceps
C. helical stone dislodger
C. micropuncture introducer
C. pacemaker
C. peelaway introducer set
C. percutaneous entry needle
C. pigtail catheter
C. rectal retractor
C. rectal speculum
C. retractor
C. stent positioner
C. straight guide wire
C. TPN catheter
C. ureteral stent
C. Urosoft stent
C. walking brace
Cook-Amplatz dilator
cookie cutter
Cook-Longdwel needle
Cooley
C. acutely-curved clamp
C. anastomosis clamp
C. anastomosis forceps
C. aortic aneurysm clamp
C. aortic cannula clamp
C. aortic clamp
C. aortic forceps
C. aortic sump tube
C. aortic vent needle
C. arterial occlusion forceps
C. arteriotomy scissors
C. atrial retractor
C. atrial valve retractor
C. auricular appendage forceps
C. bronchus clamp
C. bulldog clamp
C. cardiac tunneler
C. cardiovascular clamp
C. cardiovascular forceps
C. cardiovascular scissors
C. carotid clamp

C. carotid retractor
C. caval occlusion clamp
C. chisel
C. clamp
C. coarctation clamp
C. coarctation forceps
C. coronary dilator
C. cross-action bulldog clamp
C. CSR forceps
C. curved cardiovascular clamp
C. curved clamp
C. curved forceps
C. dilator
C. double-angled clamp
C. double-angled jaw forceps
C. femoral retractor
C. first rib shears
C. forceps
C. graft
C. graft clamp
C. graft forceps
C. graft suction tube
C. iliac clamp
C. iliac forceps
C. instrumentation
C. intracardiac suction tube
C. ligature carrier
C. mitral valve retractor
C. MPC cardiovascular retractor
C. multipurpose angled clamp
C. multipurpose clamp
C. multipurpose curved clamp
C. multipurpose forceps
C. neonatal clamp
C. neonatal instrument set
C. neonatal retractor
C. neonatal scissors
C. neonatal set case
C. neonatal sternal retractor
C. neonatal vascular clamp
C. neonatal vascular forceps
C. partial-occlusion clamp
C. patent ductus clamp
C. patent ductus forceps
C. pediatric aortic forceps
C. pediatric clamp
C. pediatric dilator

C. pediatric vascular clamp
C. peripheral vascular clamp
C. peripheral vascular forceps
C. pick
C. renal artery clamp
C. renal clamp
C. retractor
C. reverse-cut scissors
C. rib contractor
C. rib retractor
C. scissors
C. sternotomy retractor
C. subclavian clamp
C. suction tube
C. sump suction tube
C. tangential forceps
C. tangential pediatric clamp
C. tangential pediatric forceps
C. tissue forceps
C. U-suture
C. valve dilator
C. vascular clamp
C. vascular dilator
C. vascular forceps
C. vascular suction tube
C. vascular tissue forceps
C. vena caval catheter clamp
C. vena caval clamp
C. ventricular needle
C. vertricular sump
C. Vital microvascular needle holder
C. wax carver
Cooley-Anthony suction tube
Cooley-Baumgarten
C.-B. aortic clamp
C.-B. aortic forceps
Cooley-Beck
C.-B. clamp
C.-B. vessel clamp
Cooley-Derra
C.-D. anastomosis clamp
C.-D. anastomosis forceps
C.-D. clamp
Cooley-Marz sternal retractor
Cooley-Pontius
C.-P. blade

C.-P. sternal blade
C.-P. sternal shears
Cooley-Satinsky
C.-S. clamp
C.-S. multipurpose clamp
Coolidge tube
Coombs bone biopsy system
Coonrad-Morrey Total elbow
Cooper
C. argon laser
C. basal ganglia guide
C. blade fragment
C. cannula
C. chemopallidectomy cannula
C. chemopallidectomy needle
C. cryoprobe
C. disk cryostat
C. double-lumen cannula
C. endotracheal stylet
C. laser adapter
C. ligature needle
C. needle
C. pallidectomy needle
C. spinal fusion elevator
C. spinal fusion gouge
CooperVision
C. argon laser
C. I&A machine
C. laser
C. microscope
C. viscoelastic
CooperVision-Cilco
C.-C. intraocular lens
C.-C. Kelman multiflex all-PMMA intraocular lens
C.-C. Novaflex anterior chamber intraocular lens
Copal cavity varnish
Copalite
C. applicator
C. cavity varnish
Cope
C. biopsy needle
C. clamp
C. crushing clamp
C. double-ended retractor
C. gastrointestinal suture anchor set
C. lung forceps
C. mandril guide wire

Cope *(continued)*
    C. modification of a Martel intestinal clamp
    C. needle
    C. needle introducer cannula
    C. pleural biopsy needle
    C. thoracentesis needle
Cope-DeMartel clamp
Copeland
    C. anterior chamber intraocular lens
    C. electrode
    C. intraocular lens implant
    C. lens
    C. lens implant
    C. radial loop intraocular lens
    C. retinoscope
    C. reusable electrode
    C. streak retinoscope
coping
    wax up c.
copolymer stapler
copper
    c. band
    c. blade
    c. mallet
copper-clad steel needle
Copper-7 intrauterine device, Cu-7 intrauterine device
Coppridge
    C. forceps
    C. grasping forceps
    C. urethral forceps
Coratomic
    C. implantable pulse generator
    C. R-wave inhibited pacemaker
Corbett
    C. bone-cutting forceps
    C. forceps
    C. foreign body spud
Corboy
    C. hemostat
    C. needle holder
cord
    Biopac gingival retraction c.
    bipolar connection c.
    Bucy-Frazier coagulating suction cannula connection c.

    Bucy-Frazier monopolar cautery c.
    coagulating suction cannula connection c.
    connection c.
    diathermy c.
    Frazier monopolar cautery c.
    Poppen monopolar cautery c.
    Racestyptine c.
Cordes
    C. circular punch
    C. esophagoscopy forceps
    C. ethmoidal punch
    C. forceps
    C. punch forceps tip
    C. semicircular punch
    C. sphenoidal punch
    C. square punch
    C. square punch tip
Cordes-New
    C.-N. forceps
    C.-N. laryngeal punch elevator
    C.-N. laryngeal punch forceps
Cordis
    C. Atricor pacemaker
    C. catheter
    C. Chronocor pacemaker
    C. dilator
    C. Ectocor pacemaker
    C. fixed-rate pacemaker
    C. Gemini pacemaker
    C. guiding catheter
    C. Lumelec catheter
    C. Multicor pacemaker
    C. Omnicor Stanicor pacemaker
    C. Omni Stanicor Theta transvenous pacemaker
    C. pacemaker
    C. pigtail catheter
    C. Sequicor pacemaker
    C. Ventricor pacemaker
Cordis-Dow shunt adapter
cordless dermatome
Cordon Colles fracture splint
cordotomy
    c. clamp
    c. knife
core mold stent

Core-Vent implant
Corey
    C. forceps
    C. ovum forceps
    C. placental forceps
    C. tenaculum
Cor-Gel gel
Corgill bone punch
Corgill-Hartmann forceps
Corgill-Shapleigh ear curette
Coritaxic multimodal stereotaxic work station
corkscrew
    c. dural hook
    Filtzer c.
    c. hook
Corlon catheter
cornea-holding forceps
corneal
    c. bur
    c. chisel
    c. curette
    c. dissector
    c. eye implant
    c. forceps
    c. graft spatula
    c. hook
    c. implant
    c. knife
    c. knife dissector
    c. light shield
    c. marker
    c. microscope
    c. monocular loupe
    c. needle
    c. punch
    c. scissors
    c. section-enlarging scissors
    c. section scissors
    c. spud
    c. suture
    c. suture needle
    c. transplant forceps
    c. transplant scissors
    c. trephine
    c. trephine set
    c. utility forceps
cornea-splitting knife
cornea-suturing forceps
corneoscleral
    c. forceps
    c. punch

    c. scissors
    c. suturing forceps
corneoscleroconjunctival suture
corner
    c. kit
    c. retractor
Corner plug
Cornet forceps
Corning implant
Cornish wool dressing
Cornman dissecting knife
corn plane
Corometrics Medical Systems Inc. fetal monitoring system
coronary
    c. angiography analysis system
    c. artery cannula
    c. artery forceps
    c. artery probe
    c. artery scissors
    c. cannula
    c. catheter
    c. dilatation catheter
    c. dilator
    c. endarterectomy set
    c. endarterectomy spatula
    c. forceps
    c. guiding catheter
    c. perfusion cannula
    c. perfusion catheter
    c. perfusion tip
    c. scissors
    c. sinus thermodilution catheter
Coronet
    C. alloy
    C. magnet
cor pacemaker
Corpak enteral Y extension set
corrected cosmetic contact shell eye implant
Corrigan cautery
Cortac monitoring electrode
cortex
    c. extractor
    c. extractor instrument
    c. retractor
    c. screw
cortex-aspirating cannula
cortical
    c. electrode

cortical *(continued)*
>   c. pin
>   c. step drill

Cortomic pacemaker
corundum ceramic implant material
Corwin
>   C. forceps
>   C. hemostat
>   C. knife handle
>   C. tonsillar forceps
>   C. tonsillar hemostat
>   C. tonsillar hemostatic
>   forceps
>   C. wire twister

Coryllos
>   C. periosteal elevator
>   C. raspatory
>   C. retractor
>   C. rib raspatory
>   C. rib shears
>   C. shears
>   C. thoracoscpe

Coryllos-Bethune shears
Coryllos-Doyen periosteal elevator
Coryllos-Moure rib shears
Coryllos-Shoemaker rib shears
Cosman-Nashold spinal stereotaxic
>   **guide**

Cosmos
>   C. pacemaker
>   C. pulse-generator
>   pacemaker

Co-Span alloy
costal
>   c. arch retractor
>   c. elevator
>   c. periosteal elevator
>   c. periosteotome

Costa wire suture scissors
Costenbader
>   C. incision spreader
>   C. retractor

Costen-Kerrison rongeur
Costen suction tube
Coston iris needle
Coston-Trent cryo retractor
costotome
>   c. chisel
>   Tudor-Edwards c.
>   Vehmehren c.

cot
>   finger c.
>   Kenwood finger c.

O'Connor rectal finger c.
Profex finger c.
rectal finger c.
rubber finger c.

Cotrel-Dubousset instrumentation
Cottingham punch
Cottle
>   C. alar elevator
>   C. alar protector
>   C. alar retractor
>   C. angular scissors
>   C. antral chisel
>   C. biting forceps
>   C. bone crusher
>   C. bone guide
>   C. bone lever
>   C. bulldog scissors
>   C. calipers
>   C. cartilage guide
>   C. chisel
>   C. chisel osteotome
>   C. clamp
>   C. columella clamp
>   C. crossbar chisel
>   C. crossbar chisel osteotome
>   C. crossbar fishtail chisel
>   C. curved chisel
>   C. dorsal scissors
>   C. double-edged knife
>   C. double hook
>   C. dressing scissors
>   C. elevator
>   C. elevator-feeler
>   C. fishtail chisel
>   C. forceps
>   C. four-prong retractor
>   C. heavy septal scissors
>   C. hook
>   C. hook retractor
>   C. insertion forceps
>   C. knife
>   C. knife guide
>   C. lower lateral forceps
>   C. mallet
>   C. modified knife handle
>   C. nasal chisel
>   C. nasal elevator
>   C. nasal hook
>   C. nasal knife
>   C. nasal knife blade
>   C. nasal rasp
>   C. nasal scissors
>   C. nasal speculum

C. needle holder
C. osteotome
C. periosteal comb
C. periosteal elevator
C. pillar retractor
C. profilometer
C. pronged retractor
C. protected knife handle
C. rasp
C. retractor
C. scissors
C. septal elevator
C. septal speculum
C. sharp-prong retractor
C. single-blade retractor
C. single-prong tenaculum
C. skin elevator
C. skin hook
C. soft palate retractor
C. speculum
C. spicule sweeper
C. spring scissors
C. suction tube
C. tenaculum
C. tissue forceps
C. Universal nasal saw
C. Universal nasal saw
  replacement blade
C. upper lateral exposing
  retractor
C. weighted retractor
Cottle-Arruga
  C.-A. cartilage forceps
  C.-A. forceps
Cottle-Jansen
  C.-J. forceps
  C.-J. rongeur
  C.-J. rongeur forceps
Cottle-Joseph
  C.-J. hook
  C.-J. retractor
  C.-J. saw
Cottle-Kazanjian
  C.-K. bone-cutting forceps
  C.-K. cutting forceps
  C.-K. forceps
  C.-K. nasal-cutting forceps
  C.-K. nasal forceps
Cottle-MacKenty elevator
Cottle-Neivert retractor
Cottle-Walsham
  C.-W. forceps
  C.-W. septal straightener

C.-W. septum-straightening
  forceps
Cotton
  C. cartilage graft
  C. graduated dilation
    catheter
cotton
  c. applicator
  c. ball
  c. ball sponge
  c. bolster dressing
  c. carrier
  c. Duknatel suture
  c. elastic bandage
  c. elastic dressing
  c. nonabsorbable suture
  c. pledgets dressing
  c. suture
cotton-ball dressing
Cotton-Huibregtse biliary stent set
Cotton-Leung biliary stent set
Cottonoid dissector
cotton-roll-rubber-dam clamp
cotton-wadding dressing
cotton-wool bandage
Cottony Dacron suture
couching needle
coudé
  c. assist catheter
  c. bag
  c. catheter
  c. electrode
  c. fulgurating electrode
  c. hemostatic bag
  c. suction catheter
  c. urethral catheter
coudé-tip
  c.-t. catheter
  c.-t. demeure catheter
Councill
  C. basket
  C. catheter
  C. dilator
  C. retention catheter
  C. stone basket
  C. stone dislodger
  C. stone scoop
  C. ureteral dilator
  C. ureteral stone extractor
Councilman chisel
Counsellor
  C. plug
  C. vaginal mold

Coughlin

counter
Gill pressor c.
counterbore
Lloyd adapter c.
counterpressor
Acland-Bunke c.
Bruni c.
counterpulsation balloon
countersink
Count'R-Force arch brace
coupeur
capsule c.
Coupland
C. elevator
C. nasal suction tube
coupler
coupling head
Cournand
C. arterial needle
C. arteriography needle
C. catheter
C. needle
C. quadpolar catheter
Cournand-Grino
C.-G. angiography needle
C.-G. needle
Coventry stapler
cover
Accu-Flo bur-hole c.
bur hole c.
Silastic bur hole c.
Coverlet adhesive dressing
Cover-Pad dressing
Cover-Roll
C.-R. dressing
C.-R. stretch bandage
cowhorn tooth-extracting forceps
Cox
C. cytology brush
C. polypectomy snare
Coxeter
C. catheter
C. prostatic catheter
Cox-Uphoff implant
Cox-Uphoff International (CUI)
Coyne spoon
Cozean
C. angled lens forceps
C. bipolar forceps
C. implantation forceps
Cozean-McPherson
C.-M. angled lens forceps
C.-M. tying forceps

CPI
CPI Astra pacemaker
CPI Maxilith pacemaker
CPI Microthin pacemaker
CPI Minilith pacemaker
CPI pacemaker
CPI Ultra II pacemaker
CPM
continuous passive motion
CPM device
CPS
central patient station
CPS modular air cranioclast
CPS unitized air cranioclast
cps
cycles per second
CPT
CPT hip system
CPT revision tamp
CPV catheter
Crabtree
C. attic dissector
C. dissector
C. dissector pick
Crabtree-House dissector-pick
cradle
c. arm sling
cannula c.
cannula silicone support c.
silicone support c.
Crafoord
C. aortic clamp
C. arterial forceps
C. auricular clamp
C. bronchial forceps
C. clamp
C. coarctation clamp
C. coarctation forceps
C. contractor
C. forceps
C. lobectomy scissors
C. lung scissors
C. pulmonary forceps
C. retractor
C. scissors
C. thoracic scissors
Crafoord-Sellor
C.-S. auricular clamp
C.-S. hemostatic forceps
Craig
C. biopsy needle
C. forceps
C. headrest

C. headrest holder
C. nasal-cutting forceps
C. needle
C. pin
C. scissors
C. septal forceps
C. septum bone-cutting forceps
C. tonsil-seizing forceps
C. vertebral biopsy set
C. vertebral body biopsy instrument set
Craig-Sheehan retractor
Cramer wire splint
Crampton-Tsang percutaneous endoscopic biliary stent set
Crane
C. bone chisel
C. chisel
C. dental pick
C. gouge
C. mallet
C. osteotome
Craniad cup positioner
cranial
c. aneurysm clip
c. bone rongeur
c. bur
c. drill
c. forceps
c. retractor
c. rongeur
c. rongeur forceps
c. suture
cranioblade
Codman c.
Kirwan c.
cranioclast
Auvard c.
Braun c.
Codman c.
CPS modular air c.
CPS unitized air c.
Rica c.
Tarnier c.
Zweifel-DeLee c.
craniofacial
c. appliance
c. fracture appliance
cranioplastic
c. acrylic cranioplasty material
Codman c.

c. kit
c. material dressing
craniotome
DeMartel c.
Verbrugge-Souttar c.
Williams c.
craniotomy scissors
craniotribe
craniovac drain
cranio x-ray frame
cranium clip-applying forceps
Crapeau nasal snare
cravat bandage
Crawford
C. aortic retractor
C. auricular clamp
C. canaliculus probe
C. dural elevator
C. fascial forceps
C. fascial needle
C. fascial stripper
C. head fracture frame
C. head frame
C. hook
C. needle
C. retractor
C. suture ring
C. tube
Crawford-Adams
C.-A. acetabular cup
C.-A. cup
Crawford-Cooley tunneler
Crawford-Knighton forceps
cream
electroconductive c.
Ilex stoma protective c.
Synapse electrocardiographic c.
C-reamer
Concept C.-r.
Creech aortoiliac graft
Creed dissector
Creevy
C. biopsy forceps
C. bladder evacuator
C. calyx dislodger
C. calyx stone dislodger
C. dilator
C. stone dislodger
C. urethral dilator
Crego
C. elevator
C. periosteal elevator

Crego *(continued)*
    C. periosteal retractor
    C. retractor
Crego-Gigli saw
Crego-McCarroll traction bow
Cremer-Ikeda
    C.-I. papillotome
    C.-I. sphincterotome
Crenshaw
    C. caruncle clamp
    C. caruncle forceps
    C. forceps
crepe bandage
Crescent
    C. graft
    C. plaster knife
crescent
    c. broach
    c. snare
crescentic blade
Crib-O-Gram neonatal screening audiometer
Cricket
    C. disposable skin stapler
    C. stapling device
cricothyrotomy
    c. cannula
    c. trocar tube
Crigler evacuator
Crile
    C. angle retractor
    C. appendiceal clamp
    C. appendix clamp
    C. arterial forceps
    C. blade
    C. clamp
    C. cleft palate knife
    C. crushing clamp
    C. dissector
    C. forceps
    C. gall duct forceps
    C. ganglion knife
    C. gasserian ganglion dissector
    C. gasserian ganglion knife
    C. hemostat
    C. hemostatic forceps
    C. hook
    C. knife
    C. Micro-Line arterial forceps
    C. needle holder
    C. nerve hook

    C. retractor
    C. single hook
    C. spatula
    C. thyroid double-ended retractor
    C. vagotomy stripper
    C. wire passer
Crile-Barnes hemostatic forceps
Crile-Crutchfield clamp
Crile-Duval lung-grasping forceps
Crile-Murray needle holder
Crile-type clamp
Crile-Wood
    C.-W. needle holder
    C.-W. Vital needle holder
crimped
    c. Dacron prosthesis
    c. toric
crimper
    Caparosa wire c.
    c. closer forceps
    ENT wire c.
    Farrior wire c.
    c. forceps
    Francis-Gray wire c.
    Gruppe wire c.
    Juers wire c.
    McGee-Caparosa wire c.
    McGee-Priest wire c.
    McGee wire c.
    Schuknecht c.
    Schuknecht wire c.
    Sheer wire c.
    washer c.
    Wayne U. c.
    wire c.
crimping forceps
Crinotene dressing
Cripps obturator
Cristobalite investment material
Critchett eye speculum
Crites laryngeal cotton screw
Criticare sensor probe
Critikon
    C. balloon temporary pacing catheter
    C. balloon thermodilution catheter
    C. balloon-tipped end-hole catheter
    C. balloon wedge pressure catheter

C. Berman angiographic balloon catheter
C. catheter

Crockard
C. curved retractor blade
C. hard-palate retractor
C. ligament grasping forceps
C. microdissector
C. midfacial osteotomy retractor plate
C. odontoid peg-grasping forceps
C. pharyngeal retractor
C. retractor blade
C. retractor blade connector
C. small-tongue retractor blade
C. sublaminar wire guide
C. suction tube holder
C. transoral retractor body

crocodile
c. biopsy forceps
c. forceps

Cronin
C. cleft palate elevator
C. implant
C. mammary implant
C. palate knife
C. Silastic mammary prosthesis

Crosby
C. biopsy needle
C. knife

Crosby-Kugler
C.-K. biopsy capsule
C.-K. pediatric capsule

Cross
C. clamp
C. corneal bur
C. needle trocar
C. osteotome
C. scleral trephine

cross-action
c.-a. bulldog clamp
c.-a. clamp
c.-a. forceps

crossbar
c. chisel
c. chisel-osteotome
c. fishtail chisel

crossclamp

crosscut
c. bur
c. fissure bur

Crossen puncturing tenaculum forceps

cross-slot screwdriver

cross-talk pacemaker

Crotti
C. goiter retractor
C. retractor
C. thyroid retractor

Crouch corneal protector

Crowe-Davis mouth gag

Crowe-tip pin

Crowley shank

crown
Alfred Becht temporary c.
Bosworth temporary c.
Directa c.
c. drill
c. drill screw
Getz c.
Hahnenkratt temporary c.
Kontack temporary c.
PD preformed c.
RM c.
Royal c.
Safco polycarbonate c.
c. scissors
c. suture

crown-crimping pliers

Crown saw

Crozat
C. appliance
C. orthodontic wire

C-R resin syringe

crucial bandage

cruciate
c. head bone screw
c. head screw
c. ligament guide

cruciate-retaining prosthesis

cruciate-sacrificing prosthesis

cruciform
c. head bone screw
c. screwdriver

Cruickshank
C. clamp
C. entropion clamp

Crump
C. dilator
C. vessel dilator

Crump-Himmelstein dilator

161

crural
    c. hook
    c. nipper forceps
Cruricast dressing
crurotomy
    c. chisel
    c. saw
crus guide fork
crush clamp
crusher
    baby spur c.
    Berger spur c.
    bone c.
    cartilage c.
    Cottle bone c.
    DeWitt-Stetten colostomy
      spur c.
    Garlock spur c.
    Gross spur c.
    Mayo-Lovelace spur c.
    Ochsner-DeBakey spur c.
    Proud fascia c.
    Stetten spur c.
    ultrasonic stone c.
    Warthen spur c.
    Wolfson spur c.
    Wurth spur c.
crushing clamp
Crutchfield
    C. adjustable skull traction
      tongs
    C. bone drill
    C. carotid artery clamp
    C. clamp
    C. drill
    C. drill point
    C. hand drill
    C. pin
    C. skull tongs
    C. skull traction tongs
    C. tongs
    C. traction tongs
Crutchfield-Raney
    C.-R. drill
    C.-R. skull traction tong
      point
    C.-R. skull traction tongs
Cryer
    C. dental elevator
    C. Universal forceps
cryoablation catheter
Cry-O-Cadet
    Kelman C.-O.-C.

cryoenucleator
    Gallie c.
cryoextractor
    Alcon c.
    Beaver cataract c.
    Beaver disposable c.
    Bellow CO2 c.
    Frigitronics c.
    Frigitronics F-20/20
      disposable c.
    Frigitronics Mark II c.
cryogenic probe
cryogun
cryojet
    Torre c.
Cryolife valvular graft
Cryomedics colposcope
cryopencil
    Amoils c.
cryopexy
cryophake
    Keeler c.
cryoprobe
    Cooper c.
    Frigitronics c.
    intravitreal c.
    Lee c.
    Linde c.
    Sudarsky c.
cryoptor
    Thomas c.
cryoretractor
    Hartstein iris c.
cryostat
    CE-2 c.
    Cooper disk c.
cryostylet
    Tomasino c.
cryosurgical
    c. apparatus
    c. instrument
cryotherapy probe
crypt hook
cryptotome
    Blanchard c.
    Pierce c.
Crystal Tone I in-the-ear hearing aid
Crystar porcelain kit
CS
    catgut suture
CSF
    cerebrospinal fluid

CSF reservoir
CSF shunt connector forceps
CSF shunt-introducing forceps
CSF T-tube shunt
CSV Bovie electrosurgical unit
CT-10 computerized tonometer
CTI brace
CTS Relief kit
CTX needle
CU-8 needle
Cubbins
  C. bone screwdriver
  C. screw
  C. screwdriver
cube
Cuchica syringe
cuff
  aortic c.
  Astropulse c.
  atrial c.
  blood pressure c.
  blood warmer c.
  calibrated V-Lok c.
  Cardio-c.
  Childs Cardio-c.
  conductive V-Lok c.
  Ducker-Hayes nerve c.
  c. electrode
  elephant c.
  Falk vaginal c.
  Honan c.
  Honan pressure c.
  inflatable c.
  inflatable tourniquet c.
  inflatable tracheal tube c.
  Kidde tourniquet c.
  mucosal c.
  musculotendinous c.
  nerve c.
  pneumatic c.
  pressure c.
  rectal muscle c.
  reefed vaginal c.
  right atrial c.
  rotator c.
  sphygmomanometer c.
  suprahepatic caval c.
  tourniquet c.
  tracheal tube c.
  uterine c.
  vaginal c.

cuffed tube
cuff-type inactive electrode
CUI
  Cox-Uphoff International
    CUI artificial breast prosthesis
    CUI chin prosthesis
    CUI columellar implant
    CUI dorsal implant
    CUI expander
    CUI eye sphere prosthesis
    CUI gel mammary prosthesis
    CUI joint
    CUI malar implant
    CUI myringotomy tube
    CUI nasal prosthesis
    CUI rhinoplasty implant
    CUI saline mammary prosthesis
    CUI shunt
    CUI tendon prosthesis
    CUI testicular prosthesis
    CUI urological catheter
    CUI urological drain
Cu-7 intrauterine device (*var. of* Copper-7 intrauterine device)
cuirass
  c. jacket
  c. respirator
Cukier nasal forceps
Culbertson canal knife
culdoscope
  Decker fiberoptic c.
Culler
  C. eye forceps
  C. fixation forceps
  C. iris spatula
  C. iris speculum
  C. lens spoon
  C. rectus muscle hook
  C. speculum
Culley ulna splint
Cullom-Mueller adenotome
Cullom septal forceps
Culp biopsy needle
Cummings
  C. catheter
  C. four-wing catheter
  C. four-wing Malecot retention catheter
  C. nephrostomy catheter

Cummings-Pezzer
    C.-P. catheter
    C.-P. head catheter
Cunningham
    C. brace
    C. clamp
    C. incontinence clamp
Cunningham-Cotton sleeve
cup
    acetabular c.
    Alivium prosthesis c.
    APR acetabular c.
    Aufranc c.
    c. biopsy forceps
    Breinin suction c.
    Buchholz acetabular c.
    caliceal c.
    Centaur trial c.
    Chambers intrauterine c.
    Charnley c.
    Crawford-Adams c.
    Crawford-Adams
      acetabular c.
    c. curette
    dry c.
    Dual Geometry HA c.
    Duraloc acetabular c.
    ear c.
    c. forceps
    Galin silicone bleb c.
    Harris-Galante c.
    HGP II acetabular c.
    iodine c.
    c. jaw rongeur forceps
    Laing c.
    Laing concentric hip c.
    large physiological c.
    magnetic c.
    McBride c.
    McGoey-Evans c.
    McGoey-Evans acetabular c.
    McKee-Farrar c.
    McKee-Farrar acetabular c.
    MMS low-profile
      acetabular c.
    Müller-type acetabular c.
    MultiPolar bipolar c.
    nasal suction c.
    Natural-Lok acetabular c.
    New England Baptist
      acetabular c.
    Newhart-Smith c.
    O'Connor finger c.

    ocular c.
    O'Harris-Petruso c.
    Omnifit acetabular c.
    ophthalmic c.
    optic c.
    Opti-Fix acetabular c.
    Optifix acetabular c.
    c. palm manual percussor
    PCA acetabular c.
    c. pessary
    Pierce nasal c.
    c. positioner
    prostatic biopsy c.
    c. pusher header
    c. pusher shaft
    Rickham c.
    Rotalok c.
    Silastic obstetrical
      vacuum c.
    Smith-Petersen c.
    S-ROM acetabular c.
    stainless steel c.
    suction c.
    Ti-BAC acetabular c.
    Ti-BAC II acetabular c.
    Titan hip c.
    trial c.
    trial acetabular c.
    Triloc acetabular c.
    Veenema-Gusberg prostatic
      biopsy c.
    Vitallium c.
    wet c.
cup-biting forceps
cupped
    c. forceps
    c. jaw forceps
cup-shaped
    c.-s. curette forceps
    c.-s. ear forceps
    c.-s. electrode
    c.-s. forceps
    c.-s. inner ear forceps
    c.-s. middle ear forceps
Cuputi sputum collector
Curad
    C. plastic bandage
    C. plastic dressing
Curdy
    C. blade
    C. schlerotome knife
    C. sclerotome

curettage
Gynaspir vacuum c.
curette, curet
ABCH c.
Abraham rectal c.
adenoid c.
Alvis c.
Alvis eye c.
Alvis foreign body c.
Anderson c.
Angell c.
angled c.
angled ring c.
antral c.
aortic c.
apicitis c.
aspirating c.
Austin oval c.
Auto Suture c.
Ballantine uterine c.
Ballenger c.
Ballenger ethmoid c.
banjo c.
Bardic c.
Barnhill c.
Barnhill adenoid c.
Barnhill-Jones c.
Barth c.
Barth mastoid c.
bayonet c.
B-12 dental c.
Beaver c.
Beckman adenoid c.
Bellucci c.
Berlin c.
Billeau c.
Billeau ear c.
Billroth c.
biopsy c.
biopsy suction c.
Blake c.
Blake uterine c.
bone c.
Bozeman c.
Bromley uterine c.
Bronson-Ray c.
Bronson-Ray pituitary c.
Brun c.
Brun bone c.
Brun ear c.
Brun mastoid c.
Buck c.
Buck bone c.

Buck ear c.
Buck earring c.
Buck-House c.
Buck mastoid c.
Bumm c.
Bumm placental c.
Bumm uterine c.
Bunge c.
Bush intervertebral c.
Carlens c.
Carmack c.
Carmack ear c.
Carroll hook c.
Carter c.
Carter submucous c.
cervical c.
cervical biopsy c.
chalazion c.
Charnley double-ended
  bone c.
Clevedent-Lucas c.
Cloward c.
Cloward-Cone ring c.
Clyman endometrial c.
Coakley c.
Coakley antral c.
Coakley ethmoid c.
Coakley nasal c.
Coakley sinus c.
Cobb c.
Cobb bone c.
Cobb spinal c.
Cobb-style bone c.
Collin uterine c.
Concept c.
Cone c.
Cone nasal c.
Cone ring c.
Cone suction biopsy c.
Converse c.
Converse double-end c.
Converse sweeper c.
Corgill-Shapleigh ear c.
corneal c.
cup c.
cylindrical uterine c.
Daubenspeck bone c.
Daviel chalazion c.
Dawson-Yuhl c.
Dawson-Yuhl-Cone c.
DeLee c.
Dench c.
Dench ear c.

curette *(continued)*
    Dench uterine c.
    DePuy c.
    DePuy bone c.
    Derlacki c.
    Derlacki ear c.
    dermal c.
    diagnostic c.
    disk c.
    disposable vacuum c.
    double-ended c.
    double-ended bone c.
    double-ended dental c.
    double-ended stapes c.
    double-lumen c.
    down-biting c.
    Duncan c.
    Duncan endometrial c.
    Duncan endometrial
      biopsy c.
    Dunning c.
    ear c.
    elevator-c.
    embolectomy c.
    endaural c.
    endocervical c.
    endocervical biopsy c.
    endodontic c.
    endometrial c.
    endometrial biopsy c.
    endometrial biopsy
      suction c.
    endotracheal c.
    Epstein c.
    Epstein down-biting c.
    Epstein spinal fusion c.
    ethmoidal c.
    eye c.
    Farrior angulated c.
    Farrior ear c.
    Faulkner c.
    Faulkner antral c.
    Faulkner double-end ring c.
    Faulkner ethmoidal c.
    Faulkner nasal c.
    fenestration c.
    Ferguson c.
    Ferguson bone c.
    fine c.
    fine-angle c.
    Fink c.
    Fink chalazion c.
    c. forceps

    foreign body c.
    fossa c.
    Fowler c.
    Fowler double-end c.
    Fox c.
    Fox dermal c.
    Franklin-Silverman c.
    Freenseen rectal c.
    Freimuth c.
    Freimuth ear c.
    Frenckner c.
    Frenckner-Stille c.
    frontal sinus c.
    Gam-Mer spinal fusion c.
    Garcia-Rock endometrial
      biopsy c.
    Garcia-Rock endometrial
      suction c.
    Genell biopsy c.
    Gifford c.
    Gifford corneal c.
    Gillquist suction c.
    Goldman c.
    Goldstein c.
    Goodhill c.
    Goodhill double-end c.
    Govons c.
    Govons pituitary c.
    Gracey c.
    Green c.
    Green corneal c.
    Greene endocervical c.
    Greene placental c.
    Greene uterine c.
    Green uterine c.
    Gross c.
    Gross ear c.
    Guilford-Wright c.
    Guilford-Wright
      microbone c.
    Gusberg c.
    Gusberg cervical biopsy c.
    Gusberg cervical cone c.
    Gusberg endocervical c.
    Gusberg endocervical
      biopsy c.
    Halle c.
    Halle ethmoidal c.
    Halle sinus c.
    Hannon c.
    Hannon endometrial c.
    Hannon endometrial
      biopsy c.

Hardy c.
Hardy bayonet c.
Hardy modification of
  Bronson-Ray c.
Harrison c.
Harrison scarifying c.
Harrison-Shea c.
Harrison-Shea knife c.
Hartmann c.
Hartmann adenoidal c.
Hatfield bone c.
Hayden c.
Hayden tonsillar c.
Heaney c.
Heaney endometrial
  biopsy c.
Heaney uterine c.
Heath c.
Heath chalazion c.
Hebra c.
Hebra chalazion c.
Hebra corneal c.
Hibbs c.
Hibbs bone c.
Hibbs-Spratt c.
Hibbs-Spratt spinal fusion c.
Hofmeister endometrial
  biopsy c.
Holden c.
Holden uterine c.
Holtz c.
Holtz ear c.
Holtz endometrial c.
hook-type dermal c.
horizontal ring c.
Hotz c.
Hotz ear c.
Hough c.
House c.
House-Buck c.
House ear c.
House-Paparella c.
House-Paparella stapes c.
House-Saunders middle
  ear c.
House-Sheehy knife c.
House stapes c.
House tympanoplasty c.
Houtz endometrial c.
Howard spinal c.
Hunter c.
Hunter large uterine c.
Hunter uterine c.

Ingersoll c.
Ingersoll adenoid c.
Innomed c.
Innomed bone c.
intervertebral c.
irrigating c.
irrigating uterine c.
Jacobson c.
Jansen c.
Jansen bone c.
Jarit reverse adenoid c.
Jones c.
Jones adenoid c.
Jordan-Rosen c.
Juers c.
Juers ear c.
K-c.
Kelly c.
Kelly-Gray c.
Kelly-Gray uterine c.
Kerpel bone c.
Kevorkian c.
Kevorkian endocervical c.
Kevorkian endometrial c.
Kevorkian endometrial
  uterine c.
Kevorkian-Younge c.
Kevorkian-Younge biopsy c.
Kevorkian-Younge
  endocervical biopsy c.
Kevorkian-Younge uterine c.
Kezerian c.
Kirkland c.
Kos c.
Kushner-Tandatnick c.
Kushner-Tandatnick
  endometrial biopsy c.
labyrinth c.
large bowel c.
large uterine c.
Laufe aspirating c.
Laufe-Novak diagnostic c.
Laufe-Novak gynecologic c.
Laufe-Randall c.
Laufe-Randall gynecologic c.
Lempert c.
Lempert bone c.
Lempert endaural c.
Lempert fine c.
long-handle c.
loop c.
Lounsbury c.
Lounsbury placental c.

curette *(continued)*
    Luango c.
    Lucas c.
    Luer c.
    Luer bone c.
    Luongo c.
    Lynch c.
    Magielski c.
    Majewski nasal c.
    Malis c.
    Marino rotatable transsphenoidal horizontal-ring c.
    Marino rotatable transsphenoidal vertical-ring c.
    Maroon lip c.
    Martin dermal c.
    Martini bone c.
    mastoid c.
    Mayfield c.
    Mayfield spinal c.
    McCaskey c.
    McCaskey antral c.
    McElroy c.
    Meigs c.
    Meigs endometrial c.
    Meigs uterine c.
    meniscal c.
    Meyerding c.
    Meyerding saw-toothed c.
    Meyhöffer c.
    Meyhöffer chalazion c.
    microbone c.
    middle ear c.
    middle ear ring c.
    Middleton c.
    Middleton adenoid c.
    Milan uterine c.
    Miles antral c.
    Miller c.
    Misdome-Frank c.
    Moe bone c.
    Molt c.
    Mo-Mark c.
    Mosher c.
    Mosher ethmoid c.
    Moult c.
    Mueller c.
    Munchen c.
    Munchen endometrial biopsy c.
    Myles c.

    Myles antral c.
    nasal c.
    Noland-Budd c.
    Noland-Budd cervical c.
    Nordent bone c.
    Novak c.
    Novak biopsy c.
    Novak biopsy uterine c.
    Novak endometrial biopsy suction c.
    Novak gynecology biopsy c.
    Novak-Schoeckaert endometrial c.
    Novak uterine c.
    Novak uterine biopsy c.
    Novak uterine suction c.
    O'Connor double-edged c.
    Orban c.
    orthopaedic c.
    oval-window c.
    ovum c.
    Paparella c.
    Paparella angled-ring c.
    Paparella-House c.
    Paparella mastoid c.
    Paparella stapes c.
    periapical c.
    Piffard c.
    Piffard dermal c.
    Piffard dermal c. with Luer hub
    Piffard placental c.
    Pipelle-deCornier endometrial c.
    Pipelle endometrial c.
    Pipelle endometrial suction c.
    pituitary c.
    placental c.
    plastic c.
    polyvinyl c.
    Pratt c.
    Pratt antral c.
    Pratt ethmoid c.
    Pratt nasal c.
    Randall c.
    Randall biopsy c.
    Randall biopsy uterine c.
    Randall endometrial biopsy c.
    Randall endometrial biopsy suction c.
    Randall uterine c.

Randall uterine biopsy c.
Rand bayonet ring c.
Raney c.
Raney spinal fusion c.
Raney stirrup-loop c.
Ray c.
Ray pituitary c.
Read facial c.
Read oral c.
Récamier c.
Récamier uterine c.
rectal c.
Reich c.
Reich-Nechtow c.
Reich-Nechtow cervical
 biopsy c.
Reiner c.
resectoscope c.
retrograde c.
reverse-angle skid c.
reverse-curve adenoid c.
Rheinstaedter c.
Rheinstaedter flushing c.
Rheinstaedter uterine c.
Rhoton c.
Rhoton horizontal ring c.
Rhoton loop c.
Rhoton pituitary c.
Rhoton spoon c.
Rhoton vertical ring c.
Rica ear c.
Rica lipoma c.
Rica mastoid c.
Rica uterine c.
Richards c.
Richards bone c.
Richards ethmoid c.
Richards mastoid c.
Ridpath c.
Ridpath ethmoid c.
right-angle c.
rigid c.
ring c.
ring bayonet Rand c.
Rock endometrial suction c.
Rosen c.
Rosen knife c.
Rosenmüller c.
Rosenmüller fossa c.
rotatable transsphenoidal
 horizontal ring c.
rotatable transsphenoidal
 vertical ring c.

ruptured disk c.
salpingeal c.
saw-toothed c.
Scaler c.
scarifying c.
Schaeffer c.
Schaeffer ethmoid c.
Schaeffer mastoid c.
Schede c.
Schede bone c.
Schroeder c.
Schroeder uterine c.
Schuletz antral c.
Schuletz-Simmons
 ethmoidal c.
Schwartz c.
Schwartz endocervical c.
Scoville c.
Scoville ruptured disk c.
Semmes spinal c.
Semmes spinal fusion c.
serrated c.
Shambaugh adenoidal c.
Shapleigh c.
Shapleigh ear c.
Sharman c.
sharp c.
Sharp dermal c.
Shea c.
Sheehy-House c.
Sheehy-House knife c.
Simon bone c.
Simon cup uterine c.
Simones spinal c.
Simon spinal c.
Simpson c.
Simpson antral c.
Sims c.
Sims irrigating uterine c.
Sims uterine c.
sinus c.
Skeele c.
Skeele chalazion c.
Skeele corneal c.
Skeele eye c.
Skene uterine c.
Skene uterine spoon c.
skid c.
Skillern c.
Skillern sinus c.
SMIC c.
SMIC ear c.
SMIC mastoid c.

curette *(continued)*
SMIC pituitary c.
Smith-Petersen c.
soft rubber c.
sonic c.
spinal c.
spinal fusion c.
sponge ear c.
spoon c.
Sprague ear c.
Spratt c.
Spratt bone c.
Spratt ear c.
Spratt mastoid c.
stapes c.
St. Clair-Thompson c.
St. Clair-Thompson
adenoidal c.
c. sterilizing tray
stirrup-loop c.
Stiwer c.
Storz resectoscope c.
Strully c.
Strully ruptured disk c.
Stubbs c.
Stubbs adenoidal c.
submucous c.
suction c.
suction tip c.
surgical c.
Sweaper c.
Synthes facial c.
Tabb c.
Tabb ear c.
Tamsco c.
Taylor c.
Temens c.
T-handled cup c.
Thomas c.
Thomas uterine c.
Thompson c.
Thompson adenoid c.
Thorpe c.
tonsillar c.
toxemia c.
Toynbee c.
transsphenoidal c.
Uffenorde bone c.
Ulbrich wart c.
Ultra-Cut Cobb c.
uterine c.
uterine biopsy c.
uterine irrigating c.

uterine suction c.
uterine vacuum aspirating c.
(UVAC)
Vacurette suction c.
vacuum c.
Vakutage c.
vertical ring c.
V. Mueller mastoid c.
Vogel c.
Vogel adenoid c.
Vogel infant adenoid c.
Volkmann c.
Volkmann bone c.
Volkmann oval c.
Voller c.
Walker c.
Walker ring c.
Walker ruptured disk c.
Wallich c.
Walsh c.
Walsh dermal c.
Walsh hook-type dermal c.
Walton c.
Weaver chalazion c.
Weisman c.
Weisman ear c.
Weisman infant ear c.
West-Beck spoon c.
Whiting mastoid c.
Williger bone c.
Williger ear c.
Wolff dermal c.
Wright-Guilford c.
Wright-Guilford
microbone c.
Wullstein c.
Wullstein ring c.
Yankauer c.
Yankauer ear c.
Yankauer salpingeal c.
Yasargil c.
Younge endometrial c.
Younge modified
endometrial biopsy c.
Younge uterine c.
Younge uterine biopsy c.
curetting bur
Curity
C. disposable laparotomy
sponge
C. dressing
C. irrigation tray
C. leg bag

curl-back shell eye implant
Curl Cath catheter
Curon dressing
Curry
    C. cerebral needle
    C. hip nail
    C. hip nail counterbore
      with Lloyd adapter
    C. needle
    C. walking splint
Curschmann trocar
Curtis
    C. forceps
    C. tissue forceps
curved
    c. awl
    c. blade
    c. cannula
    c. cardiovascular clamp
    c. catheter
    c. chisel
    c. clamp
    c. clip
    c. cricothyrotomy cannula
    c. forceps
    c. gouge
    c. hemostat
    c. Küntscher nail system
    c. Mayo clamp
    c. meniscotome blade
    c. needle
    c. needle spud
    c. operating scissors
    c. osteotome
    c. peripheral vascular clamp
    c. suture needle
    c. tube
    c. tube stylet
    c. tying forceps
curved-8 clamp
curved-on-flat scissors
curved-tip jeweler's bipolar forceps
curvilinear chin implant
CUSA
    Cavitron ultrasonic surgical
      aspirator
Cusco vaginal speculum
Cushing
    C. aluminum cortex
      retractor
    C. aluminum retractor
    C. angled decompression
      retractor

C. angled retractor
C. bayonet tissue forceps
C. bipolar forceps
C. bipolar neurosurgical
  forceps
C. bone rongeur
C. brain depressor
C. brain forceps
C. brain retractor
C. brain spatula
C. brain spatula-spoon
C. bur
C. clamp
C. clip
C. cranial bur
C. cranial drill
C. cranial perforator
C. cranial rongeur forceps
C. decompression forceps
C. decompression retractor
C. dressing forceps
C. dressing forceps
C. drill
C. dural hook
C. dural hook knife
C. elevator
C. flat drill
C. forceps
C. gasserian ganglion hook
C. Gigli-saw guide
C. intervertebral disk
  forceps
C. intervertebral disk
  rongeur
C. laminectomy rongeur
C. little joker elevator
C. Micro Bipolar
  neurosurgical forceps
C. monopolar forceps
C. needle
C. nerve hook
C. nerve retractor
C. perforator drill
C. periosteal elevator
C. pituitary elevator
C. pituitary rongeur
C. pituitary spoon
C. raspatory
C. retractor
C. rongeur
C. self-retaining retractor
C. spatula spoon
C. S-retractor

Cushing *(continued)*
    C. S-shaped brain spatula
    C. staphylorrhaphy elevator
    C. straight retractor
    C. suture
    C. thumb forceps
    C. tissue forceps
    C. vein retractor
    C. ventricular needle
    C. Vital tissue forceps
Cushing-Brown
    C.-B. forceps
    C.-B. tissue forceps
Cushing-Gutsch
    C.-G. dressing forceps
    C.-G. tissue forceps
Cushing-Hopkins
    C.-H. elevator
    C.-H. periosteal elevator
Cushing-Kocher retractor
Cushing-Landolt
    C.-L. speculum
    C.-L. transsphenoidal
      speculum
Cushing-McKenzie clip
Cushing-Taylor carbide-jaw forceps
cushion
    Ezo denture c.
    Snug denture c.
    suture c.
cushioning suture
Cushman drain
Custodis
    C. implant
    C. suture
custom-contoured implant
cutaneous
    c. pO2 monitoring system
    c. punch
    c. suture
Cut-Blot coagulator
cutdown catheter
cuticle
    c. nipper
    c. scissors
cuticular suture
Cutinova
    C. dressing
    C. Hydro wound dressing
Cutler
    C. eye implant
    C. forceps

    C. forceps thoracoscope
    C. implant
cutout activator
cut snare wire
cutter
    adenoid c.
    AMO vitreous aspiration c.
    Bantam wire c.
    Beaver ring c.
    Breck pin c.
    Buettner-Parel c.
    Cloward-Dowel c.
    Codman wire c.
    cookie c.
    Dedo-Webb c.
    diamond pin c.
    diamond wire c.
    Doret graft c.
    double-action plate c.
    Douvas c.
    dowel c.
    Dual Geometry c.
    Expand-O-Graft c.
    fascia c.
    finger ring c.
    flat-end c.
    Gator meniscal c.
    Guilford-Wright c.
    Guilford-Wright wire c.
    Heath wire c.
    Hefty bite pin c.
    Hough Teflon c.
    Jarit pin c.
    Kirschner wire c.
    Kleinert-Kutz c.
    Kloti c.
    leather valve c.
    Lempert malleus c.
    lens glide c.
    Maguire-Harvey c.
    malleus c.
    Martin diamond wire c.
    Mashemer c.
    meniscal c.
    multiaction pin c.
    O'Malley-Heintz c.
    Parel-Crock c.
    Pendula cast c.
    plate c.
    Porter-O-Surgical c.
    ring c.'s
    rod c.
    Rogers wire c.

round-end c.
Schuknecht c.
Sheets lens c.
Sklar c.
Speck-Ange c.
stent c.
Stille cast c.
Stryker cast c.
surgical c.
suture c.
Szulc bone c.
Tolentino c.
Tolentino vitreoretinal c.
Verner-Joel c.
Vernon wire c.
vitreous c.
vitreous infusion suction c.
 (VISC)
wire c.
Wright-Guilford wire c.
Cutter-Smeloff
 C.-S. cardiac valve
  prosthesis
 C.-S. heart valve
cutting
 c. block
 c. board
 c. bur
 c. cautery
 c. Delrin block
 c. device
 c. forceps
 c. forceps tip
 c. hemostatic tonsillectome
  blade
 c. instrument
 c. loop
 c. loop electrode
 c. needle
 c. Teflon block
CVIS
 CVIS imaging device
 CVIS intravascular US
  imaging catheter
CVP
 central venous pressure catheter
 CVP catheter
 CVP system
CVS
 chorionic villus sampling
 CVS catheter
C-washer
C-wire

C. W. Mayo (*See* Mayo)
cyanoacrylate
 c. fixed orbital silicone
  sleds implant material
 c. glue
Cyberlith
 C. demand pacemaker
 C. pacemaker
CyberTach pacemaker
Cybex finger-clip pulse meter
cycler
 PD-10 peritoneal dialysis c.
cycles per second (cps)
cyclodialysis
 c. cannula
 c. spatula
cyclodiathermy needle
**Cygnet Laboratories fetal
 monitoring system**
cylinder
 Bodenham dermabrasion c.
 c. penile distendible
  prosthesis
 c. penile nondistendible
  prosthesis
 c. penile prosthesis
cylindrical
 c. bougie
 c. sponge
 c. uterine curette
cylindrical-object forceps
Cynosar catheter
cystic
 c. duct catheter clamp
 c. duct forceps
 c. duct scoop
 c. hook
cystitome [OPHTH] (*See also*
 cystotome)
 Alcon c.
 Azar c.
 Beard c.
 Capsitome c.
 Drews c.
 Drews angled c.
 formed c.
 formed non-irrigating c.
 Graefe c.
 Graefe flexible c.
 guarded c.
 guarded irrigating c.
 Holth c.
 irrigating c.

cystitome [OPHTH] *(continued)*
  irrigating short sharp c.
  Knapp c.
  knife cannula c.
  Knolle-Kelman cannulated c.
  Knolle-Kelman sharp c.
  Kratz c.
  Kratz angled c.
  Lewicky c.
  Lieppman c.
  Lieppman sharp c.
  McIntyre c.
  McIntyre guarded c.
  Nevyas double-sharp c.
  Sharp point-tip c.
  side-cutting irrigating c.
  Visitec c.
  Wheeler c.
  Wilder c.
  Worth c.
  Zawadzki c.
cystocatheter
cystodrain
Cystografin contrast material
cystometer
  Lewis recording c.
  Uroflo c.
cystopanendoscope
cystoresectoscope
  ALR c.
  anterior-posterior c.
  Damon-Julian c.
  Julian c.
cystoscope
  c. accessory
  Albarran laser c.
  Braasch direct
    catheterization c.
  Braasch-Kaplan direct
    vision c.
  Brown-Buerger c.
  Broyle retrograde c.
  Butterfield c.
  Judd c.
  Kelly c.
  Kidd c.
  Laidley double-
    catheterizing c.

  Lowsley-Peterson c.
  McCarthy-Campbell
    miniature c.
  McCarthy Foroblique
    panendoscope c.
  McCrea c.
  Miller c.
  National general purpose c.
  Nesbit c.
  Surgitek graduated c.
  Wappler c. with microlens
    optics
  Young c.
cystoscope-urethroscope adapter
cystoscopic
  c. electrode
  c. forceps
  c. fulgurating electrode
cystotome [GU] *(See also*
  cystitome)
  air c.
  Kelman c.
  Kelman air c.
  Kelman double-bladed c.
  Kelman knife c.
  Kelman knife cannula c.
  knife c.
  McIntyre reverse c.
  Mendez ultrasonic c.
  reverse c.
cystourethroscope
  ACMI c.
  microlens c.
  O'Donoghue c.
  Wappler c.
  Wappler microlens c.
Cytobrush
Cytobrush Plus
cytological brush
Czermak keratome
Czerny
  C. forceps
  C. suture
  C. tenaculum forceps
Czerny-Lembert suture

Dacron
    D. arterial prosthesis
    D. bifurcation prosthesis
    D. bolstered suture
    D. catheter
    D. graft
    D. graft clamp
    D. implant
    D. intracardiac patch
    D. knitted graft
    D. mesh
    D. pledget
    D. preclotted graft
    D. retraction tape
    D. shield
    D. stent
    D. suture
    D. tightly-woven graft
    D. traction suture
    D. tubular graft
    D. velour graft
    D. vessel prosthesis
    D. Weave Knit graft

dacryocystorhinostomy (DCR)
    d. cannula
    d. needle
    d. retractor
    d. set

Daems
    D. bronchial clamp
    D. clamp

Dagger dilator

Dahlberg hearing aid

Dahlgren
    D. iris scissors
    D. rongeur
    D. skill-cutting forceps

Dahlgren-Hudson
    D.-H. cranial forceps
    D.-H. forceps

Daicoff
    D. needle-pulling forceps
    D. vascular forceps

Daig pacemaker

Dailey fixation hook

Daily
    D. cataract needle
    D. keratome
    D. suture

Daimed leg bag

Dainer-Kaupp needle holder

Daisy irrigation-aspiration instrument

Daiwa
    D. dental needle
    D. disposable needle

Dakin
    D. catheter
    D. dressing

Dale
    D. femoral-popliteal anastomosis forceps
    D. first rib rongeur
    D. forceps
    D. rib rongeur
    D. thoracic rongeur

Dalkon shield intrauterine device

Dallas retractor

D'Allesandro
    D. clamp
    D. serial suture-holding forceps

Dall-Miles cable grip system

Dallop-type fascial prosthesis

dam drain

Damian
    D. inverter
    D. lumen finder

Damon clasp

Damon-Julian
    D.-J. cystoresectoscope
    D.-J. ring remover

Damshek
    D. needle
    D. sternal trephine

Danberg
    D. forceps
    D. iris forceps

Dan chalazion forceps

Dandy
    D. arterial forceps
    D. clamp
    D. clip
    D. forceps
    D. hemostatic forceps
    D. needle
    D. nerve hook
    D. neurosurgical scissors
    D. scalp forceps
    D. scalp hemostat

Dandy (continued)
D. scalp hemostatic forceps
D. suction tube
D. trigeminal scissors
D. ventricular needle
Dandy-Cairns
D.-C. brain needle
D.-C. ventricular needle
Dandy-Kolodny hemostatic forceps
Dan-Gradle ciliary forceps
Daniel
D. adenotome
D. clamp
D. colostomy clamp
D. double-punch laser
laparoscope
Daniels hemostatic tonsillectome
Danis retractor
Dannheim eye implant
Dann-Jennings mouth gag
Dann respirator
Dansac colostomy irrigation set
Darby surgical shoe
Dardik
D. biograft
D. umbilical graft
Darling
D. capsulotome
D. popliteal retractor
Darrach retractor
Dartigues
D. kidney-elevating forceps
D. uterine-elevating forceps
DAS single pass dialyzer
Dastoor erysiphake
Datascope
D. balloon
D. intra-aortic balloon
pump catheter
Dattner needle
Daubenspeck bone curette
Dautrey
D. chisel
D. osteotome
D. retractor
David
D. pharyngolaryngectomy
tube
D. rectal speculum
Davidoff
D. cordotomy knife
D. retractor
D. trigeminal retractor

Davidson
D. bur
D. clamp
D. collector
D. erector spinae retractor
D. forceps
D. muscle clamp
D. periosteal elevator
D. pneumothorax apparatus
D. pulmonary vessel clamp
D. pulmonary vessel forceps
D. retractor
D. scapular retractor
D. trocar
D. vessel clamp
Davidson-Mathieu-Alexander
D.-M.-A. elevator
D.-M.-A. periosteal elevator
Davidson-Mathieu rib raspatory
Davidson-Sauerbruch-Doyen elevator
Davidson-Sauerbruch rib raspatory
Daviel
D. cataract spoon
D. chalazion curette
D. chalazion knife
D. lens loupe
D. lens scoop
D. lens spoon
Davila atrial clamp
Davis
D. aneurysm clamp
D. aortic aneurysm clamp
D. bayonet forceps
D. blade
D. blade with groove
D. bone skid
D. brain retractor
D. brain spatula
D. bronchoscope
D. capsular forceps
D. catheter
D. clamp
D. coagulating forceps
D. coagulation electrode
D. conductor
D. diathermy forceps
D. dissector
D. double-ended retractor
D. electrode
D. forceps
D. foreign body spud
D. graft
D. hemostat

D. hook
D. interlocking sound
D. knife
D. knife-needle
D. lamp
D. loop stone dislodger
D. metacarpal splint
D. modified Finochietto rib spreader
D. monopolar bayonet forceps
D. monopolar forceps
D. mouth gag
D. needle
D. nerve separator
D. periosteal elevator
D. pillar retractor
D. pin
D. raspatory
D. retractor
D. rhytidectomy scissors
D. ring mouth gag
D. scalp retractor
D. self-retaininig scalp retractor
D. skid
D. spatula
D. sterilizing forceps
D. stone dislodger
D. thoracic tissue forceps
D. tonsillar needle
Davis-Bovie cautery
Davis-Crowe
    D.-C. mouth gag
    D.-C. mouth gag frame
    D.-C. tongue blade
Davis-Geck
    D.-G. eye suture
    D.-G. suture
Davol
    D. bag
    D. canal wall punch
    D. catheter
    D. dermatome
    D. drain
    D. forceps
    D. microrongeur
    D. rongeur forceps
    D. rubber catheter
    D. suction drain
    D. sump drain
    D. tube
    D. tunneler

Davol-Simon dermatome
Davy surgical button
Dawson-Yuhl
    D.-Y. curette
    D.-Y. elevator
    D.-Y. gouge
    D.-Y. impactor
    D.-Y. osteotome
    D.-Y. periosteal elevator
    D.-Y. rongeur forceps
    D.-Y. suction tube
Dawson-Yuhl-Cone curette
Dawson-Yuhl-Kerrison
    D.-Y.-K. rongeur
    D.-Y.-K. rongeur forceps
Dawson-Yuhl-Key elevator
Dawson-Yuhl-Leksell
    D.-Y.-L. rongeur
    D.-Y.-L. rongeur forceps
Day
    D. attic cannula
    D. cannula
    D. ear hook
    D. stapler
    D. tonsillar knife
DCBGS
    direct current bone growth stimulator
DCI hemolyte solution
DCP
    dynamic compression plate
DCR
    dacryocystorhinostomy
DCS
    dorsal column stimulation
    DCS implant
DDD pacemaker
    dual-sensing, dual-pacing, dual-mode pacemaker
DDI mode pacemaker
DDT lock screw insertor
dead-ender
    metal d.-e.
De Alvarez forceps
Dean
    D. antral needle
    D. antral trocar
    D. applicator
    D. blade
    D. bone rongeur
    D. bracket placer
    D. capsulotomy knife
    D. dissecting scissors

Dean *(continued)*
D. forceps
D. hemostat
D. iris knife-needle
D. MacDonald clamp
D. MacDonald gastric resection clamp
D. needle
D. periosteotome
D. rasp
D. rongeur
D. scissors
D. tonsillar forceps
D. tonsillar hemostatic forceps
D. tonsillar knife
D. tonsillar scissors
D. wash tube
Deane prosthesis
Dean-Senturia needle
Dean-Shallcross tonsil-seizing forceps
Dean-Trussler scissors
Dearor model catheter
Deaver
D. blade
D. clamp
D. operating scissors
D. pediatric retractor
D. retractor
D. scissors
D. T-drain
D. T-tube
D. tube
Deaver-type retractor
DeBakey
D. angled multipurpose clamp
D. aortic aneurysm clamp
D. aortic clamp
D. aortic exclusion clamp
D. aortic forceps
D. arterial clamp
D. Autraugrip forceps
D. blade
D. bulldog clamp
D. chest retractor
D. clamp
D. coarctation clamp
D. cross-action bulldog clamp
D. curved clamp

D. curved peripheral vascular clamp
D. dissecting forceps
D. endarterectomy scissors
D. femoral bypass tunneler
D. forceps
D. graft
D. heart valve
D. implant
D. infant and child rib spreader
D. instrumentation
D. intraluminal stripper
D. ligature carrier
D. miniature multipurpose clamp
D. multipurpose clamp
D. multipurpose forceps
D. needle
D. needle holder
D. patent ductus clamp
D. pediatric clamp
D. peripheral vascular clamp
D. pickup
D. prosthesis
D. retractor
D. right-angled multipurpose clamp
D. ring-handled bulldog clamp
D. ring-handled clamp
D. scissors
D. sidewinder aortic clamp
D. S-shaped peripheral vascular clamp
D. stitch scissors
D. suction tube
D. tangential clamp
D. tangential occlusion clamp
D. tangential occlusion forceps
D. thoracic forceps
D. thoracic tissue forceps
D. tissue forceps
D. tunneler
D. valve scissors
D. vascular clamp
D. vascular dilator
D. vascular forceps
D. vascular scissors
D. vascular tunneler

DeBakey-Adson suction tube
DeBakey-Bahnson
    D.-B. clamp
    D.-B. curved clamp
    D.-B. forceps
    D.-B. vascular clamp
DeBakey-Bainbridge
    D.-B. clamp
    D.-B. forceps
    D.-B. vascular clamp
    D.-B. vascular forceps
DeBakey-Balfour retractor
DeBakey-Beck
    D.-B. clamp
    D.-B. multipurpose forceps
DeBakey-Colovira-Rumel thoracic
  forceps
DeBakey-Cooley
    D.-C. cardiovascular forceps
    D.-C. Deaver-type retractor
    D.-C. dilator
    D.-C. forceps
    D.-C. retractor
    D.-C. valve dilator
DeBakey-Cooley-Deaver retractor
DeBakey-Crafoord vascular clamp
DeBakey-Derra
    D.-D. anastomosis clamp
    D.-D. anastomosis forceps
DeBakey-Diethrich
    D.-D. coronary artery
      forceps
    D.-D. vascular forceps
DeBakey-Harken
    D.-H. auricular clamp
    D.-H. clamp
DeBakey-Howard
    D.-H. aortic aneurysm
      clamp
    D.-H. clamp
DeBakey-Kay
    D.-K. aortic clamp
    D.-K. clamp
DeBakey-Kelly hemostatic forceps
DeBakey-Liddicoat vascular forceps
DeBakey-McQuigg-Mixter
  bronchial clamp
DeBakey-Metzenbaum scissors
DeBakey-Mixter thoracic forceps
DeBakey-Péan cardiovascular
  forceps
DeBakey-Potts scissors
DeBakey-Rankin hemostatic forceps

DeBakey-Reynolds anastomosis
  forceps
DeBakey-Rumel thoracic forceps
DeBakey-Satinsky vena caval
  clamp
DeBakey-Semb
    D.-S. clamp
    D.-S. forceps
    D.-S. ligature carrier
    D.-S. ligature carrier clamp
    D.-S. ligature-carrying
      forceps
Deboisans drain
Debove tube
debridement needle
debrider
    Sauer corneal d.
Debrisan dressing
debris-retaining acetabular reamer
decelerator
    graduated electronic d.
      (GED)
Decker
    D. fiberoptic culdoscope
    D. forceps
    D. microsurgical forceps
    D. microsurgical rongeur
    D. microsurgical scissors
    D. photoculdoscope
    D. retractor
    D. rongeur
decompression
    d. catheter
decompressive
    d. enteroclysis catheter
    d. retractor
decompressor
    Emerson-Birtheez
      abdominal d.
    Savage intestinal d.
DeCourcy
    D. clamp
    D. goiter clamp
Decubi-Care pad dressing
decubitus boot shoe
Deddish-Potts intestinal forceps
Dedo
    D. laryngoscope
    D. laser laryngoscope
    D. laser retractor
Dedo-Jako laryngoscope
Dedo-Pilling laryngoscope
Dedo-Webb cutter

Dee elbow prosthesis
deep
    d. abdominal retractor
    d. Deaver retractor
    d. ligature carrier
    d. rake retractor
    d. retractor
    d. spreader blade
deep-surgery forceps
deep-vessel forceps
Dees
    D. holder
    D. needle
    D. renal needle
    D. suture needle
defibrillator implant
deflecting
    tip d.
Defourmental
    D. forceps
    D. nasal rongeur
    D. rongeur forceps
Degnon suture
degreaser
    Cav-Clean cavity d.
Degucast alloy
Degudent alloy
Dejerine
    D. hammer
    D. percussion hammer
Dejerine-Davis percussion hammer
dekalon suture
Deklene
    D. polypropylene suture
    D. suture
Deknatel
    D. K-needle
    D. needle
    D. silk suture
    D. suture
DeKock two-way bronchial catheter
Delaborde
    D. dilator
    D. tracheal dilator
Delaborde-Trousseau tracheal
    dilator
De La Caffiniere Trapezio
    metacarpal prosthesis
DeLaginiere abdominal retractor
Delaney
    D. phrenic retractor
    D. retractor

DeLaura knee prosthesis
DeLaura-Verner knee prosthesis
De La Vega cannula
De La Vega lens pusher
delayed suture
Delbet-Reverdin needle
Delclos dilator
Delcom filling instrument
DeLee
    D. catheter
    D. cervical forceps
    D. cervix-holding forceps
    D. corner retractor
    D. curette
    D. dressing forceps
    D. fetal stethoscope
    D. forceps
    D. infant catheter
    D. laparotrachelotomy knife
    D. meconium trap aspirator
    D. obstetrical forceps
    D. ovum forceps
    D. pelvimeter
    D. retractor
    D. shuttle forceps
    D. speculum
    D. spoon tissue forceps
    D. stethoscope
    D. suction catheter
    D. tracheal catheter
    D. trap aspirator
    D. Universal retractor
    D. uterine forceps
    D. uterine-packing forceps
    D. vaginal retractor
    D. vesical retractor
DeLee-Breisky pelvimeter
DeLee-Hillis
    D.-H. fetal stethoscope
    D.-H. stethoscope
DeLee-Perce membrane perforator
DeLee-Simpson forceps
Delgado electrode
delicate
    d. forceps
    d. intervertebral disk
    rongeur
    d. needle holder
    d. operating scissors
    d. scissors
    d. thumb dressing forceps
Delima ethmoid cannula

Delitala
- D. T-nail nail
- D. T-pin

Delrin
- D. disk heart valve
- D. locking handle forceps

Delta
- D. dermatoscope
- D. external fixation frame
- D. pacemaker
- D. Recon nail
- D. Recon proximal drill guide

deluxe
- d. FIN extractor
- d. FIN pin
- d. FIN pin insertor
- d. head halter

demand pacemaker

demarcator
- flap d.

Demarest
- D. forceps
- D. septal forceps

DeMartel
- D. appendix forceps
- D. clamp
- D. conductor saw
- D. craniotome
- D. forceps
- D. neurosurgical scissors
- D. retractor
- D. scalp flap forceps
- D. scalp forceps
- D. self-retaining brain retractor
- D. suture
- D. trephine
- D. T-wire saw
- D. vascular clamp
- D. vascular scissors

DeMartel-Wolfson
- D.-W. anastomosis clamp
- D.-W. clamp
- D.-W. clamp holder
- D.-W. closing forceps
- D.-W. colon clamp
- D.-W. forceps
- D.-W. intestinal anastomotic clamp
- D.-W. intestinal clamp
- D.-W. intestinal-closing clamp
- D.-W. intestinal-closing forceps
- D.-W. intestinal-holding clamp
- D.-W. intestinal-holding forceps
- D.-W. stomach clamp

Demartel-Wolfson

Demel
- D. forceps
- D. wire clamp
- D. wire-tightening forceps
- D. wire-twisting forceps

à demeure catheter

demigauntlet
- d. bandage
- d. dressing

Demos tibial artery clamp

Demuth hip screw

Dench
- D. curette
- D. ear curette
- D. ear forceps
- D. ear knife
- D. forceps
- D. rongeur
- D. uterine curette

Denck esophagoscope

Denham pin

Denhardt-Dingman mouth gag

Denhardt mouth gag

Denholtz
- D. appliance
- D. muscle anchorage appliance

Denis Browne
- D. B. abdominal retractor blade
- D. B. adjustable-arm retractor
- D. B. cleft palate needle
- D. B. clubfoot splint
- D. B. forceps
- D. B. hip splint
- D. B. malleable copper retractor blade
- D. B. mastoid pediatric retractor blade
- D. B. mastoid retractor blade
- D. B. needle
- D. B. pediatric abdominal retractor blade

Denis Browne *(continued)*
  D. B. pediatric retractor
  D. B. pediatric retractor
    hook blade
  D. B. pediatric retractor
    oval sprocket frame
  D. B. retractor
  D. B. retractor hook blade
  D. B. retractor malleable
    wire hand
  D. B. retractor oval
    sprocket frame
  D. B. ring retractor
Denis Browne-Hendren pediatric
  retractor blade
Denker
  D. trocar
  D. tube
Denlan magnifying loupe
Dennis
  D. anastomotic clamp
  D. clamp
  D. forceps
  D. intestinal clamp
  D. intestinal forceps
Denniston dilator
Denpac porcelain powder
Densco
  D. bur
  D. dental handpiece
  D. ultrasonic scaler
Densilay alloy
Dentacolor R
Dentaflex wire
Dentaform band
dental
  d. appliance
  d. arch bar
  d. arch bar facial fracture
    appliance
  d. bur
  d. capsule
  d. cement
  d. dressing forceps
  d. drill
  d. excavator
  d. explorer
  d. forceps
  d. implant
  d. pick
  d. pliers
  d. retractor
  d. rongeur

  d. scaler
  d. wax
  d. wax carver
Dentalon R resin
dental stain remover (DSR)
dentate suture
Dentatus reamer
Dentemp filling material
Dentex acrylic
Dentifix denture repair kit
Dentlock denture adhesive
Dentloid impression material
Dentomat amalgamator
Dento-Spray oral irrigator
Dentsply
  D. alloy
  D. MVS evacuator
  D. resin
denture brush
Dentur-Eze
Dentus x-ray film
Denver
  D. connector
  D. hydrocephalus shunt
    system
  D. nasal splint
  D. pleuroperitoneal shunt
  D. reservoir
  D. shunt
  D. valve shunt
Deon hip prosthesis
De Paco implant
Depage-Janeway gastrostomy
DePalma
  D. hip prosthesis
  D. knife
  D. staple
DePaul tube
de Pezzer *(var. of* Pezzer)
depilatory dermal forceps
depolarizing electrode
depressor
  Andrews-Pynchon tongue d.
  Andrews tongue d.
  Balmer tongue d.
  Beatty tongue d.
  Blakesley tongue d.
  Boebinger tongue d.
  Bosworth tongue d.
  brain d.
  Braun uterine d.
  Braun vaginal d.
  Bruening tongue d.

Buchwald tongue d.
Chamberlain tongue d.
Colver-Dawson tongue d.
Cushing brain d.
Dorsey tongue d.
Dunn d.
Farlow tongue d.
Flynn scleral d.
Fraser d.
Granberry tongue d.
Hamilton tongue d.
Israel tongue d.
Jobson-Pynchon tongue d.
Kellogg tongue d.
Kocher d.
Layman tongue d.
Lewis tongue d.
metal tongue d.
Mullins tongue d.
O'Connor scleral d.
oral screw tongue d.
orbital d.
Pirquet tongue d.
Proetz tongue d.
Pynchon-Lillie tongue d.
Pynchon tongue d.
Schepens d.
Schepens scleral d.
Schocket scleral d.
scleral d.
Sims uterine d.
Spaide d.
Titus tongue d.
Tobold tongue d.
tongue d.
Urrets-Zavalia d.
Weder tongue d.
Weider d.
Wilder scleral d.
wood tongue d.
ZIV laryngeal d.
depth
d. check drill
d. electrode
d. gauge
Depthalon
D. monitoring electrode
DePuy
D. aeroplane splint
D. any-angle splint
D. awl
D. bolt
D. bone curette

D. cannulated reamer
D. coaptation splint
D. curette
D. drill
D. extractor
D. fracture brace
D. head halter
D. hip prosthesis with
Scuderi head
D. open-thimble splint
D. orthopaedic implant
D. pituitary rongeur
D. rainbow fracture frame
D. retractor
D. rocking leg splint
D. rolled Colles splint
D. screwdriver
D. splint
DePuy-Pott splint
DePuy-Weiss tonsillar needle
de Quervain (*See* Quervain)
Derf
D. eye needle holder
D. forceps
D. holder
D. needle holder
D. scissors
D. Vital needle holder
Derlacki
D. capsular knife
D. chisel
D. curette
D. duckbill elevator
D. ear curette
D. ear mobilizer
D. elevator
D. gouge
D. mobilizer
D. ossicle holder
Derlacki-Hough mobilizer
Derlacki-Juers head holder
Derlacki-Shambaugh chisel
Derma
D. Care dressing
D. surgical scrub soap
dermabrader
diamond d.
Iverson d.
sandpaper d.
Schumann-Schreus d.
dermacarrier
Tanner mesh graft d.
Dermacerator handpiece

Dermaclip
dermal
    d. curette
    d. elevator
    d. suture
    d. tension nonabsorbing
      suture
Dermalene
    D. polyethylene suture
    D. suture
Dermalon
    D. cuticular suture
    D. suture
Derma-Sil impression material
Dermastat
    Variable Spot D.
Dermastat II
Derma-Tattoo surgical tattoo
Dermatex compound
dermatologic ultraviolet light
dermatome
    air d.
    Bard-Parker d.
    Barker-Vacutome d.
    d. blade
    Brown d.
    Brown air d.
    Brown-Blair d.
    Castroviejo d.
    d. cement
    Concept d.
    Concept mesh grafter d.
    cordless d.
    Davol d.
    Davol-Simon d.
    DeSilva d.
    Down hand d.
    drum d.
    Duval d.
    Duval disposable d.
    Duval-Simon portable d.
    electric d.
    Goulian d.
    Hall d.
    Hood d.
    Hood manual d.
    Jordan-Day d.
    manual d.
    Meek-Wall d.
    Padgett d.
    Padgett-Hood d.
    Padgett manual d.
    Pitkin d.

    Reese d.
    Reese-Drum d.
    Reuse Expanda-graft d.
    Rica d.
    Schink d.
    Simon d.
    single-use d.
    SMIC d.
    Strempel d.
    Stryker d.
    Stryker Rolo-d.
    Tanner-Vandeput mesh d.
    Tanner-Vandeput mesh
      graft d.
    Weck d.
dermatoscope
    Delta d.
Dermicare hypoallergenic paper
** tape**
Dermicel
    D. dressing
    D. hypoallergenic cloth tape
    D. hypoallergenic knitted
      tape
    D. Montgomery strap
Dermiclear tape
Dermostat
    D. eye implant material
    D. implant
    D. orbital implant
Dermot-Pierce ball-tipped knife
DeRoaldes speculum
derotation brace
Derra
    D. anastomosis clamp
    D. aortic clamp
    D. cardiac valve dilator
    D. cardiovascular forceps
    D. clamp
    D. commissurotomy knife
    D. dilator
    D. forceps
    D. guillotine knife
    D. urethral forceps
    D. valvulotome
    D. vena caval clamp
    D. vestibular clamp
Derra-Cooley forceps
D'Errico
    D. brain spatula
    D. bur
    D. dressing forceps
    D. drill

D. enlarging bur
D. forceps
D. hypophyseal forceps
D. laminar chisel
D. laminar knife
D. laminectomy chisel
D. nerve retractor
D. nerve root retractor
D. perforating bur
D. perforating drill
D. perforator
D. periosteal elevator
D. skull trephine
D. tissue forceps
D. trephine
D. ventricular needle
D'Errico-Adson retractor
Desault
D. apparatus
D. bandage
D. dressing
Descemet punch
Deschamps
D. carrier
D. compressor
D. ligature carrier
D. ligature needle
D. needle
Deschamps-Navratil
D.-N. ligature needle
D.-N. needle
Deseigneux dilator
Deseret
D. angiocatheter
D. catheter
D. flow-directed thermodilution catheter
D. sump drain
desiccation-fulguration needle
desiccation needle
de Signeux dilator
Desilets catheter
Desilets-Hoffman
D.-H. catheter
D.-H. introducer
D.-H. micropunch introducer
D.-H. pacemaker introducer
DeSilva dermatome
Desjardins
D. dilator
D. forceps

D. gall duct probe
D. gall duct scoop
D. gallstone forceps
D. gallstone probe
D. gallstone scoop
D. kidney pedicle forceps
D. probe
Desmarres
D. cardiovascular retractor
D. chalazion forceps
D. clamp
D. corneal dissector
D. dissector
D. eye dissector
D. eye needle
D. eye speculum
D. forceps
D. iris knife
D. lid clamp
D. lid forceps
D. lid retractor
D. lid speculum
D. needle
D. paracentesis knife
D. paracentesis needle
D. retractor
D. scarifier
D. vein retractor
destructive obstetrical hook
detachable silicone balloon (DSB)
DeTakats-McKenzie
D.-M. brain clip-applying forceps
D.-M. clip-applying forceps
D.-M. forceps
detector
Clinitemp fever d.
Doplette Doppler blood flow d.
Doptone fetal pulse d.
Pendoppler ultrasonic fetal heart d.
pocket Doppler blood flow d.
detergent
Weck liquid d.
Weck-Wash d.
Detroit Receiving Hospital razor
Deucher abdominal retractor
Deune knee prosthesis
Deutschman cataract knife
Devers gall bladder tube

device

abdominal aortic counterpulsation d.
abdominal left ventricular assist d. (ALVAD)
ACMI ulcer-measuring d.
Agee 4-pin fixation d.
AICD d.
anti-siphon d.
AOR check traction d.
Aqua-Purator suction d.
Arrow-Clarke thoracentesis d.
atherectomy d.
automatic stapling d.
automatic suction d.
Auto Suture d.
Auto Suture endoscopic suction-irrigation d.
balanced traction d.
Barton traction d.
biofeedback d.
biofeedback galvanic skin response d.
Biosearch anal biofeedback d.
BIVAD centrifugal left and right ventricular assist d.
biventricular assist d. (BVAD)
blade plate fixation d.
Bosker TMI mandibular fixation d.
Bovie suction d.
Buck traction d.
Buretrol d.
Calandruccio triangular compression d.
Cameco syringe pistol aspiration d.
cardiac automatic resuscitative d. (CARD)
Cardiomemo d.
cassette cup collecting d.
CastAlert d.
Cath-Lok catheter locking d.
Cavi-Jet dental prophylaxis d.
celltrifuge d.
Chinese fingerstraps traction d.
circular stapling d.
compression d.
Concept PuddleVac floor suction d.
conductive d.
continuous passive motion d.
Copper-7 intrauterine d., Cu-7 intrauterine d.
CPM d.
Cricket stapling d.
cutting d.
CVIS imaging d.
Dalkon shield intrauterine d.
Dinamap automated blood pressure d.
distal targeting d.
Doppler d.
Doppler sound d.
double-headed P190 stapling d.
EEA stapling d.
emergency infusion d. (EID)
Erectek external erection d.
Erlangen magnetic colostomy d.
exterior pelvic d.
external vascular compression d.
EZ-Trac orthopaedic suspension d.
Finn chamber patch test d.
fixation d.
flushing d.
Fox internal fixation d.
galvanic skin response d.
Gerster traction d.
GIA stapling d.
Grass pressure-recording d.
G-suit d.
Hall intrauterine d.
halo femoral traction d.
halo hoop d.
halo traction d.
Hare splint d.
Hare traction d.
Hershey left ventricular assist d.
Heyer-Schulte d.
Hoffmann external fixation d.
Hoffmann traction d.
Hollister circumcision d.
ILA stapling d.

IMED infusion d.
infusion d.
input d.
Inspiron d.
insufflation d.
internal fixation d.
intra-aortic balloon assist d.
intracranial pressure
 monitoring d.
intramedullary d.
intramedullary fixation d.
intrauterine d. (IUD)
intrauterine contraceptive d.
 (IUCD)
Kaufman incontinence d.
Keller cephalometric d.
Kendrick extrication d.
 (KED)
Kennedy ligament
 augmentation d.
kinetic continuous passive
 motion d.
kinetic CPM d.
Laparomed cholangiogram d.
Laparomed suture-applier d.
left uterine displacement d.
 (LUD)
left ventricular assist d.
 (LVAD)
leg-holding d.
Lewis intramedullary d.
Lewis suspension d.
ligament augmentation d.
 (LAD)
linear stapling d.
Lippes loop intrauterine d.
Loewi suspension d.
LUD d.
Margulies intrauterine d.
Mazlin intrauterine d.
McAtee compression
 screw d.
McAtee olecranon d.
McCleery-Miller locking d.
mechanical d.
Medi-Breather IPPB d.
MediPort implanted
 vascular d.
metallic fixation d.
MicroTymp
 tympanometric d.
Microvasive biliary d.

Mosher Life Saver
 antichoke suction d.
Multiclip disposable ligating
 clip d.
Nemdi tweezer epilation d.
Neuropath biofeedback d.
Neurotone biofeedback d.
Nimbus Hemopump cardiac
 assist d.
Nite Train-R enuresis
 conditioning d.
Novacor left ventricular
 assist d.
Orthofix external fixation d.
Ortholav irrigation and
 suction d.
orthotic d.
output d.
ParaGard intrauterine d.
Pierce-Donachy ventricular
 assist d.
Pisces d.
Plastibell circumcision d.
Plastizote orthotic d.
PPT orthotic d.
Premium CEEA circular
 stapling d.
Progestasert intrauterine d.
prone cranial support d.
 (PCSD)
prosthetic d.
ProTrac cruciate
 reconstruction
 measurement d.
pulsatile assist d.
Resnick Tone Emitter I
 intraoral electrolarynx d.
retaining d.
Richards compression d.
right ventricular assist d.
Roger Anderson external
 skeletal fixation d.
Rosen incontinence d.
rotation d.
rotational atherectomy d.
Rudolf-Buck suturing d.
Russell traction d.
RVAD centrifugal right
 ventricular assist d.
Saf-T-Coil intrauterine d.
Sengstaken-Blakemore d.
SGIA stapling d.

device *(continued)*
    Shiley saphenous vein
       irrigation and
       pressurization d.
    Simpson directional
       coronary atherectomy d.
    Simpson PET balloon
       atherectomy d.
    SMI Surgi-Med CPM d.'s
    Smoke Controller d.
    Softepil tweezer epilation d.
    Soluset d.
    Sorbothane orthotic d.
    Spencer incontinence d.
    Spenco orthotic d.
    Spetzler MacroVac surgical
       suction d.
    Spitz-Holter flushing d.
    stapling d.
    Statak soft tissue
       attachment d.
    static topical occlusive
       hemostatic pressure d.
    stereotaxic d.
    stoma-measuring d.
    Stone clamp-locking d.
    stone-locking d.
    suction d.
    Symbion pneumatic
       assist d.
    Tatum Tee intrauterine d.
    temperature and galvanic
       skin response
       biofeedback d.
    Tenderfoot incision-
       making d.
    Thoratec biventricular
       assist d.
    Thoratec right ventricular
       assist d.
    Thoratec ventricular
       assist d.
    Throat-E-Vac suction d.
    Tibbs semi-automatic
       suturing d.
    traction d.
    Travenol infusor d.
    Universal joint d.
    Urosheath incontinence d.
    Vacuconstrictor erection d.
    vacuum erection d. (VED)
    vacuum tumescence-
       constrictor d.

    vascular/venous access d.
       (VAD)
    Venodyne pneumatic
       inflation d.
    ventricular assist d. (VAD)
    Versafix external fracture
       fixation d.
    Vidal d.
    Vidal-Ardrey modified
       Hoffman d.
    Wagner leg-lengthening d.
    Wallach freezer
       cryosurgical d.
    Wallach pencil
       cryosurgical d.
    wet-field d.
    Wizard disposable
       inflation d.
    Wolvek fixation d.
    Wright Care-TENS d.
    Zilkie d.
Devices, Ltd. pacemaker
DeVilbiss
    D. atomizer
    D. cranial forceps
    D. cranial rongeur
    D. eye irrigator
    D. forceps
    D. Mini-Dop fetal monitor
    D. nebulizer
    D. OB-Dop fetal monitor
    D. powder blower
    D. Pulmo-Aide nebulizer
       with portable air
       compressor
    D. rongeur
    D. rongeur forceps
    D. skull trephine
    D. suction pump
    D. suction tube
    D. syringe
    D. Vacu-Aide aspirator
    D. vaginal speculum
DeVilbiss-Stacy speculum
Devine-Millard-Aufricht retractor
**Devine-Millard-Frazier fiberoptic
    suction tube**
Devonshire
    D. catheter
    D. knife
    D. needle
    D. roller

Devonshire-Mack
    D.-M. cannula
    D.-M. catheter
    D.-M. clamp
    D.-M. stop
Dewald halo spinal appliance
Dewar
    D. elevator
    D. flask
DeWecker
    D. cannula
    D. eye implant
    D. forceps
    D. iris scissors
    D. scissors
    D. syringe cannula
DeWecker-Pritikin iris scissors
DeWeese
    D. axis traction forceps
    D. axis traction obstetrical
      forceps
    D. caval catheter
    D. clamp
    D. vena caval clamp
DeWeese-Hunter clip
Dewey
    D. forceps
    D. obstetrical forceps
DeWitt-Stetten colostomy spur
  crusher
Dexon
    D. absorbable synthetic
      polyglycolic acid suture
    D. II suture
    D. Plus suture
    D. polyglycolic acid mesh
    D. subcuticular suture
    D. suture
dextranomer
    d. paste
Deyerle
    D. apparatus
    D. bone graft plate
    D. component
    D. drill
    D. II plate
    D. pin
    D. plate
    D. punch
    D. screw
DG77 jet injector
DG Softgut suture
D&G suture

Diabeticorum dressing
Diaflex
    D. cytology brush
    D. dilator
    D. grasping forceps
    D. retrieval loop
    D. ureteral dilatation
      catheter
diagnostic
    d. catheter
    d. curette
    d. tube
    d. tympanometer
    d. ultrasound linear scanner
Diakart hemoperfusion cartridge
Diaket root canal cement
dialer
    IOL d.
    irrigating d.
Dialix dialyzer
Dialom bur
dial-type ophthalmodynamometer
dialysate
    d. bag
    d. preparation module
    d. tubing
dialysis catheter
dialyzer
    Asahi hollow fiber d.
    capillary flow d.
    C-Dak d.
    DAS single pass d.
    Dialix d.
    Eri-Flo d.
    Gambro-Lundia d.
    Gambro-Lundia coil d.
    Hemoclear d.
    hollow fiber capillary d.
    Idecap d.
    Nephross d.
    parallel flow d.
    Sorbiclear d.
    Terumo-Clirans d.
    twin coil d.
diameter head
diamond
    d. barrel bur
    d. blade
    d. bur
    d. dermabrader
    d. drill
    d. grip needle holder
    d. high-speed drill

diamond *(continued)*
> d. inlay bone graft
> d. knife
> d. nail
> d. pin cutter
> d. rasp
> d. wire cutter

diamond-dust bur
diamond-edge scissors
Diamond-Lite cardiovascular instrument
diamond-point suture needle
diaphanoscope
> Binner d.

diaphragm
> d. inserter
> Ortho All-Flex d.
> d. pessary
> Ramses d.
> wide seal d.

Dia pump aspirator
diathermic
> d. electrode
> d. eye electrode
> d. forceps
> d. needle
> d. retinal electrode

diathermy
> d. cord
> d. electrode
> d. forceps
> d. scissors
> underwater d.
> d. unit

diatrizoate contrast material
Dick
> D. bronchus clamp
> D. cardiac valve dilator
> D. dilator
> D. pressure clamp
> D. valve dilator

die
> pin deburring d.
> Schuknecht-Paparella wire-bending d.
> Schuknecht wire-bending d.
> wire bending d.

Diederich empyema trocar
Dieffenbach
> D. bulldog clamp
> D. clamp
> D. forceps
> D. scalpel

> D. serrefine
> D. tenotome

Dienco flowmeter
Diener forceps
Dieter
> D. forceps
> D. malleus forceps
> D. nipper

Dieter-House nipper
Diethrich
> D. aortic clamp
> D. bulldog clamp
> D. circumflex artery scissors
> D. clamp
> D. coronary artery bypass kit
> D. coronary artery scissors
> D. graft clamp
> D. kit
> D. microcoronary bulldog clamp
> D. right-angled hemostatic forceps
> D. scissors
> D. shunt clamp
> D. valve scissors

Diethrich-Hegemann scissors
Diethrich-Jackson femoral graft tunneler
Dieulafoy aspirator
Difei glasses
Digiflex cannula
digital goniometer
digitalized equipment
Digitimer pattern reversal stimulator
Digitrace home computer
Digitron dialysis chair scale
Dilamezinsert
> D. dilator
> D. penile prosthesis

Dilapan hygroscopic cervical dilator
Dilaprobe
> D. dilator
> irrigating D.
> Mixter common duct D.

dilatable bougie
dilating
> d. bougie
> d. bulb
> d. catheter
> d. forceps

d. pressure balloon catheter
d. probe
dilation, dilatation
d. balloon catheter
d. catheter
dilation-tracheobronchoscope
Edens d.-t.
dilator
achalasia d.
Alm d.
Ambler d.
American dilation system d.
American endoscopy d.
American endoscopy
  esophageal d.
American Hanks uterine d.
Amplatz d.
anal d.
aortic d.
argon vessel d.
Arnott d.
Atlee d.
Atlee uterine d.
Avenida d.
Avenida-Torres d.
Backhaus d.
Bailey d.
Bakes d.
Bakes bile duct d.
Bakes common bile duct d.
Bakes common duct d.
Bakes duct d.
Bakes gall duct d.
Bakes-Pearce d.
Bard d.
Bard urethral d.
Barnes d.
Barnes cervical d.
Barnes common duct d.
Beardsley d.
Beardsley aortic d.
Béniqué d.
Bennett common duct d.
Berens d.
Berens punctum d.
biliary balloon d.
biliary duct d.
Black-Wylie d.
Black-Wylie obstetric d.
bladder d.
Bonney cervical d.
Bossi d.
Bossi cervical d.

bougie d.
Bowman d.
Bowman lacrimal d.
Bozeman d.
Braasch ureteral d.
Bransford-Lewis d.
Bransford-Lewis ureteral d.
Brock d.
Brock cardiac d.
bronchial d.
Brown-Buerger d.
Brown-McHardy d.
Brown-McHardy air-filled
  pneumatic d.
Brown-McHardy
  pneumatic d.
Broyles d.
Broyles esophageal d.
canaliculus d.
cardiac d.
cardiac valve d.
cardioesophageal junction d.
cardiospasm d.
Castroviejo d.
Castroviejo double-end d.
Castroviejo double-end
  lacrimal d.
Castroviejo lacrimal d.
Catalano d.
d. catheter
catheter-d.
Celestin graduated d.
cervical d.
child rectal d.
Clark d.
Clark common duct d.
Clerf d.
common bile duct d.
common duct d.
Cook-Amplatz d.
Cooley d.
Cooley coronary d.
Cooley pediatric d.
Cooley valve d.
Cooley vascular d.
Cordis d.
coronary d.
Councill d.
Councill ureteral d.
Creevy d.
Creevy urethral d.
Crump d.
Crump-Himmelstein d.

dilator *(continued)*
Crump vessel d.
Dagger d.
DeBakey-Cooley d.
DeBakey-Cooley valve d.
DeBakey vascular d.
Delaborde d.
Delaborde tracheal d.
Delaborde-Trousseau
 tracheal d.
Delclos d.
Denniston d.
Derra d.
Derra cardiac valve d.
Deseigneux d.
de Signeux d.
Desjardins d.
Diaflex d.
Dick d.
Dick cardiac valve d.
Dick valve d.
Dilamezinsert d.
Dilapan hygroscopic
 cervical d.
Dilaprobe d.
disposable cervical d.
Dittel d.
Dittel uterine d.
Dittman d.
Dittsburg d.
Dotter d.
double-ended d.
Dourmashkin d.
duct d.
Eder-Puestow d.
Eder-Puestow esophageal d.
Einhorn d.
Einhorn esophageal d.
Encapsulon vessel d.
esophageal d.
esophagospasm d.
expandable cervical d.
expansile d.
Falope-ring d.
Feldbausch d.
female catheter-d.
Fenton d.
Fenton uterine d.
Ferris d.
Ferris biliary duct d.
Ferris filiform d.
fixed cervical d.
French d.

French Hanks uterine d.
French lacrimal d.
French-McRea d.
Frommer d.
frontal sinus d.
Galezowski d.
Galezowski lacrimal d.
gall duct d.
gallstone d.
Garrett d.
Garrett vascular d.
Gerbode d.
Gerbode mitral d.
Gerbode mitral
 valvulotomy d.
Gerbode valve d.
Gillquist-Oretorp-Stille d.
Glover d.
Glover modification of
 Brock aortic d.
Godelo d.
Gohrbrand d.
Gohrbrand cardiac d.
Goodell d.
Goodell uterine d.
Gouley d.
graduated Garrett d.
grooved director d.
Grüntzig balloon d.
Guggenheim-Gergoiye d.
Guyon d.
Hank-Bradley uterine d.
Hank uterine d.
Hayman d.
Hearst d.
Heath d.
Heath punctum d.
Hegar d.
Hegar-Goodell d.
Hegar rectal d.
Hegar uterine d.
Henley d.
Henning d.
Henning cardia d.
Hiebert vascular d.
Hohn vessel d.
hopkins d.
Hosford d.
Hosford double-ended
 lacrimal d.
Hosford eye d.
Hosford lacrimal d.
Hurst d.

Hurst bullet-tip d.
Hurst esophageal d.
Hurst-Maloney d.
Hurst mercury d.
Hurst mercury-filled d.
Hurst-Tucker pneumatic d.
Hurtig d.
hydrostatic d.
Iglesias d.
incision d.
infant d.
Ivinsco cervical d.
Jackson d.
Jackson bronchial d.
Jackson esophageal d.
Jackson-Mosher d.
Jackson-Mosher
  cardiospasm d.
Jackson-Plummer d.
Jackson tracheal d.
Jackson-Trousseau d.
Jewett uterine d.
Johnston d.
Johnston infant d.
Jolly d.
Jolly uterine d.
Jones d.
Jones canaliculus d.
Jones lacrimal
  canaliculus d.
Jones punctum d.
Jordan d.
Jordan wire loop d.
Kahn d.
Kahn uterine d.
Kearns d.
Kearns bladder d.
Kelly d.
Kelly orifice d.
Kelly sphincter d.
Kelly uterine d.
Keymed d.
Kleegman d.
Kohlman d.
Kohlman urethral d.
K-Pratt d.
Krol esophageal d.
Krol-Koski tracheal d.
Kron d.
Kron bile duct d.
Kron gallbladder d.
Kron gall duct d.
Laborde d.

Laborde tracheal d.
lacrimal d.
lacrimal canaliculus d.
laminaria cervical d.
laminaria seaweed
  obstetrical d.
Landau d.
laryngeal d.
Laufe cervical d.
Leader-Kohlman d.
LeFort d.
Lucchese mitral valve d.
Mahoney d.
Mahorner d.
Maloney d.
Maloney esophageal d.
Maloney mercury-filled d.
Maloney mercury-filled
  esophageal d.
Maloney tapered-tip d.
mandrin d.
Mantz d.
Mantz rectal d.
Marax d.
McCrae d.
meatal d.
Medi-Tech fascial d.
mercury-filled d.
mercury-weighted d.
Miller d.
mitral valve d.
Mixter d.
Mixter common duct
  Dilaprobe d.
Mixter irrigating
  Dilaprobe d.
Moersch cardiospasm d.
Muldoon d.
Muldoon lacrimal d.
Murphy d.
Murphy common duct d.
myocardial d.
nasal d.
Nettleship d.
Nettleship canaliculus d.
Nettleship-Wilder d.
Nettleship-Wilder lacrimal d.
olive-tipped d.
Optilume prostate
  balloon d.
Otis bougie à boule d.
Ottenheimer d.

dilator *(continued)*
Ottenheimer common
   duct d.
Outerbridge uterine d.
Palmer d.
Palmer uterine d.
Parsonnet d.
Patton d.
Patton esophageal d.
pediatric d.
pediatric rectal d.
Phillips d.
Plummer d.
Plummer esophageal d.
Plummer-Vinson d.
Plummer-Vinson
   esophageal d.
Plummer water-filled
   pneumatic esophageal d.
pneumatic d.
pneumatic balloon d.
pneumostatic d.
Potts d.
Potts expansile d.
Potts-Riker d.
Pratt d.
Pratt rectal d.
Pratt uterine d.
d. probe
probe d.
progressive d.'s
Puestow d.
punctum d.
pyloric stenosis d.
Ramstedt d.
Ramstedt pyloric stenosis d.
Ravich d.
Ravich ureteral d.
rectal d.
Reich-Nechtow d.
Richards-Moeller pneumatic
   air-filled d.
Rider-Moeller cardia d.
Rider-Moeller pneumatic d.
Rigiflex d.
Rigiflex balloon d.
Ritter d.
Ritter meatal d.
Roland d.
Rolf d.
Rolf punctum d.
Royal Hospital d.
Rubbs aortic d.

Ruedemann lacrimal d.
Russell d.
Russell hydrostatic d.
Saint Mark d.
Savary d.
Savary esophageal d.
Savary-Gilliard d.
Savary-Gilliard esophageal d.
Savary tapered
   thermoplastic d.
Scanlan vessel d.
sheath-d.
Simpson lacrimal d.
Simpson uterine d.
Sims d.
Sims uterine d.
Sinexon d.
sinus d.
Sippy d.
Sippy esophageal d.
Smedberg d.
sphincter d.
Spielberg d.
stapes d.
Starck d.
Starlinger d.
Starlinger uterine d.
Steele d.
Steele bronchial d.
Stille uterine d.
Stucker bile duct d.
Stucker gall duct d.
Szulc vascular d.
Taylor pulmonary d.
Theobald lacrimal d.
through-the-scope d.
tracheal d.
transventricular d.
Trousseau d.
Trousseau-Jackson d.
Trousseau-Jackson
   esophageal d.
Trousseau-Jackson
   tracheal d.
Trousseau tracheal d.
TTS d.
Tubbs d.
Tubbs aortic d.
Tubbs mitral valve d.
Tubbs two-bladed d.
Tucker d.
Tucker cardiospasm d.
Turner d.

two-bladed d.
ureteral d.
ureteral stone d.
urethral d.
urethral female d.
urethral male d.
urethral male follower d.
urethral meatus d.
uterine d.
vaginal d.
valve d.
Van Buren d.
Vantec d.
vascular d.
vein d.
vessel d.
VPI urethral meatal d.
Wales d.
Wales rectal d.
Walther d.
Walther urethral d.
Whylie uterine d.
Wilder d.
Wilder lacrimal d.
Williams d.
Williams lacrimal d.
wire loop d.
wire loop stapes d.
Wise d.
Wylie d.
Wylie uterine d.
Young d.
Young pediatric rectal d.
Young rectal d.
Young vaginal d.
Ziegler d.
Ziegler double-ended
  lacrimal d.
Ziegler lacrimal d.
Zipser meatal d.
dilator-catheter
  Walther d.-c.
Dilner-Doughty mouth gag
dilution container
Di-Main retractor
Dimension hip system
Dimitry
  D. chalazion trephine
  D. dacryocystorhinostomy
    trephine
  D. erysiphake
Dimitry-Bell erysiphake
Dimitry-Thomas erysiphake

**Dinamap automated blood pressure
  device**
Dingman
  D. bone-holding forceps
  D. breast dissector
  D. cartilage clamp
  D. clamp
  D. flexible retractor
  D. Flexsteel retractor
  D. forceps
  D. malleable passing needle
  D. mouth gag
  D. mouth gag frame
  D. mouth gag tongue
    depressor blade
  D. needle
  D. osteotome
  D. otoabrader
  D. otoplasty cartilage
    abrader
  D. passing needle
  D. periosteal elevator
  D. retractor
  D. wire passer
  D. zygoma elevator
  D. zygoma hook retractor
  D. zygomatic hook
Dingman-Millard mouth gag
Dingman-Pollock septal displacer
Dingman-Senn retractor
Dintenfass-Chapman knife
Dintenfass ear knife
Diode endolaser
diopter lens
diphosphonate
  methylene d. (MDP)
diploscope
Diplos pacemaker
dipstick
  Fyodorov d.
  Kelman d.
  Knolle d.
direct
  d. current bone growth
    stimulator (DCBGS)
  d. forward-vision telescope
  d. laryngoscope
  d. radial suture
Directa crown
Director
  Laser Fiber D.
director
  Brodi d.

director *(continued)*
    Doyen d.
    Dr. Quickert d.
    Durnin angled d.
    grooved d.
    Kocher goiter d.
    Kocher grooved d.
    Koenig grooved d.
    Larry rectal d.
    Leksell grooved d.
    ligature d.
    Ormco ligature d.
    Payr grooved d.
    plain-end grooved d.
    Pratt rectal d.
    probe-ended grooved d.
    Quickert grooved d.
    Stiwer grooved d.
    Toennis d.
direct-vision
    d.-v. adenotome
    d.-v. telescope
disarticulation chisel
disc *(var. of* disk)
discectomy *(var. of* diskectomy)
Dischler rectoscopic suction insert
discission
    d. blade
    d. knife
    d. needle
disclosant
    Butler Red-Cote plaque d.
discriminator
    Sweet two-point d.
    two-point d.
disimpaction forceps
disinfector
    Kestrel d.
disintegrator
    SD-1 stone d.
disk, disc
    d. curette
    d. electrode
    d. endoscope
    d. forceps
    Horico d.
    d. lens intraocular lens
    Moore d.
    Moran-Karaya d.
Diskard head halter
diskectomy, discectomy
    d. forceps

diskographic needle
dislodger
    Cook helical stone d.
    Councill stone d.
    Creevy calyx d.
    Creevy calyx stone d.
    Creevy stone d.
    Davis loop stone d.
    Davis stone d.
    Dormia d.
    Dormia stone d.
    Dormia ureteral stone d.
    Ellik loop stone d.
    Ellik stone d.
    filiform stone d.
    Gibson stone d.
    Howard-Flaherty spiral d.
    Howard-Flaherty spiral
      stone d.
    Howard spiral d.
    Howard spiral stone d.
    Howard stone d.
    Jimmy d.
    Johnson stone d.
    Levant d.
    Levant stone d.
    Mitchell ureteral stone d.
    Morton d.
    Morton stone d.
    Ortved stone d.
    Pfister-Schwartz stone d.
    Porges stone d.
    Robinson d.
    Robinson stone d.
    spiral stone d.
    stone d.
    Storz stone d.
    Tessier d.
    ureteral basket stone d.
    ureteral stone d.
    woven-loop d.
    woven-loop stone d.
    woven loop stone d.
    Wullen d.
    Wullen stone d.
    Zeiss stone d.
    Zeiss ureteral stone d.
dispenser
    Jet Vac cement d.
dispersing electrode
displacer
    air uterine d.

Dingman-Pollock septal d.
Pollock-Dingman septal d.
disposable
d. airway
d. aspiration needle
d. biopsy needle
d. catheter
d. cervical dilator
d. cystotome cannula
d. electrode
d. electrode pad
d. electrosurgical electrode
d. forceps
d. head halter
d. injection needle
d. intraluminal stapler
d. iris retractor
d. laryngoscope
d. muscle biopsy clamp
d. ocutome
d. probe
d. retractor
d. scalpel
d. sigmoidoscope
d. stone basket
d. surgical electrode
d. suturing needle
d. trephine
d. TUR drape
d. vacuum curette
d. Yankauer aspirating tube
d. Yankauer suction tube
Disposa-Loops
Disposashield
Dispos-A-Ture single-use surgical needle
Disposiquet disposable tourniquet
Disposo-Scope anoscope
Disposo-Spec disposable speculum
Dissect
Endo D.
dissecting
d. chisel
d. clamp
d. forceps
d. hook
d. probe
d. scissors
dissection
d. forceps
d. knife
d. probe

dissector
Adson d.
Allerdyce d.
Allis d.
Allis dry d.
aneurysm neck d.
Angell-James d.
Angell-James angled d.
Aspiradeps d.
aspirating d.
attic d.
Aufranc d.
Austin d.
Austin attic d.
Ball d.
Barraquer corneal d.
Beaver d.
blunt d.
Brunner d.
Brunner goiter d.
bunion d.
Butte d.
Carpenter d.
Castroviejo d.
Castroviejo corneal d.
Cavitron d.
Cherry Secto d.
Cheyne d.
Cheyne dry d.
CISA d.
Codman's Rhoton d.
Collin d.
Collin pleural d.
Colver d.
Colver tonsillar d.
corneal d.
corneal knife d.
Cottonoid d.
Crabtree d.
Crabtree attic d.
Creed d.
Crile d.
Crile gasserian ganglion d.
Davis d.
Desmarres d.
Desmarres corneal d.
Desmarres eye d.
Dingman breast d.
double-ended d.
Doyen rib d.
ear d.
Effler double-ended d.
Effler-Groves d.

dissector *(continued)*
    endarterectomy d.
    facial nerve d.
    Fager pituitary d.
    Falcao d.
    Falcao suction d.
    Feild suction d.
    Fischer d.
    Fisher tonsillar d.
    flap knife d.
    Freer d.
    Freer dural d.
    Freer elevator-d.
    Freer-Sachs d.
    Gannetta d.
    goiter d.
    Gorney d.
    Green d.
    Green corneal d.
    Green eye d.
    Haines arachnoid d.
    Hajek-Ballenger d.
    Hajek-Ballenger septal d.
    Hamrick suction d.
    Hardy d.
    Hardy pituitary d.
    Harris d.
    Hartmann tonsillar d.
    Heath d.
    Heath trephine flap d.
    Henke tonsillar d.
    Herczel d.
    Hitselberger-McElveen
      neural d.
    Holinger laryngeal d.
    Hood d.
    House d.
    House-Crabtree d.
    House-Urban d.
    House-Urban rotary d.
    House-Urban vacuum
      rotary d.
    Hunt d.
    Hunt arachnoid d.
    Hurd d.
    Hurd-Morrison d.
    Hurd tonsillar d.
    Hurd-Weder d.
    Hurd-Weder tonsillar d.
    hydrostatic d.
    Israel d.
    Israel tonsillar d.
    Jackson-Pratt d.

    Jannetta d.
    Jannetta aneurysm neck d.
    Jazbi d.
    Jazbi suction tonsillar d.
    Jazbi tonsillar d.
    Jimmy d.
    joker d.
    Judet d.
    Kennerdell-Maroon d.
    Killian d.
    King-Hurd d.
    King-Hurd tonsillar d.
    Kistner d.
    Kitner d.
    Kitner blunt d.
    Kleinert-Kutz d.
    knife d.
    Kocher d.
    Kocher goiter d.
    Kocher periosteal d.
    Kurze d.
    Kuttner d.
    laminar d.
    Lane d.
    Lang d.
    laryngeal d.
    Lemmon intimal d.
    Lewin d.
    Lewin bunion d.
    Lewin sesamoidectomy d.
    Logan d.
    Lopez-Reinke tonsillar d.
    Lothrop d.
    Lynch d.
    Lynch blunt d.
    Lynch laryngeal d.
    Lynch tonsillar d.
    MacAusland d.
    MacDonald d.
    Madden d.
    Malis d.
    Manhattan Eye and Ear
      corneal d.
    Marino rotatable
      transsphenoidal round d.
    Marino rotatable
      transsphenoidal spatula d.
    Maroon-Jannetta d.
    Martinex knife-d.
    Martinez double-ended
      corneal d.
    Mason tonsil suction d.
    McCabe facial nerve d.

McCabe flap knife d.
McElveen-Hitselberger
  neural d.
McWhinnie d.
McWhinnie tonsillar d.
microsurgical d.
Milette-Tyding d.
Miller tonsillar d.
Milligan d.
Milligan double-ended d.
Molt d.
Moorehead d.
Morrison-Hurd d.
Morrison-Hurd tonsillar d.
Mulligan d.
nasal d.
Neivert d.
nerve d.
nerve root laminectomy d.
neurosurgical d.
Oldberg d.
Olivecrona-Stille d.
Paton corneal d.
peanut d.
Peanut Secto d.
Penfield d.
Pennington septal d.
Pierce d.
Pierce submucous d.
pleural d.
Potts d.
prostatic d.
Raney d.
Rhode Island d.
Rhode Island Secto d.
Rhoton d.
Rhoton ball d.
Rhoton round d.
Rhoton spatula d.
Rienhoff d.
Rochester d.
Rochester laminar d.
Roger d.
Roger submucous d.
Rosebud d.
Rosen d.
rotary d.
rotatable transsphenoidal
  round d.
rotatable transsphenoidal
  spatula d.
round d.
Ruddy d.

Sachs-Freer d.
Schmieden-Taylor d.
Secto d.
Sens d.
septal d.
sesamoidectomy d.
Sheldon-Pudenz d.
Silverstein arachnoid d.
Silverstein auditory canal d.
Sloan d.
Sloan goiter flap d.
Smith d.
Smith tonsillar d.
Smithwick d.
Smithwick nerve d.
spatula d.
Spetzler d.
sponge d.
spud d.
square-tipped arterial d.
Stallard d.
Stallard blunt d.
Stiwer d.
Stiwer tendon d.
Stolte d.
Stolte tonsillar d.
submammary d.
submucous d.
suction d.
suction tonsillar d.
surgical d.
tissue d.
Toennis d.
Toennis-Adson d.
tonsillar d.
tonsil-suction d.
Touma d.
triangle Secto d.
Troutman corneal d.
Troutman eye d.
Troutman wave edge
  corneal d.
Truszkowski dural d.
ultrasonic d.
vascular d.
Walker d.
Walker suction tonsillar d.
Walker tonsillar d.
Walker tonsil-suction d.
Wangensteen d.
Watson-Cheyne d.
Watson-Cheyne dry d.
Weder d.

dissector *(continued)*
    West blunt d.
    West hand d.
    West plastic d.
    Wieder tonsillar d.
    Woodson double-ended d.
    Wynne-Evans tonsillar d.
    Yasargil d.
    Yoshida d.
    Yoshida aspirating
      tonsillar d.
    Yoshida tonsillar d.
    Young d.
    Young urological d.
dissector-pick
    Crabtree-House d.-p.
Distaflex dental attachment
distal
    d. femoral cutting guide
    d. slit valve catheter
    d. targeting device
distending obturator
distraction
    d. clamp
    d. hook
distractor
    femoral d.
    hook d.
Dittel
    D. dilating bougie
    D. dilator
    D. urethral bougie
    D. urethral sound
    D. uterine dilator
    D. uterine sound
Dittman dilator
Dittrich plug
Dittsburg dilator
divergent outlet forceps
diversion
    Laparostat with fiber d.
    d. stent
diverticuloscope
    Holinger-Benjamin laser d.
Diviplast impression material
Dix
    D. double-ended instrument
    D. eye spud
    D. foreign body spud
    D. gouge
    D. needle

    D. spud
    D. spud probe
Dixey spatula
Dixon
    D. blade
    D. center blade
    D. center-blade retractor
    D. flamingo forceps
Dixon-Lovelace
    D.-L. forceps
    D.-L. hemostatic forceps
Dixon-Thomas-Smith
    D.-T.-S. clamp
    D.-T.-S. colonic clamp
    D.-T.-S. intestinal clamp
Dixon-Thorpe
    D.-T. forceps
    D.-T. vitreous foreign body
      forceps
DL
  double-lumen
DLC
  double-lumen catheter
DLP
    DLP aortic root cannula
    DLP cardioplegic catheter
    DLP cardioplegic needle
DMV II contact lens remover
Doane knee retractor
Dobbhoff biliary stent
Dobbie-Trout
    D.-T. bulldog clamp
    D.-T. clamp
Docherty cheek speculum
Dockhorn retractor
docking needle
Docktor
    D. forceps
    D. needle
    D. needle forceps
    D. suture
    D. suture forceps
    D. tissue forceps
Doc's ear plug
Doctor
    D. Collins clamp
    D. Collins fracture clamp
    D. Long clamp
    D. Plymale lift fracture
      frame
Docustar fundal camera
Dodick lens-holding forceps

Dodrill forceps
Doesel-Huzly bronchoscope
dog chain retractor
Dogliotti-Gugliel mini clamp
Dogliotti valvulotome
Doherty
    D. eye implant
    D. graft
    D. implant
    D. sphere eye implant
Dohlman
    D. endoscope
    D. esophagoscope
    D. incus hook
    D. plug
Dohn-Carton brain retractor
Dohrmann-Rubin cannula
Dolan extractor
Dolley raspatory
Dolphin cord clamp
Donahoo marker
Donald clamp
Donaldson
    D. eustachian tube
    D. ventilation tube
Donald vulsellum
Donberg iris forceps
DonJoy knee brace
Donnati suture
Donnheim
    D. implant
    D. lens
donor button forceps
Dontrix gouge
Dooley nail
Doplette Doppler blood flow detector
Doppler
    D. apparatus
    D. catheter
    D. coronary catheter
    D. device
    D. flow probe
    Haemoson ultrasound D.
    Imexdop CT D.
    IntraDop intraoperative D.
    D. probe
    D. sound device
    D. stethoscope
Dopplex
    Fetal D.
Doptone fetal pulse detector
Doret graft cutter

Doriot handpiece
Dormed cranial electrotherapy stimulator
Dormia
    D. basket
    D. biliary stone basket
    D. dislodger
    D. gallstone basket
    D. stone basket
    D. stone basket catheter
    D. stone dislodger
    D. ureteral basket
    D. ureteral stone basket
    D. ureteral stone dislodger
Dornier lithotriptor
Dorrost brachial internal mammary guiding catheter
dorsal
    d. angled scissors
    d. columella implant
    d. column stimulation (DCS)
    d. column stimulator implant
    d. wrist splint with outrigger
Dorsey
    D. bayonet forceps
    D. cannula
    D. cervical foramental punch
    D. dural separator
    D. forceps
    D. needle
    D. nerve root retractor
    D. retractor
    D. screwdriver
    D. screw-holding screwdriver
    D. spatula
    D. tongue depressor
    D. transorbital leukotome
    D. ventricular cannula
Dorton self-retaining retractor
Dosick
    D. bellows assembly
    D. tunneler
dosimeter
    Rosenthal-French nebulization d.
Dos Santos aortography needle
Dos Santos lumbar aortography needle
Doss automatic percolator irrigator

Dott
- D. mouth gag
- D. retractor

Dotter
- D. caged-balloon catheter
- D. coaxial catheter
- D. dilator

Dott-Kilner mouth gag
Doubilet sphincterotome
double
- d. Becker ankle brace
- d. bridge
- d. cannula
- d. clamp
- d. clamp approximator
- d. hook
- d. Softjaw clamp
- d. Softjaw handleless clamp
- d. towel clamp

double-action
- d.-a. bone-cutting forceps
- d.-a. hump forceps
- d.-a. plate cutter
- d.-a. rongeur
- d.-a. rongeur forceps

double-angled
- d.-a. blade
- d.-a. blade plate
- d.-a. clamp
- d.-a. retractor

double-armed
- d.-a. mattress suture
- d.-a. retention suture
- d.-a. suture

double-articulated
- d.-a. bronchoscopic forceps
- d.-a. forceps tip
- d.-a. grasping forceps tip

double-band naval appliance
double-barreled needle
double-button suture
double-catheterizing
- d.-c. fin
- d.-c. sheath and obturator
- d.-c. telescope

double-channel
- d.-c. endoscope
- d.-c. irrigating bronchoscope
- d.-c. operating sheath

double-cobra retractor
double-concave
- d.-c. forceps
- d.-c. rat-tooth forceps

double-crank retractor
double-cupped forceps
double-current catheter
doubled
- d. black silk suture
- d. chromic catgut suture
- d. pursestring suture
- d. suture

double-dome reservoir
double-edged
- d.-e. knife
- d.-e. sickle knife

double-ended
- d.-e. bone curette
- d.-e. chrome probe
- d.-e. curette
- d.-e. dental curette
- d.-e. dilator
- d.-e. dissector
- d.-e. flap knife
- d.-e. needle forceps
- d.-e. nickelene probe
- d.-e. probe
- d.-e. retractor
- d.-e. root tip dental pick
- d.-e. silver probe
- d.-e. stapes curette
- d.-e. suture forceps
- d.-e. tissue forceps

double-fixation forceps
double-guarded chisel
double-headed P190 stapling device
double-J
- d.-J. indwelling catheter stent
- d.-J. silicone internal ureteral catheter stent
- d.-J. ureteral stent
- d.-J. urinary stent

double-J-stent catheter
double-lumen, dual-lumen (DL)
- d.-l. balloon stone extractor catheter
- d.-l. breast implant
- d.-l. Broviac catheter
- d.-l. cannula
- d.-l. catheter (DLC)
- d.-l. curette
- d.-l. Hickman-Broviac catheter
- d.-l. Hickman catheter
- d.-l. needle
- d.-l. Silastic catheter

double-occlusal splint
double-pigtail stent
double-pronged
    d.-p. Cottle hook
    d.-p. Fomon hook
    d.-p. fork
    d.-p. hook
double-spoon forceps
double-stop suture
double-tenaculum hook
double-tipped center-threading
  needle
double-tooth tenaculum
double-velour graft
doubly-ligated suture
Dougherty
    D. anterior chamber
      cannula
    D. anterior chamber
      irrigator
doughnut
    d. headrest
    d. pessary
Doughty tongue plate
Douglas
    D. antral trocar
    D. bag
    D. cannula
    D. ciliary forceps
    D. eye forceps
    D. forceps
    D. graft
    D. measuring plate
      pelvimeter
    D. mucosal speculum
    D. nasal scissors
    D. nasal snare
    D. nasal trocar
    D. suture
    D. suture needle
    D. tonsillar knife
    D. tonsillar snare
Dourmashkin
    D. dilator
    D. tunneled bougie
Douvas cutter
Dover
    D. abdominal belt
    D. catheter
    D. midstream urine
      collection kit

Dow Corning
    D. C. antifoam agent
      dressing
    D. C. cannula
    D. C. catheter
    D. C. external breast form
    D. C. ileal pouch catheter
    D. C. implant
dowel cutter
down-angle hook
down-biting curette
down-curved rasp
down-cutting rongeur
Downes cautery
Down hand dermatome
Downing
    D. cartilage knife
    D. cartilage scalpel
    D. clamp
    D. II laminectomy retractor
    D. retractor
    D. stapler
Downs arthroscope
Doxen mouth gag
Doyen
    D. abdominal retractor
    D. abdominal scissors
    D. bur
    D. child abdominal
      retractor
    D. clamp
    D. costal elevator
    D. director
    D. dissecting scissors
    D. electrode
    D. forceps
    D. gallbladder forceps
    D. intestinal clamp
    D. intestinal forceps
    D. myoma screw
    D. needle
    D. needle holder
    D. periosteal elevator
    D. raspatory
    D. retractor
    D. rib dissector
    D. rib elevator
    D. rib raspatory
    D. rib stripper
    D. spatula
    D. towel clamp
    D. towel forceps
    D. tumor screw

Doyen *(continued)*
  D. uterine forceps
  D. uterine vulsellum forceps
  D. vaginal retractor
  D. vaginal speculum
  D. vulsellum forceps
Doyen-Ferguson scissors
Doyen-Jansen mouth gag
Doyle vein stripper
Draeger high-vacuum erysiphake
Dragstedt
  D. graft
  D. implant
drain
  Abramson sump d.
  accordion d.
  ACMI Pezzer d.
  angle d.
  Angle-Pezzer d.
  antral d.
  Atraum with Clotstop d.
  Axiom d.
  Baker continuous flow
    capillary d.
  Bardex d.
  Bardex-Bellini d.
  Bartkiewicz two-sided d.
  Blair silicone d.
  Blake d.
  Blake silicone d.
  butterfly d.
  Chaffin-Pratt d.
  Charnley suction d.
  cigarette d.
  closed d.
  closed suction d.
  clothesline d.
  Codman lumbar external d.
  controlled d.
  craniovac d.
  CUI urological d.
  Cushman d.
  dam d.
  Davol d.
  Davol suction d.
  Davol sump d.
  Deaver T-d.
  Deboisans d.
  Deseret sump d.
  dual-sump silicone d.
  DuoDerm d.
  filtered dual sump d.
  filtered mediastinal sump d.

  d. flat kit
  fluted J-Vac d.
  flute-end right-angle d.
  Foley straight d.
  four-wing d.
  four-wing Malecot d.
  Freyer d.
  Freyer suprapubic d.
  Glove's d.
  Gomco d.
  Guibar lacrimal d.
  Hemovac d.
  Hendrickson d.
  Hendrickson supapubic d.
  Heyer-Robertson
    suprapubic d.
  Heyer-Schulte d.
  high-capacity d.
  high-capacity silicone d.
  Hollister d.
  Hysterovac d.
  Hysto-vac d.
  intercostal d.
  Jackson-Pratt d.
  Jackson-Pratt round PVC d.
  Jackson-Pratt silicone flat d.
  Jackson-Pratt silicone
    hubless flat d.
  Jackson-Pratt silicone
    round d.
  Jackson-Pratt suction d.
  Jackson-Pratt T-tube d.
  J-Vac d.
  Keith d.
  Lahey d.
  large-volume round
    silicone d.
  latex d.
  Leydig d.
  Malecot d.
  Malecot four-wing d.
  Malecot two-wing d.
  Malecot 2-wing d.
  Malecot 4-wing d.
  Mantisol d.
  Marion d.
  mediastinal d.
  mesonephric d.
  Mikulicz d.
  Mikulicz-Radecki d.
  Miller-vac d.
  Monaldi d.
  Morris d.

Morris Silastic thoracic d.
Mosher d.
Nélaton rubber tube d.
papilla d.
Penrose d.
Perma-Cath d.
Pezzer d.
Pharmaseal d.
Pharmaseal closed d.
pigtail nephrostomy d.
polyethylene d.
polyvinyl d.
Quad-Lumen d.
quarantine d.
Ragnell d.
Redivac d.
Redon d.
Reliavac d.
removal of d.
Ritter d.
Ritter suprapubic suction d.
Robertson suprapubic d.
round PVC d.
rubber d.
rubber-dam d.
rubber dam d.
Sacks biliary d.
Salem sump d.
seton d.
sheet rubber d.
Shirley sump type d.
Shirley wound d.
Silastic d.
Silastic thoracic d.
Silastic thyroid d.
silicone d.
silicone flat d.
silicone hubless flat d.
silicone round d.
silicone sump d.
silicone thoracic d.
Snyder Hemovac d.
Snyder Hemovac silicone
  sump d.
Snyder mini-Hemovac d.
soft rubber d.
Sof-Wick d.
Sovally suprapubic suction
  cup d.
spaghetti d.
stab d.
stab-wound d.
Sterivac d.

suction d.
sump d.
sump Penrose d.
suprapubic d.
suprapubic suction d.
Surgilav d.
T-d.
Teflon nasobiliary d.
thoracic d.
thyroid d.
tissue d.   *Surgidyne*
TLS d.
TLS suction d.
transnasal d.
transpapillary d.
triple-lumen sump d.
T-tube d.
T-tube d. for hysterectomy
  procedures
two-wing d.
two-wing Malecot d.
umbilical tape d.
Uni-sump d.
U-tube d.
Vacutainer d.
vacuum d.   *Varidyne*
van Sonnenberg sump d.
Vigilon d.
Wangensteen d.
Waterman sump d.
water-seal d.
water-trap d.
whistle-tip d.
Wolff d.
wolffian d.
wound d.
Wylie d.
Y-d.
Yeates d.
Younken double-lumen d.
drainage
  d. bag
  d. catheter
drain-to-wall
  d.-t.-w. suction connector
  d.-t.-w. suction tube
Drake
  D. aneurysm clip
  D. clip
**Drake-Willard hemodialysis
  machine**
Drake-Willock dialysis machine

Drape
Auto-Band Steri-D.
drape
1021 d.
3M Vi-d.
adhesive d.
adhesive plastic d.
Barrier d.
Bioclusive d.
Blair head d.
d. clamp
Convertors surgical d.
disposable TUR d.
eye d.
Eye-Pak d.
fenestrated d.
fenestrated sterile d.
gator d.
head d.
incise d.
Ioban d.
Ioban antimicrobial
  incise d.
iodophor Steri-d.
Johnson & Johnson Band-
  Aid sterile d.
3M d.
O'Connor d.
Opraflex d.
Opraflex incise d.
Op-Site d.
paper d.
plastic d.
procedure d.
Qualtex surgical d.
Rusch perineal d.
sewn-in waterproof d.
split d.
Steri-Drape d.
sterile d.
surgical d.
Surgi-Site Incise d.
Thompson d.
towel d.
Transelast surgical d.
transparent d.
TUR d.
Vi-Drape d.
V. Mueller TUR d.
Drapier needle
Dr. Bruecke aspirating tube
dreamer clamp

dressing
absorbable d.
Ace adherent d.
Ace elastic d.
Ace-Hesive d.
Ace longitudinal strips d.
Ace rubber elastic d.
acrylic resin d.
ACU-derm d.
ACU-derm wound d.
Adaptic gauze d.
Adaptic non-adherent d.
Ad-Hese-Away d.
adhesive d.
adhesive absorbent d.
Aeroplast d.
Agosteril d.
air pressure d.
Alldress multilayered
  wound d.
Allevyn d.
aloe tape d.
anorectal d.
antiseptic d.
Aquaflo d.
Aquamatic d.
Aquaphor gauze d.
ARD d.
Aureomycin gauze d.
bacitracin d.
Band-Aid d.
Barnes-Hind ophthalmic d.
barrel d.
Barton d.
Baynton d.
B-D butterfly swab d.
bias-cut stockinette d.
binocular d.
binocular eye d.
Biobrane d.
Biobrane wound d.
Bioclusive d.
Bioclusive transparent d.
Biodrape d.
Bishop-Harman d.
Blenderm surgical tape d.
BlisterFilm d.
blue sponge d.
bolus d.
bone wax d.
Borsch d.
brassiere-type d.
bulky d.

bulky compressive d.
bulky pressure d.
Bunnell d.
Bunnell-Littler d.
butterfly d.
calcium sodium alginate wound d.
Calgiswab d.
Castex rigid d.
Castmate plaster bandage d.
Cecil d.
cellophane d.
chest d.
Chick sterile d.
Chux incontinent d.
Cikloid d.
Circumpress face-lift d.
ClearSite wound d.
Clevis d.
Coban elastic d.
cocoon d.
cod liver oil-soaked strips d.
Coe-Pak periodontal d.
cohesive d.
collar d.
collodion d.
Coloplast d.
Comfeel Ulcus occlusive d.
compound d.
compression d.
Comprol d.
Contura medicated d.
Cornish wool d.
cotton-ball d.
cotton bolster d.
cotton elastic d.
cotton pledgets d.
cotton-wadding d.
Coverlet adhesive d.
Cover-Pad d.
Cover-Roll d.
cranioplastic material d.
Crinotene d.
Cruricast d.
Curad plastic d.
Curity d.
Curon d.
Cutinova d.
Cutinova Hydro wound d.
Dakin d.
Debrisan d.
Decubi-Care pad d.

demigauntlet d.
Derma Care d.
Dermicel d.
Desault d.
Diabeticorum d.
Dow Corning antifoam agent d.
Dri-Site d.
dry d.
dry-and-occlusive d.
dry pressure d.
dry sterile d. (DSD)
DuoDerm d.
DuoDerm CGF gel d.
DuoDerm porous d.
Dyna-Flex d.
elastic foam pressure d.
Elastikon d.
Elastikon wristlet d.
Elasto d.
Elastomull d.
Elastoplast d.
Elastoplast pressure d.
Elastopore d.
Enviclusive semi-occlusive adhesive film d.
Envinet gauze d.
Epigard d.
Epilock d.
Esmarch roll d.
ethylene oxide d.
Expo eye d.
Exudry d.
eye d.
EZ-Derm d.
Fastrak traction strip d.
felt d.
figure-of-eight d.
filiform d.
fine-mesh d.
finger-cot d.
fixed d.
flats of d.
Flex-Aid knuckle d.
Flex foam d.
Flexinet d.
fluff d.
fluffed gauze d.
fluffy compression d.
foam rubber d.
Foille d.
d. forceps
four-tailed d.

dressing *(continued)*
Fowler d.
Fricke d.
Fricke scrotal d.
Fuller rectal d.
Fuller shield d.
Fuller shield rectal d.
Furacin d.
Furacin gauze d.
Galen d.
Garretson d.
gauze d.
gauze stent d.
Gauztex d.
Gelfilm d.
Gelocast d.
Gibney d.
Gibson d.
Gio-occlusive d.
Glasscock d.
Glasscock ear d.
Griffin bandage lens d.
GU irrigant d.
Gypsona plaster d.
hammock d.
Harman eye d.
Harrison interlocked
  mesh d.
Hexcel cast d.
hip spica d.
Hueter perineal d.
immediate postoperative
  prosthesis d.
impermeable d.
impregnated d.
InteguDerm d.
IntraSite gel wound d.
IPOP cast d.
Ivalon d.
jacket-type chest d.
jelly d.
Jobst d.
Jobst mammary support d.
Johnson & Johnson d.
Jones d.
Kahostat wound d.
Karaya d.
Kerlix d.
Kerlix conforming
  bandage d.
Kling d.
Kling adhesive d.
Kling conform d.

Kling gauze d.
Koagamin d.
Koch-Mason d.
Koylon foam rubber d.
Larrey d.
Lister d.
Lubafax d.
Lukens bone wax d.
LYOfoam d.
LYOfoam C d.
LYOfoam wound d.
3M d.
mammary support d.
Manchu cotton d.
many-tailed d.
Martin rubber d.
mastoid d.
mechanic's waste d.
Medici aerosol adhesive
  tape remover d.
Mersilene d.
Mersilene mesh d.
Merthiolate d.
Mesalt d.
Mesalt sterile d.
Metaline d.
Microdon d.
Microfoam d.
Micropore surgical tape d.
Mitraflex multilayer
  wound d.
Mitraflex wound d.
Mitrathane wound d.
moist d.
moleskin traction hitch d.
monocular d.
monocular eye d.
Montgomery strap d.
muslin d.
mustache d.
nasal-tip d.
neoprene d.
nonadhering d.
nonadhesive d.
N-terface graft d.
Nu-Derm d.
Nu-Gauze d.
Nu-Gel d.
Nu-Gel hydrogel wound d.
Nu-wrap roll d.
occlusive d.
O'Donoghue d.
oiled silk d.

Op-Site d.
Op-Site occlusive d.
Orthoflex d.
Orthoplast d.
Ostic plaster d.
Owen cloth d.
Owen gauze d.
Oxycel d.
oxyquinoline d.
Paracine d.
paraffin d.
patch d.
peacock d.
PEG self-adhesive elastic d.
Peries medicated hygienic
  wipe d.
petrolatum d.
petrolatum gauze d.
Piedmont all-cotton
  elastic d.
plaster d.
plaster-of-Paris d.
plaster pants d.
plastic d.
pledget d.
PolyFlex traction d.
Pope halo d.
postauricular ear d.
postnasal d.
Preptic d.
Presso-Elastic d.
Pressoplast compression d.
Presso-Superior d.
pressure d.
Priessnitz d.
Primaderm d.
Primapore d.
propylene d.
protective d.
pulped muscle d.
Quadro d.
Queen Anne d.
Qwik-Clean d.
Ray-Tec d.
Red Cross adhesive d.
Release d.
Release nonadhering d.
Reston d.
Reston foam d.
Rezifilm d.
Reziplast spray-on d.
Ribble d.
Richet d.

Robert Jones d.
Robert Jones
  compressive d.
Rochester d.
roller d.
Rondic sponge d.
Rose bed d.
rubber Scan spray d.
saline d.
Sayre d.
Scan spray d.
scarlet red gauze d.
d. scissors
scrotal d.
scultetus d.
scultetus binder d.
Selofix d.
Selopor d.
semicompressive d.
semipermeable membrane d.
semipressure d.
Septisol soap d.
Septopack periodontal d.
Shah aural d.
Shantz d.
sheepskin d.
sheer spot Band-Aid d.
sheet-wadding d.
Silastic d.
silicone d.
Silverstein d.
sling d.
Sof-Rol d.
Sof-Wick d.
Sommers compression d.
Sorbsan d.
Sorbsan wound d.
spica d.
Spray Band d.
squares of d.
Sta-Tite gauze d.
stent d.
sterile d.
sterile compression d.
Steri-Strips d.
stockinette d.
Styrofoam d.
subclavian Tegaderm d.
Superflex elastic d.
Super-Trac adhesive
  traction d.
Surfasoft d.
surgical d.

dressing *(continued)*
Surgicel d.
Surgicel gauze d.
Surgifix d.
Surgiflex d.
Surgi-Pad combined d.
Surgitube d.
suspensory d.
Synthaderm d.
T-bandage d.
T-binder pressure d.
Tegaderm d.
Tegaderm occlusive d.
Tegaderm transparent d.
Tegagel nonocclusive d.
Tegasorb occlusive d.
Telfa d.
Telfa gauze d.
Telfa plastic film d.
Tenoplast elastic
  adhesive d.
Tensor elastic d.
Tes Tape d.
Thillaye d.
tie-over d.
Tomac foam rubber
  traction d.
Tomac knitted rubber
  elastic d.
transparent d.
Transpore surgical tape d.
triangular d.
tube d.
Tube-Lok tracheotomy d.
tubular d.
tulle gras d.
twill d.
Ultec d.
Uniflex d.
upper body d.
Usher Marlex mesh d.
Varick elastic d.
VariMoist d.
Vaseline d.
Vaseline gauze d.
Vaseline petroleum gauze d.
Vaseline wick d.
Velcro d.
Velcro fastener d.
Velpeau d.
Velpeau sling-d.
Velroc d.
Ventifoam traction d.

Viasorb d.
Victorian collar d.
Vi-Drape d.
Vigilon d.
Vioform d.
Vioform gauze d.
Wangensteen d.
water d.
Watson-Jones d.
Webril d.
Weck-cel d.
wet d.
wet-to-dry d.
whisk-packets d.
wick d.
wood roll d.
wound d.
wraparound d.
Xeroflo d.
Xeroform d.
Y-bandage d.
Zephyr rubber elastic d.
Zim-Flux d.
Zimocel d.
Zobec sponge d.
Zonas porous adhesive
  tape d.
Zoroc resin plaster d.
Drew clip
Drews
D. angled cystitome
D. cannula
D. capsular polisher
D. ciliary forceps
D. cystitome
D. forceps
D. inclined prism
D. intraocular forceps
D. iris retractor
D. irrigating cannula
D. lavage needle
D. suture
**Drews-Knolle reverse irrigating
  vectis**
Drew-Smythe catheter
Drews-Rosenbaum retractor
**Drews-Sato capsular fragment
  spatula**
Dreyfus
D. prosthesis forceps
D. prosthesis placement
  instrument
Dr. Gibaud thermal health support

drill

ACL d.
Acufex d.
Adson d.
Adson-Rogers perforating d.
Adson spiral d.
Adson twist d.
Aesculap d.
agility d.
air d.
Albee d.
Amico d.
anticavitation d.
Archimedean d.
ASIF twist d.
ASSI wire pass d.
automatic cranial d.
autotome d.
Bailey d.
bar d.
d. bit
bit d.
Björk d.
Björk rib d.
bone d.
bone hand d.
Bosworth d.
Bosworth crown d.
Bowen suture d.
Brunswick-Mack rotating d.
Bunnell d.
Bunnell bone d.
Bunnell hand d.
bur d.
cannulated d.
cannulated cortical step d.
Carmody d.
Carmody perforator d.
Carroll-Bunnell d.
Cebotome d.
cement eater d.
centering d.
cervical d.
Championnière bone d.
Charnley d.
Charnley centering d.
Charnley femoral condyle d.
Charnley pilot d.
Cherry d.
Cherry-Austin d.
Children's Hospital hand d.
chuck d.
Cloward d.

Cloward cervical d.
Codman d.
Codman-Shurtleff cranial d.
Codman wire pass d.
Collison d.
Collison body d.
Collison cannulated hand d.
Collison tap d.
cortical step d.
cranial d.
crown d.
Crutchfield d.
Crutchfield bone d.
Crutchfield hand d.
Crutchfield-Raney d.
Cushing d.
Cushing cranial d.
Cushing flat d.
Cushing perforator d.
dental d.
depth check d.
DePuy d.
D'Errico d.
D'Errico perforating d.
Deyerle d.
diamond d.
diamond high-speed d.
driver nail d.
extractor nail d.
fingernail d.
Fisch d.
flat d.
Galt d.
Galt hand d.
Gates-Glidden d.
glenoid d.
Gray d.
Gray bone d.
Grosse & Kempf bone d.
d. guard
d. guide
d. guide forceps
Hall d.
Hall air d.
Hall Micro-Aire d.
Hall power d.
Hall step-down d.
Hamby twist d.
hand d.
Harold Crowe d.
Harris-Smith anterior
  interbody d.
Hewson d.

drill *(continued)*
    high-speed d.
    Hudson d.
    Hudson bone d.
    Hudson cerebellar
      attachment d.
    Hudson cranial d.
    intramedullary d.
    Jacobs chuck d.
    Jordan-Day d.
    Kerr d.
    Kerr electro-torque d.
    Kerr hand d.
    Kirschner bone d.
    Kirschner wire d.
    Kodex d.
    Lentulo d.
    Lentulo spiral d.
    Light-Veley d.
    Light-Veley automatic
      cranial d.
    Light-Veley cranial d.
    Loth-Kirschner d.
    Luck d.
    Luck bone d.
    Lusskin d.
    Lusskin bone d.
    Macewen d.
    Magnuson twist d.
    Mathews d.
    Mathews hand d.
    Mathews load d.
    McKenzie d.
    McKenzie bone d.
    McKenzie cranial d.
    McKenzie perforating
      twist d.
    McKenzie perforator d.
    Michelson-Sequoia air d.
    Micro-Aire d.
    Midas Rex d.
    mini-Stryker power d.
    Minos air d.
    Mira d.
    Modny d.
    Moore d.
    Moore bone d.
    nail d.
    Neil-Moore perforator d.
    Neurain d.
    Neurairtome d.
    nipper nail d.
    Orthairtome II d.

    orthopaedic d.
    orthopaedic surgical d.
    orthopaedic Universal d.
    Osseodent surgical d.
    Osteone air d.
    ototome d.
    ototome otological d.
    Patrick d.
    Pease bone d.
    penetrating d.
    Penn d.
    perforating d.
    perforating twist d.
    perforator d.
    pilot d.
    pistol-grip hand d.
    d. point
    Portmann d.
    Ralks d.
    Ralks bone d.
    Ralks fingernail d.
    Raney d.
    Raney bone d.
    Raney cranial d.
    Raney perforator d.
    retention d.
    rib d.
    Rica bone d.
    Richards Lovejoy bone d.
    Richards pistol-grip d.
    Richmond subarachnoid
      twist d.
    Richter bone d.
    root canal d.
    scissors nail d.
    Shea d.
    Shea ear d.
    Sherman-Stille d.
    skull traction d.
    Smedberg d.
    SMIC sternal d.
    Smith d.
    spiral d.
    spiral or twist d.
    Spirec d.
    step-down d.
    Stille d.
    Stille bone d.
    Stille cranial d.
    Stille hand d.
    Stille-Sherman d.
    Stille-Sherman bone d.
    Stiwer hand d.

Stryker d.
Surgairtome air d.
surgical-orthopaedic d.
suture d.
suture hole d.
Synthes d.
tap d.
Thornwald d.
Thornwald antral d.
Treace d.
Treace stapes d.
trephine d.
Trinkle bone d.
Trinkle power d.
Trinkle Super-Cut twist d.
Trowbirdge-Campau bone d.
Trowbridge triple-speed d.
twist d.
Ullrich drill guard d.
Uniflex calibrated step d.
union broach retention d.
Universal d.
Universal two-speed
  hand d.
Vitallium d.
Warren-Mack d.
Warren-Mack rotating d.
wire d.
Wolferman d.
Wullstein d.
Zimalate d.
Zimalate twist d.
Zimmer d.
Zimmer hand d.
Zimmer-Kirschner hand d.
Zimmer Universal d.
Drinker respirator
Dri-Site dressing
drive
  spherical head hex d.
drive-extractor
  Moore hook d.-e.
driver
  Cook endoscopic curved
    needle d.
  Eby band d.
  femoral head d.
  Flatt d.
  Hall d.
  Harrington hook d.
  Jewett d.
  Ken d.
  Küntscher d.

Küntscher nail d.
K-wire d.
Massie d.
Maxi-Driver d.
McNutt d.
McReynolds d.
Milewski d.
Moore d.
Moore-Blount d.
d. nail drill
Neufeld d.
Nystroem nail d.
Nystroem-Stille d.
orthodontic band d.
ParaMax angled d.
prostatic d.
Pugh d.
Rush d.
Schneider nail d.
Sharbaro d.
surgical pin d.
tibial d.
trial d.
wire d.
Zimmer d.
Zimmer Orthair ream d.
driver-extractor
  McReynolds d.-e.
Drompp meniscotome
drop-foot
  d.-f. brace
  d.-f. splint
Dr. Quickert director
DRS composite
Dr. Twiss duodenal tube
drum
  d. dermatome
  d. elevator knife
  d. probe
  d. scraper
Drummond button
Dr. White trocar
dry
  d. cup
  d. dressing
  d. pressure dressing
  d. sterile dressing (DSD)
dry-and-occlusive dressing
Dry-Therm sterilizer
DSB
  detachable silicone balloon
DSD
  dry sterile dressing

DSR
    dental stain remover
D-syringe
D-Tach needle
Dual
    D. Geometry cutter
    D. Geometry HA cup
dual
    d. distal-lighted laryngoscope
dual-chamber
    d.-c. AV sequential
      pacemaker
    d.-c. flushing valve
    d.-c. pacemaker
dual-compartment gel-inflatable
    mammary implant
dual-lead electrode
dual-lock total hip prosthesis
dual-lumen (*var. of* double-lumen)
dual-pass pacemaker
dual-sensing, dual-pacing, dual-
    mode pacemaker (DDD
    pacemaker)
dual-sump silicone drain
Duane U-clip
Dubois decapitation scissors
Dubost valvulotome
Dubroff radial loop intraocular
    lens
Duchenne's trocar
duckbill
    d. clamp
    d. elevator
    d. forceps
    d. rongeur
    d. speculum
Ducker-Hayes nerve cuff
Ducor
    D. angiographic catheter
    D. balloon catheter
    D. cardiac catheter
duct
    d. dilator
    d. scoop
ductus clamp
Dudley
    D. rectal hook
    D. tenaculum hook
Dudley-Smith rectal speculum
Duehr-Allen eye implant
Duff debridement needle
Duffield scissors
Dufourmentel

Duggan rongeur
Duguid curved forceps
Dujovny microsuction dissection set
Duke
    D. cannula
    D. trocar
    D. tube
Dulaney
    D. antral cannula
dull
    d. retractor
    d. rotation forceps
dull-pointed forceps
dull-pronged retractor
Dulox suture
Dumas pessary
dummy sources in cesium implant
Dumon-Gilliard prosthesis
    introducer
Dumon-Harrell bronchoscope
Dumon laser-bronchoscope
Dumont
    D. dissecting forceps
    D. forceps
    D. jeweler's forceps
    D. retractor
    D. Swiss dissecting forceps
    D. thoracic scissors
    D. tweezers
Duncan
    D. curette
    D. dural film
    D. endometrial biopsy
      curette
    D. endometrial curette
    D. shoulder brace
Dundas-Grant tube
Dunhill forceps
Dunlop
    D. stripper
    D. tractor
Dunn depressor
Dunning
    D. curette
    D. elevator
duochrome test
Duocondylar knee prosthesis
duodenal
    d. clamp
    d. pin
    d. retractor
duodenofiberscope
    Olympus d.

Pentax d.
Pentax FD d.
duodenoscope
ACMI d.
d. cannula
Machida fiber-d.
Olympus d.
Olympus GIF-D d.
Pentax d.
DuoDerm
D. CGF gel dressing
D. drain
D. dressing
D. porous dressing
Duo-Drive cortical screw
Duo-Klex artificial kidney
Duo-Lock hip prosthesis
Duoloupe lens loupe
Duo-Patellar knee prosthesis
Duostat rotating hemostatic valve
Duplay
D. nasal speculum
D. tenaculum
D. tenaculum forceps
D. uterine tenaculum
D. uterine tenaculum
forceps
Duplay-Lynch nasal speculum
**Dupont distal humeral plate
system**
Dupuis cannula
Dupuy-Dutemps needle
Dupuytren
D. knife
D. suture
D. tourniquet
Dupuy-Weiss
D.-W. needle
D.-W. tonsillar needle
Durabase
D. acrylic
D. soft rebase acrylic
Duracon
D. knee component
D. knee implant
Durafill dental restorative material
Duraflow heart valve
Duragel lens
Durahue acrylic
dural
d. elevator
d. forceps
d. hook

d. implant
d. needle
d. protector
d. retractor
d. scissors
d. separator
d. substitute
d. suction retractor
d.-tenting suture
Duralay acrylic
Dura-Liner acrylic
Duralite tube
Duraloc acetabular cup
Duran annuloplasty ring
Dura Neb portable nebulizer pump
**DuraPhase semirigid penile
prosthesis**
Durapulse pacemaker
Durasoft toric
Duray-Read chisel
Duray-Wood chisel
Duredge Paufique knife
Durelon dental cement
Durham
D. needle
D. tracheostomy tube
D. tracheotomy trocar
Durnin angled director
Durogrip forceps
Duromedics bileaflet heart valve
Durotip scissors
Duryea retractor
Duthie reamer
duToit
d. shoulder staple
d. stapler
Duval
D. bag
D. dermatome
D. disposable dermatome
D. forceps
D. intestinal forceps
D. lung clamp
D. lung forceps
D. lung-grasping forceps
D. lung tissue forceps
D. tissue forceps
D. Vital intestinal forceps
Duval-Allis forceps
Duval-Collin intestinal forceps
Duval-Coryllos rib shears
Duval-Crile
D.-C. forceps

Duval-Crile *(continued)*
    D.-C. intestinal forceps
    D.-C. lung forceps
    D.-C. lung-grasping forceps
    D.-C. tissue forceps
Duval-Simon portable dermatome
Duvergier suture
DuVries needle
Duyzings clasp
DVI
    DVI pacemaker
    DVI Simpson AtheroCath
    catheter
Dworacek-Farrior canal chisel
Dwyer
    D. spinal mechanical stapler
    D. spinal screw
Dybex TENS unit
dye
    flash-lamp excited pulsed d.
    Haag-Streit fluorescein d.
    d. laser
    radiocontrast d.
Dynacor
    D. ear syringe
    D. enema cleansing kit
    D. Foley catheter
    D. leg bag
    D. suction catheter
    D. ulcer syringe

    D. vaginal irrigator set
    D. vaginal speculum
Dyna-Flex
    D.-F. dressing
    D.-F. elastic bandage
Dynaflex penile prosthesis
dynamic
    d. compression plate (DCP)
    d. penile prosthesis
    d. splint
dynamometer
    back, leg and chest d.
    Collins d.
    Harpenden handgrip d.
    Jamar d.
    orthopaedic d.
DyoCam arthroscopic video camera
Dyonics
    D. arthroscope
    D. arthroscopic instrument
    D. bur
    D. full-radius resector
    D. meniscotome
    D. needle
    D. needle scope arthroscope
    D. PS3500 drive system
    D. rod lens arthroscope
    D. rod lens laparoscope
DyoVac suction punch

E

Eagle arthroscope
ear
    e. applicator
    e. blade
    e. bougie
    e. cannula
    e. cup
    e. curette
    e. dissector
    e. forceps
    e. forceps with suction
    e. furuncle knife
    e. hook
    e. knife
    e. knife handle
    e. loop
    e. oximeter
    e. pinna prosthesis
    e. piston prosthesis
    e. polyp forceps
    e. polyp snare
    e. probe
    e. prosthesis
    e. punch forceps
    e. rasp
    e. scissors
    e. snare
    e. snare wire
    e. snare wire carrier
    e. speculum
    e. speculum holder
    e. speculum with magnifier
    e. spoon
    e. suction adapter
    e. surgery Beaver blade
    e. surgery blade
    e. syringe
ear-dressing forceps
ear-grasping forceps
Earle
    E. clamp
    E. hemorrhoidal clamp
    E. pile clamp
    E. probe
    E. rectal probe
earrings
    compression e.
Earscope otoscope
ears, nose, and throat (ENT)
Ear-Tronics hearing aid

Easi-Lav gastric lavage
East
    E. Grinstead needle
    E. Grinstead scissors
Eastman
    E. clamp
    E. cystic duct forceps
    E. dental cement
    E. forceps
    E. intestinal clamp
    E. retractor
    E. suction tube
    E. vaginal retractor
Easton cock-up splint
East-West
    E.-W. retractor
    E.-W. soft tissue retractor
Easy catheter
easy-out retractor
eater
    cement e.
Eaton
    E. nasal speculum
    E. trapezium finger joint
       replacement prosthesis
E. Benson Hood
    E. B. H. Laboratories
       esophageal tube
    E. B. H. Laboratories
       salivary bypass tube
Eber
    E. forceps
    E. holder
Eby
    E. band driver
    E. band setter
Eccentric
    E. Isotac tibial guide
    E. lock rib shears
eccentric drill guide
ECG calipers
echelon suture
Echlin
    E. duckbill rongeur
    E. laminectomy rongeur
    E. rongeur forceps
echocardiographic probe
Echols retractor
echo transponder electrode catheter
Ecker-Kazanjian forceps

Ecker-Roopenian chisel
Eckhoff forceps
ECMO
    extracorporeal membrane
      oxygenation
E-cotton bandage
Ectocor pacemaker
ectopic
    e. atrial pacemaker
    e. pacemaker
ECT pacemaker
Ectra system
Eddey parotid retractor
Edebohls
    E. clamp
    E. kidney clamp
Edelstein scissors
Edens dilation-tracheobronchoscope
Eder
    E. esophagoscope
    E. forceps
    E. gastroscope
    E. insufflator
    E. laparoscope
    E. sigmoidoscope
Eder-Bernstein gastroscope
Eder-Chamberlin gastroscope
Eder-Cohn endoscope
Eder-Hufford
    E.-H. esophagoscope
    E.-H. gastroscope
Eder-Palmer
    E.-P. gastroscope
    E.-P. semiflexible fiberoptic
      endoscope
Eder-Puestow
    E.-P. dilator
    E.-P. dilator guide
    E.-P. esophageal dilator
edge-to-edge suture
Edinburgh
    E. brain retractor
    E. retractor
    E. suture
Edna
    E. towel clamp
    E. towel forceps
Edslab
    E. catheter
    E. cholangiography catheter
    E. jaw spring clip
    E. pressure gauge

Edwards
    E. catheter
    E. clamp
    E. clip
    E. diagnostic catheter
    E. double clamp
    E. double Softjaw clamp
    E. double Softjaw handleless
      clamp
    E. handleless clamp
    E. implant
    E. parallel-jaw spring clip
    E. raspatory
    E. rectal hook
    E. seamless heart valve
    E. seamless prosthesis
    E. single clamp
    E. single Softjaw clamp
    E. single Softjaw handleless
      clamp
    E. spring clamp
    E. Teflon intracardiac
      implant
    E. Teflon intracardiac patch
      implant material
    E. Universal rod
Edwards-Carpentier aortic valve
  brush
Edwards-Verner raspatory
EEA
    end-to-end anastomosis
    EEA Auto Suture
    EEA Auto Suture stapler
    EEA disposable loading unit
    EEA stapler
    EEA stapling device
EEG
    electroencephalogram
    electroencephalograph
Effenberger
    E. contractor
    E. retractor
Effler double-ended dissector
Effler-Groves
    E.-G. cardiovascular forceps
    E.-G. dissector
    E.-G. forceps
Efos-Lite
Efteklar-Charnley hip prosthesis
Efteklar clamp
E-G alloy

Eggers
    E. contact splint
    E. plate
    E. screw
Egnell
    E. breast pump
    E. uterine aspirator
    E. vacuum extractor
egress
    e. cannula
    e. needle
Ehmke
    E. ear prosthesis
    E. platinum Teflon implant
Ehrhardt
    E. forceps
    E. lid clamp
    E. lid forceps
Eichelter-Schenk vena caval catheter
Eichen
    E. cannula
    E. irrigating cannula
Eicher
    E. chisel
    E. hip prosthesis
    E. rasp
    E. tri-fin chisel
EID
    emergency infusion device
eight-lumen
    e.-l. esophageal manometry catheter
    e.-l. manometry catheter
Eiken-Kizai hemodialysis blood tubing set
Einhorn
    E. dilator
    E. esophageal dilator
    E. tube
Einsenstein clamp
Eiselsberg ligature scissors
Eiselsberg-Mathieu needle holder
Eisenhammer speculum
Eisenstein
    E. forceps
    E. hysterectomy forceps
ejector
    Cloward dowel e.
    Johnson & Johnson saliva e.
EK-19 pad
EKG calipers

Elan electrosurgical unit
Ela pacemaker
elastic
    e. adhesive bandage
    e. bandage
    e. bougie
    e. foam bandage
    e. foam pressure dressing
    e. rubber band
    e. suture
elastic-hinge knee brace
Elastikon
    E. bandage
    E. dressing
    E. elastic tape
    E. wristlet dressing
Elast-O-Chain separator
Elasto dressing
elastomer
    American Heyer-Schulte e.
    silicone e.
Elastomull
    E. bandage
    E. dressing
    E. elastic gauze bandage
Elastoplast
    E. bandage
    E. dressing
    E. pressure dressing
Elastopore dressing
Elastorc catheter guide wire
elbow
    Coonrad-Morrey Total e.
elbowed
    e. bougie
    e. catheter
ELCA
    Excimer laser coronary angioplasty
Eldridge-Green lamp
Elecath
    E. catheter
    E. ECMO cannula
    E. pacemaker
    E. switch box
    E. thermodilution catheter
electric
    e. aspirator
    e. bed
    e. bur
    e. calipers
    e. cardiac pacemaker
    e. dermatome

electric *(continued)*
    e. laryngofissure saw
    e. probe
    e. retinoscope
electrical implant
electrically-driven bur
electricator
    e. coagulator
    e. electrosurgical unit
    National e.
Electro-Blend epilator
electrocautery
    Aspen e.
    bipolar e.
    Bovie e.
    e. cautery
    monopolar e.
    Valleylab e.
electrocoagulating biopsy forceps
electrocoagulator
electroconductive cream
electrode
    ACMI biopsy loop e.
    ACMI monopolar e.
    ACMI retrograde e.
    AE-60-I-2 implantable
      pronged unipolar e.
    AE-85-I-2 implantable
      pronged unipolar e.
    AE-60-KB implantable
      unipolar endocardial e.
    AE-85-KB implantable
      unipolar endocardial e.
    AE-60-K-10 implantable
      unipolar endocardial e.
    AE-85-K-10 implantable
      unipolar endocardial e.
    AE-60-KS-10 implantable
      unipolar endocardial e.
    AE-85-KS-10 implantable
      unipolar endocardial e.
    air-spaced e.
    angled ball-end e.
    angle-tip e.
    angular-tip e.
    angulated-blade e.
    Arrowsmith e.
    Arruga surface e.
    Arzco e.
    Aspen laparoscopic e.
    atrial e.
    ball e.
    Ballenger e.

    Ballenger follicle e.
    Ball reusable e.
    ball-tip coagulating e.
    Bard e.
    Bard-Hamm fulgurating e.
    Baumrucker e.
    bayonet-tip e.
    Beaver e.
    Beaver tail-tip e.
    Beckman stomach e.
    Berens bident e.
    biopsy loop e.
    bipolar e.
    bipolar catheter e.
    bipolar depth e.
    bipolar myocardial e.
    Birtcher e.
    biterminal e.
    blade e.
    Bovie e.
    Bovie conization e.
    Bugbee e.
    Bugbee fulgurating e.
    Buie e.
    Buie fulgurating e.
    button e.
    calomel e.
    Cambridge jelly e.
    Cameron-Miller e.
    Castroviejo e.
    Castroviejo surface e.
    e. catheter
    cautery e.
    cautery knife e.
    Cecar e.
    central terminal e.
    cerebellar e.
    cervical conization e.
    Cibis e.
    coagulating e.
    Collings e.
    Collings fulguration e.
    Collings knife e.
    CO_2mmO_2n sensor
      transcutaneous gas e.
    concentric needle e.
    conical-tip e.
    conization e.
    Copeland e.
    Copeland reusable e.
    Cortac monitoring e.
    cortical e.
    coudé e.

coudé fulgurating e.
cuff e.
cuff-type inactive e.
cup-shaped e.
cutting loop e.
cystoscopic e.
cystoscopic fulgurating e.
Davis e.
Davis coagulation e.
Delgado e.
depolarizing e.
depth e.
Depthalon monitoring e.
diathermic e.
diathermic eye e.
diathermic retinal e.
diathermy e.
disk e.
dispersing e.
disposable e.
disposable electrosurgical e.
disposable surgical e.
Doyen e.
dual-lead e.
EMG e.
ENT e.
epicardial e.
epidural e.
epilation e.
equipotential e.
ESA e.
ESA acromioplasty e.
ESA hook e.
ESA Jet Stream ball e.
ESA meniscectomy e.
ESA Smillie e.
exploring e.
external e.
eye diathermy e.
fine-needle e.
fine-wire e.
flat-tip e.
flat-wire eye e.
flexible fulgurating e.
flexible radiothermal e.
follicle e.
fulgurating e.
Galloway e.
glass pH e.
Gradle e.
Gradle needle e.
Grantham e.
Grantham lobotomy e.

Greenwald flexible
  endoscopic e.
Guyton e.
Guyton angled e.
Haiman tonsillar e.
Hamm e.
Hamm fulgurating e.
Hamm resectoscope e.
Hildreth e.
Hubbard e.
Hughes fulguration e.
Hurd e.
Hurd angular e.
Hurd bipolar diathermy e.
Hurd turbinate e.
Hyams-Timberlake wire loop
  for e.
Hymes-Timberlake e.
Iglesias e.
impedance e.
implanted e.
impregnated e.
inactive e.
indifferent e.
Innsbruck e.
intercerebral e.
e. jelly
Jewett e.
J-loop e.
Kalk e.
Karaya e.
knife e.
Kronfeld e.
Kronfeld surface e.
LaCarrere e.
lancet-shaped e.
Lane ureteral meatotomy e.
large-loop e.
Levin e.
Lifeline e.
lobotomy e.
localizing e.
loop e.
loop ball e.
Lynch e.
McCarthy e.
McCarthy coagulation e.
McCarthy diathermic
  knife e.
McCarthy fulgurating e.
McCarthy loop operating e.
McCarthy miniature loop e.
McWhinnie e.

electrode *(continued)*
- meatotomy e.
- Megadyne Fann E-Z Clean laparoscopic e.
- metal e.
- midoccipital e.
- miniature loop e.
- Moersch e.
- monopolar temporary e.
- multilead e.
- multiple-point e.
- multipurpose ball e.
- MVE-50 implantable myocardial e.
- Myerson e.
- myocardial e.
- Myowire cardiac e.
- Myowire II cardiac e.
- Nashold e.
- National cautery e.
- needle e.
- Neil-Moore e.
- Neil-Moore meatotomy e.
- Nesbit e.
- neutral e.
- New e.
- New York Hospital e.
- Nyboer esophageal e.
- ophthalmic cautery e.
- pacemaker e.
- pacing e.
- pacing wire e.
- pad e.
- panendoscope e.
- parallel-loop e.
- PE-60-I-2 implantable pronged unipolar e.
- PE-85-I-2 implantable pronged unipolar e.
- PE-60-KB implantable unipolar endocardial e.
- PE-85-KB implantable unipolar endocardial e.
- PE-60-K-10 implantable unipolar endocardial e.
- PE-85-K-10 implantable unipolar endocardial e.
- PE-85-KS-10 implantable unipolar endocardial e.
- Pischel e.
- platinum blade e.
- platinum blade meatotomy e.
- point e.
- pointed-tip e.
- proctological ball e.
- proctoscopic e.
- proctoscopic fulguration e.
- prostatic aluminum e.
- proximal e.
- punctate e.
- pyramidal e.
- Ray rhizotomy e.
- recording e.
- reference e.
- reimplanted e.
- retinal diathermy e.
- retrograde e.
- Riba electrourethrotome e.
- Ringenberg e.
- rod e.
- roller e.
- round-loop e.
- round-wire e.
- Rychener-Weve e.
- scalp e.
- Schepens e.
- Schepens surface e.
- semiflat tip e.
- Shank e.
- Shealy facet rhizotomy e.
- single-fiber EMG e.
- single-use e. (SUE)
- single-wire e.
- Skylark surface e.
- Sluder cautery e.
- Sluder-Mehta e.
- small-loop e.
- Smith e.
- Smith endoscopic e.
- spiral e.
- Stern-McCarthy e.
- stick-on e.
- stimulating e.
- Stockert cardiac pacing e.
- Storz cystoscopic e.
- Storz resectoscope e.
- straight-blade e.
- straight-point e.
- straight-tip e.
- straight-wire e.
- surface e.
- surgical e.
- Surgicraft e.
- Surgicraft pacemaker e.
- sutureless pacemaker e.

temporal e.
terminal e.
e. terminal adapter
terminal adapter e.
Timberlake e.
tissue dessication needle e.
tongue plate e.
tonsillar e.
transvenous e.
turbinate e.
Turner cystoscopic
  fulgurating e.
ultrasonic e.
underwater e.
unipolar e.
ureteral meatotomy e.
USCI pacing e.
vaginal aluminum e.
VPL e.
VPL thalamic e.
Walker e.
Walker coagulating e.
Walker ureteral
  meatotomy e.
Wappler e.
Weve e.
Williams tonsillar e.
Wilson-Cook coagulation e.
wraparound inactive e.
Wyler e.
Wyler subdural strip e.
Ziegler cautery e.
zinc ball e.
Zuker bipolar pacing e.
Zywiec e.
electrodermatome
Hood e.
Padgett e.
e. sterile blade
electrodiaphake
LaCarrere e.
Electrodyne pacemaker
electroencephalogram (EEG)
electroencephalograph (EEG)
biofeedback e.
Grass e.
Mingograf e.
electro-etching kit stencil
electrogustometer
Nagashima e.
electrohemostasis catheter
electrohydraulic lithotriptor probe

electrolysis
One-Touch e.
electrolyte solution
electromagnetic flow probe
electromucotome
Castroviejo e.
Steinhauser-Castroviejo e.
electromyogram (EMG)
electromyograph (EMG)
electromyometer
biofeedback e.
electronic
e. endoscope
e. muscle stimulator
e. stethoscope
electronic-amplified stethoscope
Electronic Artificial larynx
electronystagmograph (ENG)
Elmed-Toennis system e.
Nagashima e.
electro-oculogram (EOG)
e.-o. apparatus
electro-oculograph (EOG)
Electrorelaxor TENS unit
electroretinogram (ERG)
electroretinograph (ERG)
electroscope
Bruening e.
electrosurgical
e. biopsy forceps
e. pencil (ESP)
e. unit
electrotome
McCarthy infant e.
McCarthy miniature e.
McCarthy punctate e.
Nesbit e.
Stern-McCarthy e.
Timberlake obturator e.
Elema pacemaker
Elema-Schonander pacemaker
elephant cuff
Elevath pacemaker
elevating forceps
elevator
Abraham e.
Adson e.
Adson-Love periosteal e.
Adson periosteal e.
Alexander e.
Alexander-Farabeuf e.
Allerdyce e.
Allis periosteal e.

elevator *(continued)*
Amalgan plugger e.
Amerson bone e.
angular e.
Anthony e.
Apexo e.
Arenberg dural palpator e.
Artmann e.
Ashley cleft palate e.
Aufranc periosteal e.
Austin e.
Austin duckbill e.
Austin duckbill knife e.
Austin footplate e.
Austin right-angle e.
ball-end e.
Ballenger-Hajek e.
Ballenger septal e.
Barsky e.
Batson-Carmody e.
Behrend periosteal e.
Bellucci e.
Bennett e.
Bennett bone e.
Berry-Lambert periosteal e.
Bethune e.
Bethune periosteal e.
Blair e.
Blair cleft palate e.
blunt e.
Boies nasal e.
Boies nasal fracture e.
bone e.
Bowen periosteal e.
Bristow e.
Bristow periosteal e.
Brophy periosteal e.
Brophy tooth e.
Brown tooth e.
Cameron-Haight e.
Cameron-Haight
  periosteal e.
Cameron periosteal e.
Campbell periosteal e.
Cannon-Rochester lamina e.
Carmody-Batson e.
Carroll-Legg periosteal e.
Carroll periosteal e.
Carter submucous e.
Chandler e.
Chandler bone e.
Cheyne periosteal e.
chisel e.

Cinelli e.
Cinelli periosteal e.
cleft palate e.
clinic exolever e.
Cloward e.
Cloward periosteal e.
Cobb e.
Cobb periosteal e.
Cobb spinal e.
Cohen e.
combined wire guide
  bone e.
Converse alar e.
Converse-MacKenty e.
Converse-MacKenty
  periosteal e.
Converse periosteal e.
Cooper spinal fusion e.
Cordes-New laryngeal
  punch e.
Coryllos-Doyen periosteal e.
Coryllos periosteal e.
costal e.
costal periosteal e.
Cottle e.
Cottle alar e.
Cottle-MacKenty e.
Cottle nasal e.
Cottle periosteal e.
Cottle septal e.
Cottle skin e.
Coupland e.
Crawford dural e.
Crego e.
Crego periosteal e.
Cronin cleft palate e.
Cryer dental e.
Cushing e.
Cushing-Hopkins e.
Cushing-Hopkins
  periosteal e.
Cushing little joker e.
Cushing periosteal e.
Cushing pituitary e.
Cushing staphylorrhaphy e.
Davidson-Mathieu-
  Alexander e.
Davidson-Mathieu-Alexander
  periosteal e.
Davidson periosteal e.
Davidson-Sauerbruch-
  Doyen e.
Davis periosteal e.

Dawson-Yuhl e.
Dawson-Yuhl-Key e.
Dawson-Yuhl periosteal e.
Derlacki e.
Derlacki duckbill e.
dermal e.
D'Errico periosteal e.
Dewar e.
Dingman periosteal e.
Dingman zygoma e.
Doyen costal e.
Doyen periosteal e.
Doyen rib e.
duckbill e.
Dunning e.
dural e.
endaural e.
Farabeuf periosteal e.
Farrior-Shambaugh e.
Fay suction e.
Federspiel periosteal e.
Fibre-Lite septal e.
file e.
Fiske periosteal e.
Fomon nostril e.
Fomon periosteal e.
footplate e.
Frazier dural e.
Frazier suction e.
Freer e.
Freer double e.
Freer double-end e.
Freer periosteal e.
Freer septal e.
Friedman e.
Friedrich rib e.
Gam-Mer periosteal e.
Gillies zygoma e.
Goldman septal e.
Goodwillie periosteal e.
Gorney septal suction e.
Graham scalene e.
Guilford-Wright drum e.
Guilford-Wright duckbill e.
Haberman suction e.
Hajek-Ballenger e.
Hajek-Ballenger septal e.
Halle e.
Halle septal e.
Hamrick e.
Hamrick suction e.
Hargis periosteal e.
Harper periosteal e.

Harrington spinal e.
Hatt golf-stick e.
Hayden palate e.
Hedblom e.
Hedblom costal e.
Henner e.
Henner endaural e.
Herczel e.
Herczel periosteal e.
Herczel raspatory e.
Herczel rib e.
Hibbs chisel e.
Hibbs costal e.
Hibbs periosteal e.
Hibbs spinal fusion
   chisel e.
Hoen periosteal e.
Hopkins-Cushing
   periosteal e.
Hough spatula e.
House e.
House ear e.
House endaural e.
House stapes e.
House Teflon-coated e.
Howorth e.
Hu-Friedy e.
Hulka-Kenwick uterine e.
Hurd e.
Hurd septal e.
Iowa University e.
Iowa University
   periosteal e.
Jackson perichondrial e.
Jacobson counter-pressure e.
Jannetta angular e.
Jannetta duckbill e.
Jarit periosteal e.
Jordan e.
Jordan canal e.
Jordan-Rosen e.
Joseph-Killian septal e.
Joseph nasal e.
Joseph periosteal e.
Kennerdell-Maroon e.
Kennerdell-Maroon
   duckbill e.
Key e.
Key periosteal e.
Killian septal e.
Kilner e.
Kinsella e.
Kinsella periosteal e.

elevator *(continued)*
    Kirmisson e.
    Kirmisson periosteal e.
    Kleesattel e.
    Kleinert-Kutz e.
    Kocher e.
    Kocher periosteal e.
    Koenig e.
    Kos e.
    Krego e.
    Ladd e.
    laminar e.
    Lamont e.
    Lane e.
    Lane periosteal e.
    Lange bone e.
    Langenbeck e.
    Langenbeck periosteal e.
    Lee-Cohen septal e.
    Lempert e.
    Lempert heavy e.
    Lempert narrow e.
    Lewis periosteal e.
    Lindholm-Stille e.
    Logan periosteal e.
    long back-handed e.
    Louisville e.
    Love-Adson e.
    Love-Adson periosteal e.
    Lowis periosteal e.
    L-shaped e.
    Luongo septal e.
    MacDonald periosteal e.
    MacKenty-Converse periosteal e.
    MacKenty periosteal e.
    MacKenty septal e.
    Magielski e.
    Malis e.
    Matson-Alexander e.
    Matson rib e.
    McCollough e.
    McGee canal e.
    Melt e.
    MGH periosteal e.
    Miller-Apexo e.
    Miller dental e.
    Molt e.
    Molt periosteal e.
    Monks malar e.
    Moore bone e.
    Moorehead e.
    mucosal e.
    Murphy-Lane bone e.
    narrow e.
    Neurological Institute periosteal e.
    Norcross periosteal e.
    Nordent oral surgery e.
    Norrbacka bone e.
    Ohl periosteal e.
    orthopaedic e.
    orthopaedic shoulder e.
    Overholt e.
    Overholt periosteal e.
    Pace periosteal e.
    palatorrhaphy e.
    Paparella duckbill e.
    Pennington e.
    Pennington septal e.
    periosteal e.
    Perkins e.
    Phemister raspatory e.
    Pierce e.
    Polcyn e.
    Pollock sweetheart periosteal e.
    Pollock zygoma e.
    Poppen e.
    Poppen periosteal e.
    Potts dental e.
    Presbyterian Hospital e.
    Presbyterian Hospital staphylorrhaphy e.
    Proctor mucosal e.
    Quervain e.
    Raney periosteal e.
    Ray-Parsons-Sunday staphylorrhaphy e.
    Read periosteal e.
    Rhoton e.
    Rhoton general purpose e.
    Rica nasal periosteale.
    Richards Cobb spinal e.
    Richardson periosteal e.
    right-angle e.
    Rissler periosteal e.
    Rochester e.
    Roger e.
    Roger septal e.
    Rosen angular e.
    Rowe bone e.
    Rubin-Lewis periosteal e.
    Rudderman "Frelevator" fragment e.
    Sabbatsberg septum e.

Sauerbruch-Frey rib e.
Sayre e.
Sayre double-end
  periosteal e.
Sayre periosteal e.
Scheer knife e.
Schuknecht e.
Scott-McCracken e.
Sebileau e.
Sédillot e.
Sédillot periosteal e.
septal e.
Sewall ethmoidal e.
Sewall mucoperiosteal
  periosteal e.
Shambaugh e.
Shambaugh-Derlacki e.
Shambaugh-Derlacki
  duckbill e.
Shambaugh narrow e.
Shea e.
Shea long back-handed e.
Silverstein dural e.
skin e.
skull e.
SMIC periosteal e.
Smith-Petersen e.
Sokolec e.
Somers uterine e.
Spurling periosteal e.
stapes e.
staphylorrhaphy e.
Steele periosteal e.
Stille-Langenbeck e.
Stille periosteal e.
Stolte-Stille e.
Story orbital e.
suction e.
Sunday staphylorrhaphy e.
Suraci hook e.
Suraci zygoma hook e.
Tabb e.
Tabb ear e.
Tarlov nerve e.
Tenzel e.
Tenzel double-end
  periosteal e.
Tenzel periosteal e.
Tobolsky e.
Traquair e.
Traquair periosteal e.
Tronzo e.
Turner cord e.

Turner periosteal e.
Urquhart periosteal e.
uterine e.
von Langenbeck
  periosteal e.
Walker submucous e.
Ward periosteal e.
Warwick James e.
Watson-Jones e.
West blunt e.
Willauer-Gibbon e.
Willauer-Gibbon
  periosteal e.
Williger e.
Winter e.
Woodson e.
Woodson dental
  periosteal e.
Wright-Guilford drum e.
Wurzelheber dental e.
zygoma e.
elevator-displacer
  Goldman septal e.-d.
elevator-dissector
  Allerdyce e.-d.
elevator-feeler
  Cottle e.-f.
elevator-knife
  Paparella drum e.-k.
elevator-retractor
  nostril e.-r.
  Storz orbital e.-r.
**El Gamal coronary bypass
  catheter**
El Gamal guiding catheter
Elgiloy
  E. frame of prosthetic value
  E. lead-tip pacemaker
  E. pacemaker
Elgiloy-Heifitz aneurysm clip
Elias lid retractor
eliminator
  Osher iris tuck e.
  torque e.
Elite pacemaker
Ellik
  E. bladder evacuator
  E. evacuator
  E. kidney stone basket
  E. loop stone dislodger
  E. meatotome
  E. resectoscope
  E. sound

Ellik *(continued)*
  E. stone basket
  E. stone dislodger
Ellik-Shaw obturator
Elliot
  E. corneal trephine
  E. femoral condyle holder
  E. knee plate
  E. trephine
  E. trephine handle
Elliott
  E. blade plate
  E. forceps
  E. gallbladder forceps
  E. hemostatic forceps
  E. obstetrical forceps
Ellis
  E. buttress plate
  E. eye needle holder
  E. foreign body spud
  E. holder
  E. needle holder
  E. needle probe
  E. probe
  E. spud
Ellison
  E. fixation staple
  E. glenoid rim punch
Ellman rotary scaler
Ellsner gastroscope
Elmar artificial kidney
Elmed
  E. diagnostic laparoscope
  E. hysteroscope
  E. operating laparoscope
Elmed-Toennis system electronystagmograph
ELP femoral prosthesis
Elsberg
  E. brain-exploring cannula
  E. cannula
  E. ventricular cannula
Elschnig
  E. capsular forceps
  E. cataract knife
  E. cataract spoon
  E. cyclodialysis forceps
  E. cyclodialysis spatula
  E. fixation forceps
  E. forceps
  E. lens scoop
  E. lens spoon
  E. lid retractor

  E. pterygium knife
  E. retractor
  E. scoop
  E. secondary membrane forceps
  E. tissue-grasping forceps
Elschnig-O'Brien
  E.-O. fixation forceps
  E.-O. forceps
  E.-O. tissue-grasping forceps
Elschnig-O'Connor
  E.-O. fixation forceps
  E.-O. forceps
Elsie-Brown otoabrader
embolectomy
  e. catheter
  e. curette
embryotome
  obstetrical decapitating e.
emergency infusion device (EID)
Emerson
  E. Birtheez abdominal decompressor
  E. bronchoscope
  E. postoperative ventilator
  E. pump
  E. respirator
  E. vein stripper
Emerson-Segal Medimizer demand nebulizer
Emesay suture button
Emesco handpiece
EMG
  electromyogram
  electromyograph
  EMG electrode
Emiks heart valve
Emir
  E. razor
  E. razor blade
Emmet
  E. forceps
  E. hemostatic bag
  E. needle
  E. obstetrical forceps
  E. obstetrical retractor
  E. ovarian trocar
  E. probe
  E. retractor
  E. tenaculum
  E. tenaculum hook
  E. trocar
  E. uterine probe

E. uterine scissors
E. uterine tenaculum hook
Emmet-Gellhorn pessary
Emmet-Murphy needle
EMPI Neuropacer TENS unit
Encapsulon
E. epidural catheter
E. sheath introducer
E. vessel dilator
encased screw
en chemise catheter
encircling
e. band
e. clip
Encor pacemaker
endarterectomy
e. dissector
e. scissors
e. spatula
e. stripper set
endaural
e. curette
e. elevator
e. retractor
e. speculum
e. surgery chisel
end-cutting reamer
Ender
E. nail
E. pin
E. rod
end-hole
e.-h. catheter
e.-h. pigtail catheter
Endo
E. Clip ML/Surgiport
System pack
E. Dissect
E. Grasp
E. Grasp grasper
E. rotating knee joint
prosthesis
E. shears
E. zoom lens camera
endocamera
Polaroid instant e.
Endocam video camera system
endocapsular artificial lens
intraocular lens
endocardial
e. balloon lead
e. bipolar pacemaker

e. cardiac lead
e. pacemaker
endocardiograph
endocervical
e. biopsy curette
e. curette
e. probe
endocervicometer scope
Endoclip applier
endocoagulator
endodiathermy
endodontic
e. broach
e. curette
e. file
e. pin
e. plugger
e. reamer
e. sealer
endoesophageal tube
endo-GIA surgical clip
endo-illuminator
Grieshaber e.-i.
endo-irrigator
Endo-Lase C02 laser
endolaser
Diode e.
e. probe
Endoloop chromic ligature suture
instrument
endoluminal stent
endolymphatic shunt tube
introducer
endometrial
e. biopsy curette
e. biopsy set
e. biopsy suction curette
e. curette
e. forceps
e. implant
e. polyp forceps
endometriotic implant
end-on mattress suture
endo-osseous
e.-o. dental implant
e.-o. implant
endo-otoprobe
Gherini-Kaufman e.-o.
Horn e.-o.
Maloney e.-o.
Endopap endometrial sampler

Endopath
> E. disposable surgical trocar
> E. ES endoscopic stapler

Endo-P-Probe

endoprosthesis
> Austin Moore curved e.
> Austin Moore straight-
> stem e.
> Averett head and neck e.
> biliary e.
> Centrax e.
> Centrax bipolar e.
> Leinbach head and neck e.
> Matchett-Brown hip e.
> metatarsophalangeal e.
> Proctor-Livingston e.
> Ring-Derlan TM biliary e.
> Schneider-Wallstent e.
> Thompson e.
> Wilson-Cook e.

endoscope
> ACMI e.
> battery-powdered e.
> Cilco ophthalmic e.
> disk e.
> Dohlman e.
> double-channel e.
> Eder-Cohn e.
> Eder-Palmer semiflexible
> fiberoptic e.
> electronic e.
> end-viewing e.
> fiberoptic e.
> flexible e.
> Foroblique e.
> forward-viewing e.
> French-McCarthy e.
> Fujinon e.
> Fujinon EVE video e.
> Fujinon EVG-F upper GI
> video e.
> Fujinon flexible e.
> Fujinon flexible lower GI e.
> Fujinon UGI-FP e.
> GIF-HM e.
> GIF-XQ e.
> Hamou e.
> Haslinger e.
> JFB III e.
> Kelly e.
> Lowsley-Peterson e.
> Machida flexible e.
> McCarthy e.

> mother-daughter e.
> Needlescoper e.
> Olympus e.
> Olympus OES flexible e.
> Olympus Pre-OES flexible e.
> Ono loupe for e.
> oral e.
> pediatric e.
> Pentax e.
> Pentax flexible e.
> Pentax side-viewing e.
> rigid e.
> Rockey e.
> Satelite ear e.
> semiflexible e.
> semirigid e.
> side-viewing e.
> TJF e.
> Toshiba video e.
> video e.
> Welch Allyn video e.
> Wolf e.

endoscopic
> e. BICAP probe
> e. biopsy forceps
> e. electrode handle
> e. grasping forceps
> e. heat probe
> e. irrigator
> e. retrograde
> cholangiopancreatography
> (ERCP)
> e. suture-cutting forceps
> e. telescope

endoskeletal prosthesis

endospeculum
> e. forceps
> Kogan e.

Endostat
> E. calibration pod insert
> E. fiber stripper

Endo-Suction sinus microstat set

endotracheal
> e. catheter
> e. catheter forceps
> e. curette
> e. tube
> e. tube brush
> e. tube forceps

endotriptor stone-crushing basket
end-over-end running suture
EndoVideo-Five endoscopic camera

Endslip denture adhesive
end-to-end anastomosis (EEA)
Endura dressing forceps
Endur bonding material
Enduron acetabular liner
end-viewing endoscope
Enemette enema cleansing kit
Enertrax pacemaker
ENG
    electronystagmograph
Engelmann thigh splint
Engel-May nail
Engel plaster saw
Engh porous metal hip prosthesis
Englehardt femoral prosthesis
English
    E. clamp
    E. forceps
    E. hospital reflex percussor
    E. lock
    E. MacIntosh fiberoptic
    laryngoscope blade
    E. nail nipper
    E.-pattern clamp
    E. tissue forceps
English-McNab shoulder prosthesis
Engstrom respirator
Enhanced Torque 8F guiding
  catheter
EnhanCement gun
Enker
    E. brain retractor
    E. self-retaining brain
    retractor
enlarging bur
Ennis forceps
ENT
    ears, nose, and throat
    ENT bite block
    ENT electrode
    ENT speculum
    ENT wire crimper
Entera Flo spike set
Frenta enteral feeding bag
enteroscope
    Goldberg MPC operative e.
enterostomy clamp
enterotomy scissors
Entract dilation and occlusion
  catheter
entropion, entropium
    e. clamp
    e. forceps

enucleation
    e. compressor
    e. scissors
    e. scoop
    e. spoon
enucleator
    Hardy e.
    Hardy bayonet e.
    Marino rotatable
    transsphenoidal e.
    Rhoton e.
    rotatable transsphenoidal e.
    transsphenoidal e.
    Young prostatic e.
Enviclusive semi-occlusive adhesive
  film dressing
Envinet gauze dressing
Envisan
    E. cleaning pad scrub soap
    E. dextranomer pad
    E. dextranomer paste
    E. wound cleaning paste
    scrub soap
EOG
    electro-oculogram
    electro-oculograph
epicardial
    e. electrode
    e. lead
    e. pacemaker
    e. retractor
epidural electrode
Epigard dressing
epiglottis retractor
epilation, epilating
    e. electrode
    e. forceps
    e. needle
epilator
    Electro-Blend e.
    Epilot high-frequency
    needle-type e.
    high-frequency tweezer-
    type e.
    Removatron e.
    Super Epitron high-
    frequency e.
    Thermaderm e.
    Trichodemolus e.
Epilatron hair-removal machine
Epilock dressing
Epilot high-frequency needle-type
  epilator

episcleral forceps
episiotomy scissors
epistaxis balloon
Epoxylite dental resin cement
Eppendorfer
    E. biopsy forceps
    E. biopsy punch forceps
    E. cardiac catheter
    E. catheter
    E. cervical biopsy forceps
    E. punch
Epstein
    E. blade
    E. collar stud acrylic lens
    E. curette
    E. down-biting curette
    E. hammer
    E. hemilaminectomy blade
    E. intraocular lens
    E. lens implant
    E. needle
    E. osteotome
    E. posterior chamber lens
    E. rasp
    E. spinal fusion curette
Epstein-Copeland lens
EPTFE
    expanded
    polytetrafluoroethylene
        EPTFE graft prosthesis
        EPTFE sutures
        EPTFE vascular suture
Equen-Neuffer laryngeal knife
Equen stomach magnet
equipment
    digitalized e.
equipotential electrode
Equisetene suture
eraser
    e. cautery
    hemastatic e.
eraser-tip cautery
erbium-YAG laser
ERCP
    endoscopic retrograde
    cholangiopancreatography
        ERCP cannula
        ERCP catheter
Erectaid penile prosthesis
Erectek external erection device
erector spinae retractor

ERG
    electroretinogram
    electroretinograph
Ergo
    E. bipolar forceps
    E. irrigation system
    E. micro-aspirator
ergometry
    bicycle e.
Erhardt
    E. clamp
    E. ear speculum
    E. eyelid forceps
    E. forceps
    E. lid clamp
    E. lid forceps
Eric-aid prosthesis
Erich
    E. arch bar
    E. arch malleable bar
    E. biopsy forceps
    E. dental arch bar
    E. facial fracture appliance
    E. facial fracture frame
    E. forceps
    E. laryngeal biopsy forceps
    E. maxillary splint
    E. nasal splint
    E. swivel
Erich-Winter arch bar
Erickssson-Stille carotid clamp
Eric Lloyd
    E. L. extractor
    E. L. introducer
Eri-Flo dialyzer
Eriksson
    E. guide
    E. muscle cannula
Eriksson-Paparella holder
ERI-Lyte hemodialysis concentrate
erisophake (var. of erysiphake)
Erlangen
    E. magnetic colostomy
        device
    E. set
Ermold needle holder
Ernst radium applicator
eroder
    facet e.
Erosa
    E. amnioscope
    E. disposable hypodermic
    needle

Erosa-Spec vaginal speculum
erthmoidomaxillary suture
erysiphake, erisophake
  Barraquer e.
  Bell e.
  Castroviejo e.
  Dastoor e.
  Dimitry e.
  Dimitry-Bell e.
  Dimitry-Thomas e.
  Draeger high-vacuum e.
  Esposito e.
  Falcao e.
  Flayol-Grant e.
  Floyd-Grant e.
  Harken e.
  Harrington e.
  Johnson e.
  Johnson-Bell e.
  Kara e.
  L'Esperance e.
  L'Esperance right-angle e.
  Maumenee e.
  Maumenee-Park e.
  New York e.
  nucleus e.
  Nugent e.
  Nugent-Green-Dimitry e.
  Post-Harrington e.
  right-angle e.
  Sakler e.
  Searcy e.
  Searcy oval cup e.
  Simcoe nucleus e.
  Storz-Bell e.
  Viers e.
  Welsh e.
  Welsh rubber bulb e.
  Welsh Silastic e.
Erythroflex catheter
ESA
  ESA acromioplasty electrode
  ESA electrode
  ESA hook electrode
  ESA Jet Stream ball
    electrode
  ESA meniscectomy electrode
  ESA Smillie electrode
escape pacemaker
E-Series
  E.-S. bipolar forceps
  E.-S. forceps
  E.-S. micro-infertility kit

  E.-S. needle holder
  E.-S. scissors
ESI
  ESI bite block
  ESI laryngoscope
  ESI sigmoidoscope
ESKA Jonas silicone-silver penile
  prosthesis
Esmarch
  E. bandage
  E. bandage scissors
  E. plaster knife
  E. plaster shears
  E. probe
  E. probe with Myrtle leaf
    end
  E. roll dressing
  E. scissors
  E. tin bullet probe
  E. tourniquet
esophageal
  e. airway
  e. balloon
  e. balloon catheter
  e. dilating flexible metal
    spiral tip
  e. dilating set
  e. dilator
  e. forceps
  e. manometry catheter
  e. mercury-filled bougie
  e. motility perfused catheter
  e. prosthesis
  e. retractor
  e. scissors
  e. stent
  e. tapered mercury-filled
    bougie
esophagofiberscope
  Olympus e.
esophagoscope
  ACMI e.
  ACMI fiberoptic e.
  ballooning e.
  Blom-Singer e.
  Boros e.
  Broyles e.
  Bruening e.
  Brunings e.
  Chevalier Jackson e.
  child e.
  Denck e.
  Dohlman e.

esophagoscope *(continued)*
    Eder e.
    Eder-Hufford e.
    Eutaw-Hoffman e.
    fiberoptic e.
    Foregger rigid e.
    Foroblique e.
    Foroblique fiberoptic e.
    full-lumen e.
    Haslinger e.
    Holinger e.
    Holinger child e.
    Holinger infant e.
    Hopkins rod-lens e.
    Hufford e.
    infant e.
    Jackson e.
    Jackson full-lumen e.
    Jasbee e.
    Jesberg e.
    Jesberg oval e.
    Jesberg upper e.
    J-scope e.
    Kalk e.
    Lell e.
    LoPresti fiberoptic e.
    Moersch e.
    Mosher e.
    Moure e.
    Olympus e.
    optical e.
    oval e.
    oval-open e.
    pediatric e.
    Roberts e.
    Roberts folding e.
    Roberts-Jesberg e.
    Roberts oval e.
    Sam Roberts e.
    Schindler e.
    Schindler optical e.
    standard full-lumen e.
    Storz e.
    Storz operating e.
    Storz optical e.
    Storz pediatric e.
    Tesberg e.
    Tucker e.
    Universal e.
    upper e.
    Yankauer e.
esophagoscopic
    e. cannula

    e. catheter
    e. forceps
esophagospasm dilator
ESP
    electrosurgical pencil
Esposito erysiphake
Esquire dental sterilizer
Esser
    E. graft
    E. implant
    E. prosthesis
Essig arch bar
Essrig
    E. dissecting scissors
    E. forceps
    E. tissue forceps
Estecar prosthesis
esthesiometer
    manual e.
Estilux
    E. dental restorative
    material
    E. ultraviolet system
Estridge ventricular needle
Etch-Master
    E.-M. electrolyte solution
    E.-M. electronic stencil
    E.-M. felt pad
    E.-M. kit
ether bed
Ethibond
    E. polyester suture
    E. suture
Ethicon
    E. clip
    E. Polytef paste prosthesis
    E. silk suture
    E. suture
    E. TG Plus needle
    E. TGW needle
Ethicon-Atraloc suture
Ethiflex
    E. retention suture
    E. suture
Ethilon
    E. nylon suture
    E. suture
Ethi-pack suture
ethmoidal
    e. chisel
    e. curette
    e. forceps
    e. punch

ethmoid-cutting forceps
Ethox rectal tube
Ethridge
    E. forceps
    E. hysterectomy forceps
Ethrone
    E. implant
    E. implant material
    E. prosthesis
ethylene oxide dressing
E-type dental implant
Eucotone monitor
EUE tonsillar snare
European in-the-bag lens
Euroton hearing aid
eustachian
    e. bougie
    e. bur
    e. catheter
    e. filiform set
    e. probe
Eutaw-Hoffman esophagoscope
euthyscope
evacuator
    Bard e.
    Bigelow e.
    bladder e.
    Creevy bladder e.
    Crigler e.
    Dentsply MVS e.
    Ellik e.
    Ellik bladder e.
    Hutch e.
    ice clot e.
    Iglesias e.
    Kennedy-Cornwell bladder e.
    Laufe portable uterine e.
    McCarthy e.
    McKenna Tide-Ur-Ator e.
    oval-window piston e.
    Sklar e.
    Snyder Hemovac e.
    Thompson e.
    Timberlake e.
    Toomey bladder e.
    e. tubing
Evacupack disposable suction
  cannister
Evans
    E. forceps
    E. tissue forceps
    E. Vital tissue forceps

Eve-Neivert
    E.-N. tonsillar wire
Everclear laryngeal mirror
Everest alloy
Everett forceps
Evermed catheter
eversor
    Roveda e.
everter
    Berens lid e.
    Berke double-end lid e.
    lid e.
    Luther-Peter lid e.
    Pess lid e.
    Siniscal-Smith lid e.
    Strubel lid e.
    Vail lid e.
    Walker lid e.
everting
    e. interrupted suture
    e. suture
Eves-Neivert tonsillar snare
Eves tonsillar snare
Evoport auditory evoked potential
  system
Ewald
    E. elbow prosthesis
    E. forceps
    E. gastroscope
    E. tissue forceps
    E. tube
Ewald-Hensler arthroscopic punch
Ewald-Hudson
    E.-H. brain forceps
    E.-H. clamp
    E.-H. dressing forceps
    E.-H. tissue forceps
Ewald-Walker knee implant
E wildcat orthodontic wire
Ewing
    E. capsular forceps
    E. eye implant
    E. forceps
    E. lid clamp
EWSCL
    extended wear soft contact lens
Exakta Varex gastrocamera
examination retractor
examining
    e. arthroscope
    e. gastroscope
    e. hysteroscope
    e. lamp

examining *(continued)*
    e. spotlight
    e. telescope
excavator
    Austin e.
    Clev-Dent e.
    dental e.
    Farrior e.
    Farrior oval-window e.
    Farrior oval-window piston
      gauge e.
    fenestration e.
    Henry Schein e.
    Hough e.
    Hough oval-window e.
    Hough-Saunders e.
    Hough whirlybird e.
    House e.
    House-Hough e.
    Lempert e.
    Merlis obstetrical e.
    middle ear e.
    Nordent e.
    oval-window e.
    Paparella-Hough e.
    PD e.
    Schuknecht e.
    Schuknecht whirlybird e.
    sinus tympani e.
    SMIC e.
    stapes e.
    whirlybird e.
    whirlybird stapes e.
Excell
    E. polishing point
    E. polishing wheel
exchanger
    heat e.
exchange wire
Excimer
    E. cool laser
    E. laser
    E. laser coronary
      angioplasty (ELCA)
exclusion clamp
exenteration
    e. forceps
    e. spoon
Exmoor plastics aural grommet
Exo-bed tractor
exolever forceps

exophthalmometer
    Hertel e.
    Luedde e.
exoplant
Exo-static overhead tractor
expandable
    e. blade
    e. breast implant
    e. cervical dilator
expanded polytetrafluoroethylene
   (EPTFE)
expanded polytetrafluoroethylene
   sutures
expander
    CUI e.
    Ormco orthodontic arch-e.
    Radovan tissue e.
    self-inflating tissue e.
    surgical skin graft e.
Expander mammary implant
   material
expanding reamer
Expand-O-Graft cutter
expansile dilator
expansion screw
explant
    silicone e.
explorer
    dental e.
    Nordent e.
    operative e.
    SMIC e.
    Steri-Probe e.
exploring
    e. cannula
    e. electrode
    e. needle
Expo eye dressing
expressor
    Arruga e.
    Arruga lens e.
    Bagley-Wilmer e.
    Bagley-Wilmer lens e.
    Berens e.
    Berens lens e.
    follicle e.
    follicle lid e.
    Fyodorov lens e.
    Goldmann e.
    Heath e.
    Heath follicle lid e.
    Heath lid e.
    Hess e.

Hess tonsillar e.
Hosford meibomian
    gland e.
intracapsular lens e.
iris e.
Kirby e.
Kirby hook e.
Kirby intracapsular lens e.
Kirby intracapsular lens e.
    with cylindrical separator
Kirby intracapsular lens e.
    with double-ball separator
Kirby intracapsular lens e.
    with flat separator
Kirby intracapsular
    separator lens e. with
    curved zonular separator
Kirby lens e.
lens e.
lid e.
Medallion lens e.
nucleus e.
Osher nucleus stab e.
Rizzuti eye e.
Rizzuti iris e.
Rizzuti lens e.
Smith e.
Smith lens e.
Smith lid e.
Smith lid lens e.
tonsillar e.
Verhoeff e.
Verhoeff lens e.
Wilmer-Bagley e.
Wilmer-Bagley iris e.
Wilmer-Bagley lens e.

Express PTCA catheter
extended
    e. anatomical high-profile
        malar implant
    e. wear soft contact lens
        (EWSCL)
extender
    rear-tip e.
extension
    e. apparatus
    bifurcated drain e.
    e. bone clamp
    e. bow
    e. clamp
    Hudson cerebellar e.
    Jackson-Pratt bifurcated
        drain e.

Linx guide wire e.
    e. tube
exterior pelvic device
external
    e. asynchronous pacemaker
    e. auditory larynx
    e. breast prosthesis
    e. catheter
    e. demand pacemaker
    e. electrode
    e. functional neuromuscular
        stimulator
    e. pacemaker
    e. transthoracic pacemaker
    e. vascular compression
        device
    e. vein stripper
external-internal pacemaker
externally-controlled noninvasive
    programmed stimulation
    pacemaker
externofrontal retractor
extracapsular eye forceps
extrachromic suture
extracorporeal
    e. membrane oxygenation
        (ECMO)
    e. membrane oxygenation
        system
    e. pump
extracting forceps
extraction hook
extractor
    Andrews comedo e.
    ball e.
    Bellows cryoextractor e.
    Bilos pin e.
    Bird modified vacuum e.
    Bird vacuum e.
    broach e.
    cataract rotoextractor e.
    Cherry screw e.
    cloverleaf pin e.
    comedo e.
    cortex e.
    Councill ureteral stone e.
    deluxe FIN e.
    DePuy e.
    Dolan e.
    Egnell vacuum e.
    Eric Lloyd e.
    femoral trial e.
    fetal head e.

extractor *(continued)*
fetal vacuum e.
food e.
Gill-Welsh cortex e.
Glassman stone e.
Hallach comedo e.
head e.
Intraflex intramedullary pin e.
Jarit comedo e.
Jewett bone e.
Kobayashi vacuum e.
Küntscher e.
Lewicky cortex e.
Lloyd nail e.
magnetic e.
Malström vacuum e.
Massie e.
McDermott e.
McNutt e.
McReynolds e.
Mignon cataract e.
Mityvac e.
Mityvac vacuum e.
Moore-Blount e.
Moore hooked e.
Moore nail e.
Murless fetal head e.
Murless head e.
e. nail drill
Roto-extractor e.
Rush e.
Rutner stone e.
Saalfeld comedo e.
Schamberg e.
Schamberg comedo e.
Silastic cup e.
Simcoe cortex e.
Smith-Petersen e.
Southwick screw e.
stem e.
Torpin vectis e.
Troutman cataract e.
Unna comedo e.
ureteral stone e.
Walsh cortex e.
Walton comedo e.
Welsh cortex e.
Wilson-Cook eight-wire basket stone e.
Zimmer e.
Extrafil breast implant

extramedullary
e. alignment arch
e. alignment guide
extraoral appliance
extrusion
e. balloon catheter
e. needle
exudate disposal bag
Exudry dressing
eye
artificial e.
e. bandage
e. blade
e. calipers
e. curette
e. diathermy electrode
e. drape
e. dressing
e. and ear cannula
e. forceps
e. implant
e. instrument rack tray
e. knife
e. magnet
e. needle holder
e. needle holder forceps
e. occluder
e. pad
e. patch
e. probe
probe with e.
e. protector
e. retractor
e. scissors
e. shield
e. spears
e. speculum
e. sphere implant
e. stitch scissors
e. surgery blade
e. suture
e. suture forceps
e. suture scissors
eyed
e. needle
e. probe
e. suture needle
eye-dressing forceps
eye-fixation forceps
eyeglass hearing aid
eyeknife blade

eyeless
    e. atraumatic suture needle
    e. needle
    e. suture needle
eyelet clasp
eyelid
    e. forceps
    e. retractor
Eye-Pak drape
E-Z
    E-Z guide

    E-Z M barium contrast
      material
    E-Z syringe
EZ-Derm dressing
E-Z-EM
    E-Z-EM biopsy needle
    E-Z-EM cut biopsy needle
Ezo denture cushion
EZ Temp thermometer
**EZ-Trac orthopaedic suspension
device**

F

Fabian screw
Fabry coagulator
face
    f. rest
    f. shield
    f. shield headband
facebow
    Kinematic f.
    Ortho-Yomy f.
    Rickett f.
face-lift
    f.-l. marker
    f.-l. retractor
    f.-l. scissors
facet
    f. eroder
    f. rasp
facial
    f. fracture appliance
    f. fracture appliance dental arch bar
    f. fracture appliance swivel
    f. nerve dissector
    f. nerve knife
    f. nerve stimulator
Facit uterine polyp forceps
Faden suture
Fager pituitary dissector
Fahey-Compere pin
Fahey pin
Fairdale orthodontic appliance
Falcao
    F. dissector
    F. erysiphake
    F. fixation forceps
    F. suction dissector
Falcone rongeur
Falcon filter
Falk
    F. appendectomy spoon
    F. clamp
    F. forceps
    F. lion-jaw forceps
    F. needle
    F. retractor
    F. vaginal cuff
    F. vaginal cuff clamp
    F. vaginal retractor
fallopian
    f. cannula

    f. catheter
    f. tube forceps
Falope
    F. ring
    F. tubal sterilization ring
Falope-ring
    F.-r. applicator
    F.-r. dilator
    F.-r. tubal occlusion band
false suture
Fansler
    F. anoscope
    F. proctoscope
    F. rectal speculum
Fansler-Ives anoscope
Fanta speculum
Farabeuf
    F. bone clamp
    F. bone-holding forceps
    F. double-ended retractor
    F. forceps
    F. periosteal elevator
    F. raspatory
    F. retractor
    F. rugine
    F. saw
Farabeuf-Collin raspatory
Farabeuf-Lambotte
    F.-L. bone clamp
    F.-L. bone forceps
    F.-L. bone-holding clamp
    F.-L. bone-holding forceps
    F.-L. clamp
    F.-L. forceps
Faraci punch
Faraci-Skillern sphenoid punch
Faraday shield
Farah cystoscopic needle
far-and-near suture
Farenheit and centigrade flat bath thermometer
Farkas urethral speculum
Farlow
    F. tongue depressor
    F. tonsillar snare
Farlow-Boettcher snare
Farmingdale retractor
far-near suture

Farnham
  F. forceps
  F. nasal-cutting forceps
Farnsworth test
Faro coolbeam lamp
Farr
  F. retractor
  F. self-retaining retractor
  F. spring retractor
  F. wire retractor
Farrell applicator
Farrington
  F. forceps
  F. nasal polyp forceps
  F. septal forceps
Farrior
  F. angulated curette
  F. anterior footplate pick
  F. applicator
  F. blunt palpator
  F. bur
  F. ear curette
  F. ear speculum
  F. excavator
  F. footplate pick
  F. forceps
  F. mushroom raspatory
  F. otoplasty knife
  F. oval speculum
  F. oval-window excavator
  F. oval-window pick
  F. oval-window piston
    gauge excavator
  F. posterior footplate pick
  F. septal cartilage stripper
    knife
  F. sickle knife
  F. speculum
  F. suction applicator
  F. triangular knife
  F. wire crimper
  F. wire-crimping forceps
Farrior-Derlacki chisel
Farrior-Dworacek canal chisel
Farrior-Joseph
  F.-J. bayonet saw
  F.-J. saw
Farrior-McHugh ear knife
Farrior-Shambaugh elevator
Farris tissue forceps
far suture
Fasanella
  F. cannula

  F. double-ended retractor
  F. iris retractor
  F. lacrimal cannula
  F. retractor
fascia
  f. cutter
  f. lata heart valve
  f. lata implant
  f. lata prosthesis
  f.l stripper
fascial
  f needle
  f snare
fasciatome
  Lane f.
  Luck f.
  Masson f.
  Moseley f.
Fasplint
FAST
  flow-assisted, short-term
    FAST balloon catheter
    FAST right heart
      cardiovascular catheter
Fastcure denture repair material
Fasteeth denture adhesive
Fastlok implantable staple
Fast-Pass lead pacemaker
Fastrak traction strip dressing
Fat-O-Meter skinfold calipers
fat-pad retractor
faucet aspirator
faucial
  f. catheter
  f. eustachian catheter
Fauer peritoneal clamp
Faulkner
  F. antral chisel
  F. antral curette
  F. chisel
  F. curette
  F. double-end ring curette
  F. ethmoidal curette
  F. nasal curette
  F. trocar
  F. trocar chisel
Faulkner-Browne chisel
Faure
  F. biopsy forceps
  F. forceps
  F. peritoneal forceps
  F. uterine biopsy forceps

Fauvel
- F. forceps
- F. laryngeal forceps

Favaloro
- F. atrial retractor
- F. clamp
- F. coronary scissors
- F. ligature carrier
- F. proximal anastomsis clamp
- F. scissors
- F. self-retaining sternal retractor

Favaloro-Morse sternal retractor
Favaloro-Semb ligature carrier
Favorite clamp
Fay
- F. suction elevator
- F. suction elevator suction tube

Fazio-Montgomery cannula
Fazioplast
Fearon tracheoscope
Feaster
- F. Dualens intraocular lens
- F. dual-placement intraocular lens
- F. lens hook
- F. lens manipulator

feather
- f. clamp
- f. knife
- f. scalpel

Feather carbon breakable blade
feathered extended malar implant
Fechner intraocular lens
Federov (*var. of* Fyodorov)
Federspiel
- F. cheek retractor
- F. needle
- F. periosteal elevator
- F. scissors

feeder
- Brecht f.

feeding gastrostomy
feeler
- O'Donoghue cartilage f.

Fehland
- F. clamp
- F. intestinal clamp
- F. intestinal forceps
- F. right-angled colon clamp

Feilchenfeld
- F. forceps
- F. splinter forceps

Feild
- F. retractable blade assembly
- F. suction dissector

Feild-Lee biopsy needle
Fein
- F. antral trocar
- F. antral trocar needle
- F. cannula
- F. needle

Feldbausch dilator
Feldman
- F. lip retractor
- F. radial keratotomy marker
- F. retractor

Feldstein blepharoplasty clip
Fell-O'Dwyer apparatus
Fell sucker tip
felt dressing
female
- f. catheter
- f. catheter-dilator
- f. sound

femoral
- f. artery cannula
- f. broach
- f. clamp
- f. condyle
- f. distractor
- f. drill bit
- f. guide tip
- f. guiding catheter
- f. head driver
- f. impactor
- f. neck retractor
- f. notch guide
- f. perfusion cannula
- f. shaft reamer
- f. stem
- f. trial extractor

femorofemoral crossover prosthesis
fence splint
fenestra implant
fenestrated
- f. blade forceps
- f. catheter
- f. clip
- f. cup biopsy forceps
- f. Drake clip
- f. drape

243

fenestrated *(continued)*
  f. forceps
  f. Moore-type femoral stem
  f. stem
  f. sterile drape
fenestration
  f. bur
  f. curette
  f. excavator
  f. hook
fenestrator
  Montgomery tracheal f.
  Rosen f.
fenestrometer
  Guilford-Wright f.
  Paparella f.
  Rosen f.
  Wright-Guilford f.
Fenger
  F. gallbladder probe
  F. gall duct probe
  F. gallstone probe
  F. probe
  F. spiral gallstone probe
Fenlin total shoulder system
Fenton
  F. bolt
  F. bulldog vulsellum
  F. dilator
  F. tibial bolt
  F. uterine dilator
Ferciot
  F. tip-toe splint
  F. wire guide
Ferguson
  F. abdominal scissors
  F. accessory eye implant
  F. angiotribe
  F. angiotribe forceps
  F. basket
  F. bone clamp
  F. bone curette
  F. bone-holding forceps
  F. curette
  F. esophageal probe
  F. forceps
  F. gall duct scoop
  F. gallstone scoop
  F. implant
  F. mouth gag
  F. needle
  F. probe
  F. retractor

F. round-body needle
F. scissors
F. stone basket
F. suture needle
F. tenaculum forceps
F. tubular vaginal speculum
F. uterine scissors
F. vaginal speculum
Ferguson-Ackland mouth gag
Ferguson-Brophy mouth gag
Ferguson-Frazier suction tube
Ferguson-Gwathmey mouth gag
Ferguson-Metzenbaum scissors
Ferguson-Moon
  F.-M. rectal retractor
  F.-M. retractor
Fergusson
  F. speculum
  F. tubular vaginal speculum
Fernstroem bladder retractor
Fernstroem-Stille retractor
Ferris
  F. biliary duct dilator
  F. colporrhaphy forceps
  F. common duct scoop
  F. dilator
  F. disposable bone marrow
    aspiration needle
  F. filiform dilator
  F. forceps
  F. Robb tonsillar knife
  F. Smith bone-biting forceps
  F. Smith cup-jaw rongeur
    forceps
  F. Smith cup rongeur
    forceps
  F. Smith disk rongeur
  F. Smith forceps
  F. Smith fragment forceps
  F. Smith-Gruenwald rongeur
  F. Smith-Halle bur
  F. Smith-Halle sinus bur
  F. Smith intervertebral disk
    rongeur
  F. Smith-Kerrison disk
    rongeur
  F. Smith-Kerrison
    laminectomy rongeur
  F. Smith-Kerrison punch
  F. Smith-Kerrison rongeur
  F. Smith-Kerrison rongeur
    forceps

F. Smith Lyman
  periosteotome
F. Smith needle holder
F. Smith orbital retractor
F. Smith pituitary rongeur
F. Smith punch
F. Smith retractor
F. Smith rongeur
F. Smith-Sewall orbital
  retractor
F. Smith-Sewall retractor
F. Smith-Spurling
  intervertebral disk forceps
F. Smith-Spurling rongeur
F. Smith-Takahashi forceps
F. Smith-Takahashi rongeur
F. Smith tissue forceps
Ferrolite crown remover
ferrule clamp
Ferszt
  F. dissecting hook
  F. ligature passer
fetal
  f. head extractor
  f. stethoscope
  f. substantia nigra implant
  f. vacuum extractor
Fetal Dopplex
Fetalert fetal heart monitor
Fetasonde fetal monitoring system
fetoscope
Fett carpal prosthesis
Feuerstein
  F. drainage tube
  F. split ventilation tube
FFP
  flexible fluoropolymer
FG diamond bur
fiber
  f. cleaver
  laser f.
  Laserscope disposable
    Endostat f.
  f. mallet
  SLT FiberTact/Contact
    laser f.
fibergastroscope
fiberglass
  f. graft
  f. staff
fiberoptic
  f. anoscope
  f. arthroscope

f. bronchoscope
f. cable
f. cable adapter
f. endoscope
f. esophagoscope
f. gastroscope
f. hysteroscope
f. laryngoscope
f. light carrier
f. light pipe
f. light projector
f. light source
f. loupe
f. microscope
f. otoscope
f. oximeter catheter
f. probe
f. proctosigmoidoscope
f. retractor
f. right-angle telescope
f. sheath
f. sigmoidoscope
f. slide laryngoscope
f. suction tube
f. surgical field illuminator
f. telescope
f. vaginal speculum
fiberscope
  Hirschowitz f.
  Hirschowitz
    gastroduodenal f.
  Olympus f.
  Pentax f.
  side-viewing f.
Fibrel gelatin matrix implant
Fibre-Lite septal elevator
fibroid hook
Fichman suture-cutting forceps
field
  Graefe electric f.
Field tourniquet
figure-of-eight
  f.-o.-e. bandage
  f.-o.-e. dressing
  f.-o.-e. suture
filament suture
file
  Aagesen f.
  bone f.
  Charnley trochanter f.
  f. elevator
  endodontic f.
  Hedstrom f.

Surgilase fiber

file *(continued)*
Kleinert-Kutz bone f.
K root canal f.
Miller bone f.
Nordent bone f.
orthopaedic bone f.
orthopaedic surgical f.
pulp canal f.
Putti bone f.
root canal f.
scrub f.
SMIC bone f.
SMIC periodontal f.
S root canal f.
surgical f.
filiform
f. bougie
f. bougie probe
f. catheter
f. dressing
f. follower
f. guide
LeFort f.
Rusch f.
f. stone dislodger
filiform-tipped catheter
Fillauer
F. bar
F. night splint
filler
paste f.
spiral f.
film
Accufilm articulating f.
Accu-Flo dural f.
Dentus x-ray f.
Duncan dural f.
MDS Truspot articulating f.
3TC x-ray f.
Filshie clip
filter
Adams kidney stone f.
arterial f.
bird's nest f.
bird's nest IVC f.
BTF-37 arterial blood f.
Cook f.
Falcon f.
Gianturco-Roehm bird's nest vena caval f.
Greenfield f.
Greenfield IVC f.
Holter in-line shunt f.

Interface arterial blood f.
Jostra arterial blood f.
Kim-Ray Greenfield vena cava f.
K-37 pediatric arterial blood f.
f. maintainer
Medi-Tech IVC f.
Millex f.
Millipore f.
Mobin-Uddin vena cava f.
Monomer f.
Nalzene f.
f. needle
Simon-Nitinol f.
Simon-Nitinol inferior vena caval f.
Swank high-flow arterial blood f.
Vena-Tech dual vena caval f.
William Harvey arterial blood f.
filtered
f. dual sump drain
f. mediastinal sump drain
Filtzer
F. corkscrew
F. interbody rasp
fin
convertible f.
double-catheterizing f.
final-cut acetabular reamer
finder
Carabelli lumen f.
Damian lumen f.
Hedwig lumen f.
lumen f.
Tucker vertebrated lumen f.
Findley folding pessary
Fine
F. scissors
F. suture-tying forceps
fine
f. arterial forceps
f. chromic suture
f. curette
f. forceps
f. needle
f. silk suture
f. suture
fine-angle curette

Fine-Castroviejo
  F.-C. forceps
  F.-C. suturing forceps
fine-dissecting forceps
Fine-Gill corneal knife
fine-line tissue marker
fine-mesh dressing
fine-needle electrode
Finesse
  F. guiding catheter
  F. large-lumen guiding
    catheter
fine-tissue forceps
fine-tooth
  f.-t. clamp
  f.-t. forceps
fine-wire electrode
finger
  f. circumference gauge
  f. cot
  f. cot splint
  f. extension clockspring
    splint
  f. goniometer
  f. joint implant
  mechanical f.
  f. muscle tester
  f. plate
  f. prosthesis
  Quire automatic f.
  f. rake retractor
  f. retractor
  f. ring cutter
  f. ring saw
  f. splint
finger-cot dressing
fingernail drill
Finite dental glazing compound
Fink
  F. chalazion curette
  F. cul-de-sac cannula
  F. curette
  F. fixation forceps
  F. forceps
  F. irrigator
  F. lacrimal retractor
  F. laryngoscope
  F. muscle hook
  F. retractor
  F. tendon tucker
  F. tendon-tucker forceps

Fink-Jameson
  F.-J. forceps
  F.-J. oblique muscle forceps
Fink-Rowland keratome
Fink-Scobie hook
Fink-Weinstein syringe
Finn chamber patch test device
finned-stem punch
Finney
  F. penile implant
  F. prosthesis
Finney-Flexirod prosthesis
Finnoff
  F. laryngoscope
  F. sinus transilluminator
  F. transilluminator
Finochietto
  F. arterial clamp
  F. bronchus clamp
  F. clamp
  F. clamp carrier
  F. forceps
  F. hand retractor
  F. infant rib contractor
  F. infant rib retractor
  F. laminectomy retractor
  F. laminectomy retractor
    blade
  F. lobectomy forceps
  F. needle
  F. needle holder
  F. retractor
  F. rib retractor
  F. rib spreader
  F. scissors
  F. spreader
  F. thoracic forceps
Finochietto-Burford
  F.-B. rib contractor
  F.-B. rib spreader
**Finochietto-Geissendorfer rib
  retractor**
Finochietto-Stille rib spreader
Finsen
  F. retractor
  F. tracheal hook
  F. wound hook
Finsterer
  F. myringotomy split tube
  F. suction tube
  F. suture
Firlene eye magnet
Firmdent denture adhesive

247

first rib shears | fixator

first rib shears
Firtel broach
Fisch
- F. bone drill irrigator
- F. cutting bur
- F. drill
- F. dural hook
- F. dural retractor
- F. microcrurotomy scissors

Fischer
- F. cannula
- F. dissector
- F. needle
- F. pneumothoracic needle
- F. silicone ventricular cannula
- F. sterilizing storage rack

Fischl
- F. dissecting forceps
- F. forceps

Fischmann angiotribe forceps
Fish
- F. antral probe
- F. cannula
- F. forceps
- F. grasping forceps
- F. infusion cannula
- F. inlet
- F. nasal-dressing forceps
- F. nasal forceps
- F. nasal-grasping forceps
- F. sinus probe

Fisher
- F. advancement forceps
- F. bed
- F. brace
- F. cannula
- F. capsular forceps
- F. double-ended retractor
- F. eye needle
- F. eye spoon
- F. fenestrated lid retractor
- F. forceps
- F. iris forceps
- F. knife
- F. lid retractor
- F. needle
- F. retractor
- F. solid-blade retractor
- F. spoon
- F. spoon needle spoon
- F. spud
- F. tape board

- F. tonsillar dissector
- F. tonsillar knife
- F. tonsillar retractor
- F. ventricular cannula

Fisher-Arlt
- F.-A. forceps
- F.-A. iris forceps

fisherman's pliers
Fisher-Nugent retractor
Fisher-Smith spatula
fishhook needle
fish-mouth suture
fishtail
- f. chisel
- f. spatula
- f. spatula raspatory

Fiske periosteal elevator
Fisk tractor
fissure bur
fistular
- f. hook
- f. needle
- f. probe
- f. scissors

fit
- interference f.

Fitch obturator
Fitzgerald
- F. aortic aneurysm clamp
- F. aortic aneurysm forceps
- F. forceps

Fitzpatrick suction tube
Fitzwater
- F. forceps
- F. ligature carrier
- F. peanut sponge-holding forceps

fixation
- f. apparatus
- f. bandage
- f. base
- f. button
- f. device
- f. forceps
- f. hook
- OrthoSorb pin f.
- f. pin
- f. ring
- f. suture
- f. twist hook

fixator
- Ace-Fischer external f.
- articulated external f.

248

Bay external f.
hex-fix external f.
Hoffmann external f.
Pennig dynamic wrist f.
Stuhler-Heise f.
fixed
f. appliance
f. arch bar
f. cervical dilator
f. dressing
fixed-focus scope
fixed-rate
f.-r. asynchronous atrial pacemaker
f.-r. asynchronous ventricular pacemaker
f.-r. pacemaker
Fixodent denture adhesive
Flagg
F. laryngoscope
F. stainless steel laryngoscope blade
flamingo
f. antrostomy forceps
f. forceps
Flanagan spinal fusion gouge
flange
Callahan f.
Scuderi-Callahan f.
flanged Teflon tube
Flannery ear speculum
flap
bladder f.
f. demarcator
f. knife
f. knife dissector
flared spinal rod
flash
f. tray
flash-lamp excited pulsed dye
flask
Dewar f.
flat
f. bottom reservoir
f. brain spatula support
f. drill
f. eye bandage
f. needle spud
f. spatula
f. spatula needle
f. spud
f. suture
f. tenotomy hook

flat-blade-tipped catheter
Flateau
F. oval punch
F. oval tip
flat-end cutter
flats of dressing
Flatt
F. driver
F. finger prosthesis
flattened irrigating cannula
flat-tip electrode
flat-wire eye electrode
flavine wool mold
Flaxedil suture
Flayol-Grant erysiphake
Fleming
F. conization instrument
F. conization instrument blade
Fletcher
F. dressing forceps
F. forceps
F. sponge forceps
F. tonsillar knife
Fletcher-Pierce cannula
Fletcher-Suit polyp forceps
Fletcher-Van Doren
F.-V. D. forceps
F.-V. D. sponge-holding forceps
F.-V. D. uterine forceps
F.-V. D. uterine polyp forceps
Fletching femoral hernia implant material
Fleurant bladder trocar
Flexacryl hard rebase acrylic
Flex-Aid knuckle dressing
Flexcon lens
Flex-E-Z wax
Flex foam dressing
flexible
f. aortic clamp
f. arm
f. blade osteotome
f. bronchoscope
f. catheter
f. Dualens implant
f. endoscope
f. fluoropolymer (FFP)
f. fluoropolymer contact lens
f. foreign body forceps

flexible *(continued)*
  f. fulgurating electrode
  f. gastroscope
  f. injection needle
  f. metal catheter
  f. nasopharyngoscope
  f. optical biopsy forceps
  f. probe
  f. pump
  f. radiothermal electrode
  f. reamer
  f. retractor
  f. retractor extension arm
  f. retractor pressure clamp
  f. retractor sliding clamp
  f. rod penile implant
  f. shaft retractor
  f. sigmoidoscope
  f. sound
  f. vascular clamp
flexible-loop
  f.-l. anterior chamber
    intraocular lens
  f.-l. posterior chamber
    intraocular lens
flexible-tip J-guide wire
flexible-wire bundle reamer
Flexicair
  F. bed
  F. low-air-loss bed
**Flexicath silicone subclavian
  cannula**
Flexicon gauze bandage
Flexi-Flate
  F.-F. II penile implant
  F.-F. penile implant
  F.-F. penile prosthesis
Flexiflo
  F. enteral feeding tube
  F. gastrostomy tube
  F. gastrostomy tube enteral
    delivery system
  F. Sachs-Veni tube
  F. Stomate gastrostomy
    tube
  F. suction feeding tube
  F. tap-fill enteral tube
  F. Taptainer tube
  F. tube
Flexilite
  F. conforming elastic
    bandage
  F. gauze bandage

Flexinet dressing
Flexi-rod
  F.-r. II penile implant
  F.-r. penile prosthesis
Flexiscope arthroscope
Flexistone impression material
Flexitone suture
Flexi-Ty vessel band
Flex-O-Jet aspirator
Flexon
  F. steel suture
  F. suture
flexor hinge hand splint brace
Flexo wax
Flexsol
Flexsteel
  F. retractor
  F. ribbon retractor
Flextip catheter
Flieringa
  F. fixation ring
  F. ring
  F. scleral ring
Flieringa-Legrand fixation ring
Flint glass speculum
floating
  f. catheter
  f. disk heart valve
  f. shoulder socket
floor-standing surgical light
floppy guide wire
**Florex medical compression
  stockings**
Florida brace
Flo-Switch
  Medi-Tech HP F.-S.
flotation catheter
Flourotip cannula
flow-assisted, short-term (FAST)
flow-directed
  f.-d. balloon cardiovascular
    catheter
  f.-d. balloon-tipped catheter
  f.-d. catheter
  f.-d. thermodilution catheter
Flowers mandibular glove
flowmeter
  Dienco f.
  mini-Wright peak f.
  Statham f.
flow-oximetry catheter
flow probe
flow-regulator clamp

Floyd
    F. loop cannula
    F. needle
    F. pneumothorax injection
    needle
Floyd-Barraquer
    F.-B. speculum
    F.-B. wire speculum
Floyd-Grant erysiphake
fluff dressing
fluffed gauze dressing
fluffy compression dressing
Fluhrer
    F. bullet probe
    F. rectal probe
fluid
    cerebrospinal f. (CSF)
fluid-filled catheter
fluorescence-guided "smart" laser
Fluorescite syringe
fluoroscopic foreign body forceps
Fluoro Tip ERCP cannula
flushing
    f. device
    f. reservoir
    f. valve
flute
    f. cannula
    f. needle
fluted
    f. J-Vac drain
    f. nail
    f. reamer
    f. stem punch
flute-end right-angle drain
Fluvog
    F. irrigator
    F. irrigator-aspirator
Flynn scleral depressor
Flynt
    F. aortography needle
    F. needle
foam
    f. rubber dressing
    f. rubber stent
    f. rubber vaginal stent
FoaMTrac traction bandage
Foerger airway
Foerster
    F. abdominal retractor
    F. abdominal ring retractor
    F. capsulotomy knife

    F. enucleation snare
    F. eye forceps
    F. eye forceps
    F. forceps
    F. gallbladder forceps
    F. iris forceps
    F. sponge forceps
    F. sponge-holding forceps
    F. surgical support brassiere
    F. tissue forceps
    F. uterine forceps
Foerster-Ballenger forceps
Foerster-Bauer sponge-holding
    forceps
Foerster-Mueller forceps
Foerster-Van Doren sponge-holding
    forceps
Fogarty
    F. arterial embolectomy
    catheter
    F. arterial irrigation catheter
    F. balloon
    F. balloon biliary catheter
    F. balloon catheter
    F. biliary balloon probe
    F. biliary probe
    F. bulldog clamp-applying
    forceps
    F. calibrator
    F. catheter
    F. clamp
    F. dilation catheter
    F. embolus catheter
    F. forceps
    F. gallstone catheter
    F. Hydragrip clamp
    F. insert
    F. irrigation catheter
    F. occlusion catheter
    F. probe
    F. venous irrigation catheter
    F. venous thrombectomy
    catheter
Fogarty-Chin
    F.-C. catheter
    F.-C. clamp
    F.-C. extrusion balloon
    catheter
    F.-C. peripheral dilatation
    catheter
Fogarty-Hydragrip insert
Fogarty-Softjaw insert

foil
    f. carrier
    Shimstock occlusion f.
Foille dressing
Folatex catheter
folding
    f. approximating clamp
    f. blade
    f. laryngoscope
    f. lens
fold-over finger splint
Foley
    F. acorn-bulb catheter
    F. bag
    F. balloon catheter
    F. catheter
    F. cone-tip catheter
    F. forceps
    F. hemostatic bag
    F. straight drain
    F. vas isolation forceps
Foley-Alcock
    F.-A. bag
    F.-A. bag catheter
    F.-A. catheter
    F.-A. hemostatic bag
follicle
    f. electrode
    f. expressor
    f. lid expressor
follower
    filiform f.
    Rusch f.
Foltz
    F. catheter
    F. flushing reservoir
    F. needle
Foltz-Overton cardiac catheter
Fomon
    F. angular scissors
    F. chisel
    F. chisel guard
    F. double-edge knife
    F. hook
    F. hook retractor
    F. knife
    F. lower lateral scissors
    F. nasal chisel
    F. nasal hook
    F. nasal rasp
    F. nasal retractor
    F. nostril elevator
    F. nostril retractor

    F. osteotome
    F. periosteal elevator
    F. periosteotome
    F. rasp
    F. retractor
    F. saber-back scissors
    F. scissors
    F. upper lateral scissors
Fonix hearing aid
food extractor
foot
    f. holder
    f. stool
footplate, foot plate
    f. chisel
    f. elevator
    f. hook
    f. pick
foramen-plugging forceps
Forbes
    F. eosphageal speculum
    F. uterine-dressing forceps
force fulcrum retractor
forceps
    Abbott-Mayfield f.
    Abernaz strut f.
    abscess f.
    Absolok f.
    Acland microvascular clamp-
      applying f.
    ACMI f.
    ACMI Martin f.
    ACMI Martin endoscopy f.
    Acufex curved basket f.
    Acufex rotary basket f.
    Acufex straight f.
    Acufex straight basket f.
    Adair f.
    Adair-Allis f.
    Adair-Allis tissue f.
    Adair breast tenaculum f.
    Adair breast tissue
      tenaculum f.
    Adair tenaculum f.
    Adair tissue f.
    Adair tissue-holding f.
    Adair uterine f.
    Adair uterine tenaculum f.
    adenoid f.
    Adler f.
    Adler bone f.
    Adler-Kreutz f.
    Adler punch f.

adnexal f.
Adson f.
Adson arterial f.
Adson bayonet dressing f.
Adson-Biemer f.
Adson bipolar f.
Adson brain f.
Adson-Brown f.
Adson-Brown tissue f.
Adson-Callison f.
Adson-Callison tissue f.
Adson clip-applying f.
Adson clip-introducing f.
Adson cranial rongeur f.
Adson dressing f.
Adson drill guide f.
Adson hemostatic f.
Adson hypophyseal f.
Adson-Mixter f.
Adson-Mixter neursurgical f.
Adson monopolar f.
Adson scalp clip-applying f.
Adson straight bipolar f.
Adson thumb f.
Adson tissue f.
Adson tooth f.
Adson Vital tissue f.
advancement f.
Aesculap f.
Akins valve re-do f.
Alabama University f.
Alabama University
  utility f.
Alderkreutz f.
Alderkreutz tissue f.
Alexander dressing f.
Alexander-Farabeuf f.
Allen f.
Allen intestinal f.
Allen intestinal
  anastomosis f.
Allen uterine f.
alligator f.
alligator crimper f.
alligator ear f.
alligator grasping f.
alligator jaws f.
alligator nasal f.
Allis f.
Allis-Abramson breast
  biopsy f.
Allis-Adair f.
Allis-Adair intestinal f.

Allis-Adair tissue f.
Allis-Coakley f.
Allis-Coakley tonsillar f.
Allis-Coakley tonsil-seizing f.
Allis delicate tissue f.
Allis-Duval f.
Allis intestinal f.
Allis Micro-Line pediatric f.
Allis-Ochsner f.
Allis-Ochsner tissue f.
Allis-Ochsner tonsillar f.
Allis pediatric f.
Allis thoracic f.
Allis tissue f.
Allis tissue-holding f.
Allis-Willauer f.
Allis-Willauer tissue f.
Almeida f.
Alvis f.
Alvis fixation f.
Ambrose eye f.
Amdur lid f.
Amenabar capsular f.
AMO phacoemulsification
  lens-folder f.
anastomosis f.
Andrews f.
Andrews-Hartmann f.
Andrews-Hartmann
  rongeur f.
Andrews tonsillar f.
Andrews tonsil-seizing f.
aneurysm f.
Angell-James
  hypophysectomy f.
Angell-James punch f.
Angell-James reverse-action
  hypophysectomy f.
angiotribe f.
angled f.
angled stone f.
angled suture-carrying f.
angulated f.
Anis f.
Anis capsulotomy f.
Anis corneal f.
Anis corneoscleral f.
Anis intraocular lens f.
Anis microsurgical tying f.
Anis straight corneal f.
Anis tying f.
anterior f.
anterior capsule f.

forceps *(continued)*
anterior resection
  intestinal f.
anterior segment f.
Anthony-Fisher f.
antral f.
aortic f.
aortic aneurysm f.
aortic occlusion f.
Apfelbaum f.
Apfelbaum bipolar f.
applicator f.
applying f.
approximation f.
Archer f.
Archer splinter f.
Arrow articulation paper f.
Arrowsmith-Clerf pin-
  closing f.
Arrowsmith fixation f.
Arruga capsular f.
Arruga curved f.
Arruga curved capsular f.
Arruga-Gill f.
Arruga-McCool f.
Arruga-McCool capsular f.
Arruga tip f.
arterial f.
Arthro Force basket
  cutting f.
Arthur splinter f.
articulation paper f.
Artilk f.
Asch f.
Asch nasal-straightening f.
Asch septal f.
Asch septum-straightening f.
Ashby f.
Ashby fluoroscopic f.
Ashby fluoroscopic foreign
  body f.
Ash dental f.
Ash septum-straightening f.
ASSI f.
ASSI bipolar coagulating f.
Athens f.
atraumatic f.
atraumatic tissue f.
atraumatic visceral f.
aural f.
auricular appendage f.
Austin f.
Auto Suture f.

Autraugrip f.
Autraugrip tissue f.
Auvard-Zweifel f.
axis-traction f.
Ayers f.
Ayers chalazion f.
Azar intraocular f.
Azar lens f.
Azar lens-holding f.
Azar tying f.
Azar utility f.
Babcock f.
Babcock-Beasley f.
Babcock intestinal f.
Babcock lung-grasping f.
Babcock thoracic tissue f.
Babcock thoracic tissue-
  holding f.
Babcock tissue f.
Babcock Vital atraumatic f.
Babcock Vital intestinal f.
Babcock Vital tissue f.
baby Adson f.
baby Allis f.
baby Crile f.
baby dressing f.
baby hemostatic f.
baby intestinal tissue f.
baby Lane f.
baby Lane bone-holding f.
baby Mikulicz f.
baby Mixter f.
baby mosquito f.
baby Overholt f.
baby tissue f.
backbiting f.
Backhaus f.
Backhaus towel f.
Bacon f.
Bacon cranial f.
Bacon cranial rongeur f.
Baer f.
Baer bone-cutting f.
Bahnson-Brown f.
Bailey f.
Bailey aortic valve-cutting f.
Bailey chalazion f.
Bailey-Williamson f.
Bailey-Williamson
  obstetrical f.
Bainbridge f.
Bainbridge hemostatic f.
Bainbridge intestinal f.

Bainbridge resection f.
Bainbridge thyroid f.
Baird f.
Baird chalazion f.
Baker f.
Baker tissue f.
Ball f.
Ballantine f.
Ballantine hysterectomy f.
Ballantine-Peterson f.
Ballantine-Peterson
  hysterectomy f.
Ballenger f.
Ballenger-Foerster f.
Ballenger hysterectomy f.
Ballenger sponge f.
Ballenger sponge-holding f.
Ballenger tonsillar f.
Ballenger tonsil-seizing f.
Bane f.
Bane rongeur f.
Bangerter f.
Bangerter muscle f.
Bardeleben bone-holding f.
Bard-Parker f.
Bard-Parker transfer f.
Barkan f.
Barkan iris f.
Barlow f.
Barnes-Crile f.
Barnes-Crile hemostatic f.
Barnes-Hill f.
Barnes-Simpson f.
Barnes-Simpson obstetrical f.
Baron f.
Barraquer f.
Barraquer ciliary f.
Barraquer conjunctival f.
Barraquer corneal utility f.
Barraquer fixation f.
Barraquer-Katzin f.
Barraquer mosquito f.
Barraquerry cilia f.
Barraquer suture f.
Barraquer-Troutman f.
Barraquer-Troutman
  corneal f.
Barraquer-von Mandach
  clot f.
Barraya f.
Barraya tissue f.
Barrett f.
Barrett-Allen f.

Barrett-Allen placental f.
Barrett-Allen uterine f.
Barrett-Allen uterine-
  elevating f.
Barrett intestinal f.
Barrett lens f.
Barrett-Murphy f.
Barrett-Murphy intestinal f.
Barrett placental f.
Barrett tenacular f.
Barrett uterine tenaculum f.
Barrie-Jones f.
Barrie-Jones angled
  crocodile f.
Barron alligator f.
Barron seizing alligator
  hemorrhoidal f.
Barsky f.
Barton f.
Barton obstetrical f.
basket f.
basket-cutting f.
basket-punch f.
basket-type crushing f.
Bauer f.
Bauer dissecting f.
Bauer sponge f.
Baumberger f.
Baumgartner f.
Baum-Hecht f.
Baum-Hecht tarsorrhaphy f.
Bausch articulation paper f.
bayonet f.
bayonet bipolar f.
bayonet bipolar
  electrosurgical f.
bayonet molar f.
Bead f.
Bead ethmoidal f.
beaked cowhorn f.
bean f.
Beardsley f.
bearing-seating f.
Beasley-Babcock f.
Beasley-Babcock tissue f.
Beaupre f.
Beaupre ciliary f.
Beaupre epilation f.
Bechert f.
Bechert-McPherson angled
  tying f.
Bechert-McPherson tying f.
Beck f.

forceps *(continued)*
Beebe f.
Beebe hemostatic f.
Beebe wire-cutting f.
Beer f.
Beer ciliary f.
Behen ear f.
Behrend cystic duct f.
Bellucci f.
Bellucci ear f.
Benaron f.
Benaron scalp-rotating f.
Bengolea f.
Bengolea arterial f.
Bennell f.
Bennett ciliary f.
Bennett epilation f.
Berens f.
Berens capsular f.
Berens corneal transplant f.
Berens muscle f.
Berens muscle clamp f.
Berens muscle recession f.
Berens recession f.
Berger f.
Berger biopsy f.
Bergeron pillar f.
Bergh ciliary f.
Berghmann-Foerster
   sponge f.
Bergman f.
Bergman tissue f.
Berke f.
Berke ciliary f.
Berkeley f.
Berke ptosis f.
Bernard uterine f.
Berne f.
Berne nasal f.
Bernhard towel f.
Berry f.
Berry uterine-elevating f.
Best f.
Best common duct stone f.
Best gallstone f.
Best stone f.
Bettman-Noyes f.
Bevan f.
Bevan gallbladder f.
Bevan hemostatic f.
Beyer f.
Beyer rongeur f.
B-H f.

Bigelow f.
Billroth f.
Billroth tumor f.
Billroth uterine tumor f.
Bill traction handle f.
Binkhorst lens f.
biopsy f.
biopsy punch f.
biopsy specimen f.
bipolar f.
bipolar coagulating f.
bipolar coagulation-suction f.
bipolar coaptation f.
bipolar cutting f.
bipolar eye f.
bipolar irrigating f.
bipolar suction f.
bipolar transsphenoidal f.
Bircher-Ganske f.
Bircher-Ganske meniscal f.
Bireks dissecting f.
Birkett f.
Birkett hemostatic f.
Bishop-Harman f.
Bishop-Harman dressing f.
Bishop-Harman eye
   dressing f.
Bishop-Harman foreign
   body f.
Bishop-Harman iris f.
Bishop-Harman tissue f.
Bishop tendon tucker f.
Bishop tissue f.
biting f.
Björk diathermy f.
Björk-Stille diathermy f.
bladder f.
bladder specimen f.
Blade-Wilde ear f.
Blake f.
Blake dressing f.
Blake ear f.
Blake embolus f.
Blake gallstone f.
Blakesley f.
Blakesley ethmoidal f.
Blakesley septal f.
Blakesley septal bone f.
Blakesley septal
   compression f.
Blakesley-Wilde ear f.
Blakesley-Wilde nasal f.
Blalock f.

Blalock-Kleinert f.
Blanchard f.
Blanchard hemorrhoidal f.
Bland cervical traction f.
Bland vulsellum f.
Blaydes f.
Blaydes angled-lens f.
Blaydes corneal f.
Blaydes lens-holding f.
Block-Potts intestinal f.
Blohmka tonsillar f.
Bloodwell f.
Bloodwell-Brown f.
Bloodwell tissue f.
Bloodwell vascular f.
Bloodwell vascular tissue f.
Bloomberg lens f.
Blum f.
Blumenthal uterine
  dressing f.
Boer craniotomy f.
Boerma obstetrical f.
Boettcher f.
Boettcher arterial f.
Boettcher pulmonary
  artery f.
Boettcher-Schmidt f.
Boettcher tonsillar f.
Boettcher tonsillar artery f.
Boies f.
Boies cutting f.
Bolton f.
Bonaccolto f.
Bonaccolto capsule
  fragment f.
Bonaccolto jeweler's f.
Bonaccolto new cup jaws f.
Bonaccolto utility f.
Bonaccolto utility pickup f.
Bond f.
Bond placental f.
bone-biting f.
bone-cutting f.
bone-cutting double-action f.
bone-holding f.
bone-splitting f.
Bonn f.
Bonn European suturing f.
Bonney f.
Bonney tissue f.
Bonn iris f.
Bonn peripheral
  iridectomy f.

Bonn suturing f.
Bores f.
Bores corneal fixation f.
Bores U-shaped f.
Boston Lying-In cervical f.
Boston Lying-In cervical-
  grasping f.
Botvin f.
Botvin iris f.
Botvin vulsellum f.
Bovie coagulating f.
Bovino scleral-spreading f.
Bowen suction loose
  body f.
box-joint f.
Boys-Allis f.
Boys-Allis tissue f.
Boys-Allis tissue-holding f.
Bozeman f.
Bozeman-Douglas dressing f.
Bozeman dressing f.
Bozeman LR dressing f.
Bozeman LR packing f.
Bozeman LR uterine-
  dressing f.
Bozeman packing f.
Bozeman uterine f.
Bozeman uterine-dressing f.
Bozeman uterine-packing f.
B-P transfer f.
Braasch f.
Braasch bladder specimen f.
Bracken f.
Bracken fixation f.
Bracken-Forkas corneal f.
Bracken iris f.
Bracken scleral fixation f.
Bracken tissue-grasping f.
Bradford f.
Bradford thyroid f.
Bradford thyroid traction f.
Bradford thyroid traction
  vulsellum f.
brain f.
brain dressing f.
brain spatula f.
brain tissue f.
brain tumor f.
Braithwaite f.
Brand f.
Brand passing f.
Brand shunt-introducing f.
Brand tendon f.

forceps *(continued)*
 Brand tendon-holding f.
 Brand tendon-pulling f.
 Brand tendon-tunneling f.
 Braun f.
 Braun tenaculum f.
 Braun uterine tenaculum f.
 breast tenaculum f.
 Brenner f.
 Bridge f.
 Bridge deep-surgery f.
 Bridge hemostatic f.
 Bridge intestinal f.
 Brigham f.
 Brigham brain tumor f.
 Brigham dressing f.
 Brigham thumb tissue f.
 Brigham tissue f.
 broad-blade f.
 Brock biopsy f.
 bronchial f.
 bronchial biopsy f.
 bronchial-grasping f.
 bronchoscopic f.
 bronchoscopic biopsy f.
 bronchoscopic oval-cup
  biopsy f.
 bronchoscopic rotation f.
 bronchus f.
 bronchus-grasping f.
 Brophy f.
 Brophy dressing f.
 Brophy tissue f.
 Brown f.
 Brown-Adson f.
 Brown-Adson tissue f.
 Brown-Bahnson f.
 Brown-Bahnson bayonet f.
 Brown-Buerger f.
 Brown side-grasping f.
 Brown side-grasping tissue f.
 Brown-Swan f.
 Brown thoracic f.
 Brown tissue f.
 Broyles f.
 Broyles optical f.
 Bruening f.
 Bruening-Citelli f.
 Bruening cutting-tip f.
 Bruening ethmoid
  exenteration f.
 Bruening nasal-cutting
  septal f.
 Bruening septal f.
 Bruening f. stylet
 Brunner f.
 Brunner intestinal f.
 Brunner sigmoid
  anastomosis f.
 Brunner tissue f.
 Brunschwig f.
 Brunschwig arterial f.
 Brunschwig visceral f.
 Bryant nasal f.
 Buck foreign body f.
 Buerger-McCarthy f.
 Buerger-McCarthy bladder f.
 Buie f.
 Buie biopsy f.
 Buie rectal f.
 Buie specimen f.
 bulldog f.
 bulldog clamp-applying f.
 bullet f.
 Bumpus f.
 Bumpus specimen f.
 Bunim f.
 Bunim urethral f.
 Bunker f.
 Bunker modification of
  Jackson laryngeal f.
 Burch f.
 Burch biopsy f.
 Burford f.
 Burford coarctation f.
 Burnham f.
 Burnham biopsy f.
 Burns f.
 Burns bone f.
 Butler bayonet f.
 Cairns f.
 Cairns-Dandy hemostasis f.
 Cairns dissection f.
 Cairns hemostatic f.
 Calibri f.
 Callahan f.
 Callahan scleral fixation f.
 Callison-Adson tissue f.
 Campbell f.
 Campbell ligature-carrier f.
 Campbell ureteral f.
 Campbell ureteral
  catheter f.
 Campbell urethral
  catheter f.
 Cane f.

Cane bone-holding f.
cannulated f.
cannulated bronchoscopic f.
capsular f.
capsule fragment f.
capsule-grasping f.
capsulorrhexis f.
capsulotomy f.
caput f.
Carb-Bite tissue f.
carbide-jaw f.
Cardio-Grip iliac f.
Cardio-Grip tissue f.
cardiovascular f.
cardiovascular tissue f.
Cardona f.
Cardona corneal
  prosthesis f.
Cardona threading lens f.
Carlens f.
Carmalt f.
Carmalt arterial f.
Carmalt hemostatic f.
Carmalt hysterectomy f.
Carmalt splinter f.
Carmalt thoracic f.
Carmody f.
Carmody-Brophy f.
Carmody thumb tissue f.
Carmody tissue f.
carotid artery f.
Carrel hemostatic f.
Carrel mosquito f.
Carroll-Adson f.
Carroll-Adson dural f.
Carroll bone-holding f.
Carroll tendon-passing f.
Carroll tendon-pulling f.
cartilage f.
cartilage-holding f.
caruncle f.
Caspar f.
Caspar alligator f.
Cassidy-Brophy f.
Cassidy-Brophy dressing f.
Castaneda f.
Castaneda-Mixter f.
Castaneda suture tag f.
Castaneda vascular f.
Castroviejo f.
Castroviejo-Arruga f.
Castroviejo-Arruga
  capsular f.

Castroviejo bay f.
Castroviejo capsular f.
Castroviejo-Colibri f.
Castroviejo-Colibri corneal f.
Castroviejo corneoscleral f.
Castroviejo corneoscleral
  suture f.
Castroviejo cross-action
  capsule f.
Castroviejo fixation f.
Castroviejo-Furness corneal-
  holding f.
Castroviejo-Simpson f.
Castroviejo suture f.
Castroviejo transplant f.
Castroviejo transplant-
  grafting f.
Castroviejo tying f.
Catalano f.
Catalano capsular f.
Catalano corneoscleral f.
Catalano tying f.
catheter f.
catheter-introducing f.
Cavanaugh-Wells tonsillar f.
cephalic blade f.
cervical f.
cervical biopsy f.
cervical biopsy punch f.
cervical grasping f.
cervical hemostatic f.
cervical punch f.
cervical traction f.
cesarean f.
Chamberlen f.
Chamberlen obstetrical f.
Championnière f.
Chandler f.
Chandler iris f.
Chandler spinal-
  perforating f.
Chang bone-cutting f.
Chaput f.
Chaput tissue f.
Charnley f.
Charnley-Riches arterial f.
Charnley suture f.
Cheatle sterilizing f.
Cheron f.
Cheron dressing f.
Cheron uterine dressing f.
Cherry f.
Cherry-Adson f.

forceps *(continued)*
Cherry-Kerrison f.
Cherry-Kerrison laminectomy
  rongeur f.
Cherry-Kerrison rongeur f.
Chester f.
Chester sponge f.
Chevalier Jackson f.
Chevalier Jackson
  bronchoesophagoscopy f.
chicken-bill rongeur f.
Child f.
Child clip-applying f.
Child intestinal f.
Children's Hospital f.
Children's Hospital
  dressing f.
Children's Hospital
  intestinal f.
Childs-Phillips f.
Chimani pharyngeal f.
Choyce f.
Choyce intraocular lens f.
Choyce lens f.
Choyce lens-inserting f.
Christopher-Stille f.
Chubb tonsillar f.
Cicherelli f.
Cicherelli rongeur f.
Cilco lens f.
ciliary f.
cilia suture f.
circular cup bronchoscopic
  biopsy f.
Citelli f.
Citelli-Bruening ear f.
Citelli rongeur f.
Civiale f.
clamp f.
Clark f.
Clark capsule fragment f.
Clark-Guyton f.
Clark-Verhoeff f.
Clark-Verhoeff capsular f.
Clayman f.
Clayman corneal f.
Clayman-Kelman intraocular
  lens f.
Clayman lens f.
Clayman lens-holding f.
Clayman lens-inserting f.
Clayman-McPherson tying f.
Clayman suturing f.

cleft palate f.
Clemetson uterine f.
Clerf f.
Clevedent f.
Cleveland bone-cutting f.
clip f.
clip-applying f.
clip-applying f.
clip-applying aneurysm f.
clip-introducing f.
clip-removing f.
closed iris f.
closer f.
closing f.
clot f.
coagulating f.
coagulating-suction f.
coagulation f.
Coakley f.
Coakley-Allis f.
Coakley-Allis tonsillar f.
Coakley tonsillar f.
coaptation f.
coarctation f.
Cobaugh eye f.
Codman fallopian tube f.
Codman ovary f.
Cohan corneal f.
Cohan corneal utility f.
Cohen nasal-dressing f.
cold cup f.
cold cup biopsy f.
Colibri f.
Colibri corneal f.
Colibri corneal utility f.
Colibri eye f.
Colibri-Pierce f.
Colibri-Storz f.
Colibri-Storz corneal f.
College f.
Coller f.
Coller arterial f.
Coller hemostatic f.
Colley tissue f.
Colley traction f.
Collier f.
Collier-Crile f.
Collier-Crile hemostatic f.
Collier-DeBakey f.
Collier-DeBakey
  hemostatic f.
Collier hemostatic f.
Collin f.

Collin dressing f.
Collin-Duval f.
Collin-Duval-Crile
  intestinal f.
Collin-Duval intestinal f.
Collin intestinal f.
Collin lung-grasping f.
Collin mucous f.
Collin ovarian f.
Collin-Pozzi uterine f.
Collin tissue f.
Collin tongue f.
Collin tongue-seizing f.
Collin uterine-elevating f.
Collis f.
Collis-Maumenee corneal f.
Collis micro-utility f.
Coloviras-Rummel
  thoracic f.
Colver f.
Colver-Coakley f.
Colver-Coakley tonsillar f.
Colver tonsillar f.
Colver tonsillar pillar-
  grasping f.
Colver tonsil-seizing f.
common duct-holding f.
common duct stone f.
common McPherson f.
compression f.
Cone f.
Cone wire-twisting f.
conjunctival f.
conjunctival fixation f.
connector f.
Cook flexible biopsy f.
Cooley f.
Cooley anastomosis f.
Cooley aortic f.
Cooley arterial occlusion f.
Cooley auricular
  appendage f.
Cooley-Baumgarten aortic f.
Cooley cardiovascular f.
Cooley coarctation f.
Cooley CSR f.
Cooley curved f.
Cooley-Derra anastomosis f.
Cooley double-angled jaw f.
Cooley graft f.
Cooley iliac f.
Cooley multipurpose f.
Cooley neonatal vascular f.

Cooley patent ductus f.
Cooley pediatric aortic f.
Cooley peripheral
  vascular f.
Cooley tangential f.
Cooley tangential
  pediatric f.
Cooley tissue f.
Cooley vascular f.
Cooley vascular tissue f.
Cope lung f.
Coppridge f.
Coppridge grasping f.
Coppridge urethral f.
Corbett f.
Corbett bone-cutting f.
Cordes f.
Cordes esophagoscopy f.
Cordes-New f.
Cordes-New laryngeal
  punch f.
Corey f.
Corey ovum f.
Corey placental f.
Corgill-Hartmann f.
cornea-holding f.
corneal f.
corneal transplant f.
corneal utility f.
cornea-suturing f.
corneoscleral f.
corneoscleral suturing f.
Cornet f.
coronary f.
coronary artery f.
Corwin f.
Corwin tonsillar f.
Corwin tonsillar
  hemostatic f.
Cottle f.
Cottle-Arruga f.
Cottle-Arruga cartilage f.
Cottle biting f.
Cottle insertion f.
Cottle-Jansen f.
Cottle-Jansen rongeur f.
Cottle-Kazanjian f.
Cottle-Kazanjian bone-
  cutting f.
Cottle-Kazanjian cutting f.
Cottle-Kazanjian nasal f.
Cottle-Kazanjian nasal-
  cutting f.

forceps *(continued)*

Cottle lower lateral f.
Cottle tissue f.
Cottle-Walsham f.
Cottle-Walsham septum-
straightening f.
cowhorn tooth-extracting f.
Cozean angled lens f.
Cozean bipolar f.
Cozean implantation f.
Cozean-McPherson angled
lens f.
Cozean-McPherson tying f.
Crafoord f.
Crafoord arterial f.
Crafoord bronchial f.
Crafoord coarctation f.
Crafoord pulmonary f.
Crafoord-Sellor hemostatic f.
Craig f.
Craig nasal-cutting f.
Craig septal f.
Craig septum bone-cutting f.
Craig tonsil-seizing f.
cranial f.
cranial rongeur f.
cranium clip-applying f.
Crawford fascial f.
Crawford-Knighton f.
Creevy biopsy f.
Crenshaw f.
Crenshaw caruncle f.
Crile f.
Crile arterial f.
Crile-Barnes hemostatic f.
Crile-Duval lung-grasping f.
Crile gall duct f.
Crile hemostatic f.
Crile Micro-Line arterial f.
crimper f.
crimper closer f.
crimping f.
Crockard ligament
grasping f.
Crockard odontoid peg-
grasping f.
crocodile f.
crocodile biopsy f.
cross-action f.
Crossen puncturing
tenaculum f.
crural nipper f.
Cryer Universal f.

CSF shunt connector f.
CSF shunt-introducing f.
Cukier nasal f.
Culler eye f.
Culler fixation f.
Cullom septal f.
cup f.
cup biopsy f.
cup-biting f.
cup jaw rongeur f.
cupped f.
cupped jaw f.
cup-shaped f.
cup-shaped curette f.
cup-shaped ear f.
cup-shaped inner ear f.
cup-shaped middle ear f.
curette f.
Curtis f.
Curtis tissue f.
curved f.
curved-tip jeweler's
bipolar f.
curved tying f.
Cushing f.
Cushing bayonet tissue f.
Cushing bipolar f.
Cushing bipolar
neurosurgical f.
Cushing brain f.
Cushing-Brown f.
Cushing-Brown tissue f.
Cushing cranial rongeur f.
Cushing decompression f.
Cushing dressing f.
Cushing dressing f.
Cushing-Gutsch dressing f.
Cushing-Gutsch tissue f.
Cushing intervertebral
disk f.
Cushing Micro Bipolar
neurosurgical f.
Cushing monopolar f.
Cushing-Taylor carbide-
jaw f.
Cushing thumb f.
Cushing tissue f.
Cushing Vital tissue f.
Cutler f.
cutting f.
cylindrical-object f.
cystic duct f.
cystoscopic f.

Czerny f.
Czerny tenaculum f.
Dahlgren-Hudson f.
Dahlgren-Hudson cranial f.
Dahlgren skill-cutting f.
Daicoff needle-pulling f.
Daicoff vascular f.
Dale f.
Dale femoral-popliteal
  anastomosis f.
D'Allesandro serial suture-
  holding f.
Danberg f.
Danberg iris f.
Dan chalazion f.
Dandy f.
Dandy arterial f.
Dandy hemostatic f.
Dandy-Kolodny
  hemostatic f.
Dandy scalp f.
Dandy scalp hemostatic f.
Dan-Gradle ciliary f.
Dartigues kidney-elevating f.
Dartigues uterine-elevating f.
Davidson f.
Davidson pulmonary
  vessel f.
Davis f.
Davis bayonet f.
Davis capsular f.
Davis coagulating f.
Davis diathermy f.
Davis monopolar f.
Davis monopolar bayonet f.
Davis sterilizing f.
Davis thoracic tissue f.
Davol f.
Davol rongeur f.
Dawson-Yuhl-Kerrison
  rongeur f.
Dawson-Yuhl-Leksell
  rongeur f.
Dawson-Yuhl rongeur f.
De Alvarez f.
Dean f.
Dean-Shallcross tonsil-
  seizing f.
Dean tonsillar f.
Dean tonsillar hemostatic f.
DeBakey f.
DeBakey aortic f.
DeBakey Autraugrip f.

DeBakey-Bahnson f.
DeBakey-Bainbridge f.
DeBakey-Bainbridge
  vascular f.
DeBakey-Beck
  multipurpose f.
DeBakey-Colovira-Rumel
  thoracic f.
DeBakey-Cooley f.
DeBakey-Cooley
  cardiovascular f.
DeBakey-Derra
  anastomosis f.
DeBakey-Diethrich coronary
  artery f.
DeBakey-Diethrich
  vascular f.
DeBakey-Diethrick f.
DeBakey dissecting f.
DeBakey-Kelly hemostatic f.
DeBakey-Liddicoat
  vascular f.
DeBakey-Mixter thoracic f.
DeBakey multipurpose f.
DeBakey-Péan
  cardiovascular f.
DeBakey-Rankin
  hemostatic f.
DeBakey-Reynolds
  anastomosis f.
DeBakey-Rumel thoracic f.
DeBakey-Semb f.
DeBakey-Semb ligature-
  carrying f.
DeBakey tangential
  occlusion f.
DeBakey thoracic f.
DeBakey thoracic tissue f.
DeBakey tissue f.
DeBakey vascular f.
Decker f.
Decker microsurgical f.
Deddish-Potts intestinal f.
deep-surgery f.
deep-vessel f.
Defourmental f.
Defourmental rongeur f.
DeLee f.
DeLee cervical f.
DeLee cervix-holding f.
DeLee dressing f.
DeLee obstetrical f.
DeLee ovum f.

forceps *(continued)*
    DeLee shuttle f.
    DeLee-Simpson f.
    DeLee spoon tissue f.
    DeLee uterine f.
    DeLee uterine-packing f.
    delicate f.
    delicate thumb dressing f.
    Delrin locking handle f.
    Demarest f.
    Demarest septal f.
    DeMartel f.
    DeMartel appendix f.
    DeMartel scalp f.
    DeMartel scalp flap f.
    DeMartel-Wolfson f.
    DeMartel-Wolfson closing f.
    DeMartel-Wolfson intestinal-closing f.
    DeMartel-Wolfson intestinal-holding f.
    Demel f.
    Demel wire-tightening f.
    Demel wire-twisting f.
    Dench f.
    Dench ear f.
    Denis Browne f.
    Dennis f.
    Dennis intestinal f.
    dental f.
    dental dressing f.
    depilatory dermal f.
    Derf f.
    Derra f.
    Derra cardiovascular f.
    Derra-Cooley f.
    Derra urethral f.
    D'Errico f.
    D'Errico dressing f.
    D'Errico hypophyseal f.
    D'Errico tissue f.
    Desjardins f.
    Desjardins gallstone f.
    Desjardins kidney pedicle f.
    Desmarres f.
    Desmarres chalazion f.
    Desmarres lid f.
    DeTakats-McKenzie f.
    DeTakats-McKenzie brain clip-applying f.
    DeTakats-McKenzie clip-applying f.
    DeVilbiss f.
    DeVilbiss cranial f.
    DeVilbiss rongeur f.
    DeWecker f.
    DeWeese axis traction f.
    DeWeese axis traction obstetrical f.
    Dewey f.
    Dewey obstetrical f.
    Diaflex grasping f.
    diathermic f.
    diathermy f.
    Dieffenbach f.
    Diener f.
    Dieter f.
    Dieter malleus f.
    Diethrich right-angled hemostatic f.
    dilating f.
    Dingman f.
    Dingman bone-holding f.
    disimpaction f.
    disk f.
    diskectomy f.
    disposable f.
    dissecting f.
    dissection f.
    divergent outlet f.
    Dixon flamingo f.
    Dixon-Lovelace f.
    Dixon-Lovelace hemostatic f.
    Dixon-Thorpe f.
    Dixon-Thorpe vitreous foreign body f.
    Docktor f.
    Docktor needle f.
    Docktor suture f.
    Docktor tissue f.
    Dodick lens-holding f.
    Dodrill f.
    Donberg iris f.
    donor button f.
    Dorsey f.
    Dorsey bayonet f.
    double-action bone-cutting f.
    double-action hump f.
    double-action rongeur f.
    double-articulated bronchoscopic f.
    double-concave f.
    double-concave rat-tooth f.
    double-cupped f.
    double-ended needle f.

double-ended suture f.
double-ended tissue f.
double-fixation f.
double-spoon f.
Douglas f.
Douglas ciliary f.
Douglas eye f.
Doyen f.
Doyen gallbladder f.
Doyen intestinal f.
Doyen towel f.
Doyen uterine f.
Doyen uterine vulsellum f.
Doyen vulsellum f.
dressing f.
Drews f.
Drews ciliary f.
Drews intraocular f.
Dreyfus prosthesis f.
drill guide f.
duckbill f.
Duguid curved f.
dull-pointed f.
dull rotation f.
Dumont f.
Dumont dissecting f.
Dumont jeweler's f.
Dumont Swiss dissecting f.
Dunhill f.
Duplay tenaculum f.
Duplay uterine tenaculum f.
dural f.
Durogrip f.
Duval f.
Duval-Allis f.
Duval-Collin intestinal f.
Duval-Crile f.
Duval-Crile intestinal f.
Duval-Crile lung f.
Duval-Crile lung-grasping f.
Duval-Crile tissue f.
Duval intestinal f.
Duval lung f.
Duval lung-grasping f.
Duval lung tissue f.
Duval tissue f.
Duval Vital intestinal f.
ear f.
ear-dressing f.
ear-grasping f.
ear polyp f.
ear punch f.
Eastman f.

Eastman cystic duct f.
Eber f.
Echlin rongeur f.
Ecker-Kazanjian f.
Eckhoff f.
Eder f.
Edna towel f.
Effler-Groves f.
Effler-Groves
  cardiovascular f.
Ehrhardt f.
Ehrhardt lid f.
Eisenstein f.
Eisenstein hysterectomy f.
electrocoagulating biopsy f.
electrosurgical biopsy f.
elevating f.
Elliott f.
Elliott gallbladder f.
Elliott hemostatic f.
Elliott obstetrical f.
Elschnig f.
Elschnig capsular f.
Elschnig cyclodialysis f.
Elschnig fixation f.
Elschnig-O'Brien f.
Elschnig-O'Brien fixation f.
Elschnig-O'Brien tissue-
  grasping f.
Elschnig-O'Connor f.
Elschnig-O'Connor
  fixation f.
Elschnig secondary
  membrane f.
Elschnig tissue-grasping f.
Emmet f.
Emmet obstetrical f.
endometrial f.
endometrial polyp f.
endoscopic biopsy f.
endoscopic grasping f.
endoscopic suture-cutting f.
endospeculum f.
endotracheal catheter f.
endotracheal tube f.
Endura dressing f.
English f.
English tissue f.
Ennis f.
entropion f.
epilation f.
episcleral f.
Eppendorfer biopsy f.

forceps *(continued)*
    Eppendorfer biopsy punch f.
    Eppendorfer cervical
      biopsy f.
    Ergo bipolar f.
    Erhardt f.
    Erhardt eyelid f.
    Erhardt lid f.
    Erich f.
    Erich biopsy f.
    Erich laryngeal biopsy f.
    E-Series f.
    E-Series bipolar f.
    esophageal f.
    esophagoscopic f.
    Essrig f.
    Essrig tissue f.
    ethmoidal f.
    ethmoid-cutting f.
    Ethridge f.
    Ethridge hysterectomy f.
    Evans f.
    Evans tissue f.
    Evans Vital tissue f.
    Everett f.
    Ewald f.
    Ewald-Hudson brain f.
    Ewald-Hudson dressing f.
    Ewald-Hudson tissue f.
    Ewald tissue f.
    Ewing f.
    Ewing capsular f.
    exenteration f.
    exolever f.
    extracapsular eye f.
    extracting f.
    eye f.
    eye-dressing f.
    eye-fixation f.
    eyelid f.
    eye needle holder f.
    eye suture f.
    Facit uterine polyp f.
    Falcao fixation f.
    Falk f.
    Falk lion-jaw f.
    fallopian tube f.
    Farabeuf f.
    Farabeuf bone-holding f.
    Farabeuf-Lambotte f.
    Farabeuf-Lambotte bone f.
    Farabeuf-Lambotte bone-
      holding f.

Farnham f.
Farnham nasal-cutting f.
Farrington f.
Farrington nasal polyp f.
Farrington septal f.
Farrior f.
Farrior wire-crimping f.
Farris tissue f.
Faure f.
Faure biopsy f.
Faure peritoneal f.
Faure uterine biopsy f.
Fauvel f.
Fauvel laryngeal f.
Fehland intestinal f.
Feilchenfeld f.
Feilchenfeld splinter f.
fenestrated f.
fenestrated blade f.
fenestrated cup biopsy f.
Ferguson f.
Ferguson angiotribe f.
Ferguson bone-holding f.
Ferguson tenaculum f.
Ferris f.
Ferris colporrhaphy f.
Ferris Smith f.
Ferris Smith bone-biting f.
Ferris Smith cup-jaw
  rongeur f.
Ferris Smith cup rongeur f.
Ferris Smith fragment f.
Ferris Smith-Kerrison
  rongeur f.
Ferris Smith-Spurling
  intervertebral disk f.
Ferris Smith-Takahashi f.
Ferris Smith tissue f.
Fichman suture-cutting f.
fine f.
fine arterial f.
Fine-Castroviejo f.
Fine-Castroviejo suturing f.
fine-dissecting f.
Fine suture-tying f.
fine-tissue f.
fine-tooth f.
Fink f.
Fink fixation f.
Fink-Jameson f.
Fink-Jameson oblique
  muscle f.
Fink tendon-tucker f.

Finochietto f.
Finochietto lobectomy f.
Finochietto thoracic f.
Fischl f.
Fischl dissecting f.
Fischmann angiotribe f.
Fish f.
Fisher f.
Fisher advancement f.
Fisher-Arlt f.
Fisher-Arlt iris f.
Fisher capsular f.
Fisher iris f.
Fish grasping f.
Fish nasal f.
Fish nasal-dressing f.
Fish nasal-grasping f.
Fitzgerald f.
Fitzgerald aortic
  aneurysm f.
Fitzwater f.
Fitzwater peanut sponge-
  holding f.
fixation f.
flamingo f.
flamingo antrostomy f.
Fletcher f.
Fletcher dressing f.
Fletcher sponge f.
Fletcher-Suit polyp f.
Fletcher-Van Doren f.
Fletcher-Van Doren sponge-
  holding f.
Fletcher-Van Doren
  uterine f.
Fletcher-Van Doren uterine
  polyp f.
flexible foreign body f.
flexible optical biopsy f.
fluoroscopic foreign body f.
Foerster f.
Foerster-Ballenger f.
Foerster-Bauer sponge-
  holding f.
Foerster eye f.
Foerster eye f.
Foerster gallbladder f.
Foerster iris f.
Foerster-Mueller f.
Foerster sponge f.
Foerster sponge-holding f.
Foerster tissue f.
Foerster uterine f.

Foerster-Van Doren sponge-
  holding f.
Fogarty f.
Fogarty bulldog clamp-
  applying f.
Foley f.
Foley vas isolation f.
foramen-plugging f.
Forbes uterine-dressing f.
foreign body f.
foreign body cystoscopy f.
foreign body eye f.
forward-grasping f.
Foss f.
Foss cardiovascular f.
Foss clamp f.
Foss intestinal clamp f.
Foster-Ballenger f.
Fox bipolar f.
Fox tissue f.
fragment f.
Francis f.
Francis chalazion f.
Frangenheim f.
Frangenheim biopsy
  punch f.
Frangenheim hook f.
Fränkel f.
Fränkel cutting-tip f.
Fränkel double-articulated-
  tip f.
Fränkel esophagoscopy f.
Fränkel laryngeal f.
Fränkel tampon f.
Frankfeldt f.
Frankfeldt grasping f.
Fraser f.
Freer-Gruenwald f.
Freer-Gruenwald punch f.
Freer septal f.
French-pattern f.
Fricke arterial f.
Friedman rongeur f.
Friedman taper-jaw
  rongeur f.
Fry nasal f.
Fuchs f.
Fuchs capsular f.
Fuchs capsulotomy f.
Fuchs extracapsular f.
Fuchs iris f.
Fujinon f.
Fujinon biopsy f.

forceps *(continued)*
    Fulpit f.
    Fulpit tissue f.
    Furness f.
    Furness cornea-holding f.
    Furness polyp f.
    Gabriel Tucker f.
    galeal f.
    gallbladder f.
    gall duct f.
    gallstone f.
    Gambale-Merrill bone-cutting f.
    Gam-Mer bone-cutting f.
    Gardner hysterectomy f.
    Garland f.
    Garland hysterectomy f.
    Garrigue f.
    Garrigue uterine-dressing f.
    Garrison f.
    Gaskin fragment f.
    gastrointestinal f.
    Gauss hemostatic f.
    Gavin-Miller f.
    Gavin-Miller colon f.
    Gavin-Miller intestinal f.
    Gavin-Miller tissue f.
    Gaylor f.
    Gaylor biopsy f.
    Gaylor uterine biopsy f.
    Gaylor uterine specimen f.
    Geissendorfer f.
    Geissendorfer uterine f.
    Gelfilm f.
    Gelfoam f.
    Gelfoam pressure f.
    Gellhorn f.
    Gellhorn biopsy punch f.
    Gellhorn uterine biopsy f.
    Gelpi f.
    Gelpi hysterectomy f.
    Gelpi-Lowrie f.
    Gelpi-Lowrie hysterectomy f.
    Gemini f.
    Gemini gall duct f.
    Gemini hemostatic f.
    Gemini Mixter f.
    Gemini thoracic f.
    general tissue f.
    general wire f.
    Gerald f.
    Gerald Bayonet microbipolar neurosurgical f.
    Gerald bipolar f.
    Gerald brain f.
    Gerald dressing f.
    Gerald straight microbipolar neurosurgical f.
    Gerald tissue f.
    Gerbode f.
    Gerbode cardiovascular tissue f.
    GI f.
    GIA f.
    Gifford f.
    Gifford fixation f.
    Gifford iris f.
    Gilbert f.
    Gilbert cystic duct f.
    Gill f.
    Gill-Chandler iris f.
    Gill curved iris f.
    Gillespie obstetrical f.
    Gill-Fuchs f.
    Gill-Fuchs capsular f.
    Gill-Hess f.
    Gill-Hess iris f.
    Gillies f.
    Gillies dissecting f.
    Gillies tissue f.
    Gill incision-spreading f.
    Gill iris f.
    Gillquist-Oretorp-Stille f.
    Gill-Safar f.
    Gill-Welsh capsular f.
    Ginsberg f.
    Ginsberg tissue f.
    Girard f.
    Girard corneoscleral f.
    Glassman f.
    Glassman-Allis f.
    Glassman-Allis common duct-holding f.
    Glassman-Allis intestinal f.
    Glassman-Allis miniature intestinal f.
    Glassman-Allis noncrushing common duct f.
    Glassman-Allis noncrushing intestinal f.
    Glassman-Allis noncrushing tissue-holding f.
    Glassman-Babcock f.
    Glassman noncrushing pickup f.
    Glassman pickup f.

Glenn diverticular f.
Glenner f.
Glenner hysterectomy f.
Glenner vaginal
  hysterectomy f.
globular object f.
Glover f.
Glover anastomosis f.
Glover coarctation f.
Glover curved f.
Glover infundibular
  rongeur f.
Glover patent ductus f.
Glover rongeur f.
Glover spoon-shaped f.
goiter f.
goiter-seizing f.
goiter vulsellum f.
Gold f.
Gold deep-surgery f.
Gold hemostatic f.
Goldman-Kazanjian f.
Goldman-Kazanjian nasal f.
Gomco f.
Good f.
Goodhill f.
Goodhill tonsillar f.
Goodhill tonsillar artery f.
Goodhill tonsillar
  hemostatic f.
Good obstetrical f.
Goodyear-Gruenwald f.
Gordon f.
Gordon bead f.
Gordon ciliary f.
Gordon uterine f.
Gordon uterine vulsellum f.
Gordon vulsellum f.
Gradle f.
Gradle ciliary f.
Graefe f.
Graefe curved iris f.
Graefe dressing f.
Graefe eye f.
Graefe eye-dressing f.
Graefe eye-fixation f.
Graefe fixation f.
Graefe iris f.
Graefe nonmagnetic
  fixation f.
Graefe straight iris f.
Graefe tissue f.
Graefe tissue-grasping f.

Grafco Halsted f.
grasping f.
grasping biopsy f.
grasping tripod f.
Gray f.
Gray arterial f.
Gray cystic duct f.
Gray gall duct f.
Grayton f.
Grayton corneal f.
Grazer blepharoplasty f.
Green f.
Green-Armytage f.
Green-Armytage
  hemostatic f.
Green chalazion f.
Greene tube-holding f.
Green fixation f.
Green suction tube f.
Green tissue-grasping f.
Greenwood f.
Greenwood bipolar f.
Greenwood bipolar
  coagulation-suction f.
Greenwood coagulation f.
Gregory f.
Greven alligator f.
Grey Turner f.
Grieshaber f.
Grieshaber iris f.
Griffiths-Brown f.
grooved tying f.
Gross f.
Gross dressing f.
Gross hyoid-cutting f.
Gross sponge f.
Grotting f.
Gruenwald f.
Gruenwald bayonet-
  dressing f.
Gruenwald-Bryant f.
Gruenwald-Bryant nasal f.
Gruenwald-Bryant nasal-
  cutting f.
Gruenwald dissecting f.
Gruenwald dressing f.
Gruenwald Durogrip f.
Gruenwald ear f.
Gruenwald-Jansen f.
Gruenwald-Love f.
Gruenwald-Love
  neurosurgical f.
Gruenwald nasal-cutting f.

forceps *(continued)*

Gruenwald nasal-dressing f.
Gruenwald tissue f.
Gruppe f.
Gruppe wire-crimping f.
Gruppe wire prosthesis-
crimping f.
Guggenheim adenoidal f.
guide f.
Guilford-Wright f.
guillotome f.
Guist f.
Guist fixation f.
Gunderson muscle f.
Gunderson recession f.
Gunnar-Hey roller f.
Gusberg uterine f.
Gutgemann auricular
appendage f.
Gutglass f.
Gutglass cervix
hemostatic f.
Gutglass hemostatic
cervical f.
Gutierrez-Najar grasping f.
Guyton f.
Guyton-Clark f.
Guyton-Clark capsule
fragment f.
Guyton-Noyes f.
Guyton-Noyes fixation f.
Guyton suturing f.
Haberer gastrointestinal f.
Haberer-Gili f.
Haberer intestinal f.
Hagenbarth clip f.
Hagenbarth clip-applying f.
Haig Ferguson obstetrical f.
Haig obstetrical f.
Hajek f.
Hajek antral punch f.
Hajek-Koffler f.
Hajek-Koffler sphenoidal f.
Hakler f.
Hale f.
Hale obstetrical f.
Halifax placement f.
Hallberg f.
hallux f.
Halsey f.
Halsey mosquito f.
Halsted f.
Halsted arterial f.
Halsted curved mosquito f.
Halsted hemostatic f.
Halsted Micro-Line
arterial f.
Halsted mosquito
hemostatic f.
Halsted-Swanson tendon-
passing f.
Hamby f.
Hamby clip-applying f.
Hamilton f.
Hamilton deep-surgery f.
hammer f.
Hank-Dennen obstretical f.
Hannahan f.
Hardy Bayonet neurosurgical
bipolar f.
Hardy bipolar f.
Hardy dressing f.
Hardy microbipolar f.
harelip f.
Harken f.
Harken cardiovascular f.
Harken-Cooley f.
Harman f.
Harman fixation f.
Harms f.
Harms microtying f.
Harms suture-tying f.
Harms-Tubingen f.
Harms-Tubingen tying f.
Harms tying f.
Harms utility f.
Harms vessel f.
Harrington f.
Harrington clamp f.
Harrington lung-grasping f.
Harrington-Mayo f.
Harrington-Mayo tissue f.
Harrington-Mixter f.
Harrington-Mixter clamp f.
Harrington-Mixter
thoracic f.
Harrington thoracic f.
Harrington thoracic
clamp f.
Harrington vulsellum f.
Harris f.
Harris angled suture-
carrying f.
Harris suture-carrying f.
Hartmann f.
Hartmann alligator f.

Hartmann-Citelli f.
Hartmann-Citelli alligator f.
Hartmann-Citelli ear
  punch f.
Hartmann-Corgill ear f.
Hartmann ear f.
Hartmann ear-dressing f.
Hartmann ear polyp f.
Hartmann-Gruenwald
  nasal f.
Hartmann-Gruenwald nasal-
  cutting f.
Hartmann hemostatic f.
Hartmann-Herzfeld f.
Hartmann-Herzfeld ear f.
Hartmann mosquito f.
Hartmann mosquito
  hemostatic f.
Hartmann nasal-cutting f.
Hartmann nasal-dressing f.
Hartmann nasal polyp f.
Hartmann-Noyes nasal-
  dressing f.
Hartmann-Proctor ear f.
Hartmann tonsillar punch f.
Hartmann uterine biopsy f.
Hartmann-Weingärtner ear f.
Hartmann-Wullstein f.
Hartmann-Wullstein ear f.
Haslinger tip f.
Hawk-Dennen f.
Hawkins f.
Hawkins cervical biopsy f.
Hawks-Dennen f.
Hawks-Dennen obstetrical f.
Hayes anterior resection f.
Hayes anterior resection
  intestinal f.
Hayes Martin f.
Hayes-Olivecrona f.
Hayes-Olivecrona clip f.
Hayton-Williams f.
Healy f.
Healy gastrointestinal f.
Healy intestinal f.
Healy suture-removing f.
Healy uterine biopsy f.
Heaney f.
Heaney hysterectomy f.
Heaney-Kantor f.
Heaney-Kantor
  hysterectomy f.
Heaney-Rezek f.

Heaney-Simon f.
Heaney-Simon
  hysterectomy f.
Heaney-Stumf f.
Heaney tissue f.
Heath f.
Heath chalazion f.
Heath clip-removing f.
Heath nasal f.
Hecht fascia lata f.
Heermann f.
Heermann alligator f.
Heermann alligator ear f.
Heermann ear f.
Hegenbarth f.
Hegenbarth clip f.
Hegenbarth clip-applying f.
Hegenbarth-Michel clip-
  applying f.
Hegenbarth wound clip-
  applying f.
Heidelberg f.
Heidelberg fixation f.
Heiming kidney stone f.
Heiss f.
Heiss arterial f.
Heiss hemostatic f.
Heiss vulsellum f.
Heller biopsy f.
hemoclip-applying f.
hemorrhoidal f.
hemostatic f.
hemostatic cervical f.
hemostatic neurosurgical f.
hemostatic tissue f.
hemostatic tonsillar f.
hemostatic tracheal f.
hemostatis clip-applying f.
Hendren f.
Hendren cardiovascular f.
Hendren pediatric f.
Henke f.
Henke punch f.
Henrotin f.
Henrotin uterine
  vulsellum f.
Henrotin vulsellum f.
Henry ciliary f.
Herff f.
Herff membrane-
  puncturing f.
Herget f.
Herget biopsy f.

forceps *(continued)*
   Herman f.
   Hermann bone-holding f.
   Herrick f.
   Herrick kidney f.
   Herrick kidney pedicle f.
   Hertel f.
   Hertel kidney stone f.
   Hertel rigid dilator stone f.
   Hertel rigid kidney stone f.
   Hertel stone f.
   Herzfeld f.
   Herzfeld ear f.
   Herz meniscal f.
   Herz tendon f.
   Hess f.
   Hess-Barraquer f.
   Hess-Barraquer iris f.
   Hessburg lens f.
   Hessburg lens-inserting f.
   Hess capsular f.
   Hess capsular iris f.
   Hess-Gill f.
   Hess-Gill eye f.
   Hess-Gill iris f.
   Hess-Horwitz f.
   Hess-Horwitz iris f.
   Hess iris f.
   Hevesy polyp f.
   Heyman f.
   Heyman-Knight nasal dressing f.
   Heyman nasal f.
   Heyman nasal-cutting f.
   Heywood-Smith dressing f.
   Heywood-Smith gallbladder f.
   Heywood-Smith sponge-holding f.
   Hibbs f.
   Hibbs biting f.
   Hibbs bone-cutting f.
   Hibbs bone-holding f.
   high f.
   Hildebrandt uterine f.
   Hildebrandt uterine hemostatic f.
   Hildyard f.
   Hildyard nasal f.
   Himalaya dressing f.
   Hinderer cartilage f.
   Hinderer cartilage-holding f.
   Hirschman f.

   Hirschman hemorrhoidal f.
   Hirschman jeweler's f.
   Hirschman lens f.
   Hirschman lens-inserting f.
   Hirst f.
   Hirst-Emmet obstetrical f.
   Hirst-Emmet placental f.
   Hirst obstetrical f.
   Hodge f.
   Hodge obstetrical f.
   Hoen f.
   Hoen alligator f.
   Hoen bayonet f.
   Hoen dressing f.
   Hoen grasping f.
   Hoen hemostatic f.
   Hoen scalp f.
   Hoen scalp hemostatic f.
   Hoen tissue f.
   Hoffmann f.
   Hoffmann ear f.
   Hoffmann ear punch f.
   Hoffmann-Pollock f.
   holding f.
   Holinger f.
   Holinger specimen f.
   hollow-object f.
   Holmes f.
   Holmes fixation f.
   Holth f.
   Holth punch f.
   Holzbach f.
   Holzbach hysterectomy f.
   hook f.
   Hopkins f.
   Hopkins aortic f.
   Horsley f.
   Horsley bone-cutting f.
   Horsley-Stille bone-cutting f.
   Hosemann f.
   Hosemann choledochus f.
   Hosford-Hicks transfer f.
   Hoskin f.
   Hospital arterial f.
   hot biopsy f.
   hot flexible f.
   Hough f.
   Hough alligator f.
   House f.
   House alligator f.
   House alligator crimper f.
   House alligator grasping f.
   House alligator strut f.

House cup f.
House-Dieter eye f.
House ear f.
House Gelfoam pressure f.
House grasping f.
House miniature f.
House oval-cup f.
House pressure f.
House strut f.
House-Wullstein f.
House-Wullstein cup f.
House-Wullstein ear f.
House-Wullstein oval-cup f.
Houspian clip-applying f.
Howard f.
Howard closing f.
Howard tonsillar f.
Howard tonsil-ligating f.
Hoxworth f.
Hoyt f.
Hoyt deep-surgery f.
Hoytenberger tissue f.
Hoyt hemostatic f.
Hubbard f.
Hubbard corneoscleral f.
Huber f. handle
Hudson f.
Hudson brain f.
Hudson cranial f.
Hudson cranial rongeur f.
Hudson dressing f.
Hudson rongeur f.
Hudson tissue f.
Hudson tissue-dressing f.
Hufnagel f.
Hufnagel mitral valve f.
Hufnagel mitral valve-
  holding f.
Hulka clip f.
Hulka-Kenwick f.
Hulka-Kenwick uterine-
  elevating and f.
Hulka-Kenwick uterine-
  manipulating f.
Hulka tenaculum f.
hump f.
Hunt f.
Hunt chalazion f.
Hunter splinter f.
Hunt tumor f.
Hunt vessel f.
Hunt-Yasargil pituitary f.
Hurd f.

Hurd bone f.
Hurdner tissue f.
Hurd septal f.
Hurd septal bone-cutting f.
Hurd septum-cutting f.
Hurteau f.
Hyde f.
Hyde corneal f.
hyoid-cutting f.
hypogastric artery f.
hypophyseal f.
hypophysectomy f.
hysterectomy f.
iliac f.
Iliff blepharochalasis f.
IMA f.
Imperatori f.
Imperatori laryngeal f.
implant f.
implantation f.
infant biopsy f.
infundibular f.
infundibular rongeur f.
Ingraham-Fowler clip-
  applying f.
inlet f.
insertion f.
instrument-grasping f.
instrument-handling f.
insulated f.
insulated bayonet f.
insulated monopolar f.
insulated tissue f.
intervertebral disk f.
intervertebral disk
  rongeur f.
intestinal f.
intestinal anastomosis f.
intestinal closing f.
intestinal holding f.
intestinal tissue f.
intestinal tissue-holding f.
intracapsular lens f.
intraocular f.
intraocular irrigating f.
intraocular lens f.
intrathoracic f.
introducing f.
Iowa f.
Iowa membrane f.
Iowa membrane-
  puncturing f.
Iowa-Mengert membrane f.

forceps *(continued)*
    Iowa State f.
    Iowa State fixation f.
    iris f.
    iris bipolar f.
    iris tissue f.
    isolation f.
    I-tech intraocular foreign
        body f.
    I-tech splinter f.
    I-tech tying f.
    Jackson f.
    Jackson alligator f.
    Jackson alligator grasping f.
    Jackson approximation f.
    Jackson biopsy f.
    Jackson broad-blade
        staple f.
    Jackson button f.
    Jackson cross-action f.
    Jackson cup round-punch f.
    Jackson cylindrical-object f.
    Jackson double-concave rat-
        tooth f.
    Jackson double-prong f.
    Jackson down-jaw f.
    Jackson dull-pointed f.
    Jackson endoscopic f.
    Jackson fenestrated meat f.
    Jackson fenestrated peanut-
        grasping f.
    Jackson forward-grasping f.
    Jackson head-holding f.
    Jackson hemostatic f.
    Jackson hollow-object f.
    Jackson infant f.
    Jackson infant biopsy f.
    Jackson laryngeal f.
    Jackson laryngeal
        applicator f.
    Jackson laryngeal basket f.
    Jackson laryngeal-dressing f.
    Jackson laryngeal-grasping f.
    Jackson laryngeal punch f.
    Jackson laryngeal ring-
        rotation f.
    Jackson laryngofissure f.
    Jackson papilloma f.
    Jackson punch f.
    Jackson ring-jaw f.
    Jackson ring-rotation f.
    Jackson rotation f.
    Jackson sharp-pointed f.

    Jackson side-curved f.
    Jackson sister-hook f.
    Jackson square-specimen f.
    Jackson tendon f.
    Jackson tracheal f.
    Jackson tracheal
        hemostatic f.
    Jackson triangular-punch f.
    Jacob f.
    Jacobs biopsy f.
    Jacobson f.
    Jacobson bipolar f.
    Jacobson dressing f.
    Jacobson hemostatic f.
    Jacobson microdressing f.
    Jacobson mosquito f.
    Jacob uterine vulsellum f.
    Jacob vulsellum f.
    Jaffe suturing f.
    Jager meniscal f.
    Jako f.
    Jako laryngeal f.
    Jako microlaryngeal f.
    Jako microlaryngeal cup f.
    Jako microlaryngeal
        grasping f.
    Jameson f.
    Jameson muscle f.
    Jameson muscle recession f.
    Jameson recession f.
    Jameson strabismus f.
    Jameson tracheal muscle f.
    James wound
        approximation f.
    Jannetta f.
    Jannetta alligator grasping f.
    Jannetta bayonet f.
    Jannetta microbayonet f.
    Jansen f.
    Jansen bayonet f.
    Jansen bayonet dressing f.
    Jansen bayonet ear f.
    Jansen bayonet nasal f.
    Jansen dissecting f.
    Jansen dressing f.
    Jansen ear f.
    Jansen-Gruenwald f.
    Jansen-Middleton f.
    Jansen-Middleton nasal-
        cutting f.
    Jansen-Middleton septal f.
    Jansen-Middleton
        septotomy f.

Jansen-Middleton septum-
  cutting f.
Jansen monopolar f.
Jansen-Mueller f.
Jansen nasal-dressing f.
Jansen-Struyken f.
Jansen-Struyken septal f.
Jansen thumb f.
Jarcho f.
Jarcho tenaculum f.
Jarcho uterine tenaculum f.
Jarit f.
Jarit-Allis tissue f.
Jarit brain f.
Jarit-Crafoord f.
Jarit-Dandy f.
Jarit-Liston bone-cutting f.
Jarit microsuture tying f.
Jarit mosquito f.
Jarit sterilizer f.
Jarit tendon-pulling f.
Jarit tube-occluding f.
Jarit wire-pulling f.
Jarvis f.
Jarvis hemorrhoidal f.
Javerts placental f.
Javerts polyp f.
Jayles f.
Jensen f.
Jensen intraocular lens f.
Jensen lens f.
Jensen lens-inserting f.
Jervey f.
Jervey iris f.
Jesberg f.
Jesberg grasping f.
jeweler's f.
jeweler's bipolar f.
jeweler's pickup f.
Johns Hopkins f.
Johns Hopkins
  gallbladder f.
Johns Hopkins gall duct f.
Johns Hopkins hemostatic f.
Johns Hopkins occluding f.
Johns Hopkins serrefine f.
Johnson f.
Johnson brain tumor f.
Johnson ptosis f.
Johnson thoracic f.
Jones f.
Jones hemostatic f.
Jones IMA f.

Jones towel f.
Joplin f.
Joplin bone-holding f.
Jordan strut f.
Judd f.
Judd-Allis f.
Judd-Allis intestinal f.
Judd-Allis tissue f.
Judd-DeMartel f.
Judd-DeMartel gallbladder f.
Judd strabismus f.
Judd suture f.
Juers f.
Juers crimper f.
Juers-Lempert f.
Juers-Lempert rongeur f.
Juers lingual f.
jugum f.
Julian f.
Julian-Damian thoracic f.
Julian splenorenal f.
Julian thoracic f.
Julian thoracic artery f.
Julian thoracic hemostatic f.
jumbo biopsy f.
Jurasz f.
Jurasz laryngeal f.
Kadesky f.
Kahler biopsy f.
Kahler bronchial f.
Kahler bronchial biopsy f.
Kahler bronchoscopic f.
Kahler bronchus-grasping f.
Kahler laryngeal f.
Kahler laryngeal biopsy f.
Kahler polyp f.
Kahn f.
Kahn tenaculum f.
Kalman f.
Kalman occluding f.
Kalman tube-occluding f.
Kalt f.
Kalt capsule f.
Kansas University corneal f.
Kantor f.
Kantrowitz f.
Kantrowitz dressing f.
Kantrowitz thoracic f.
Kantrowitz tissue f.
Kapp f.
Kapp applying f.
Kapp-Beck f.
Karp aortic punch f.

forceps *(continued)*
    Katzin-Barraquer f.
    Katzin-Barraquer Colibri f.
    Katzin-Barraquer corneal f.
    Kaufman f.
    Kaufman ENT f.
    Kaufman insulated f.
    Kaufman insulated
      monopolar f.
    Kazanjian f.
    Kazanjian bone-cutting f.
    Kazanjian-Cottle f.
    Kazanjian cutting f.
    Kazanjian nasal f.
    Kazanjian nasal-cutting f.
    Kazanjian nasal hump f.
    Kazanjian nasal hump-
      cutting f.
    Kelly f.
    Kelly arterial f.
    Kelly dressing f.
    Kelly-Gray uterine f.
    Kelly hemostatic f.
    Kelly-Murphy f.
    Kelly-Murphy hemostatic f.
    Kelly-Murphy hemostatic
      uterine vulsellum f.
    Kelly ovum f.
    Kelly placental f.
    Kelly polypus f.
    Kelly-Rankin f.
    Kelly tissue f.
    Kelly urethral f.
    Kelman f.
    Kelman implantation f.
    Kelman intraocular f.
    Kelman irrigator f.
    Kelman-McPherson f.
    Kelman-McPherson
      corneal f.
    Kelman-McPherson
      microtying f.
    Kelman-McPherson suture f.
    Kelman-McPherson tissue f.
    Kelman-McPherson tying f.
    Kennedy f.
    Kennedy uterine
      vulsellum f.
    Kennedy vulsellum f.
    Kennerdell bayonet f.
    Kent f.
    keratotomy f.

    Kern f.
    Kern bone-holding f.
    Kern-Lane bone-holding f.
    Kerrison f.
    Kerrison rongeur f.
    Kevorkian f.
    Kevorkian biopsy f.
    Kevorkian uterine biopsy f.
    Kevorkian-Younge f.
    Kevorkian-Younge biopsy f.
    Kevorkian-Younge cervical
      biopsy f.
    Kevorkian-Younge uterine
      biopsy f.
    Khodadad f.
    Khodadad microclip f.
    kidney f.
    kidney-elevating f.
    kidney pedicle f.
    kidney stone f.
    Killian f.
    Killian-Jameson f.
    Killian septal f.
    Killian septal compression f.
    King-Prince f.
    King-Prince recession f.
    Kingsley f.
    Kingsley grasping f.
    King tissue f.
    Kirby f.
    Kirby-Arthus fixation f.
    Kirby-Bracken iris f.
    Kirby corneoscleral f.
    Kirby eye tissue f.
    Kirby fixation f.
    Kirby intracapsular lens f.
    Kirby iris f.
    Kirby lens f.
    Kirby tissue f.
    Kirkpatrick f.
    Kirkpatrick tonsillar f.
    Kirschner-Ullrich f.
    Kirwan-Adson ophthalmic
      bipolar f.
    Kirwan coaptation
      ophthalmic bipolar f.
    Kirwan iris curved
      ophthalmic bipolar f.
    Kirwan iris straight
      ophthalmic bipolar f.
    Kirwan jeweler's curved
      ophthalmic bipolar f.

Kirwan jeweler's insulated straight ophthalmic bipolar f.
Kirwan Nadler-style coaptation ophthalmic bipolar f.
Kirwan-Tenzel ophthalmic bipolar f.
Kitner f.
Kitner goiter f.
Kitner thyroid-packing f.
Kjelland f.
Kjelland-Barton f.
Kjelland-Luikart f.
Kjelland-Luikart obstetrical f.
KleenSpec f.
Kleinert-Kutz bone-cutting f.
Kleinert-Kutz rongeur f.
Kleinert-Kutz tendon-passing f.
Kleinert-Kutz tendon retriever f.
Kleppinger f.
Kleppinger bipolar f.
KLI f.
KLI bipolar f.
KLI monopolar f.
Knapp f.
Knapp-Luer trachoma f.
Knapp trachoma f.
Knight f.
Knight nasal f.
Knight nasal-cutting f.
Knight nasal septum-cutting f.
Knighton-Crawford f.
Knight polyp f.
Knight septal f.
Knight septum-cutting f.
Knight-Sluder f.
Knight Sluder nasal f.
Knight turbinate f.
Knolle lens implantation f.
Knolle-Shepard lens f.
Knolle-Volker lens-holding f.
knot-holding f.
Kocher f.
Kocher arterial f.
Kocher hemostatic f.
Kocher intestinal f.
Kocher kidney-elevating f.

Kocher Micro-Line intestinal f.
Kocher-Ochsner f.
Kocher-Ochsner hemostatic f.
Koeberlé f.
Koenig vascular f.
Koerte gallstone f.
Koffler f.
Koffler-Lillie f.
Koffler-Lillie septal f.
Koffler septal f.
Koffler septal bone f.
Kogan endospeculum f.
Kolb f.
Kolb bronchial f.
Kolodny f.
Korte gallstone f.
Kos crimper f.
Kraff intraocular utility f.
Kraff lens-inserting f.
Kraff-Osher lens f.
Kraff suturing f.
Kraff tying f.
Kraff-Utrata intraocular utility f.
Kramer f.
Kratz lens-inserting f.
Krause f.
Krause biopsy f.
Krause esophagoscopy f.
Krause punch f.
Krause Universal f.
Kremer fixation f.
Kronfeld f.
Kronfeld micropin f.
Kronfeld suturing f.
Krönlein hemostatic f.
K/S-Allis f.
Kuhne coverglass f.
Kuhnt f.
Kuhnt capsular f.
Kuhnt fixation f.
Kulvin-Kalt f.
Kulvin-Kalt iris f.
Kurze f.
Kurze microbiopsy f.
Kurze micrograsping f.
Kurze pickup f.
Küstner uterine tenaculum f.
Kwapis interdental f.
Laborde f.

forceps *(continued)*
Lahey f.
Lahey arterial f.
Lahey-Babcock f.
Lahey dissecting f.
Lahey gall duct f.
Lahey goiter-seizing f.
Lahey goiter vulsellum f.
Lahey hemostatic f.
Lahey lock arterial f.
Lahey-Péan f.
Lahey-Sweet dissecting f.
Lahey tenaculum f.
Lahey thoracic f.
Lahey thyroid tenaculum f.
Lahey thyroid tissue
  traction f.
Lahey thyroid traction f.
Lahey thyroid traction
  vulsellum f.
Lahey traction f.
Lajeune hemostatic f.
Lambert f.
Lambert chalazion f.
Lambert-Kay anastomosis f.
Lambotte f.
Lambotte bone-holding f.
Lambotte fibular f.
laminectomy rongeur f.
Lancaster-O'Connor f.
lancet-shaped biopsy f.
Landers vitrectomy lens f.
Landon f.
Lane f.
Lane bone f.
Lane bone-holding f.
Lane gastrointestinal f.
Lane intestinal f.
Lane tissue f.
Lange approximation f.
Langenbeck f.
Langenbeck bone-holding f.
Lang iris f.
laparoscopic f.
Laplace f.
Larsen tendon f.
laryngeal f.
laryngeal applicator f.
laryngeal basket f.
laryngeal biopsy f.
laryngeal bronchial
  grasping f.
laryngeal curette f.

laryngeal grasping f.
laryngeal punch f.
laryngeal rotation f.
laryngeal sponging f.
laryngofissure f.
laser microlaryngeal cup f.
laser microlaryngeal
  grasping f.
Laser ovary f.
Lauer f.
Laufe f.
Laufe-Barton-Kjelland
  obstetrical f.
Laufe-Barton-Kjelland-Piper
  obstetrical f.
Laufe-Barton obstetrical f.
Laufe divergent outlet f.
Laufe obstetrical f.
Laufe-Piper f.
Laufe-Piper obstetrical f.
Laufe-Piper uterine polyp f.
Laufe polyp f.
Laufe uterine polyp f.
Laufman f.
Laval advancement f.
Lawrence f.
Lawrence deep f.
Lawrence deep-surgery f.
Lawrence hemostatic f.
Lawton f.
Lawton-Schubert biopsy f.
Lawton-Wittner cervical
  biopsy f.
Lazar microsuction f.
Leader f.
Leader vas isolation f.
Leahey marginal
  chalazion f.
Leahey suture f.
Leasure nasal f.
Leaver sclerotomy f.
Lebsche f.
Lebsche sternal punch f.
Lee delicate hemostatic f.
Lees arterial f.
Lees nontraumatic f.
Lefferts f.
Lefferts bone-cutting f.
Leigh f.
Leigh capsular f.
Leigh right-handed f.
Lejeune f.
Lejeune thoracic f.

Leksell f.
Leksell rongeur f.
Leland-Jones f.
Lemmon-Russian f.
Lemoine f.
Lempert f.
Lempert rongeur f.
lens f.
lens implantation f.
lens loop f.
Leonard f.
Leonard deep f.
Leonard deep-surgery f.
Leo Schwartz
   multipurpose f.
Leo Schwartz sponge-
   holding f.
Leriche f.
Leriche hemostatic f.
Leriche tissue f.
LeRoy clip-applying f.
LeRoy infant clip-
   applying f.
Lester f.
Lester fixation f.
Levenson tissue f.
Levora fixation f.
Levret f.
Lewin f.
Lewin bone-holding f.
Lewin spinal-perforating f.
Lewis f.
Lewis septal f.
Lewis tonsillar hemostatic f.
Lewis ureteral stone
   isolation f.
Lewkowitz f.
Lewkowitz lithotomy f.
Lewkowitz ovum f.
Lewkowitz placental f.
Lexer tissue f.
Leyro-Diaz f.
Leyro-Diaz thoracic f.
lid f.
Lieberman f.
Lieberman-Pollock f.
Lieberman-Pollock double
   corneal f.
Lieberman suturing f.
Lieberman tying f.
Lieb-Guerry f.
ligamenta flava f.
ligament-grasping f.

ligature f.
ligature-carrying f.
ligature-carrying aneurysm f.
Lillehei f.
Lillehei valve f.
Lillehei valve-grasping f.
Lillie f.
Lillie intestinal f.
Lillie intestinal tissue f.
Lillie-Killian f.
Lillie-Killian septal f.
Lillie-Killian septal bone f.
Lillie tissue-holding f.
Lindsay-Rea f.
lingual f.
Linnartz f.
Linn-Graefe iris f.
lion-jaw f.
lion-jaw bone-holding f.
Lister f.
Lister conjunctival f.
Liston f.
Liston bone-cutting f.
Liston-Key-Horsley f.
Liston-Littauer bone-
   cutting f.
Liston-Stille f.
Liston-Stille bone-cutting f.
Liston-Stille double-action
   bone-cutting f.
lithotomy f.
Litt f.
Littauer f.
Littauer bone-cutting f.
Littauer ciliary f.
Littauer ear f.
Littauer ear-dressing f.
Littauer ear polyp f.
Littauer-Liston f.
Littauer-Liston bone-
   cutting f.
Littauer nasal-dressing f.
Littauer-West cutting f.
Littlewood f.
Littlewood tissue f.
Livingston f.
Llobera f.
Llobera fixation f.
Lloyd-Davis occlusion f.
lobe f.
lobectomy f.
lobe-grasping f.
lobe-holding f.

forceps *(continued)*
    Lobell f.
    Lobell splinter f.
    Lobenstein-Tarnier f.
    Lockwood f.
    Lockwood-Allis f.
    Lockwood-Allis intestinal f.
    Lockwood-Allis tissue f.
    Lockwood intestinal f.
    Lockwood tissue f.
    Lombard-Beyer f.
    Lombard-Beyer rongeur f.
    London f.
    London tissue f.
    Long f.
    Long hysterectomy f.
    Long Island f.
    Long Island College
      Hospital f.
    Long Island College
      Hospital placental f.
    long-jaw basket f.
    long tissue f.
    Long f. with teeth
    loop-type snare f.
    loop-type stone-crushing f.
    loose body f.
    loose body suction f.
    Lordan chalazion f.
    Lore f.
    Lore subglottic f.
    Lore suction tip-holding f.
    Lore suction tube-holding f.
    Lore tendon grip f.
    Lorna nonperforating
      towel f.
    Lothrop f.
    Lothrop ligature f.
    Love-Gruenwald f.
    Love-Gruenwald alligator f.
    Love-Gruenwald pituitary f.
    Love-Kerrison f.
    Love-Kerrison rongeur f.
    Lovelace f.
    Lovelace bladder f.
    Lovelace gallbladder
      traction f.
    Lovelace hemostatic f.
    Lovelace hemostatic
      tissue f.
    Lovelace lung f.
    Lovelace lung-grasping f.
    Lovelace thyroid-traction f.

Lovelace thyroid-traction
    vulsellum f.
Lovelace tissue f.
Lovelace traction lung f.
Lovelace traction tissue f.
low f.
Löw-Beer f.
Löwenberg f.
lower f.
lower gall duct f.
lower lateral f.
Lowis intervertebral disk f.
Lowis IV disk rongeur f.
Lowman f.
Lowman bone-holding f.
Lowsley f.
Lowsley grasping f.
Lowsley-Luc f.
Lowsley prostatic f.
Lowsley prostatic lobe-
    holding f.
Luc f.
Lucae f.
Lucae bayonet dressing f.
Lucae bayonet ear f.
Lucae bayonet tissue f.
Lucae dissecting f.
Lucae dressing f.
Lucae ear f.
Luc ethmoidal f.
Luc nasal-cutting f.
Luc septal f.
Luc septum-cutting f.
Luer f.
Luer hemorrhoidal f.
Luer rongeur f.
Luer-Whiting f.
Luer-Whiting rongeur f.
Luikart f.
Luikart-Bill f.
Luikart-Kjelland f.
Luikart-Kjelland
    obstetrical f.
Luikart-McLane f.
Luikart-Simpson f.
Luikart-Simpson
    obstetrical f.
lung f.
lung-grasping f.
lung tissue f.
Lutz f.
Lutz septal f.
Lutz septal ridge f.

Lutz septal ridge-cutting f.
Lynch f.
Lynch cup-shaped curette f.
Lynch laryngeal f.
Lyon f.
MacGregor f.
MacGregor conjunctival f.
Machemer diamond-
dusted f.
MacKenty f.
MacKenty tissue f.
MacQuigg-Mixter f.
Madden f.
Madden-Potts f.
Madden-Potts intestinal f.
Madden-Potts tissue f.
Magielski f.
Magielski coagulating f.
Magielski-Heermann f.
Magielski-Heermann strut f.
Magielski tonsillar f.
Magielski tonsil-seizing f.
Magill f.
Magill catheter f.
Magill catheter-introducing f.
Magill endotracheal f.
Magill endotracheal
cathether-introducing f.
Maier f.
Maier dressing f.
Maier polyp f.
Maier sponge f.
Maier uterine f.
Maier uterine-dressing f.
Mailler colon f.
Mailler cut-off f.
Mailler intestinal f.
Mailler rectal f.
Maingot hysterectomy f.
Malis f.
Malis angled-up bipolar f.
Malis bipolar coagulation f.
Malis bipolar cutting f.
Malis bipolar irrigating f.
Malis cup f.
Malis-Jensen f.
Malis-Jensen bipolar f.
Malis titanium
microsurgical f.
malleus f.
mammary-coronary tissue f.
Manhattan Eye and Ear
suturing f.

Mann f.
Manning f.
Mansfield f.
March-Barton f.
Marcuse f.
marginal chalazion f.
Markwalder f.
Marshik f.
Marshik tonsillar f.
Marshik tonsil-seizing f.
Martin f.
Martin bipolar
coagulation f.
Martin cartilage f.
Martin meniscal f.
Martin nasopharyngeal f.
Martin nasopharyngeal
biopsy f.
Martin thumb f.
Martin tissue f.
Martin uterine tenaculum f.
Maryan f.
Maryan biopsy punch f.
Masterson hysterectomy f.
Mastin goiter f.
Mastin muscle f.
Mastin muscle tissue f.
mastoid rongeur f.
Mathieu foreign body f.
Mathieu tongue f.
Mathieu tongue-seizing f.
Mathieu urethral f.
Maumenee f.
Maumenee-Colibri f.
Maumenee-Colibri corneal f.
Maumenee corneal f.
Maumenee cross-action
capsular f.
Maumenee straight-action
capsule f.
Maumenee tissue f.
Max f.
Max Fine f.
Max Fine tying f.
maxillary disimpaction f.
maxillary fracture f.
Mayer f.
Mayfield f.
Mayfield aneurysm f.
Mayfield applying f.
Mayo f.
Mayo-Blake gallstone f.
Mayo-Blake stone f.

forceps *(continued)*

Mayo bone-cutting f.
Mayo-Harrington f.
Mayo kidney f.
Mayo kidney pedicle f.
Mayo-Ochsner f.
Mayo-Péan f.
Mayo-Péan hemostatic f.
Mayo-Robson f.
Mayo-Robson
  gastrointestinal f.
Mayo-Robson intestinal f.
Mayo-Russian f.
Mayo-Russian
  gastrointestinal f.
Mayo-Russian tissue f.
Mayo tissue f.
Mayo ureter isolation f.
Mazzacco flexible lens f.
Mazzariello-Caprini stone f.
McCarthy f.
McCarthy-Alcock f.
McCarthy-Alcock
  hemostatic f.
McCarthy visual f.
McCarthy visual
  hemostatic f.
McClintock placental f.
McClintock uterine f.
McCoy f.
McCoy septal f.
McCoy septum-cutting f.
McCravey f.
McCullough f.
McCullough strabismus f.
McCullough suture f.
McCullough suture-tying f.
McCullough suturing f.
McCullough utility f.
McGannon f.
McGannon lens f.
McGee-Paparella f.
McGee-Paparella wire-
  crimping f.
McGee-Priest f.
McGee-Priest-Paparella f.
McGee-Priest-Paparella
  closure f.
McGee-Priest-Paparella
  crimper-f.
McGee-Priest wire-closure f.
McGee-Priest wire-
  crimping f.

McGee wire-closure f.
McGee wire-crimping f.
McGill f.
McGivney hemorrhoidal f.
McGravey f.
McGravey tissue f.
McGregor f.
McGregor conjunctival f.
McGuire f.
McGuire marginal
  chalazion f.
McHenry f.
McHenry tonsillar f.
McHenry tonsillar artery f.
McIndoe f.
McIndoe bone-cutting f.
McIndoe dissecting f.
McIndoe dressing f.
McIndoe rongeur f.
McIntosh f.
McIntosh suture-holding f.
McKay f.
McKay ear f.
McKenzie f.
McKenzie brain clip-
  applying f.
McKenzie brain clip-
  cutting f.
McKenzie clip-applying f.
McKenzie clip-introducing f.
McKenzie grasping f.
McLane-Luikart
  obstetrical f.
McLane obstetrical f.
McLane pile f.
McLane-Tucker-Kjelland f.
McLane-Tucker-Luikart f.
McLane-Tucker obstetrical f.
McLean capsular f.
McLean ophthalmological f.
McLearie bone f.
McNealey-Glassman-
  Mixter f.
McNealey-Glassman-Mixter
  ligature-carrying
  aneurysm f.
McNealey-Glassman-
  Babcock f.
McPherson f.
McPherson angled f.
McPherson angled bipolar f.
McPherson-Castroviejo f.
McPherson corneal f.

McPherson curved bipolar
iris f.
McPherson irrigating f.
McPherson lens f.
McPherson microbipolar f.
McPherson microcorneal f.
McPherson micro-iris f.
McPherson micropin f.
McPherson microsuture f.
McPherson-Pierse f.
McPherson-Pierse
microcorneal f.
McPherson-Pierse
microsuturing f.
McPherson straight
bipolar f.
McPherson straight bipolar
iris f.
McPherson suture-tying f.
McPherson suturing f.
McPherson tying f.
McQuigg f.
McQuigg-Mixter f.
McQuigg-Mixter bronchial f.
McWhorter tonsillar f.
Meacham-Scoville f.
meat f.
meat-grasping f.
mechanical f.
mechanical finger f.
Medicon f.
Medicon-Jackson f.
Medicon-Jackson rectal f.
Medicon-Packer mosquito f.
Medicon wire-twister f.
medium f.
Meeker f.
Meeker artery f.
Meeker deep-surgery f.
Meeker gallbladder f.
Meeker hemostatic f.
Meeker intestinal f.
meibomian f.
meibomian expressor f.
membrane f.
membrane-puncturing f.
Mendel ligature f.
Mengert membrane-
puncturing f.
meniscal basket f.
Merlin stone f.
Merriam f.
Merz hysterectomy f.

Metzel-Wittmoser f.
Metzenbaum f.
Metzenbaum tonsillar f.
Metzenbaum-Tydings f.
MGH f.
MGH uterine vulsellum f.
MGH vulsellum f.
Michel f.
Michel clip-applying f.
Michel clip-removing f.
Michel suture clip-
applying f.
Michel tissue f.
Michel wound clip f.
Michel wound clip-
applying f.
Michel wound clip-
removing f.
Michigan f.
Michigan intestinal f.
Michigan University
intestinal f.
Micrins f.
micro-Allis f.
micro-arterial f.
microbayonet f.
microbiopsy f.
microbipolar f.
microbronchoscopic
grasping f.
microbronchoscopic tissue f.
microclamp f.
microclip f.
microcorneal f.
microcup f.
microcup pituitary f.
microdissecting f.
microdressing f.
micro-extractor f.
micro-Halstead arterial f.
microlaryngeal cup-shaped f.
microlaryngeal grasping f.
Micro-Line arterial f.
microneedle holder f.
microneurosurgical f.
micropin f.
Microsnap hemostatic f.
microsurgical f.
microsurgical biopsy f.
microsurgical grasping f.
microsurgical tying f.
microsuture-tying f.
Microtek cupped f.

forceps *(continued)*
  microtip f.
  microtip bipolar jeweler's f.
  microtissue f.
  microtying f.
  microtying eye f.
  micro-utility f.
  microvascular f.
  microvascular clamp-applying f.
  microvascular tying f.
  middle ear f.
  middle ear strut f.
  Mikulicz f.
  Mikulicz peritoneal f.
  Mikulicz tonsillar f.
  Milex f.
  Miller f.
  Miller articulating f.
  Miller bayonet f.
  Miller rectal f.
  Millin f.
  Millin capsular f.
  Millin capsule-grasping f.
  Millin ligature-guiding f.
  Millin lobe-grasping f.
  Millin prostatectomy f.
  Millin T-shaped f.
  Mill-Rose biopsy f.
  Mills mammary-coronary tissue f.
  Mills saphenous-aortic tissue f.
  Mills tissue f.
  miniature intestinal f.
  mini-micro f.
  Mitchell-Diamond f.
  Mitchell-Diamond biopsy f.
  mitral f.
  mitral valve-holding f.
  Mixter f.
  Mixter arterial f.
  Mixter baby hemostatic f.
  Mixter full-curve f.
  Mixter gallbladder f.
  Mixter gall duct f.
  Mixter gallstone f.
  Mixter hemostatic f.
  Mixter-McQuigg f.
  Mixter mosquito f.
  Mixter-O'Shaughnessy f.
  Mixter-O'Shaughnessy dissecting f.
  Mixter-O'Shaughnessy hemostatic f.
  Mixter-O'Shaughnessy ligature f.
  Mixter-Paul arterial f.
  Mixter-Paul hemostatic f.
  Mixter pediatric f.
  Mixter pediatric hemostatic f.
  Mixter thoracic f.
  Mixter thoracic clamp f.
  Moberg f.
  Moberg-Stille f.
  modified Younge f.
  Moehle f.
  Moehle corneal f.
  Moersch f.
  Moersch bronchoscopic f.
  Moersch bronchoscopic specimen f.
  Molt f.
  Molt pedicle f.
  Monod punch f.
  monopolar f.
  monopolar coagulating f.
  monopolar insulated f.
  Montenovesi cranial f.
  Montenovesi cranial rongeur f.
  Moody f.
  Moody fixation f.
  Moore f.
  Moore lens f.
  Moore lens-implanting f.
  Moore lens-inserting f.
  Morgenstein blunt f.
  Moritz-Schmidt f.
  Moritz-Schmidt laryngeal f.
  Morris f.
  Morson f.
  Mosher f.
  Mosher ethmoid punch f.
  mosquito f.
  mosquito hemostatic f.
  Mount f.
  Mount intervertebral disk f.
  Mount intervertebral disk rongeur f.
  Mount-Mayfield f.
  Mount-Mayfield aneurysm f.
  Mount-Olivecrona f.
  mouse-tooth f.
  Moynihan f.

Moynihan gall duct f.
Moynihan intestinal f.
Moynihan kidney pedicle f.
Moynihan-Navratil f.
Moynihan towel f.
MPC coagulation f.
Muck f.
Muck tonsillar f.
mucous f.
Mueller f.
Mueller-Markham patent
  ductus f.
Muir hemorrhoidal f.
Muldoon meibomian f.
multipurpose f.
multitoothed cartilage f.
Mundie f.
Mundie placental f.
Murless head extractor f.
Murphy f.
Murphy-Péan hemostatic f.
Murphy tonsillar f.
Murray f.
muscle f.
Museholdt f.
Museholdt nasal-dressing f.
Museux f.
Museux-Collins uterine
  vulsellum f.
Museux tenaculum f.
Museux uterine f.
Museux uterine vulsellum f.
Museux vulsellum f.
Musial tissue f.
Mustarde f.
Myerson f.
Myerson bronchial f.
Myerson laryngeal f.
Myerson miniature laryngeal
  biopsy f.
Myles f.
Myles hemorrhoidal f.
Myles nasal f.
Myles nasal-cutting f.
Nadler bipolar coaptation f.
Naegele f.
Naegele obstetrical f.
nail-extracting f.
nasal f.
nasal alligator f.
nasal bone f.
nasal cartilage-holding f.
nasal-cutting f.

nasal-dressing f.
nasal-grasping f.
nasal hump-cutting f.
nasal insertion f.
nasal lower lateral f.
nasal needle holder f.
nasal-packing f.
nasal polyp f.
nasal septal f.
nasopharyngeal biopsy f.
Natvig wire-twister f.
needle f.
needle-holder f.
Negus f.
Negus-Green f.
Negus tonsillar f.
Nelson f.
Nelson lung f.
Nelson lung-dissecting f.
Nelson lung tissue f.
Nelson-Martin f.
Nelson tissue f.
neonatal vascular f.
nephrolithotomy f.
Neubauer f.
Neubauer foreign body f.
Neubauer vitreous micro-
  extractor f.
Neubuser tubal-seizing f.
neurosurgical f.
neurosurgical dressing f.
neurosurgical ligature f.
neurosurgical suction f.
neurosurgical tissue f.
neurovascular f.
Neuwirth-Palmer f.
Nevins f.
Nevins dressing f.
Nevins tissue f.
Nevyas lens f.
New f.
New biopsy f.
Newman f.
Newman tenaculum f.
Newman uterine f.
Newman uterine
  tenaculum f.
New Orleans f.
New Orleans Eye and
  Ear f.
New tissue f.
New York Eye and Ear f.

forceps *(continued)*
New York Eye and Ear
 fixation f.
New York Eye and Ear
 Hospital fixation f.
Nicola f.
Niedner f.
Niedner dissecting f.
NIH mitral valve f.
NIH mitral valve-grasping f.
Niro wire-twister f.
Nisbet eye f.
Nisbet fixation f.
Nissen f.
Nissen cystic f.
Nissen gall duct f.
Nissen hassux f.
Noble f.
Noble iris f.
noncrushing f.
noncrushing common
 duct f.
noncrushing intestinal f.
noncrushing pickup f.
noncrushing tissue-holding f.
nonfenestrated f.
nonmagnetic f.
nonmagnetic dressing f.
nonmagnetic tissue f.
nonperforating towel f.
nonslipping f.
nontoothed f.
nontraumatizing f.
nontraumatizing visceral f.
Nordan-Colibri f.
Nordan tying f.
Norris sponge f.
Norwood f.
Noto dressing f.
Noto ovum f.
Noto polypus f.
Noto sponge f.
Noto sponge-holding f.
Novak fixation f.
Noyes f.
Noyes ear f.
Noyes nasal f.
Noyes nasal-dressing f.
Nugent f.
Nugent fixation f.
Nugent superior rectus f.
Nugent utility f.
Nugowski f.

Nussbaum intestinal f.
Nyhus-Potts intestinal f.
Nystroem tumor f.
Oberhill obstetrical f.
O'Brien f.
O'Brien-Elschnig f.
O'Brien-Elschnig fixation f.
O'Brien fixation f.
obstetrical f.
occluding f.
Ochsner f.
Ochsner arterial f.
Ochsner-Dixon f.
Ochsner-Dixon arterial f.
Ochsner hemostatic f.
Ockerblad f.
O'Connor f.
O'Connor biopsy f.
O'Connor-Elschnig
 fixation f.
O'Connor eye f.
O'Connor grasping f.
O'Connor iris f.
O'Connor lid f.
O'Dell spicule f.
odontoid peg-grasping f.
O'Gawa-Castroviejo f.
O'Gawa-Castroviejo tying f.
O'Gawa suture f.
O'Gawa suture-fixation f.
O'Gawa tying f.
Ogura f.
O'Hanlon f.
O'Hara f.
Oldberg f.
Oldberg intervertebral
 disk f.
Oldberg pituitary rongeur f.
Olivecrona f.
Olivecrona aneurysm f.
Olivecrona rongeur f.
Olivecrona-Toennis f.
Olivecrona-Toennis clip-
 applying f.
Olympus alligator-jaw
 endoscopic f.
Olympus basket-type
 endoscopic f.
Olympus biopsy f.
Olympus endoscopic
 biopsy f.
Olympus hot biopsy f.

Olympus magnetic
 extractor f.
Olympus minisnare f.
Olympus pelican-type
 endoscopic f.
Olympus rat-tooth
 endoscopic f.
Olympus rubber-tip
 endoscopic f.
Olympus shark-tooth
 endoscopic f.
Olympus tripod-type
 endoscopic f.
Olympus W-shaped
 endoscopic f.
Ombrédanne f.
optical biopsy f.
oral f.
oral rongeur f.
Orr f.
Orr gall duct f.
orthopaedic f.
O'Shaughnessy f.
O'Shaughnessy arterial f.
Osher bipolar coaptation f.
Osher capsular f.
Osher conjunctival f.
Osher foreign body f.
Osher haptic f.
Osher superior rectus f.
ossicle-holding f.
Ossoff-Karlan laser f.
Ostrum f.
Ostrum antral punch-tip f.
Ostrum punch f.
otologic cup f.
Otto f.
Otto tissue f.
Oughterson f.
outlet f.
oval cup f.
ovary f.
Overholt f.
Overholt dissecting f.
Overholt-Geissendörfer f.
Overholt-Geissendörfer
 arterial f.
Overholt-Geissendörfer
 hemostatic f.
Overholt-Mixter dissecting f.
Overstreet f.
Overstreet endometrial
 polyp f.

Overstreet polyp f.
ovum f.
Pace-Potts f.
Packer mosquito f.
packing f.
Page f.
Page tonsillar f.
Palmer biopsy f.
Palmer biopsy drill f.
Palmer cutting f.
Palmer-Drapier f.
Palmer grasping f.
Pang f.
Pang biopsy f.
Pang nasopharyngeal f.
Pang nasopharyngeal
 biopsy f.
Panje-Shagets
 tracheoesophageal fistula f.
papilloma f.
parametrium f.
Parker fixation f.
Parker-Kerr f.
Park lens implantation f.
partial occlusion f.
passing f.
patent ductus f.
Paterson brain clip f.
Paterson laryngeal f.
Paton f.
Paton corneal f.
Paton corneal transplant f.
Paton extra-delicate f.
Patterson f.
Patterson bronchoscopic f.
Patterson bronchoscopic
 biopsy f.
Patterson specimen f.
Paufique f.
Paufique suturing f.
Paulson infertility
 microtissue f.
Paulson infertility
 microtying f.
Pauwels fracture f.
Payne-Ochsner f.
Payne-Ochsner arterial f.
Payne-Péan f.
Payne-Péan arterial f.
Payne-Rankin f.
Payne-Rankin arterial f.
Payr f.
Payr pylorus f.

forceps *(continued)*
Péan f.
Péan arterial f.
Péan GI f.
Péan hemostatic f.
Péan hysterectomy f.
Péan intestinal f.
Péan sponge f.
peanut f.
peanut-fenestrated f.
peanut-grasping f.
peanut sponge-holding f.
peapod bead-type f.
peapod intervertebral disk f.
pediatric f.
pedicle f.
Peers towel f.
Peet f.
Peet mosquito f.
Peet splinter f.
pelican biopsy f.
Pelkmann foreign body f.
Pelkmann gallstone f.
Pelkmann sponge f.
Pelkmann uterine f.
Pelkmann uterine-dressing f.
pelvic reduction f.
pelvic tissue f.
Pemberton f.
Penfield f.
Penfield suture f.
Penfield watchmaker f.
Penn-Anderson fixation f.
Pennington f.
Pennington hemorrhoidal f.
Pennington hemostatic f.
Pennington tissue f.
Pennington tissue-grasping f.
Percy f.
Percy intestinal f.
Percy tissue f.
Percy-Wolfson gallbladder f.
Perdue tonsillar hemostat f.
perforating f.
peripheral blood vessel f.
peripheral iridectomy f.
peripheral vascular f.
peritoneal f.
Perritt f.
Perritt double-fixation f.
Perritt double-fixation
  suture f.
Perritt fixation f.

Perritt lens f.
Perritt lens implantation f.
Perry f.
Peter-Bishop f.
Peters tissue f.
Peyman-Green vitreous f.
Peyman vitreous-grasping f.
Pfau f.
Pfau polypus f.
Pfister-Schwartz basket f.
phalangeal f.
Phaneuf f.
Phaneuf arterial f.
Phaneuf hysterectomy f.
Phaneuf peritoneal f.
Phaneuf uterine artery f.
Phaneuf vaginal f.
Phillips f.
Phillips fixation f.
Phillips swan neck f.
phimosis f.
Phipps f.
phrenicectomy f.
physician's pickup f.
physician's splinter f.
pickup f.
pickup noncrushing f.
Pierse f.
Pierse Colibri f.
Pierse Colibri corneal
  utility f.
Pierse Colibri-type
  corneal f.
Pierse Colibri utility f.
Pierse corneal f.
Pierse corneal Colibri-
  type f.
Pierse fixation f.
Pierse-Hoskins f.
Pierse-type Colibri f.
Pierse-type fine f.
Pierse-type skeleton f.
Pigott f.
Pike jawed f.
pile f.
pillar f.
pillar-grasping f.
Pilling f.
Pilling-Liston bone utility f.
pin-bending f.
pinch f.
pin-seating f.
Piper f.

Piper obstetrical f.
Pischel f.
Pischel micropin f.
Pitanguy f.
Pitha f.
Pitha foreign body f.
Pitha urethral f.
pituitary f.
pituitary rongeur f.
placement f.
placenta previa f.
plain f.
plain splinter f.
plain sterilizer f.
plain thumb f.
plain tissue f.
plane iris f.
plastic f.
plastic suture-removal f.
plate-holding f.
platform f.
pleurectomy f.
Pley f.
Pley capsular f.
Plondke uterine f.
Plondke uterine-elevating f.
point f.
Polk placental f.
Polk sponge f.
Pollock f.
Pollock double corneal f.
polyp f.
polypus f.
Poppen f.
Poppen intervertebral
  disk f.
Porter f.
Porter duodenal f.
Post f.
posterior f.
postnasal sponge f.
Potta coarctation f.
Potter sponge f.
Potter tonsillar f.
Potts f.
Potts bronchial f.
Potts bulldog f.
Potts coarctation f.
Potts fixation f.
Potts intestinal f.
Potts-Nevins dressing f.
Potts patent ductus f.
Potts-Smith f.

Potts-Smith dressing f.
Potts-Smith monopolar f.
Potts-Smith tissue f.
Potts thumb f.
Poutasse f.
Poutasse renal artery f.
Pozzi tenaculum f.
Pratt f.
Pratt hemostatic f.
Pratt-Smith f.
Pratt-Smith hemostatic f.
Pratt-Smith tissue-grasping f.
Pratt tissue f.
Pratt tissue-grasping f.
Pratt T-shaped f.
Pratt T-shaped hemostatic f.
Pratt vulsellum f.
Prentiss f.
prepuce f.
Presbyterian Hospital f.
Presbyterian Hospital tube-
  occluding f.
pressure f.
Preston ligamentum
  flavum f.
Price-Thomas f.
Price-Thomas bronchial f.
Price-Thomas bronchus f.
Primbs suturing f.
Prince f.
Prince advancement f.
Prince muscle f.
Prince trachoma f.
proctological f.
proctological grasping f.
proctological polyp f.
Proctor phrenectomy f.
Proctor phrenicectomy f.
prostatectomy f.
prostatic f.
prostatic lobe f.
prostatic lobe-holding f.
protological biopsy f.
Proud adenoidectomy f.
Providence arterial f.
Providence Hospital f.
Providence Hospital
  arterial f.
Providence Hospital
  classic f.
Providence Hospital
  hemostatic f.
ptosis f.

forceps *(continued)*
    pulmonary arterial f.
    pulmonary vessel f.
    punch f.
    Puntenney f.
    Puntenney tying f.
    Puntowicz arterial f.
    QSA dressing f.
    Quervain f.
    Quervain cranial f.
    Quervain cranial rongeur f.
    Quevedo f.
    Quevedo conjunctival f.
    Quire f.
    Quire finger f.
    Quire foreign body f.
    Quire mechanical finger f.
    Raaf f.
    Raaf-Oldberg intervertebral disk f.
    Raimondi f.
    Raimondi scalp f.
    Raimondi scalp hemostatic f.
    Ralks f.
    Ralks ear f.
    Ralks splinter f.
    Ralks wire-cutting f.
    Rampley f.
    Rampley sponge f.
    Rand f.
    Randall f.
    Randall kidney stone f.
    Randall stone f.
    Raney f.
    Raney clip f.
    Raney clip-applying f.
    Raney rongeur f.
    Raney scalp clip f.
    Raney scalp clip-applying f.
    Raney straight coagulating f.
    Rankin f.
    Rankin arterial f.
    Rankin-Crile f.
    Rankin-Crile hemostatic f.
    Rankin hemostatic f.
    Rankow f.
    Rapp f.
    Rappazzo intraocular foreign body f.
    Rappazzo intraocular lens f.
    Ratliff-Blake f.
    Ratliff-Blake gallstone f.
    Ratliff-Mayo f.
    Ratliff-Mayo gallstone f.
    Ratliff-Mayo stone f.
    rat-tooth f.
    rat-tooth grasping f.
    Ray f.
    Ray kidney stone f.
    reach-and-pin f.
    Read f.
    recession f.
    rectal f.
    rectal biopsy f.
    Reese f.
    Reese advancement f.
    Reese muscle f.
    regular f.
    regular f. with teeth
    Reich-Nechtow f.
    Reich-Nechtow hypogastric artery f.
    Reich-Nechtow hysterectomy f.
    Reill f.
    Reiner-Knight f.
    Reiner-Knight ethmoid-cutting f.
    Reinhoff f.
    Reisinger f.
    Reisinger lens f.
    Reisinger lens-extracting f.
    renal artery f.
    Resano sigmoid f.
    resection intestinal f.
    retrieval f.
    Reul coronary f.
    reverse-action hypophysectomy f.
    Rezek f.
    Rhoton f.
    Rhoton-Adson dressing f.
    Rhoton-Adson tissue f.
    Rhoton bayonet bipolar f.
    Rhoton bipolar f.
    Rhoton cup f.
    Rhoton-Cushing f.
    Rhoton-Cushing dressing f.
    Rhoton-Cushing tissue f.
    Rhoton dressing f.
    Rhoton dural f.
    Rhoton grasping f.
    Rhoton microcup f.
    Rhoton microdissecting f.
    Rhoton microtying f.

Rhoton microvascular f.
Rhoton ring tumor f.
Rhoton-Tew bipolar f.
Rhoton tissue f.
Rhoton transsphenoidal
  bipolar f.
Rhoton tumor f.
Rhoton tying f.
Riba-Valeira f.
rib rongeur f.
Rica-Adson f.
Rica clip-applying f.
Rica hemostatic f.
Rich f.
Richards f.
Richards Andrews f.
Richards tonsil-grasping f.
Richards tonsillar f.
Richards tonsil-seizing f.
Riches diathermy f.
Richmond f.
Richter f.
Richter-Heath f.
Richter-Heath clip f.
Richter-Heath clip-
  removing f.
Richter-Heath suture-
  removing f.
Richter suture clip-
  removing f.
ridge f.
Ridley f.
Rienhoff arterial f.
Rigenberg f.
right-angle f.
rigid biopsy f.
rigid kidney stone f.
ring f.
Ringenberg ear f.
Ringenberg stapedectomy f.
ring-rotation f.
Ripstein f.
Ripstein arterial f.
Ripstein tissue f.
Ritch-Krupin Denver eye
  valve insertion f.
Ritter f.
Rizzuti double-prong f.
Rizzuti scleral f.
Rizzuti scleral fixation f.
Rizzuti superior rectus f.
Rizzuti-Verhoeff f.
Rizzutti f.

Rizzutti-Furness cornea-
  holding f.
Robb f.
Robb sponge-holding f.
Robb tonsillar f.
Robb tonsillar sponge f.
Roberts f.
Roberts arterial f.
Roberts bronchial f.
Roberts bronchial biopsy f.
Roberts hemostatic f.
Robertson f.
Robertson tonsillar f.
Robertson tonsil-seizing f.
Roberts-Singley dressing f.
Roberts-Singley thumb f.
Robson intestinal f.
Rochester f.
Rochester-Carmalt f.
Rochester-Carmalt
  hemostatic f.
Rochester-Carmalt
  hysterectomy f.
Rochester-Davis f.
Rochester-Ewald f.
Rochester-Ewald tissue f.
Rochester gallstone f.
Rochester-Harrington f.
Rochester-Mixter f.
Rochester-Mixter arterial f.
Rochester-Mixter gall
  duct f.
Rochester-Müller f.
Rochester-Ochsner f.
Rochester-Ochsner
  hemostat f.
Rochester oral f.
Rochester-Péan f.
Rochester-Péan hemostatic f.
Rochester-Péan
  hysterectomy f.
Rochester-Rankin f.
Rochester-Rankin arterial f.
Rochester-Rankin
  hemostatic f.
Rochester-Russian f.
Rochester tissue f.
Rockey f.
Roeder f.
Roeder towel f.
Roeltsch f.
Roger f.
Roger hysterectomy f.

forceps *(continued)*

Roger vascular-toothed hysterectomy f.
Rogge sterilizing f.
Rolf f.
Rolf jeweler's f.
Rolf utility f.
roller f.
rongeur f.
Ronis cutting f.
Rose disimpaction f.
rotating f.
rotation f.
Roubaix f.
round punch f.
Rovenstine f.
Rovenstine catheter-introducing f.
Rowe f.
Rowe bone-drilling f.
Rowe disimpaction f.
Rowe-Killey f.
Rowe maxillary f.
Rowland f.
Rowland double-action f.
Rowland double-action hump f.
Rowland hump f.
Rowland nasal hump f.
Royce f.
rubber-dam clamp f.
rubber-shod f.
Rubgy deep-surgery f.
Rudd Clinic f.
Rudd Clinic hemorrhoidal f.
Ruel f.
Rugby f.
Rugby deep-surgery f.
Rugelski arterial f.
Rumel f.
Rumel dissecting f.
Rumel hemostatic f.
Rumel lobectomy f.
Rumel thoracic f.
Rumel thoracic artery f.
Rumel thoracic-dissecting f.
Ruskin f.
Ruskin bone-cutting f.
Ruskin bone-splitting f.
Ruskin-Liston f.
Ruskin-Liston bone-cutting f.
Ruskin rongeur f.

Ruskin-Rowland f.
Russell f.
Russell-Davis f.
Russell hysterectomy f.
Russian f.
Russian-Péan f.
Russian thumb f.
Russian tissue f.
Russ-model tumor f.
Russ-model vascular f.
Rycroft tying f.
Sachs f.
Sachs tissue f.
Saenger ovum f.
Saenger placental f.
Sajou laryngeal f.
Sam Roberts f.
Sam Roberts bronchial f.
Sam Roberts bronchial biopsy f.
Samuels f.
Samuels hemoclip-applying f.
Sanders f.
Sanders-Castroviejo f.
Sanders vasectomy f.
Sandt suture f.
Sandt utility f.
Santy f.
Santy dissecting f.
Santy ring-end f.
saphenous-aorta tissue f.
Saqalain dressing f.
Sarot f.
Sarot arterial f.
Sarot intrathoracic f.
Sarot pleurectomy f.
Satinsky f.
Satinsky tangential occlusion f.
Satterlee advancement f.
Satterlee muscle f.
Sauer f.
Sauerbruch f.
Sauerbruch pickup f.
Sauerbruch rib rongeur f.
Sauer outer ring f.
Sauer suture f.
Sauer suturing f.
Sawtell f.
Sawtell arterial f.
Sawtell-Davis f.

Sawtell-Davis tonsillar
  hemostat f.
Sawtell gallbladder f.
Sawtell hemostatic f.
Sawtell tonsillar f.
Sawtell tonsillar artery f.
scalp f.
scalp clip f.
scalp clip-applying f.
Scanlan laproscopic f.
Scanzoni f.
Schaaf foreign body f.
Schaedel towel f.
Schanzioni craniotomy f.
Scharff bipolar f.
Schatz utility f.
Scheer crimper f.
Scheie-Graefe f.
Scheie-Graefe fixation f.
Scheinmann f.
Scheinmann
  esophagoscopy f.
Scheinmann laryngeal f.
Schepens f.
Schick f.
Schindler f.
Schindler peritoneal f.
Schlesinger f.
Schlesinger cervical punch f.
Schlesinger intervertebral
  disk f.
Schlesinger meniscus-
  grasping f.
Schmidt hemostatic f.
Schmidt-Rumpler f.
Schnidt f.
Schnidt gall duct f.
Schnidt-Rumpler f.
Schnidt thoracic f.
Schnidt tonsillar f.
Schnidt tonsillar
  hemostatic f.
Schoenberg f.
Schoenberg intestinal f.
Schoenberg uterine f.
Schoenberg uterine-
  elevating f.
Schroeder f.
Schroeder-Braun f.
Schroeder-Braun uterine f.
Schroeder tenaculum f.
Schroeder tissue f.

Schroeder uterine
  tenaculum f.
Schroeder uterine
  vulsellum f.
Schroeder-Van Doren
  tenaculum f.
Schroeder vulsellar f.
Schubert f.
Schubert biopsy f.
Schubert biopsy punch f.
Schubert cervical biopsy f.
Schubert uterine biopsy f.
Schubert uterine biopsy
  punch f.
Schubert uterine
  tenaculum f.
Schumacher f.
Schumacher biopsy f.
Schutz f.
Schwartz f.
Schwartz clip-applying f.
Schwartz obstetrical f.
Schwartz temporary vessel
  clamp-applying f.
Schweigger f.
Schweigger capsular f.
Schweigger extracapsular f.
Schweizer f.
Schweizer cervix-holding f.
Schweizer uterine f.
scissors f.
sclerectomy punch f.
Scobee-Allis f.
Scoville f.
Scoville brain f.
Scoville brain spatula f.
Scoville clip-applying f.
Scoville-Greenwood f.
Scoville-Greenwood Bayonet
  neurosurgical bipolar f.
Scoville-Hurteau f.
screw-holding f.
Scudder f.
Scudder intestinal f.
Scuderi f.
Scuderi bipolar
  coagulating f.
Searcy f.
Searcy capsular f.
Segond f.
Segond hysterectomy f.
Segond-Landau
  hysterectomy f.

forceps *(continued)*

Segond tumor f.
Seiffert f.
Seiffert esophagoscopy f.
Seiffert laryngeal f.
seizing f.
Seletz f.
Seletz foramen-plugging f.
self-opening f.
self-retaining bone f.
Selman f.
Selman nonslip tissue f.
Selman peripheral blood vessel f.
Selman tissue f.
Selman vessel f.
Selverstone f.
Selverstone embolus f.
Selverstone intervertebral disk f.
Selverstone intervertebral disk rongeur f.
Semb f.
Semb bone-cutting f.
Semb bone-holding f.
Semb dissecting f.
Semb-Ghazi f.
Semb-Ghazi dissecting f.
Semb ligature f.
Semb ligature-carrying f.
Semb rongeur f.
Semken f.
Semken bipolar f.
Semken dressing f.
Semken infant f.
Semken microbipolar neurosurgical f.
Semken thumb f.
Semken tissue f.
Semmes dural f.
Senn f.
Senning f.
Senning cardiovascular f.
Senturia f.
septal f.
septal bone f.
septal compression f.
septal ridge f.
septum-cutting f.
septum-straightening f.
sequestrum f.
serrated f.
serrefine f.

Sewall f.
Sewall brain clip-applying f.
Seyfert f.
Shaaf f.
Shaaf eye f.
Shaaf foreign body f.
Shallcross f.
Shallcross cystic duct f.
Shallcross-Dean gall duct f.
Shallcross gallbladder f.
Shallcross hemostatic f.
Shallcross nasal f.
Shallcross nasal-packing f.
shark-tooth f.
sharp-pointed f.
Sharpshay-Healy laryngeal alligator f.
Sharpshay-Healy laryngeal-cutting f.
Sharpshay-Healy laryngeal-grasping f.
Shearer f.
Shearer chicken-bill f.
Shearer rongeur f.
sheathed flexible gastric f.
Sheehy f.
Sheehy ossicle-holding f.
Sheets lens f.
Sheets lens-inserting f.
Sheets-McPherson angled f.
Sheets-McPherson tying f.
Sheinmann laryngeal f.
Shepard f.
Shepard bipolar f.
Shepard curved intraocular lens f.
Shepard intraocular lens f.
Shepard intraocular lens-inserting f.
Shepard intraocular utility f.
Shepard lens f.
Shepard lens-inserting f.
Shepard-Reinstein intraocular lens f.
Shepard tying f.
short-tooth f.
Shuppe biting f.
Shuster f.
Shuster suture f.
Shuster tonsillar f.
Shute f.
Shutt f.
Shutt Aggressor f.

Shutt alligator f.
Shutt blunt tip f.
Shutt B-scoop f.
Shutt grasping f.
shuttle f.
Shutt Mini-Aggressor f.
Shutt minitip f.
Shutt retrograde f.
Shutt shovel nose f.
Shutt suction f.
side-curved f.
side-cutting basket f.
side-grasping f.
side-grasping tissue f.
Siegler f.
Siegler biopsy f.
sigmoidoscope biopsy f.
Silcock dissection f.
Silver f.
Silver endaural f.
Simcoe implantation f.
Simcoe lens f.
Simcoe lens implant f.
Simcoe lens-inserting f.
Simcoe nucleus f.
Simcoe nucleus intraocular
  removal f.
Simcoe posterior chamber f.
Simcoe posterior chamber
  lens f.
Simcoe superior rectus f.
Simons stone-removing f.
Simpson f.
Simpson-Braun obstetrical f.
Simpson-Luikart f.
Simpson-Luikart
  obstetrical f.
Simpson obstetrical f.
Sims-Maier sponge and
  dressing f.
single-tooth f.
Singley f.
Singley intestinal f.
Singley intestinal tissue f.
Singley tissue f.
Singley-Tuttle f.
Singley-Tuttle dressing f.
Singley-Tuttle intestinal f.
Singley-Tuttle tissue f.
Sinskey f.
Sinskey intraocular lens f.
Sinskey-McPherson f.
Sinskey microtying f.

Sinskey-Wilson f.
Sinskey-Wilson foreign
  body f.
sinus biopsy f.
Sisson f.
Sisson hemostatic f.
sister hook f.
Skene f.
Skene tenaculum f.
Skene uterine f.
Skene uterine tenaculum f.
Skene uterine vulsellum f.
Skene vulsellum f.
Skillern f.
Skillern phimosis f.
Skillman f.
Skillman arterial f.
Skillman hemostatic f.
Skillman mosquito f.
Skillman mosquito
  hemostatic f.
Skillman prepuce f.
skin f.
sleeve-spreading f.
sleeve-spreading dilating f.
sliding capsular f.
Sluder-Ballenger tonsillar
  punch f.
small bone-cutting f.
small bone-holding f.
small joint f.
Smart f.
Smart chalazion f.
Smart nonslipping
  chalazion f.
Smellie obstetrical f.
Smith f.
Smith grasping f.
Smith lion-jaw f.
Smith obstetrical f.
Smith-Petersen f.
Smithwick f.
Smithwick clip-applying f.
Smithwick-Hartmann f.
smooth dressing f.
smooth tissue f.
smooth-tooth f.
Snellen f.
Snellen entropion f.
Snyder f.
Snyder deep-surgery f.
Somers f.
Somers uterine f.

forceps *(continued)*
    Somers uterine-elevating f.
    Songer tonsillar f.
    Soonawalla vasectomy f.
    Sparta micro-iris f.
    specimen f.
    speculum f.
    Spence f.
    Spence-Adson f.
    Spence-Adson clip-introducing f.
    Spencer f.
    Spencer chalazion f.
    Spence rongeur f.
    Spencer plication f.
    Spencer-Wells f.
    Spencer-Wells arterial f.
    Spencer-Wells chalazion f.
    Spencer-Wells hemostatic f.
    Spero f.
    Spero meibomian f.
    Spero meibomian expressor f.
    Spetzler f.
    sphenoidal punch f.
    spicule f.
    spinal-perforating f.
    spinal rongeur f.
    spiral f.
    splinter f.
    splitting f.
    sponge f.
    sponge-and-dressing f.
    sponge-holding f.
    sponging f.
    spoon-shaped f.
    spring-handled f.
    Spurling f.
    Spurling intervertebral disk f.
    Spurling-Kerrison f.
    Spurling-Kerrison rongeur f.
    Spurling rongeur f.
    Spurling tissue f.
    square specimen f.
    squeeze-handle f.
    SSW f.
    Stamm bone-cutting f.
    standard f.
    standard arterial f.
    stapedectomy f.
    stapes f.
    staple f.

    Stark vulsellum f.
    Starr f.
    Starr fixation f.
    Staude f.
    Staude-Jackson tenaculum f.
    Staude-Moore f.
    Staude-Moore tenaculum f.
    Staude-Moore uterine f.
    Staude-Moore uterine tenaculum f.
    Staude tenaculum f.
    Staude uterine tenaculum f.
    Stavis fixation f.
    St. Clair f.
    St. Clair-Thompson f.
    St. Clair-Thompson abscess f.
    St. Clair-Thompson adenoidal f.
    St. Clair-Thompson peritonsillar abscess f.
    Steinmann intestinal f.
    Steinmann intestinal-grasping f.
    sterilizing f.
    sternal punch f.
    Stern-Castroviejo f.
    Stern-Castroviejo locking f.
    Stern-Castroviejo suturing f.
    Stevens f.
    Stevens fixation f.
    Stevens iris f.
    Stevenson f.
    Stevenson cupped-jaw f.
    Stevenson grasping f.
    Stevenson microsurgical f.
    Stieglitz splinter f.
    Stille f.
    Stille-Adson f.
    Stille-Babcock f.
    Stille-Barraya intestinal f.
    Stille-Barraya intestinal-grasping f.
    Stille-Barraya vascular f.
    Stille-Björk f.
    Stille-Crafoord f.
    Stille-Crile f.
    Stille gallstone f.
    Stille-Halsted f.
    Stille-Horsley f.
    Stille-Horsley bone-cutting f.
    Stille-Horsley rib f.
    Stille kidney f.

Stille kidney pedicle f.
Stille-Liston f.
Stille-Liston bone f.
Stille-Liston bone-cutting f.
Stille-Liston rib-cutting f.
Stille-Luer f.
Stille-Luer rongeur f.
Stille rongeur f.
Stille-Russian f.
Stille tissue f.
Stille-Waugh f.
Stiwer biopsy f.
Stiwer bone-holding f.
Stiwer dressing f.
Stiwer sponge f.
Stiwer tissue f.
St. Martin f.
St. Martin eye f.
St. Martin suturing f.
Stone f.
stone f.
Stone clamp-applying f.
stone-crushing f.
stone-extraction f.
stone-grasping f.
Stone intestinal f.
Stoneman f.
Stone tissue f.
Storey f.
Storey gall duct f.
Storey-Hillar dissecting f.
Storey thoracic f.
Storey thoracic
  hemostatic f.
Storz f.
Storz biopsy f.
Storz-Bonn f.
Storz-Bonn suturing f.
Storz bronchoscopic f.
Storz ciliary f.
Storz curved f.
Storz cystoscopic f.
Storz esophagoscopic f.
Storz grasping biopsy f.
Storz kidney stone f.
Storz miniature f.
Storz nasopharyngeal
  biopsy f.
Storz optical biopsy f.
Storz sinus biopsy f.
Storz stone-crushing f.
Storz stone-extraction f.
strabismus f.

straight f.
straight coagulating f.
straight-end cup f.
straight single tenaculum f.
straight-tip jeweler's
  bipolar f.
Strassburger tissue f.
Strassmann uterine f.
Strassmann uterine-
  elevating f.
Stratte f.
Streli f.
Strelinger catheter-
  introducing f.
Stringer f.
Stringer catheter-
  introducing f.
Stringer newborn throat f.
Struempel f.
Struempel ear f.
Struempel ear alligator f.
Struempel ear punch f.
Struempel-Voss ethmoidal f.
Struempel-Voss nasal f.
Strully dressing f.
Strully tissue f.
strut f.
Struyken f.
Struyken ear f.
Struyken nasal f.
Struyken nasal-cutting f.
Struyken turbinate f.
St. Vincent f.
St. Vincent tube-clamping f.
St. Vincent tube-occluding f.
Styles f.
subglottic f.
suction f.
suction tube-holding f.
Suker iris f.
superior rectus f.
Sutherland vitreous f.
suture f.
suture-carrying f.
suture clip f.
suture clip-applying f.
suture clip-removing f.
suture-holding f.
suture-pulling f.
suture-removing f.
suture-spreading f.
suture tag f.
suture and tying f.

forceps *(continued)*
    suture-tying f.
    suture-tying platform f.
    suturing f.
    Swan-Brown arterial f.
    Sweet f.
    Sweet clip-applying f.
    Sweet dissecting f.
    Sweet ligature f.
    Syark vulsellum f.
    synovium biopsy f.
    Szuler f.
    Szuler vascular f.
    Szultz corneal f.
    tack-and-pin f.
    Takahashi f.
    Takahashi cutting f.
    Takahashi ethmoidal f.
    Takahashi nasal f.
    Takahashi neurosurgical f.
    tampon f.
    Tamsco f.
    tangential f.
    taper-jaw rongeur f.
    Tarnier f.
    Tarnier axis-traction f.
    Tarnier obstetrical f.
    Taylor f.
    Taylor-Cushing dressing f.
    Taylor dissecting f.
    Taylor tissue f.
    Teale f.
    Teale tenaculum f.
    Teale uterine f.
    Teale uterine vulsellum f.
    Teale vulsellum f.
    Tekno f.
    temporary clip-applying f.
    temporary vessel clamp-
      applying f.
    tenaculum f.
    tendon f.
    tendon-holding f.
    tendon-passing f.
    tendon-pulling f.
    tendon-tunneling f.
    Tennant f.
    Tennant-Colibri corneal f.
    Tennant intraocular lens f.
    Tennant lens f.
    Tennant lens-inserting f.
    Tennant-Maumenee f.

    Tennant-Troutman superior
      rectus f.
    Tennant tying f.
    Tenzel f.
    Tenzel bipolar f.
    Terson f.
    Terson capsular f.
    Terson extracapsular f.
    Tessier disimpaction
      device f.
    Thackray dental f.
    Theurig sterilizer f.
    Thomas f.
    Thomas shot compression f.
    Thomas uterine tissue-
      grasping f.
    Thompson hip prosthesis f.
    Thompson rasp f.
    Thoms f.
    Thoms-Allis f.
    Thoms-Allis intestinal f.
    Thoms-Allis tissue f.
    Thoms-Gaylor f.
    Thoms-Gaylor f.
    Thoms-Gaylor biopsy f.
    Thoms-Gaylor uterine f.
    Thoms-Gaylor uterine
      biopsy f.
    Thoms tissue f.
    Thoms tissue-grasping f.
    thoracic f.
    thoracic artery f.
    thoracic hemostatic f.
    thoracic tissue f.
    Thorek gallbladder f.
    Thorek-Mixter f.
    Thorek-Mixter gallbladder f.
    Thorek-Mixter gall duct f.
    Thornton episcleral f.
    Thornton fixation f.
    Thornton incision-
      spreading f.
    Thornton intraocular f.
    Thorpe f.
    Thorpe conjunctival f.
    Thorpe conjunctival
      fixation f.
    Thorpe corneal f.
    Thorpe corneoscleral f.
    Thorpe cup-jaw f.
    Thorpe foreign body f.
    Thorpe suture-spreading f.
    Thrasher intraocular f.

three-armed basket f.
three-prong grasping f.
three-prong sterilizer f.
throat f.
thumb f.
thumb-dressing f.
thumb tissue f.
Thurston-Holland
  fragment f.
thyroid f.
thyroid traction f.
Tickner f.
Tickner tissue f.
Tiemann bullet f.
Tiley dressing f.
Tilley-Henckel f.
Tischer biopsy f.
Tischler f.
Tischler cervical f.
Tischler cervical biopsy f.
Tischler cervical biopsy
  punch f.
Tischler-Morgan biopsy f.
tissue f.
tissue-dressing f.
tissue-grasping f.
tissue-holding f.
titanium bipolar f.
Tivnen f.
Tivnen tonsillar f.
Tivnen tonsil-seizing f.
Tobey f.
Tobey ear f.
Tobold f.
Tobold-Fauvel grasping f.
Tobold laryngeal f.
Toennis-Adson f.
Toennis tumor-grasping f.
Tomac f.
tongue f.
tongue-holding f.
tongue-seizing f.
tonsil-holding f.
tonsillar f.
tonsillar abscess f.
tonsillar artery f.
tonsillar hemostatic f.
tonsillar needle holder f.
tonsillar pillar grasping f.
tonsillar punch f.
tonsil-ligating f.
tonsil-seizing f.
tonsil-suturing f.

Tooke corneal f.
Toomey f.
toothed f.
toothed thumb f.
toothed tissue f.
tooth-extracting f.
toothless f.
Torchia capsular f.
Torchia-Colibri f.
Torchia lens implantation f.
Torchia microbipolar f.
Torchia tissue f.
Torchia tying f.
Torres cross-action f.
torsion f.
towel f.
towel clip f.
Tower f.
Tower muscle f.
Townley f.
Townley tissue f.
tracheal f.
tracheal hemostatic f.
trachoma f.
traction f.
transfer f.
transphenoidal f.
transplant-grafting f.
transsphenoidal bipolar f.
triangular punch f.
Troeltsch f.
Troeltsch ear f.
Troeltsch ear-dressing f.
Troeltsch nasal-dressing f.
Trotter f.
Trousseau f.
Trousseau dilating f.
Troutman f.
Troutman-Barraquer f.
Troutman-Barraquer
  Colibri f.
Troutman-Barraquer
  corneal f.
Troutman-Barraquer corneal
  utility f.
Troutman-Barraquer iris f.
Troutman corneal f.
Troutman-Llobera f.
Troutman-Llobera fixation f.
Troutman-Llobera
  Flieringa f.
Troutman microsurgery f.
Troutman rectal f.

forceps *(continued)*
    Troutman superior rectus f.
    Trush grasping f.
    Trylon hemostatic f.
    T-shaped f.
    T-shaped angled f.
    tube f.
    tube-occluding f.
    tubing clamp f.
    Tubinger gall stone f.
    tubular f.
    Tucker f.
    Tucker bead f.
    Tucker hallux f.
    Tucker-McLane f.
    Tucker-McLane axis-
      traction f.
    Tucker-McLane-Luikart f.
    Tucker-McLane obstetrical f.
    Tucker reach-and-pin f.
    Tucker tack-and-pin f.
    Tudor-Edwards f.
    Tuffier f.
    Tuffier artery traction f.
    tumor f.
    turbinate f.
    Turnbull f.
    Turnbull adhesions f.
    Turner-Babcock tissue f.
    Turner-Warwick-Adson f.
    Turner-Warwick stone f.
    Turrell f.
    Turrell biopsy f.
    Turrell rectal biopsy f.
    Turrell specimen f.
    Turrell-Wittner rectal f.
    Turrell-Wittner rectal
     biopsy f.
    Tuttle f.
    Tuttle dressing f.
    Tuttle obstetrical f.
    Tuttle-Singley thoracic f.
    Tuttle thoracic f.
    Tuttle thumb f.
    Tuttle tissue f.
    Twisk f.
    two-stream irrigating f.
    two-toothed f.
    Tydings f.
    Tydings-Lakeside f.
    Tydings-Lakeside tonsillar f.
    Tydings-Lakeside tonsil-
     seizing f.
    Tydings tonsillar f.
    Tydings tonsil-seizing f.
    tying f.
    tympanoplasty f.
    Tyrrell foreign body f.
    Ullrich f.
    Ullrich-Aesculap f.
    Ullrich bone-holding f.
    Ullrich dressing f.
    Ullrich small bone-
     holding f.
    Ullrich-St. Gallen f.
    Universal f.
    University f.
    University of Kansas f.
    University of Kansas
     corneal f.
    University of Michigan
     Mixter f.
    University of Michigan
     Mixter thoracic f.
    upbiting f.
    upbiting biopsy f.
    upbiting cup f.
    upcurved basket f.
    Uppsala gall duct f.
    Urbantschitsch f.
    Urbantschitsch nasal f.
    ureteral f.
    ureteral catheter f.
    ureteral isolation f.
    ureteral stone f.
    ureteral stone isolation f.
    U-shaped f.
    uterine f.
    uterine artery f.
    uterine biopsy f.
    uterine biopsy punch f.
    uterine-dressing f.
    uterine-elevating f.
    uterine-holding f.
    uterine-manipulating f.
    uterine-packing f.
    uterine polyp f.
    uterine specimen f.
    uterine tenaculum f.
    uterine vulsellum f.
    utility f.
    Utrata f.
    Utrata capsulorrhexis f.
    vaginal f.
    vaginal hysterectomy f.
    valve redo f.

Van Buren f.
Van Buren bone-holding f.
Van Buren sequestrum f.
Vanderbilt f.
Vanderbilt arterial f.
Vanderbilt deep-vessel f.
Vanderbilt hemostatic f.
Vanderbilt University
  hemostatic f.
Vanderbilt University
  vessel f.
Vander Pool sterilizer f.
Van Doren f.
Van Doren uterine f.
Van Doren uterine biopsy
  punch f.
Van Mandach capsule
  fragment and clot f.
Vannas fixation f.
Van Ruben f.
Van Struyken f.
Van Struyken nasal f.
Van Struyken nasal-
  cutting f.
Vantage tube-occluding f.
Vantec grasping f.
Varco f.
Varco gallbladder f.
Varco thoracic f.
vari-angle temporary clip-
  applying f.
vascular f.
vascular and needle-
  pulling f.
vascular tissue f.
vasectomy f.
vas isolation f.
Vaughn sterilizer f.
vectis f.
vectis cesarean f.
vectis cesarean section f.
vena caval f.
Verbrugge f.
Verbrugge bone-holding f.
Verhoeff f.
Verhoeff capsular f.
Verhoeff cataract f.
vessel f.
vessel clip-applying f.
vessel pediatric f.
vessel peripheral f.
Vick-Blanchard f.

Vick-Blanchard
  hemorrhoidal f.
Victor-Bonney f.
Vigger-5 eye f.
Virtus f.
Virtus splinter f.
viscera-holding f.
visceral f.
vise f.
visual hemostatic f.
Vital f.
Vital Adson tissue f.
Vital Babcock tissue f.
Vital Cushing tissue f.
Vital Duval intestinal f.
Vital Evans pelvic tissue f.
Vital general tissue f.
Vital intestinal f.
Vital lung-grasping f.
Vital needle holder f.
Vital Potts-Smith f.
Vital tissue f.
Vital Wangensteen tissue f.
vitreous-grasping f.
V. Mueller biopsy f.
V. Mueller bone-cutting f.
V. Mueller laser Adson
  tissue f.
V. Mueller laser Backhaus
  towel f.
V. Mueller laser Crile
  micro-arterial f.
V. Mueller laser micro-
  Allis f.
V. Mueller laser Rhoton
  microtying f.
V. Mueller laser Singley
  tissue f.
V. Mueller nonperforating
  towel f.
V. Mueller tying f.
V. Mueller-Vital laser
  Babcock f.
V. Mueller-Vital laser Potts-
  Smith f.
Vogler hysterectomy f.
Vogt f.
Vogt toothed capsular f.
vomer f.
vomer septal f.
von Mandach f.
von Petz f.

forceps *(continued)*

Voris-Oldberg intervertebral disk f.
Voris-Wester f.
Vorse tube-occluding f.
Vorse-Wester f.
VPI-Ambrose resectoscope f.
vulsellum f.
Wachtenfeldt f.
Wachtenfeldt clip-applying f.
Wachtenfeldt clip-removing f.
Wadsworth lid f.
Wagensteen tissue f.
Wainstock eye f.
Waldeau f.
Waldeau fixation f.
Waldenstrom laryngeal f.
Waldeyer f.
Waldron f.
Walker f.
Wallace cesarean f.
Walsh f.
Walsham f.
Walsham nasal f.
Walsham septal f.
Walsham septum-straightening f.
Walsh tissue f.
Walter f.
Walter splinter f.
Walther f.
Walther tissue f.
Walton f.
Walton-Allis tissue f.
Walton-Liston f.
Walton meniscal f.
Walton-Schubert f.
Walton-Schubert uterine biopsy f.
Walzl hysterectomy f.
Wangensteen f.
Wangensteen intestinal f.
Wangensteen tissue f.
Warthen f.
watchmaker f.
Watson f.
Watson angular f.
Watson tonsil-seizing f.
Watson-Williams f.
Watson-Williams ethmoid-biting f.
Watson-Williams nasal f.
Watson-Williams polyp f.
Watzke f.
Watzke sleeve-spreading f.
Waugh-Brophy f.
Waugh dissection f.
Waugh dressing f.
Waugh tissue f.
wave-tooth f.
Weaver f.
Weaver chalazion f.
Weck f.
Weck-Harms f.
Weck hysterectomy f.
Weck rectal biopsy f.
Weck towel f.
Weck uterine biopsy f.
Weeks eye f.
Weiger-Zollner f.
Weil f.
Weil-Blakesley ethmoidal f.
Weil ear f.
Weil ethmoidal f.
Weiner uterine biopsy f.
Weingartner f.
Weingartner ear f.
Weis chalazion f.
Weisenbach f.
Weisman f.
Weisman uterine tenaculum f.
Welch Allyn f.
Welch Allyn anal biopsy f.
Weller cartilage f.
Weller meniscal f.
Wells f.
Welsh f.
Welsh ophthalmological f.
Welsh pupil spreader-retractor f.
Wertheim f.
Wertheim-Cullen f.
Wertheim-Cullen compression f.
Wertheim-Cullen hysterectomy f.
Wertheim-Cullen kidney pedicle f.
Wertheim-Cullen pedicle f.
Wertheim hysterectomy f.
Wertheim-Navratil f.
Wertheim uterine f.
Wertheim vaginal f.
Westermark f.

Westermark-Stille f.
Westermark uterine
  dressing f.
Westmacott f.
Westmacott dressing f.
West nasal-dressing f.
Westphal f.
Westphal gall duct f.
Westphal hemostatic f.
Wheeler plaque f.
Wheeler vessel f.
White f.
White-Lillie f.
White-Lillie tonsillar f.
White-Lillie tonsil-seizing f.
White-Oslay f.
White-Oslay prostatic f.
White-Oslay prostatic lobe-
  holding f.
White-Smith f.
White tonsillar f.
White tonsillar hemostatic f.
White tonsil-seizing f.
Wickman uterine f.
Wiener hysterectomy f.
Wies f.
Wies chalazion f.
Wiet otologic cup f.
Wikstroem f.
Wikstroem arterial f.
Wilde f.
Wilde-Blakesley f.
Wilde-Blakesley ethmoidal f.
Wilde ear f.
Wilde ethmoidal f.
Wilde ethmoidal
  exenteration f.
Wilde intervertebral disk f.
Wilde laminectomy f.
Wilde nasal-cutting f.
Wilde nasal-dressing f.
Wilder dilating f.
Wilde septal f.
Wilde-Troeltsch f.
Willauer-Allis f.
Willauer-Allis thoracic f.
Willauer-Allis thoracic
  tissue f.
Willauer-Allis tissue f.
Willauer intrathoracic f.
Willett f.
Willett placental f.
Willett placenta previa f.

Willett scalp flap f.
Williams f.
Williamsburg f.
Williams diskectomy f.
Williams gastrointestinal f.
Williams intestinal f.
Williams splinter f.
Williams tissue f.
Williams uterine f.
Williams vessel-holding f.
Wills Hospital f.
Wills Hospital
  ophthalmology f.
Wills Hospital utility f.
Wills utility f.
Wills utility eye f.
Wilmer iris f.
Wilson-Cook biopsy f.
Wilson-Cook bronchoscope
  biopsy f.
Wilson-Cook colonoscope
  biopsy f.
Wilson-Cook gastroscope
  biopsy f.
Wilson-Cook grasping f.
Wilson-Cook hot biopsy f.
Wilson-Cook retrieval f.
Wilson-Cook tripod
  retrieval f.
Wilson vitreous foreign
  body f.
Winter-Nassauer placental f.
Winter ovum f.
wire-closure f.
wire-crimping f.
wire prosthesis-crimping f.
wire-pulling f.
wire-twisting f.
Wittner f.
Wittner uterine biopsy f.
Wolf biopsy f.
Wolf biting-basket f.
Wolf curved-basket f.
Wolfe cataract delivery f.
Wolfe eye f.
Wolfe uterine cuff f.
Wolfson f.
Woodward f.
Woodward hemostatic f.
Woodward-Potts intestinal f.
Woodward thoracic artery f.
Woodward thoracic
  hemostatic f.

forceps *(continued)*
    Worth f.
    Worth advancement f.
    Worth muscle f.
    Worth strabismus f.
    wound f.
    wound-clip f.
    Wright-Rubin f.
    Wrigley f.
    W-shape f.
    Wullstein f.
    Wullstein ear f.
    Wullstein-House f.
    Wullstein-Paparella f.
    Wullstein tympanoplasty f.
    Wylie f.
    Wylie tenaculum f.
    Wylie uterine f.
    Wylie uterine tenaculum f.
    X-long cement f.
    Yankauer f.
    Yankauer ethmoidal f.
    Yankauer ethmoid-cutting f.
    Yankauer-Little f.
    Yankauer-Little tube f.
    Yasargil f.
    Yasargil alligator-type f.
    Yasargil angled f.
    Yasargil applying f.
    Yasargil arterial f.
    Yasargil bayonet-shaped f.
    Yasargil bipolar f.
    Yasargil clip-applying f.
    Yasargil microvessel clip applying f.
    Yasargil neurosurgical bipolar f.
    Yasargil straight f.
    Yeoman f.
    Yeoman biopsy f.
    Yeoman rectal biopsy f.
    Yeoman uterine f.
    Yeoman-Wittner rectal f.
    Yeoman-Wittner rectal biopsy f.
    Young f.
    Younge f.
    Younge-Kevorkian f.
    Younge uterine f.
    Younge uterine biopsy f.
    Young intestinal f.
    Young lobe f.
    Young prostatectomy f.
    Young prostatic f.
    Young rubber-jaws f.
    Young tongue f.
    Young tongue-holding f.
    Young tongue-seizing f.
    Young uterine f.
    Zeeifel angiotribe f.
    Zenker f.
    Zenker dissecting and ligature f.
    Zeppelin obstetrical f.
    Ziegler f.
    Ziegler ciliary f.
    Zimmer-Hoen f.
    Zimmer-Schlesinger f.
    Zollinger f.
    Zollinger multipurpose tissue f.

Ford
    F. clamp
    F. Hospital ventricular cannula

Ford-Deaver retractor

forearm reduction unit

Foregger
    F. bronchoscope
    F. laryngoscope
    F. rigid esophagoscope

foreign
    f. body curette
    f. body cystoscopy forceps
    f. body eye forceps
    f. body forceps
    f. body loop
    f. body needle
    f. body probe
    f. body screw
    f. body spud

fork
    crus guide f.
    double-pronged f.
    Gardiner-Brown neurological tuning f.
    f. hammer
    Hardy f.
    Hardy implant f.
    Hartmann tuning f.
    Jacobson f.
    Jannetta double-pronged f.
    Jarit tuning f.
    Leasure tuning f.
    magnesium tuning f.
    McCabe crus guide f.

neurological tuning f.
Okonek-Yasargil tumor f.
Penn tuning f.
Penn tuning f.
3-prong f.
Ralks tuning f.
Rhoton 3-prong f.
Rica tuning f.
Riverbank Laboratories
  tuning f.
Rydel-Seiffert tuning f.
SMIC tuning f.
tuning f.
form
Amoena breast f.
breast f.
Dow Corning external
  breast f.
Spenco external breast f.
Trulife silicone breast f.
Yours Truly asymmetrical
  external breast f.
formaldehyde catgut suture
Formatray mandibular splint
formed
f. cystitome
f. non-irrigating cystitome
Formex barium catheter
FormFlex
F. formacresal lens
F. intraocular lens
Foroblique
F. bronchoscope
F. endoscope
F. esophagoscope
F. fiberoptic esophagoscope
F. lens
F. microlens resectoscope
F. panendoscope
F. resectoscope
F. telescope
Forrester
F. brace
F. cervical collar brace
F. clamp
F. head halter
F. head splint
F. spray
Fort urethral bougie
forty-day chromic catgut suture
forward-grasping forceps
forwarding probe
forward-viewing endoscope

Foss
F. anterior resection clamp
F. bifid gallbladder retractor
F. bifid retractor
F. biliary retractor
F. cardiovascular clamp
F. cardiovascular forceps
F. clamp
F. clamp forceps
F. forceps
F. gallbladder retractor
F. intestinal clamp
F. intestinal clamp forceps
F. retractor
fossa curette
Foster
F. bed
F. enucleation snare
F. fracture frame
F. scissors
F. snare
F. turning fracture frame
Foster-Ballenger
F.-B. forceps
F.-B. nasal speculum
Fothergill suture
Fotofil
F. activator light
F. dental restorative
  material
Fouli tourniquet
fountain
xenon cold light f.
Fountain design prosthesis
four-by-fours (4x4s)
four-eye catheter
four-flanged nail
four-footed lens lens
four-legged cage heart valve
four-piece intraocular lens
four-point
f.-p. cervical brace
f.-p. fixation intraocular
  lens
four-prong
f.-p. finger speculum
f.-p. finger splint
f.-p. retractor
four-tailed
f.-t. bandage
f.-t. dressing
four-wing
f.-w. catheter

four-wing *(continued)*
  f.-w. drain
  f.-w. Malecot drain
  f.-w. Malecot retention
    catheter
Fowler
  F. curette
  F. double-end curette
  F. dressing
  F. self-retaining retractor
  F. urethral sound
Fowler-Zollner knife
Fox
  F. balloon
  F. bipolar forceps
  F. clavicular splint
  F. conformer
  F. curette
  F. dermal curette
  F. eye implant
  F. eyelid implant
  F. eye shield
  F. eye speculum
  F. hydrostatic irrigator
  F. implant
  F. internal fixation device
  F. postnasal balloon
  F. prosthesis
  F. sphere eye implant
  F. sphere implant
  F. tissue forceps
Fox-Blazina prosthesis
Frackelton
  F. fascial needle
  F. needle
  F. wire threader
Frac-Sur
  F.-S. apparatus
  F.-S. appliance
  F.-S. splint
  F.-S. unit
fraction
  MB f.
Fractomed splint
Fractura
  F. Flex bandage
  F. Flex elastic bandage
fracture
  f. appliance
  f. band
  f. bar
  f. bed
  f. chisel

  f. frame
  f. splint
fracture-banding apparatus
Fraenkel *(var. of* Fränkel)
Fragen
  F. anterior commissure
    microlaryngoscope
  F. carrier
  F. laryngoscope
  F. laryngoscope fiberoptic
    light
fragment
  Cooper blade f.
  f. forceps
fragmentation probe
Frahm carver
Frahur
  F. cartilage clamp
  F. clamp
  F. scissors
frame
  Ace-Fischer f.
  Alexian Brothers overhead
    fracture f.
  Andrews f.
  A-f. orthosis
  arch bars f.
  Balkan fracture f.
  Böhler-Braun fracture f.
  Böhler reducing fracture f.
  Bradford fracture f.
  Braun f.
  Buck extension f.
  Charest head f.
  Charest head fracture f.
  Cole hyperextension
    fracture f.
  Colles external fixation f.
  cranio x-ray f.
  Crawford head f.
  Crawford head fracture f.
  Davis-Crowe mouth gag f.
  Delta external fixation f.
  Denis Browne pediatric
    retractor oval sprocket f.
  Denis Browne retractor oval
    sprocket f.
  DePuy rainbow fracture f.
  Dingman mouth gag f.
  Doctor Plymale lift
    fracture f.
  Elgiloy f. of prosthetic
    value

Danis-Weber

Erich facial fracture f.
Foster fracture f.
Foster turning fracture f.
fracture f.
Goldthwait fracture f.
Goligher retractor f.
Granberry hyperextension
  fracture f.
halo fracture f.
halo head f.
head f.
Heffington lumbar seat
  spinal surgery f.
Herzmark fracture f.
Hibbs fracture f.
hyperextension fracture f.
Irby head f.
Janes fracture f.
Jewett f.
Joseph septal f.
laminectomy f.
Leivers mouth gag f.
Leksell f.
Leksell stereotaxic f.
Lex-Ton lumbar
  laminectomy f.
Malcolm-Rand cranial x-
  ray f.
mouth gag f.
occluding fracture f.
overhead fracture f.
pediatric retractor oval
  sprocket f.
Pittsburgh pelvic triangular
  external f.
Pittsburgh triangular f.
Putti f.
quadraplegic standing f.
Rainbow fracture f.
Rand-Malcolm cranial x-
  ray f.
reducing fracture f.
Relton-Hall f.
retractor f.
retractor oval sprocket f.
Richards Colles fracture f.
Russell f.
Slatis f.
Stryker CircOlectric
  fracture f.
Stryker turning fracture f.
Thomas fracture f.

Thompson hyperextention
  fracture f.
trial fracture f.
Vasocillator fracture f.
Vidal-Hoffman fixator f.
Whitman fracture f.
Wilson f.
Wilson spinal f.
Wingfield fracture f.
Young rubber dam
  fracture f.
Zimcode traction f.
Zimmer fracture f.
Framer tendon-passing needle
Francer porcelain powder
Franceschetti corneal trephine
Francis
  F. chalazion forceps
  F. forceps
  F. knife spud
Francis-Gray wire crimper
Francke needle
Franco triflange ventilation tube
Frangenheim
  F. biopsy punch forceps
  F. forceps
  F. hook forceps
  F. hook punch
  F. laparoscope
Fränkel, Fraenkel, Frankel
  F. appliance
  F. cutting-tip forceps
  F. double-articulated-tip
    forceps
  F. esophagoscopy forceps
  F. forceps
  F. head band
  F. laryngeal forceps
  F. sinus probe
  F. speculum
  F. tampon forceps
Frankfeldt
  F. diathermy snare
  F. forceps
  F. grasping forceps
  F. hemorrhoidal needle
  F. needle
  F. rectal snare
  F. rectal snare bushing for
    stem
  F. rectal snare hinged-loop
    wire

Frankfeldt *(continued)*
  F. rectal snare insulated
    stem
  F. sigmoidoscope
  F. snare
Franklin
  F. liver puncture needle
  F. malleable retractor
  F. retractor
Franklin-Silverman
  F.-S. biopsy cannula
  F.-S. biopsy needle
  F.-S. cannula
  F.-S. curette
  F.-S. needle
  F.-S. prostatic needle
  F.-S. urologic biopsy needle
Franz
  F. abdominal retractor
  F. retractor
Fraser
  F. depressor
  F. forceps
  F. suction tube
Frater
  F. intracardiac retractor
  F. retractor
Frazier
  F. aspirating tube
  F. brain-exploring cannula
  F. brain-exploring trocar
  F. brain suction tube
  F. Britetrac nasal suction
    tube
  F. cannula
  F. cerebral retractor
  F. cordotomy hook
  F. cordotomy knife
  F. disposable suction tube
  F. dural elevator
  F. dural hook
  F. dural scissors
  F. dural separator
  F. exploring cannula
  F. fiberoptic suction tube
  F. laminectomy retractor
  F. lighted retractor
  F. modified suction tube
  F. monopolar cautery cord
  F. nasal suction tube
  F. needle
  F. nerve hook

  F. obturator aspirating
    suction tube
  F. osteotome
  F. pituitary capsulectomy
    knife
  F. retractor
  F. skin hook
  F. suction
  F. suction cannula
  F. suction elevator
  F. suction tip
  F. suction tube
  F. suction tube obturator
  F. ventricular cannula
  F. ventricular needle
Frazier-Adson
  F.-A. clamp
  F.-A. osteoplastic clamp
  F.-A. osteoplastic flap clamp
Frazier-Fay retractor
Frazier-Ferguson
  F.-F. aspirating tube
  F.-F. ear suction tube
  F.-F. suction tube
Frazier-Paparella
  F.-P. mastoid suction tube
  F.-P. mastoid tube
  F.-P. suction tube
Frazier-Sachs clamp
Frederick
  F. needle
  F. pneumothoracic needle
Fredricks mammary prosthesis
free
  f. implant
  f. ligature suture
Freedom
  F. dental unit
  F. external catheter
Freeman
  F. Blue-Max cannula
  F. capsular polisher
  F. clamp
  F. face-lift retractor
  F. positioning cannula
  F. retractor
  F. rhytidectomy scissors
  F. transorbital leukotome
Freeman-Samuelson knee prosthesis
Freeman-Schepens scissors
Freeman-Swanson knee prosthesis
Freenseen
  F. liver biopsy needle

F. rectal curette
F. ultrasound needle
Freer
F. bone chisel
F. chisel
F. dissector
F. double elevator
F. double-end elevator
F. dural dissector
F. dural retractor
F. elevator
F. elevator-dissector
F. lacrimal chisel
F. nasal chisel
F. nasal gouge
F. nasal knife
F. nasal spatula
F. periosteal elevator
F. periosteotome
F. retractor
F. septal elevator
F. septal forceps
F. septal knife
F. skin hook
F. skin retractor
F. spatula
F. submucous chisel
F. submucous knife
F. submucous retractor
Freer-Gruenwald
F.-G. forceps
F.-G. punch forceps
Freer-Ingal
F.-I. nasal knife
F.-I. submucous knife
Freer-Sachs dissector
Freestyle CAPD catheter adapter
free-tie suture
Freiberg
F. hip retractor
F. nerve root retractor
F. retractor
F. traction tractor
Freiburg
F. biopsy set
F. mediastinoscope
Freidenwald-Guyton snare
Freidrich-Ferguson retractor
Freimuth
F. curette
F. ear curette
Frejka splint
Frekatheter vena caval catheter

French
F. angiographic catheter
F. brain retractor
F. catheter
F. chisel
F. curve out-of-plane catheter
F. dilator
F. Foley catheter
F. Hanks uterine dilator
F. in-plane guiding catheter
F. JR4 Schneider catheter
F. lacrimal dilator
F. lock
F. MBIH catheter
F. mushroom-tip catheter
F. needle
F. red-rubber Robinson catheter
F. retractor
F. Robinson catheter
F. SAL catheter
F. scoop
F. sheath
F. Silastic Foley catheter
F. sound
F. spring-eye needle
F. S-shaped brain retractor
F. S-shaped retractor
F. stent
F. suture
F. tripolar His catheter
5-French
5-F. angiographic catheter
5-F. stiff catheter
French-eye
F.-e. needle
F.-e. needle holder
F.-e. Vital needle holder
French-McCarthy endoscope
French-McRea dilator
French-pattern
F.-p. forceps
F.-p. lacrimal probe
F.-p. osteotome
F.-p. raspatory
F.-p. spatula
French-Stern-McCarthy retractor
Frenckner curette
Frenckner-Stille
F.-S. curette
F.-S. punch

Fresenius
F. dialysis machine
F. Euro-Collins kit
Fresgen frontal sinus probe
Fresnel
F. lens
F. lens pusher
F. nystagmus glasses
F. nystagmus spectacles
Frey
F. eye implant
F. tunneled eye implant
Freyer
F. drain
F. suprapubic drain
Frey-Freer bur
Frey-Sauerbruch rib shears
Fricke
F. arterial forceps
F. bandage
F. dressing
F. scrotal dressing
friction lock pin
Frieberg cartilage knife
Friederich-Ferguson retractor
Friedman
F. bone rongeur
F. clip
F. elevator
F. knife guide
F. olive-tip vein stripper
F. perineal retractor
F. rasp
F. retractor
F. rongeur
F. rongeur forceps
F. tantalum clip
F. taper-jaw rongeur forceps
F. vaginal retractor
F. vein stripper
F. visual field analyzer
Friedman-Hruby lens
Friedman-Otis
F.-O. bougie
F.-O. bougie à boule
Friedrich
F. clamp
F. raspatory
F. rib elevator
Friedrich-Petz
F.-P. clamp
F.-P. machine resector

Friend catheter
Friend-Hebert catheter
Friesner ear knife
Frigitronics
F. colposcope
F. cryoextractor
F. cryoprobe
F. disposable cryosurgical stylet
F. F-20/20 disposable cryoextractor
F. Mark II cryoextractor
F. nitrous oxide cryosurgery apparatus
F. probe
Frimberger-Karpiel
F.-K. 12 O'Clock papillotome
F.-K. 12 O'Clock sphincterotome
Fritsch
F. abdominal retractor
F. catheter
F. retractor
Fritz
F. aspirator
F. needle
frog-leg splint
Frohm mouth gag
Froimson splint
Frommer dilator
frontal
f. sinus cannula
f. sinus chisel
f. sinus curette
f. sinus dilator
f. sinus probe
f. sinus rasp
f. sinus wash tube
f. suture
f. zygomatic suture
frontalis snare
front build-up eye implant
frontoethmoidal suture
frontolacrimal suture
frontomalar suture
frontonasal suture
frontoparietal suture
frontosphenoid suture
frontozygomatic suture
Frost suture
Fruehevald splint

Frye
- F. aspirator
- F. portable aspirator

Frykholm
- F. bone rongeur
- F. goniometer

Fry nasal forceps

Fuchs
- F. capsular forceps
- F. capsulotomy forceps
- F. extracapsular forceps
- F. forceps
- F. iris forceps
- F. keratome
- F. surgical stool
- F. two-way syringe

Fuji
- F. cavity varnish
- F. dental cement

Fujica camera

Fujinon
- F. biopsy forceps
- F. diagnostic laparoscope
- F. endoscope
- F. EVE video endoscope
- F. EVG-F upper GI video endoscope
- F. flexible endoscope
- F. flexible lower GI endoscope
- F. flexible sigmoidoscope
- F. forceps
- F. operating laparoscope
- F. UGI-FP endoscope

Fulcast alloy
fulgurating electrode
full-curved clamp
full-dimpled lucite eye implant

Fuller
- F. perianal shield
- F. rectal dressing
- F. shield
- F. shield dressing
- F. shield rectal dressing
- F. silicone sponge

full-hand splint
full-lumen esophagoscope
full-occlusal splint
full-radius resector
full-thickness implant

fully
- f. automatic atrioventricular Universal dual-channel pacemaker
- f. automatic pacemaker

Fulpit
- F. forceps
- F. tissue forceps

Fulton
- F. laminectomy rongeur
- F. mouth gag
- F. pediatric scissors
- F. retractor

Ful-Vue
- F.-V. ophthalmoscope
- F.-V. spot retinoscope
- F.-V. streak retinoscope

functional fracture brace

fundal
- f. camera
- f. laser lens

funduscope
fundus-retinal camera
funicular suture
Funsten supination splint

Furacin
- F. dressing
- F. gauze dressing
- F. gauze holder

Furlong tendon stripper
Furlow cylinder passer

Furness
- F. anastomosis clamp
- F. catheter
- F. clamp
- F. cornea-holding forceps
- F. forceps
- F. polyp forceps
- F. suture

Furness-Clute
- F.-C. anastomosis clamp
- F.-C. clamp
- F.-C. duodenal clamp
- F.-C. pin

Furness-McClure-Hinton clamp
furrier's suture
fusiform bougie

Futch
- F. antral cannula
- F. cannula

Futuro wrist brace

311

Fyodorov, Federov, Fydorov, Fyoderov
  F. dipstick
  F. eye implant
  F. four-loop iris clip intraocular lens
  F. implant
  F. intraocular lens
  F. lens expressor
  F. lens implant
  F. type II intraocular lens
  F. type II lens implant
  F. type I intraocular lens
  F. type I lens implant
Fyodorov-Sputnik FFP contact intraocular lens

Gabarro
    G. board
    G. plate skin retractor
    G. retractor
Gabriel
    G. proctoscope
    G. syringe
    G. Tucker bougie
    G. Tucker forceps
gaff
gag
    Boettcher-Jennings mouth g.
    Boyle-Davis mouth g.
    Brophy mouth g.
    Brown-Davis mouth g.
    Brown-Fillebrown-Whitehead
      mouth g.
    Brown-Whitehead mouth g.
    Collis mouth g.
    Crowe-Davis mouth g.
    Dann-Jennings mouth g.
    Davis-Crowe mouth g.
    Davis mouth g.
    Davis ring mouth g.
    Denhardt-Dingman mouth g.
    Denhardt mouth g.
    Dilner-Doughty mouth g.
    Dingman-Millard mouth g.
    Dingman mouth g.
    Dott-Kilner mouth g.
    Dott mouth g.
    Doxen mouth g.
    Doyen-Jansen mouth g.
    Ferguson-Ackland mouth g.
    Ferguson-Brophy mouth g.
    Ferguson-Gwathmey
      mouth g.
    Ferguson mouth g.
    Frohm mouth g.
    Fulton mouth g.
    Green mouth g.
    Green-Sewall mouth g.
    Hayton-Williams mouth g.
    Heister mouth g.
    Hewitt mouth g.
    Hibbs mouth g.
    Jansen mouth g.
    Jansen-Sluder mouth g.
    Jennings Loktite mouth g.

    Jennings mouth g.
    Jennings-Skillern mouth g.
    Kilner-Dott mouth g.
    Kilner mouth g.
    Lane mouth g.
    Lange mouth g.
    Leivers mouth g.
    Lewis mouth g.
    Maunder oral screw
      mouth g.
    McDowell mouth g.
    McIvor mouth g.
    McKesson mouth g.
    Mithoefer-Jansen mouth g.
    Molt mouth g.
    mouth g.
    Negus mouth g.
    Newkirk mouth g.
    oral screw mouth g.
    oral speculum mouth g.
    palate-type mouth g.
    Proetz-Jansen mouth g.
    Proetz mouth g.
    Pynchon mouth g.
    Ralks-Davis mouth g.
    Rew-Wyly mouth g.
    Roser-Koenig mouth g.
    Roser mouth g.
    Seeman-Seiffert mouth g.
    side mouth g.
    Sluder-Ferguson mouth g.
    Sluder-Jansen mouth g.
    Sydenham mouth g.
    Thackray mouth g.
    Trousseau mouth g.
    Wesson mouth g.
    Whitehead-Jennings
      mouth g.
    Whitehead mouth g.
    Wolf Loktite mouth g.
    Wolf mouth g.
Gaillart-Arlt suture
gaiter brace
Galand in-the-bag lens
**Galand-Knolle modified J-loop
    intraocular lens**
Galante hip prosthesis
Galaxy pacemaker
galeal forceps

Galen
   G. bandage
   G. dressing
Galetti articulator
Galezowski
   G. dilator
   G. lacrimal dilator
Galin
   G. intraocular lens implant
   G. lens spatula
   G. silicone bleb cup
gall
   g. duct dilator
   g. duct forceps
   g. duct probe
   g. duct scoop
Gall-Addison uterine manipulator
Gallagher
   G. antral rasp
   G. bipolar mapping probe
   G. probe
   G. trocar
gallbladder
   g. aspirator
   g. bed
   g. cannula
   g. forceps
   g. retractor
   g. ring clamp
   g. scissors
   g. scoop
   g. spoon
Gallie
   G. cryoenucleator
   G. fascial needle
   G. needle
   G. tendon passer
Galloway electrode
gallows
   Killian suspension g.
Gallows splint
gallows-type retractor
gallstone
   g. basket
   g. dilator
   g. forceps
   g. probe
   g. scoop
Galt
   G. drill
   G. hand drill
   G. skull trephine
   G. trephine

Galton ear whistle
galvanic
   g. probe
   g. skin response (GSR)
   g. skin response device
Galveston
   G. metacarpal brace
   G. splint
Gambale-Merrill bone-cutting forceps
Gambee suture
Gambro
   G. catheter
   G. dialyzer holder
   G. hemodialyzer
   G. hemofiltration system
   G. system
Gambro-Lundia
   G.-L. coil dialyzer
   G.-L. dialyzer
gamma camera
Gam-Mer
   G.-M. aneurysm clamp
   G.-M. bipolar coagulator
   G.-M. bone-cutting forceps
   G.-M. bur
   G.-M. chuck
   G.-M. clip applier
   G.-M. gouge
   G.-M. groover
   G.-M. medial esophageal retractor
   G.-M. minimallet
   G.-M. miniosteotome
   G.-M. nerve hook
   G.-M. oblique raspatory
   G.-M. occipital retractor
   G.-M. occlusion clamp
   G.-M. periosteal elevator
   G.-M. rasp
   G.-M. rongeur
   G.-M. spinal fusion curette
   G.-M. vise
Gamophen
   G. scrub soap
   G. suture
Gandhi knife
Gandy clamp
ganglion
   g. injection needle
   g. scissors
Gannetta dissector

Gans
    G. cannula
    G. cyclodialysis cannula
    G. eye cannula
Gant
    G. clamp
    G. gallbladder retractor
    G. probe
    G. rectal probe
Ganz-Edwards coronary infusion catheter
Ganzfeld stimulator
Garceau
    G. bougie
    G. catheter
    G. ureteral catheter
Garcia
    G. aortic clamp
    G. classic aortic clamp
    G. endometrial biopsy set
Garcia-Ibanez
    G.-I. M picture camera
    G.-I. super 8 camera
Garcia-Novito eye implant
Garcia-Rock
    G.-R. endometrial biopsy curette
    G.-R. endometrial suction curette
Gard-all boot shoe
Gardiner-Brown neurological tuning fork
Gardlok neurosurgical sponge
Gardner
    G. bone chisel
    G. chisel
    G. headrest
    G. hysterectomy forceps
    G. needle
    G. needle holder
    G. skull clamp
    G. skull clamp pin
    G. suture needle
Gardner-Wells
    G.-W. headrest
    G.-W. skull tongs
    G.-W. traction tongs
    G.-W. traction tongs screw
Garfield-Holinger laryngoscope
Gariel pessary
Garland
    G. clamp
    G. forceps

    G. hysterectomy clamp
    G. hysterectomy forceps
Garlock spur crusher
Garren-Edwards gastric balloon
Garretson
    G. bandage
    G. dressing
Garrett
    G. dilator
    G. peripheral vascular retractor
    G. retractor
    G. vascular dilator
    G. vein passer
Garrigue
    G. forceps
    G. uterine-dressing forceps
    G. vaginal retractor
    G. vaginal speculum
    G. weighted vaginal speculum
Garrison forceps
Garron spatula
garter
    Goffman eye g.
Garter shield
Gartner tonometer
gas
    g. insufflator
    g. laser
Gaskell clamp
Gaskin fragment forceps
Gass
    G. cannula
    G. cataract-aspirating cannula
    G. cervical punch
    G. corneoscleral punch
    G. dye applicator
    G. neurosurgical light
    G. retinal detachment cannula
    G. retinal detachment hook
    G. scleral marker
    G. sclerotomy punch
    G. vitreous-aspirating cannula
gastric
    g. balloon
    g. bubble
    g. clamp
    g. resection retractor

gastrocamera
    Bolex g.
    Exakta Varex g.
    Olympus g.
Gastroccult
gastroenterostomy
    g. catheter
    g. clamp
gastrofiberscope
    Pentax FG g.
Gastrografin contrast material
gastrointestinal (GI)
    g. anastomosis (GIA)
    g. clamp
    g. forceps
    g. needle
    g. surgical gut suture
    g. surgical linen suture
    g. surgical silk suture
gastroplasty stapler
Gastroport
Gastroscan motility system
gastroscope
    ACMI g.
    ACMI examining g.
    Benedict g.
    Benedict operating g.
    Bernstein g.
    Cameron g.
    Cameron omni-angle g.
    Chevalier Jackson g.
    Eder g.
    Eder-Bernstein g.
    Eder-Chamberlin g.
    Eder-Hufford g.
    Eder-Palmer g.
    Ellsner g.
    Ewald g.
    examining g.
    fiberoptic g.
    flexible g.
    GFC g.
    GTF-A g.
    GTF Olympus g.
    Herman-Taylor g.
    Hirschowitz g.
    Housset-Debray g.
    Janeway g.
    Jenning-Streifeneder g.
    Kelling g.
    Krentz g.
    Mancke flex-rigid g.
    Olympus g.
    Pentax g.
    peroral g.
    Schindler g.
    Sielaff g.
    Taylor g.
    Tomenius g.
    Universal g.
    Wolf-Henning g.
    Wolf-Knittlingen g.
    Wolf-Schindler g.
gastrostomy
    Beck g.
    g. button
    Depage-Janeway g.
    feeding g.
    Glassman g.
    Kader g.
    Partipilo g.
    percutaneous endoscopic g.
     (PEG)
    g. plug
    Russell percutaneous
     endoscopic g.
    Ssabanejeu-Frank g.
    Stamm g.
    Witzel g.
Gastrovist contrast medium
Gatch bed
gate
    g. clamp
    g. clip
Gates-Glidden drill
gator drape
Gator meniscal cutter
Gatron
    G. nerve stimulator
    G. stimulator
Gaubatz rib retractor
Gauderer-Ponsky PEG
Gau gastric balloon
gauge
    anterior chamber g.
    Austin g.
    bone screw depth g.
    Broggi-Kelman dipstick g.
    calibrated depth g.
    Charnley socket-size g.
    Cloward depth g.
    Cloward L-W g.
    Cloward spanner g.
    depth g.
    Edslab pressure g.
    finger circumference g.

Harris femoral head g.
Knolle lens g.
manual dermatome
thickness g.
measuring g.
Mendez degree g.
Neumann depth g.
orthopaedic depth g.
oval piston g.
Pilling Excalibur g.
pinwheel sensation g.
pressure g.
screw depth g.
Shepard depth g.
Shepard incision depth g.
Stahl lens g.
Tinnant g.
Gauje curved chisel
Gaulian knife guide
gauntlet bandage
Gauss hemostatic forceps
Gauthier retractor
Gauvain brace
gauze
absorbable g.
absorbent g.
g. bandage
g. dissector sponge
g. dressing
KBM absorbent g.
Oxycel g.
g. packer
g. pad carrier
g. pattern scissors
g. rosebud sponge
g. scissors
g. sponge
g. stent
g. stent dressing
surgical steel g.
Surgicel g.
tantalum g.
g. tissue bag
White Plume absorbent g.
Gauztex
G. bandage
G. dressing
Gavin-Miller
G.-M. clamp
G.-M. colon forceps
G.-M. forceps
G.-M. intestinal forceps
G.-M. tissue forceps

Gavriliu gastric tube
Gaylor
G. biopsy forceps
G. forceps
G. uterine biopsy forceps
G. uterine specimen forceps
GBH bypass tube
G-C
G-C filling instrument
G-C polishing strip
G-C "SMOOTH CUT"
diamond point
G-C syringe
G-C Vest investment
material
G-C wax carver
GC
general closure
GC needle
GE
GE pacemaker
GE Rudischhauser
articulating paper
Geckeler screw
GED
graduated electronic decelerator
Geenen
G. biliary cytology brush
G. Endotorque guide wire
G. graduated dilation
catheter
G. pancreatic stent
Gehrung pessary
Geiger cautery
Geissendorfer
G. forceps
G. rib retractor
G. uterine forceps
gel
Aquasonic g.
Betadine g.
Carrington wound g.
Cor-Gel g.
Hurricaine g.
Lectrosonic g.
Liqui-Cor g.
Poh disclosing g.
Topax g.
Gel-Clean
Geldmacher tendon-passing probe
gel-filled
g.-f. implant
g.-f. prosthesis

Gelfilm
- G. dressing
- G. forceps
- G. retinal implant
- G. retinal orbital implant

Gelfoam
- G. forceps
- G. pledget
- G. pressure forceps
- G. punch

Gellhorn
- G. biopsy punch forceps
- G. forceps
- G. pessary
- G. uterine biopsy forceps
- G. uterine biopsy punch

Gellquist scissors
Gelocast dressing
Gelpi
- G. abdominal retractor
- G. forceps
- G. hysterectomy forceps
- G. perineal retractor
- G. retractor
- G. self-retaining retractor
- G. vaginal retractor

Gelpi-Lowrie
- G.-L. forceps
- G.-L. hysterectomy forceps

gel-saline
- g.-s. mammary implant
- g.-s. Surgitek mammary prosthesis

Gely suture
Gembase dental cement
Gemcem dental cement
Gemcore dental cement
Gemini
- G. clamp
- G. forceps
- G. gall duct forceps
- G. hemostatic forceps
- G. hip
- G. Mixter forceps
- G. pacemaker
- G. syringe
- G. thoracic forceps

Genell biopsy curette
general
- g. closure (GC)
- g. closure needle
- g. closure suture
- g. eye surgery suture
- g. probe
- g. retractor
- g. tissue forceps
- g. utility scissors
- g. wire forceps

General Electric pacemaker
generator
- Coratomic implantable pulse g.
- Grass visual pattern g.
- Maxilith pacemaker pulse g.
- Medtronic pulse g.
- Microlith pacemaker pulse g.
- Minilith pacemaker pulse g.
- multiprogrammable pulse g.
- Optima pulse g.
- Radionics lesion g.
- Radionics radiofrequency lesion g.
- Radionics stimulus g.
- Spectrax SXT pulse g.
- Stilith implantable cardiac pulse g.
- ventricular demand pulse g.
- Vivalith II pulse g.

Genesis total knee system
Genga bandage
Genisis
- G. dual-chamber pacemaker
- G. pacemaker

Gensini
- G. catheter
- G. Teflon catheter

gentian violet marking pen
Gentle-Flo suction catheter
Geomedic knee prosthesis
Geometric total knee prosthesis
Georgiade
- G. breast prosthesis
- G. visor halo fixation apparatus

Gerald
- G. Bayonet microbipolar neurosurgical forceps
- G. bipolar forceps
- G. brain forceps
- G. clamp
- G. dressing forceps
- G. forceps
- G. straight microbipolar neurosurgical forceps
- G. tissue forceps

Gerber space maintainer
Gerbode
  G. cardiovascular tissue
    forceps
  G. dilator
  G. forceps
  G. mitral dilator
  G. mitral valvulotomy
    dilator
  G. modified Burford rib
    spreader
  G. patent ductus clamp
  G. spreader
  G. sternal retractor
  G. valve dilator
  G. valvulotome
Gergoyie-Guggenheim olive
Gergoyie olive
Germain needle holder
Germa-medica scrub soap
German lock
Germicide C.R.I. scrub soap
Gerow Small-Carrion penile
  implant
Gerster
  G. bone clamp
  G. fracture appliance
  G. traction bar
  G. traction device
Gerzog
  G. bone hammer
  G. ear knife
  G. mallet
  G. nasal speculum
Gerzog-Ralks knife
Gesco
  G. aspirator
  G. catheter
Getz
  G. crown
  G. root canal pin
  G. rubber base
Geuder
  G. corneal needle
  G. implanter
  G. keratoplasty needle
GFC gastroscope
GFH alloy
Ghajar guide
Ghazi rib retractor
Gherini-Kaufman endo-otoprobe

GHM
  GHM KLE II x-ray film
    holder
  GHM polishing strip
GI
  gastrointestinal
  GI clamp
  GI forceps
  GI pop-off silk suture
  GI silk suture
GIA
  gastrointestinal anastomosis
  GIA forceps
  GIA II loading unit
  GIA staple
  GIA stapler
  GIA stapling device
Giannestras turnbuckle
Giannini needle holder
Gianturco
  G. stent
  G. suture
Gianturco-Roehm bird's nest vena
  caval filter
Gianturco-Rosch bilary Z stent
Giardet corneal scissors
Gibbon
  G. catheter
  G. indwelling ureteral stent
  G. ureteral stent
  G. urethral catheter
Gibbs eye punch
Gibney
  G. bandage
  G. dressing
Gibson
  G. anterior chamber
    irrigator
  G. dressing
  G. splint
  G. stone dislodger
  G. suture
Gibson-Balfour
  G.-B. abdominal retractor
  G.-B. retractor
Gibson-Cooke sweat test apparatus
Gibson-Ross board
Giertz
  G. rib guillotine
  G. rib shears
Giertz-Stille rib shears
Giesy ureteral dilatation balloon

319

Gifford
 G. corneal applicator
 G. corneal curette
 G. curette
 G. fixation forceps
 G. forceps
 G. holder
 G. iris forceps
 G. mastoid retractor
 G. retractor
 G. scalp retractor
Gifford-Jansen mastoid retractor
GIF-HM endoscope
GIF-XQ endoscope
Gigator hemorehoidal ligator
Gigli
 G. saw
 G. solid-handle saw
 G. spiral saw wire
 G. wire saw
Gigli-saw
 G.-s. blade
 G.-s. guide
 G.-s. handle
Gilbert
 G. balloon catheter
 G. catheter
 G. cystic duct forceps
 G. forceps
 G. pediatric balloon
  catheter
 G. pediatric catheter
 G. plug sealing catheter
 G. prosthesis
Gilbert-Graves speculum
Gilbert-type Bardex Foley catheter
Gilfillan humeral prosthesis
Giliberty acetabular prosthesis
Gill
 G. biopsy brush
 G. blade
 G. corneal knife
 G. curved iris forceps
 G. double irrigating-
  aspirating cannula
 G. forceps
 G. incision spreader
 G. incision-spreading forceps
 G. iris forceps
 G. iris knife
 G. irrigating-aspirating
  cannula
 G. needle

 G. pressor counter
 G. respirator
 G. sinus cannula
 G. ureteral brush biopsy kit
Gill-Chandler iris forceps
Giller hearing aid
Gillespie obstetrical forceps
Gillette brace
Gill-Fuchs
 G.-F. capsular forceps
 G.-F. forceps
Gill-Hess
 G.-H. forceps
 G.-H. iris forceps
 G.-H. mules
Gillies
 G. bone hook
 G. dissecting forceps
 G. dural hook
 G. forceps
 G. horizontal dermal suture
 G. implant
 G. nasal hook
 G. needle holder
 G. prosthesis
 G. single-hook skin retractor
 G. skin hook
 G. suture scissors
 G. tissue forceps
 G. zygoma elevator
 G. zygoma hook
Gillies-Converse skin hook
Gillies-Dingman hook
Gillmore needle
Gillquist
 G. suction curette
 G. suction tube
Gillquist-Oretorp-Stille
 G.-O.-S. dilator
 G.-O.-S. forceps
 G.-O.-S. knife
 G.-O.-S. needle holder
 G.-O.-S. probe
**Gillquist-Stille arthroplasty suction
 tube**
Gill-Safar forceps
Gill-Welsh
 G.-W. aspirating cannula
 G.-W. cannula
 G.-W. capsular forceps
 G.-W. capsular polisher
 G.-W. cortex extractor

G.-W. curette capsular polisher
G.-W. double-barreled irrigating-aspirating cannula
G.-W. double cannula
G.-W. irrigating-aspirating cannula
G.-W. irrigating cannula
G.-W. lens loupe
G.-W. olive-tip cannula
G.-W. scissors
G.-W. Vannas angled microscissors
Gill-Welsh-Morrison lens loupe
Gill-Welsh-Vannas
G.-W.-V. capsulotomy scissors
G.-W.-V. scissors
Gilmer dental splint
Gilmore probe
Gil-Vernet
G.-V. lumbotomy retractor
G.-V. renal retractor
G.-V. renal sinus retractor
G.-V. retractor
gingival clamp
gingivectomy knife
Ginsberg
G. forceps
G. tissue forceps
Gio-occlusive dressing
Girard
G. anterior chamber needle
G. cannula
G. corneoscleral forceps
G. forceps
G. irrigating cannula
G. keratoprosthesis prosthesis
G. needle
G. probe
G. scleral expander ring
G. synechia spatula
Girard-Swan
G.-S. knife-needle
G.-S. needle
G.-S. needle-knife
Girdner probe
girth hitch
Gissane spike nail
Givner eye retractor
glabellar rasp
Glandosane synthetic saliva

Glaser
G. laminectomy retractor
G. retractor
Glasgow-pattern rongeur
Glass
G. abdominal retractor
G. liver-holding clamp
G. retractor
glass
g. bead sterilizer
g. pH electrode
g. retracting rod
semifinished g.
g. sphere eye implant
g. sphere implant
g. vaginal plug
Worst corneal contact g.
Glasscock
G. dressing
G. ear dressing
G. scissors
Glasscock-House knife
glasses
Difei g.
Fresnel nystagmus g.
Grafco magnifying g.
magnifying g.
nystagmus g.
presbyopia g.
Glassman
G. anterior resection clamp
G. basket
G. brush
G. clamp
G. forceps
G. gastroenterostomy clamp
G. gastrointestinal clamp
G. gastrostomy
G. intestinal clamp
G. liver-holding clamp
G. noncrushing anterior resection clamp
G. noncrushing clamp
G. noncrushing gastroenterostomy clamp
G. noncrushing gastrointestinal clamp
G. noncrushing pickup forceps
G. pickup forceps
G. stone extractor
G. thin-point scissors

Glassman-Allis
  G.-A. clamp
  G.-A. common duct-holding forceps
  G.-A. forceps
  G.-A. intestinal forceps
  G.-A. miniature intestinal forceps
  G.-A. noncrushing common duct forceps
  G.-A. noncrushing intestinal forceps
  G.-A. noncrushing tissue-holding forceps
Glassman-Babcock forceps
Glattelast compression pantyhose
Glaucotest
Gleason
  G. headband
  G. rasp
  G. speculum
Glegg nasal polyp snare
Glenn diverticular forceps
Glenner
  G. forceps
  G. hysterectomy forceps
  G. retractor
  G. vaginal hysterectomy forceps
  G. vaginal retractor
glenoid
  g. alignment peg
  g. drill
  g. drill guide
  g. fin broach
  g. fin guide
  g. fixation screw
  g. implant base impactor
  g. metal tray
glide
  Hessburg intraocular lens g.
  intraocular lens g.
  Pearce intraocular g.
  Sheets g.
  Sheets eye g.
  Sheets intraocular g.
  g. wire
Glidewire guide wire
Glisson snare
globe prolapsus pessary
Glomark fluorescent skin marker

glove
  Flowers mandibular g.
  Tactylon surgical g.'s
Glove-n-Gel
  G.-n-G. amniotome
  G.-n-G. amniotomy kit
Glover
  G. anastomosis forceps
  G. auricular-appendage clamp
  G. auricular clamp
  G. bulldog clamp
  G. clamp
  G. coarctation clamp
  G. coarctation forceps
  G. curved clamp
  G. curved forceps
  G. dilator
  G. forceps
  G. infundibular rongeur forceps
  G. modification of Brock aortic dilator
  G. patent ductus clamp
  G. patent ductus forceps
  G. rongeur
  G. rongeur forceps
  G. spoon anastomosis clamp
  G. spoon clamp
  G. spoon-shaped clamp
  G. spoon-shaped forceps
  G. suction tube
  G. vascular clamp
Glover-DeBakey clamp
Glover's suture
Glover-Stille clamp
Glover-type bulldog clamp
gloves
Glove's drain
Gluck rib shears
glue
  cyanoacrylate g.
glue-in suture
glutaraldehyde-tanned bovine graft
glycerine syringe
GM alloy
Gobin-Weiss loop
Godelo dilator
Godiva wax
Goebel-Stoeckel snare

Goelet
    G. double-ended retractor
    G. retractor
Goethe suture
Goffman
    G. blue eye garter shield
    G. eye garter
    G. occluder
goggle
    stenopaic g.
Gohrbrand
    G. cardiac dilator
    G. dilator
    G. valvulotome
Goidnich bone plate
goiter
    g. clamp
    g. dissector
    g. forceps
    g. hook
    g. ligature carrier
    g. retractor
    g. scissors
    g. vulsellum forceps
goiter-seizing forceps
Golaski-UMI vascular prosthesis
Gold
    G. deep-surgery forceps
    G. forceps
    G. hemostatic forceps
    G. pessary
gold
    g. ear marker
    g. eye implant
    g. implant
    g. ring
    g. sphere eye implant
    g. weight and wire spring
      implant material
Goldbacher
    G. anoscope
    G. anoscope speculum
    G. needle
    G. proctoscope
    G. rectal needle
Goldberg
    G. MPC mediastinoscope
    G. MPC operative
      enteroscope
Goldblatt clamp
Golden Retriever
Goldman [ENT]
    G. bar

    G. cartilage punch
    G. chisel
    G. curette
    G. guarded chisel
    G. guillotine nerve knife
    G. knife guide
    G. saw
    G. septal elevator
    G. septal elevator-displacer
    G. septal scissors
    G. Universal nerve hook
Goldman-Fox gum scissors
Goldman-Kazanjian
    G.-K. forceps
    G.-K. nasal forceps
    G.-K. rongeur
Goldmann [OPHTH]
    G. applanation tonometer
    G. contact lens
    G. expressor
    G. goniolens
    G. knife needle
    G. multimirrored lens
      implant
    G. perimeter
    G. three-mirror gonioscopy
      lens
Gold-Mules eye implant
Goldstein
    G. anterior chamber
      cannula
    G. anterior chamber-
      irrigating cannula
    G. anterior chamber
      irrigator
    G. cannula
    G. curette
    G. irrigating cannula
    G. lacrimal cannula
    G. lacrimal sac retractor
    G. retractor
    G. septal speculum
Goldthwait
    G. bar
    G. brace
    G. fracture appliance
    G. fracture frame
golf-club
    g.-c. knife spud
    g.-c. spud
golf tee-shaped polyvinyl prosthesis
Golgi apparatus

Goligher
    G. modification of the
        Berkeley-Bonney retractor
    G. retractor
    G. retractor frame
    G. speculum
    G. sternal-lifting retractor
Gomco
    G. aspirator
    G. bloodless circumcision
        clamp
    G. circumcision clamp
    G. drain
    G. forceps
    G. portable suction
        aspirator
    G. suction aspirator
    G. suction tube
    G. umbilical cord clamp
    G. uterine aspirator
Gomco-Bell clamp
Gomez
    G. gastric retractor
    G. retractor
gonad shield
Gonin-Amsler marker
goniolaser
    Thorpe 4-mirror g.
goniolens
    Cardona focalizing g.
    Goldmann g.
    PF Lee pediatric g.
    Thorpe 4-mirror g.
goniometer
    Carroll finger g.
    Conzett g.
    digital g.
    finger g.
    Frykholm g.
    Grafco g.
    International standard g.
    Jarit finger g.
    Mottgen g.
    orthopaedic g.
    Osborne g.
    Thole g.
    Tomac g.
    Universal g.
    Zimmer g.
gonioprism
    Posner g.
    Posner diagnostic g.

    Posner surgical g.
    Swan-Jacob g.
gonioscope
    Heine g.
    Maine g.
    Nevada g.
    Thorpe surgical g.
    University of Michigan g.
goniotomy knife
Gonnin-Amsler scleral marker
Gooch
    G. mastoid retractor
    G. retractor
    G. splint
Good
    G. antral rasp
    G. forceps
    G. obstetrical forceps
    G. retractor
    G. tonsillar scissors
Goodale-Lubin
    G.-L. cardiac catheter
    G.-L. catheter
Goode
    G. T-tube
    G. tube
Goodell
    G. dilator
    G. uterine dilator
Goodfellow
    G. cannula
    G. frontal sinus cannula
Goodhill
    G. cautery
    G. curette
    G. double-end curette
    G. forceps
    G. hook
    G. knife
    G. prosthesis
    G. retractor
    G. strut introducer
    G. tonsillar artery forceps
    G. tonsillar forceps
    G. tonsillar hemostat clamp
    G. tonsillar hemostatic
        forceps
Goodhill-Down knife
**Goodhill-Pynchon tonsillar suction
    tube**
Goodlite super headlight
Good-Reiner scissors
Goodwillie periosteal elevator

Goodwin
  G. bone clamp
  G. clamp
Goodyear
  G. retractor
  G. tonsillar knife
  G. tonsillar retractor
Goodyear-Gruenwald forceps
gooseneck chisel
Goot-Lite headband
Gordh needle
Gordon
  G. bead forceps
  G. ciliary forceps
  G. forceps
  G. uterine forceps
  G. uterine vulsellum forceps
  G. vulsellum forceps
Gore-Tex
  G.-T. cardiovascular patch
  G.-T. catheter
  G.-T. graft
  G.-T. peritoneal catheter
  G.-T. prosthesis
  G.-T. shunt
  G.-T. soft tissue patch
  G.-T. surgical membrane
  G.-T. suture
  G.-T. vascular graft
  G.-T. vascular implant
gorget
  Anthony g.
  Teale g.
Gorlin
  G. catheter
  G. pacing catheter
Gorney
  G. dissector
  G. rhytidectomy scissors
  G. rubber band applicator
  G. septal suction elevator
Gorsch
  G. needle
  G. sigmoidoscope
gossamer silk suture
Gossert self-retaining retractor
Gosset
  G. abdominal retractor
  G. appendectomy retractor
  G. retractor
  G. self-retaininig retractor
Gosteyer punch

Gott
  G. cannula
  G. implant
  G. low-profile prosthesis
  G. shunt
  G. tube
Gott-Daggett heart valve prosthesis
Gottesman splash shield
Gottschalk
  G. aspirator
  G. middle ear aspirator
  G. nasostat
  G. transverse saw
Goudet uterine scoop
Gouffon hip pin
annular gouge
gouge
  Alexander g.
  Alexander bone g.
  Alexander mastoid g.
  Andrews g.
  Andrews mastiod g.
  annular g.
  antral g.
  Army bone g.
  Army-pattern bone g.
  Aufranc arthroplasty g.
  Ballenger g.
  Bishop g.
  Bishop mastoid g.
  Boley dental g.
  bone g.
  Bowen g.
  Bowls septal g.
  Campbell arthroplasty g.
  Capner g.
  Cave scaphoid g.
  Charnley g.
  Chermel bone g.
  Cobb g.
  Cobb spinal g.
  Codman g.
  Codman bone g.
  concave g.
  Cooper spinal fusion g.
  Crane g.
  curved g.
  Dawson-Yuhl g.
  Derlacki g.
  Dix g.
  Dontrix g.
  Flanagan spinal fusion g.
  Freer nasal g.

gouge *(continued)*
    Gam-Mer g.
    Guy g.
    Hibbs g.
    Hibbs bone g.
    Hibbs spinal fusion g.
    hip arthroplasty g.
    Hoen laminar g.
    Holmes cartilage g.
    Hough g.
    hump g.
    Kezerian g.
    Killian g.
    Kuhnt g.
    Lahey Clinic spinal fusion g.
    Lexer g.
    Lexer mini g.
    Lillie g.
    long-handle offset g.
    Lucas g.
    Mannerfelt g.
    Martin hip g.
    mastoid g.
    Meyerding g.
    Meyerding curved g.
    Moe g.
    Moore g.
    Moore spinal fusion g.
    Morgenstein g.
    Murphy g.
    nasal g.
    Neivert rocking g.
    Newport cartilage g.
    Nicola g.
    orthopaedic g.
    Parkes hump g.
    Partsch g.
    Partsch bone g.
    Petanguy-McIndoe g.
    Pilling g.
    Putti arthroplasty g.
    Rica g.
    Rica mastoid g.
    Richards Cobb spinal g.
    Richards Hibbs g.
    Rowen spinal fusion g.
    Rubin g.
    Schuknecht g.
    semicircular g.
    SMIC g.
    SMIC mastoid g.
    Smith-Petersen g.
    Smith-Petersen arthrosplasty g.
    Smith-Petersen bone g.
    spinal fusion g.
    Stacke g.
    Stille g.
    Stille bone g.
    Stille-pattern bone g.
    Stille-Stiwer g.
    surgical g.
    swan-neck g.
    Todd foreign body g.
    Trough g.
    Turner spinal g.
    Tworek Universal g.
    Ultra-Cu /Hibbs g.
    Ultra-Cut Cobb spinal g.
    Ultra-Cut Hibbs g.
    U.S. Army g.
    Walton g.
    Walton foreign body g.
    Watson-Jones g.
    West bone g.
    West nasal g.
    Zielke scoliosis g.

Gould
    G. PentaCath 5-lumen thermodilution catheter
    G. suture

Goulet retractor

Gouley
    G. catheter
    G. dilator
    G. tunneled urethral sound
    G. whalebone filiform catheter

Goulian
    G. blade
    G. dermatome

Goutz catheter

Govons
    G. curette
    G. pituitary curette

grabber
    meniscal suture g.

Graber appliance

Gracey curette

gradient index lens

Gradle
    G. ciliary forceps
    G. corneal trephine
    G. electrode
    G. eyelid retractor

G. forceps
G. needle electrode
G. retractor
G. stitch scissors
graduated
g. catheter
g. electronic decelerator (GED)
g. Garrett dilator
graduated-size catheter
Gradwhol sternal bone marrow aspirator
Graefe
G. cataract knife
G. cataract spoon
G. curved iris forceps
G. cystitome
G. cystitome knife
G. dressing forceps
G. electric field
G. eye-dressing forceps
G. eye-fixation forceps
G. eye forceps
G. eye speculum
G. fixation forceps
G. flexible cystitome
G. forceps
G. hook
G. instrument
G. iris forceps
G. iris hook
G. iris knife
G. iris needle
G. knife-needle
G. mules
G. needle
G. nonmagnetic fixation forceps
G. scarifier
G. speculum
G. strabismus hook
G. straight iris forceps
G. tissue forceps
G. tissue-grasping forceps
Graether
G. collar button
G. collar buttonhook
G. collar-button iris retractor
G. collar-button retractor
G. mushroom hook
G. retractor
Graf cervical cordotomy knife

Grafco
G. breast pump
G. cannula
G. colostomy bag
G. cotton tip applicator
G. eye shield
G. goniometer
G. Halsted forceps
G. head mirror
G. ileostomy bag
G. incontinence clamp
G. laryngeal mirror
G. magnet
G. magnifying glasses
G. Martin laryngectomy tube
G. ophthalmoscope
G. otoscope
G. pelvic traction belt
G. percussion hammer
G. perineal lamp
G. pinwheel
G. seizure stick
G. tourniquet
G. tracheal tube brush
G. umbilical cord clamp
G. x-ray apron
graft
accordion g.
acrylic g.
Albee bone g.
albumin-coated vascular g.
aldehyde-tanned bovine g.
autologous fat g.
AV Gore-Tex g.
Banks bone g.
Bard g.
Bard PTFE g.
B-B g.
Berens g.
bifurcated vascular g.
Bionit vascular g.
BioPolyMeric femoropopliteal bypass g.
BioPolyMeric vascular g.
Blair-Brown g.
g. board
Bonfiglio bone g.
Boplant g.
Boyd bone g.
Braun g.
Braun-Wangensteen g.
brephoplastic g.

graft *(continued)*
Brett bone g.
B-W g.
cable g.
Calcitite bone g.
Campbell g.
g. clamp
Codivilla g.
Cooley g.
Cotton cartilage g.
Creech aortoiliac g.
Crescent g.
Cryolife valvular g.
Dacron g.
Dacron knitted g.
Dacron preclotted g.
Dacron tightly-woven g.
Dacron tubular g.
Dacron velour g.
Dacron Weave Knit g.
Dardik umbilical g.
Davis g.
DeBakey g.
diamond inlay bone g.
Doherty g.
double-velour g.
Douglas g.
Dragstedt g.
Esser g.
fiberglass g.
glutaraldehyde-tanned
  bovine g.
Gore-Tex g.
Gore-Tex vascular g.
Hemashield collagen-
  enhanced g.
IMA g.
Impra Flex vascular g.
Impra microporous PTFE
  vascular g.
Impra vascular g.
Inclan g.
Ionescu-Shiley pericardial
  valve g.
Ivalon g.
Jeb g.
Kebab g.
Kiel g.
knitted g.
Koenig g.
Krause-Wolfe g.
latex sponge g.
Lee g.

Lo-Por vascular g.
lyophilized g.
mandril g.
Mangoldt epithelial g.
Marlex mesh g.
Marqez-Gomez
  conjunctival g.
Marquez-Gomez
  conjunctival g.
McFarland tibial g.
McMaster bone g.
Meadox Microvel g.
Meadox Microvel double-
  velour Dacron g.
Meadox vascular g.
g. measuring instrument
Mediform dural g.
Mersilene g.
mesh g.
methyl methacrylate g.
Meyerding bone g.
Microknit patch g.
Microknit vascular g.
Microvel g.
Millesi interfascicular g.
Milliknit g.
Mules g.
Nicholl bone g.
Nicoll bone g.
N-terface g. dressing
Ollier g.
Ollier-Thiersch g.
Ostrup vascularized rib g.
Padgett g.
Padgett mesh skin g.
Paladon g.
Papineau bone g.
paraffin g.
patch g.
Paufique g. knife
Peri-Guard vascular g.
Phemister g.
Phemister onlay bone g.
pigskin g.
plasma TFE vascular g.
Plexiglas g.
Plystan g.
polyethylene g.
Poly-Plus Dacron
  vascular g.
polytetrafluoroethylene g.
polyurethane g.
polyvinyl g.

porcine g.
preclotted g.
Proplast g.
prosthetic g.
PTFE Gore-Tex g.
Rastelli g.
Rehne skin g. knife
Reverdin g.
Ruese bone g.
Sauvage Bionit g.
Sauvage Dacron g.
seamless g.
Seddon nerve g.
Shea vein g. scissors
Sheen tip g.
Shiley Tetraflex vascular g.
sieve g.
Silastic g.
Silovi saphenous vein g.
Siloxane g.
Solvang g.
Speed osteotomy g.
sponge g.
spongiosa bone g.
St. Jude composite valve g.
g. suction tube
Supramid g.
Thiersch g.
tube g.
tunnel g.
Varivas R vein g.
Velex woven Dacron
  vascular g.
Vitagraft vascular g.
Wesolowski bypass g.
Wesolowski Teflon g.
Wolfe g.
Wölfe-Krause g.
Graft Assist graft holder
Graham
  G. blunt hook
  G. Clark silicone sponge
  G. dural hook
  G. nerve hook
  G. pediatric scissors
  G. rib contractor
  G. scalene elevator
  G. scissors
Graham-Kerrison punch
Gram cannula
Granberry
  G. finger traction bow

  G. hyperextension fracture
    frame
  G. splint
  G. tongue depressor
Grandon cortex extractor set
granny knot suture
Grant
  G. abdominal aortic
    aneurysm clamp
  G. aortic aneurysm clamp
  G. clamp
  G. dural separator
  G. gallbladder retractor
  G. holder
  G. needle holder
  G. retractor
Grantham
  G. electrode
  G. lobotomy electrode
  G. lobotomy needle
grasper
  atraumatic g.
  Endo Grasp g.
  Hansen g.
  Hasson g.
  loose body g.
grasping
  g. biopsy forceps
  g. clamp
  g. forceps
  g. forceps tip
  g. instrument
  g. tripod forceps
Grass
  G. electroencephalograph
  G. pressure-recording device
  G. visual pattern generator
grater
  acetabular g.
  g.-type reamer with
    Zimmer-Hudson shank
Graves
  G. bivalve speculum
  G. Britetrac vaginal
    speculum
  G. open-side vaginal
    speculum
  G. speculum
  G. vaginal speculum
gravity
  g. assist system
  g. infusion cannula

Gray
- G. arterial forceps
- G. bone drill
- G. clamp
- G. cystic duct forceps
- G. drill
- G. forceps
- G. gall duct forceps

Grayton
- G. corneal forceps
- G. forceps

Grazer blepharoplasty forceps

Great
- G. Ormand Street tracheostomy tube
- G. Ormond Street pediatric tracheostomy tube

great toe implant

Greck ileostomy bag

Green
- G. automatic corneal trephine
- G. bulldog clamp
- G. calipers
- G. cataract knife
- G. chalazion forceps
- G. clamp
- G. corneal curette
- G. corneal dissector
- G. corneal marker
- G. curette
- G. dissector
- G. eye calipers
- G. eye dissector
- G. eye needle holder
- G. eye shield
- G. fixation forceps
- G. forceps
- G. goiter retractor
- G. holder
- G. lens scoop
- G. lens spatula
- G. lid clamp
- G. mouth gag
- G. muscle hook
- G. needle holder
- G. optical crater marker
- G. pendulum scalpel
- G. retractor
- G. spatula
- G. stabismus tucker
- G. strabismus hook
- G. suction tube forceps
- G. suction tube-holding clamp
- G. tissue-grasping forceps
- G. uterine curette

green
- g. braided suture
- g. laser
- g. monofilament polygliconate suture

Green-Armytage
- G.-A. forceps
- G.-A. hemostatic forceps
- G.-A. polythene rod
- G.-A. reamer
- G.-A. syringe

Greenberg
- G. instrument holder
- G. Maxi-Vise adapter
- G. retractor
- G. Universal retractor

Greene
- G. endocervical curette
- G. goiter retractor
- G. needle
- G. placental curette
- G. retractor
- G. thyroid retractor
- G. tube-holding forceps
- G. uterine curette

Greenfield
- G. filter
- G. IVC filter
- G. needle

Green-Gould needle

Green-Kenyon
- Green-Kenyon corneal marker
- Green-Kenyon marker

Green-Sewall mouth gag

Greenwald flexible endoscopic electrode

Greenwood
- G. bipolar coagulation-suction forceps
- G. bipolar forceps
- G. coagulation forceps
- G. forceps
- G. spinal trephine

Gregg cannula

Gregory
- G. baby profunda clamp
- G. bulldog clamp
- G. carotid bulldog clamp

G. clamp
G. external clamp
G. forceps
G. stay suture
G. stay suture clamp
G. vascular miniature clamp
Greiling gastroduodenal tube
Greven alligator forceps
Grey-Hess screen
Grey Turner forceps
grid
    Amsler g.
    Bernell g.
Grierson stripper
Grieshaber
G. blade
G. corneal needle
G. corneal trephine
G. endo-illuminator
G. eye needle
G. eye needle holder
G. forceps
G. global control tubing set
G. holder
G. iris forceps
G. iris needle
G. keratome
G. knife
G. needle
G. needle holder
G. ophthalmic needle
G. retractor
G. spring wire retractor
G. trephine
G. wire retractor
Griffin bandage lens dressing
Griffiths-Brown forceps
Grigor fiber light guide catheter
grinder
    skin g.
GRIN lens
Grizzard
G. cannula
G. subretinal cannula
Groenholm
G. lid retractor
G. retractor
Groff electrosurgical knife
Grollman
G. catheter
G. pigtail catheter
Gromley-Russell cannula

grommet
    Exmoor plastics aural g.
    Shah g.
    Shepard g.
    Silastic g.
    Szulc g.
    Twardon g.
grooved
    g. director
    g. director dilator
    g. silicone sponge
    g. tying forceps
groover
    Alway g.
    Gam-Mer g.
groove suture
Groshong
G. catheter
G. double-lumen catheter
G. dual-lumen catheter
Gross
G. brain spatula
G. clamp
G. coarctation clamp
G. coarctation occlusion clamp
G. curette
G. dressing forceps
G. ductus spreader
G. ear curette
G. ear hook
G. ear spoon
G. ear spud
G. forceps
G. hyoid-cutting forceps
G. iris retractor
G. occluding clamp
G. patent ductus retractor
G. probe
G. retractor
G. sponge forceps
G. spur crusher
Grosse
Grosse & Kempf
G. & K. bone drill
G. & K. femoral nail
G. & K. tibial nail
Gross-Pomeranz-Watkins
G.-P.-W. atrial retractor
G.-P.-W. retractor
Grotena
G. abdominal belt

Grotena *(continued)*
  G. abdominal support
  G. lumbar belt
Grotting forceps
Grover
  G. Atra-grip clamp
  G. auricular appendage
    clamp
  G. clamp
Gruber
  G. bougie
  G. ear speculum
  G. speculum
Gruca
  G. hip reamer
  G. spring
Gruening eye magnet
Gruentzig *(var. of* Grüntzig)
Gruenwald
  G. bayonet-dressing forceps
  G. dissecting forceps
  G. dressing forceps
  G. Durogrip forceps
  G. ear forceps
  G. forceps
  G. nasal-cutting forceps
  G. nasal-dressing forceps
  G. nasal punch
  G. pituitary rongeur
  G. punch
  G. retractor
  G. tissue forceps
Gruenwald-Bryant
  G.-B. forceps
  G.-B. nasal-cutting forceps
  G.-B. nasal forceps
Gruenwald-Jansen forceps
Gruenwald-Love
  G.-L. forceps
  G.-L. intervertebral disk
    rongeur
  G.-L. neurosurgical forceps
Grundelach punch
Grüntzig, Gruentzig
  G. arterial balloon catheter
  G. balloon
  G. balloon angiography
    catheter
  G. balloon catheter
  G. balloon dilator
  G. catheter
  G. catheter
  G. D dilating catheter

  G. D-G dilating catheter
  G. Dilaca catheter
  G. 20-30 dilating catheter
  G. femoral stiffening
    cannula
  G. G dilating catheter
  G. S dilating catheter
  G. steerable catheter
Gruppe
  G. forceps
  G. wire crimper
  G. wire-crimping forceps
  G. wire prosthesis
  G. wire prosthesis-crimping
    forceps
GSB
  GSB elbow prosthesis
  GSB knee prosthesis
G-11 scrub soap
G.S.I. scrub soap
GSR
  galvanic skin response
G-suit device
GTF-A gastroscope
GTF Olympus gastroscope
GTS trephine
guard
  Albany eye g.
  BandageGuard half-leg g.
  cannula g.
  CastGuard g.
  Cloward cervical drill g.
  Codman skull perforator g.
  drill g.
  Fomon chisel g.
  Hansen keratome g.
  Horsley g.
  intracardiac sucker g.
  Joseph g.
  Peri-Guard g.
  Peri-Guard vascular graft g.
  pin g.
  plastic mouth g.
  Rubin-Wright forceps g.
  Somatics mouth g.
  Storz Teflon forceps g.
  tip g.
  tooth g.
  Ullrich drill g.
  Wright-Rubin forceps g.
guarded
  g. chisel

g. cystitome
g. irrigating cystitome
Guardian pacemaker
Gudebrod suture
Guedel
    G. airway
    G. blade
    G. laryngoscope
    G. laryngoscope blade
    G. rubber airway
Guedel-Negus laryngoscope
Guepar knee prosthesis
Guest needle
Guggenheim
    G. adenoidal forceps
    G. scissors
Guggenheim-Gergoiye dilator
Guggenheim-Schuknecht scissors
Guibar lacrimal drain
Guibor
    G. canaliculus intubation
      set
    G. Expo eye bubble
    G. Expo eye bubble shield
    G. Expo flat eye bandage
    G. tube
guide
    acetabular angle g.
    acetabular cup peg drill g.
    acetabular shell g.
    Acufex g.
    Acufex alignment g.
    Adson drill g.
    Adson Gigli-saw g.
    AGC dual-pivot resection g.
    antirotation g.
    Argon spring g.
    Bailey g.
    Bailey Gigli-saw g.
    Barraquer wire g.
    Béniqué catheter g.
    Blair Gigli-saw g.
    bone g.
    Borchard Gigli-saw g.
    bougie g.
    Bow & Arrow cannulated
      drill g.
    Caldwell g.
    cartilage g.
    catheter g.
    g. catheter
    CCK femoral stem
      provisional g.

chamfer g.
Clayman g.
Clayman intraocular g.
Cloward g.
Cloward guard g.
Codman g.
Cone g.
Cooper basal ganglia g.
Cosman-Nashold spinal
  stereotaxic g.
Cottle bone g.
Cottle cartilage g.
Cottle knife g.
Crockard sublaminar wire g.
cruciate ligament g.
Cushing Gigli-saw g.
Delta Recon proximal
  drill g.
distal femoral cutting g.
drill g.
eccentric drill g.
Eccentric Isotac tibial g.
Eder-Puestow dilator g.
Eriksson g.
extramedullary alignment g.
E-Z g.
femoral notch g.
Ferciot wire g.
filiform g.
g. forceps
Friedman knife g.
Gaulian knife g.
Ghajar g.
Gigli-saw g.
glenoid drill g.
glenoid fin g.
Goldman knife g.
Guyon catheter g.
Guyon curved catheter g.
hand-held drill g.
Harrison forked-type
  strut g.
Harris precoat neck
  osteotomy g.
Hewson ligament drill g.
House strut g.
House wire g.
House wire strut g.
humeral cutting g.
IM/EM tibial resection g.
Interson biopsy needle g.
intramedullary g.
Iowa pudendal needle g.

guide *(continued)*
Iowa trumpet needle g.
Iowa trumpet pudendal
needle g.
Jonesco bone wire g.
Kazanjian g.
LeFort filiform g.
ligature g.
Lipscomb-Anderson drill g.
L-resection g.
Lunderquist-Ring torque g.
measuring g.
MOD femoral drill g.
Modny g.
Morrissey Gigli-saw g.
Mumford Gigli-saw g.
needle g.
Neivert knife g.
Oshukova collapsible
bougie g.
Palmer cruciate ligament g.
patellar drill g.
patellar reamer g.
patellar resection g.
g. pin
pin g.
Poppen Gigli-saw g.
protector g.
ProTrac ACL tibial g.
ProTrac alignment g.
ProTrac endoscopic ACL
drill g.
Puddu drill g.
pudendal block needle
and g.
pudendal needle g.
punch g.
Rand-Wells
pallidothalmomectomy g.
Raney Gigli-saw g.
Raney saw g.
rear-entry ACL drill g.
Rhinelander g.
Richards drill g.
Savary-Gilliard wire g.
Scanlan ligature g.
scaphoid screw g.
Schlesinger Gigli-saw g.
Slidewire extension g.
Stader pin g.
Stewart cruciate ligament g.
Stewart ligament g.
Stille Gigli-saw g.

stoma-centering g.
straight catheter g.
surgical instrument g.
g. suture
telescoping g.
tissue anchor g. (TAG)
Todd stereotaxic g.
Todt-Heyer cannula g.
Tracer wire g.
trumpet needle g.
Tucker vertebrated g.
Tworek screw g.
Unis Universal g.
Urbanski strut g.
Uslenghi drill g.
Van Buren catheter g.
Van Buren curve
catheter g.
Wilson-Cook standard
wire g.
wire g.
g. wire (*See* wire)
wire and drill g.
wire speculum wire g.
guider
NL3 g.
Medi-Tech guide wire
guiding
g. cannula
g. catheter
g. catheter with side hole
Guild-Pratt rectal speculum
Guilford
G. brace
G. scissors
**Guilford-Schuknecht wire-cutting
scissors**
Guilford-Wright
G.-W. bivalve speculum
G.-W. bur
G.-W. bur saw
G.-W. clip
G.-W. crurotomy knife
G.-W. curette
G.-W. cutter
G.-W. cutting block
G.-W. double-edged knife
G.-W. drum elevator
G.-W. duckbill elevator
G.-W. elevator flap knife
G.-W. elevator knife
G.-W. fenestrometer
G.-W. flap knife

G.-W. footplate pick
G.-W. forceps
G.-W. incudostapedial knife
G.-W. meatal retractor
G.-W. microbone curette
G.-W. middle ear
   instrument
G.-W. prosthesis
G.-W. roller knife
G.-W. scissors
G.-W. stapes pick
G.-W. suction tube
G.-W. suction tube clip
G.-W. Teflon wire piston
G.-W. wire cutter
Guilford-Wullstein bur saw
guillotine
   g. adenotome
   Ballenger-Sluder g.
   Giertz rib g.
   Lilienthal rib g.
   Myles g.
   Poppers tonsillar g.
   g. scissors
   Sluder-Sauer tonsillar g.
   Sluder tonsillar g.
   SMIC tonsillar g.
   tonsillar g.
   Van Osdel g.
   Zipster rib g.
guillotome forceps
GU irrigant dressing
Guist
   G. enucleation scissors
   G. eye implant
   G. eye speculum
   G. fixation forceps
   G. forceps
   G. sphere eye implant
Guist-Black eye speculum
Guleke bone rongeur
Gullstrand
   G. lens loupe
   G. ophthalmoscope
Gullstrand-Zeiss lens loupe
gum
   Brophy g.
Gum Machine oral irrigator
gun
   caulking g.
   clip g.
   EnhanCement g.
   Mentor injector g.

Miltex g.
seam-sealer g.
surgical stapling g.
Gundelach punch
Gunderson
   G. muscle forceps
   G. recession forceps
Gunnar-Hey roller forceps
Gunning jaw splint
Gunston-Hult knee prosthesis
Gunston polycentric knee
   prosthesis
Gusberg
   G. cervical biopsy curette
   G. cervical cone curette
   G. curette
   G. endocervical biopsy
      curette
   G. endocervical biopsy
      punch
   G. endocervical curette
   G. hysterectomy clamp
   G. uterine forceps
Gussenbauer
   G. clamp
   G. suture
Gustilo-Kyle total hip
gustometer
gut
   g. chromic suture
   g. clamp
   g. plain suture
   g. suture
Gutgeman
   G. auricular appendage
      clamp
   G. clamp
Gutgemann auricular appendage
   forceps
Gutglass
   G. cervix hemostatic forceps
   G. forceps
   G. hemostat
   G. hemostatic cervical
      forceps
Guthrie
   G. eye-fixation hook
   G. fixation hook
   G. hook
   G. iris hook
   G. retractor
   G. skin hook
Gutierrez-Najar grasping forceps

gutta-percha point
Gutter speculum
Guttmann
  G. obstetrical retractor
  G. retractor
  G. vaginal retractor
  G. vaginal speculum
Guy
  G. gouge
  G. tenotomy knife
guy
  g. steading suture
  g. suture
Guyon
  G. catheter guide
  G. clamp
  G. curved catheter guide
  G. dilating bougie
  G. dilating sound
  G. dilator
  G. exploratory bougie
  G. kidney clamp
  G. ureteral catheter
  G. urethral sound
  G. vessel clamp
Guyon-Benique urethral sound
Guyon-Péan
  G.-P. clamp
  G.-P. vessel clamp
Guyton
  G. angled electrode

  G. corneal trephine
  G. electrode
  G. forceps
  G. scissors
  G. suture
  G. suturing forceps
Guyton-Clark
  G.-C. capsule fragment
    forceps
  G.-C. forceps
Guyton-Friedenwald suture
Guyton-Lundsgaard sclerotome
Guyton-Noyes
  G.-N. fixation forceps
  G.-N. forceps
Guyton-Park
  G.-P. eye speculum
  G.-P. speculum
Guzman-Blanco epiglottic retractor
Gwathmey
  G. hook
  G. suction tube
GX cephalometer
Gyn-A-Lite vaginal speculum
Gynaspir vacuum curettage
Gynefold
  G. prolapse pessary
  G. retrodisplacement pessary
Gynosampler endometrial aspirator
Gypsona plaster dressing

H

HA
  hydroxyapatite
Haab
  H. after-cataract knife
  H. eye magnet
  H. knife needle
  H. needle
  H. needle knife
Haag-Streit
  H.-S. fluorescein dye
  H.-S. pacemeter
  H.-S. slit lamp
Haberer
  H. gastrointestinal forceps
  H. intestinal clamp
  H. intestinal forceps
  H. spatula
Haberer-Gili forceps
Haberman suction elevator
**HA-biointegrated dental implant
  system**
Hackett sacral belt
Hader dental attachment
Haeggstrom antral trocar
Haemoson ultrasound Doppler
Haering
  H. esophageal prosthesis
  H. tube
Haftelast self-adhering bandage
Hagan surface suction tube
Hagar probe
Hagedorn
  H. needle
  H. suture needle
Hagenbarth
  H. clip-applying forceps
  H. clip forceps
Hagfer needle holder
Hagie
  H. pin
  H. T-stack
  H. wrench
Haglund
  H. plaster scissors
  H. spreader
  H. vaginal speculum
Haglund-Stille
  H.-S. plaster spreader
  H.-S. vaginal speculum

Hagner
  H. bag
  H. bag catheter
  H. catheter
  H. hemostatic bag
  H. urethral bag
Hahn cannula
Hahnenkratt
  H. aspirator
  H. backing
  H. dental clasp
  H. lingual bar
  H. matrix band
  H. orthodontic wire
  H. retainer
  H. root canal pin
  H. root canal post
  H. temporary crown
Haidinger brush
Haig
  H. Ferguson obstetrical
    forceps
  H. obstetrical forceps
Haight
  H. baby retractor
  H. pediatric rib spreader
  H. pulmonary retractor
  H. retractor
  H. rib retractor
  H. rib spreader
Haight-Finochietto
  H.-F. retractor
  H.-F. rib retractor
  H.-F. rib spreader
Haik
  H. eye implant
  H. implant
Haiman tonsillar electrode
Haimovici arteriotomy scissors
Haines arachnoid dissector
Haitz canaliculus punch
Hajek
  H. antral punch forceps
  H. antral retractor
  H. antral rongeur
  H. cannula
  H. chisel
  H. downbiting rongeur
  H. forceps
  H. lip retractor

Hajek *(continued)*
   H. mallet
   H. retractor
   H. septal chisel
   H. sphenoidal punch
     forceps
   H. upbiting rongeur
Hajek-Ballenger
   H.-B. dissector
   H.-B. elevator
   H.-B. septal dissector
   H.-B. septal elevator
Hajek-Claus rongeur
Hajek-Koffler
   H.-K. forceps
   H.-K. laminectomy rongeur
   H.-K. reversible punch
   H.-K. rongeur
   H.-K. sphenoidal forceps
   H.-K. sphenoidal punch
   H.-K. sphenoidal rongeur
Hajek-Skillern
   H.-S. punch
   H.-S. sphenoidal punch
Hakansson
   H. bone rongeur
   H. rongeur
Hakansson-Olivecrona rongeur
Hakim
   H. catheter
   H. shunt
   H. valve system
Hakko Dwellcath catheter
Hakler forceps
Halberg indirect ophthalmoscope
Hale
   H. forceps
   H. obstetrical forceps
half-curved clamp
half-hitch suture
half-moon retractor
half ring
Halifax
   H. fine adjustment
     instrument
   H. interlaminar clamp kit
   H. placement forceps
   H. wrench
Hall
   H. air drill
   H. arthrotome
   H. bur
   H. dermatome

   H. double-hole spinal
     stapler
   H. drill
   H. driver
   H. intrauterine device
   H. mandibular implant
     system
   H. mastoid bur
   H. Micro-Aire drill
   H. modified Moe hook
   H. modular acetabular
     reamer system
   H. Neurairtome with Smith
     perforator
   H. Orthairtome
   H. power drill
   H. sacral anchor
   H. screwdriver
   H. self-holding introducer
   H. spinal screw
   H. step-down drill
Hallach comedo extractor
Hallberg forceps
Hall-Chevalier stripper
Halle
   H. bone bur
   H. bur
   H. chisel
   H. curette
   H. dural knife
   H. elevator
   H. ethmoidal curette
   H. nasal speculum
   H. needle
   H. septal elevator
   H. septal needle
   H. sinus curette
   H. trigeminus knife
   H. vascular spatula
Halle-Tieck nasal speculum
Hall-Fish hyfrecator
Hall-Kaster
   H.-K. heart valve
   H.-K. tilting-disk valve
     prosthesis
Hallman tunneler
Hallpike-Blackmore ear microscope
hallux forceps
halo
   h. femoral traction device
   h. fracture frame
   h. head frame
   h. hoop device

h. retractor
h. traction device
h. tractor
Twin Cities Lo-Profile h.
Halo CO₂ laser system
halogen
h. coaxial ophthalmoscope
h. ophthalmoscope
h. otoscope
Halogen Lite set
Halogen transilluminator
Halsey
H. forceps
H. mosquito forceps
H. needle
H. needle holder
H. Vital needle holder
Halsey-Webster needle holder
Halsted
H. arterial forceps
H. clamp
H. curved mosquito forceps
H. forceps
H. hemostat
H. hemostatic forceps
H. interrupted mattress
suture
H. mattress suture
H. Micro-Line arterial
forceps
H. mosquito hemostat
H. mosquito hemostatic
forceps
H. mules
H. strabismus scissors
Halsted-Swanson tendon-passing
forceps
halter
Cerva crane h.
deluxe head h.
DePuy head h.
Diskard head h.
disposable head h.
Forrester head h.
head h.
neck-wrap h.
Repro head h.
standard head h.
Upper 7 model head h.
Zimfoam head h.
Zimmer head h.
Zyler head h.
Hamas upper limb prosthesis

Hamblin minimagnet
Hamburger-Brennan-Mahorner
thyroid retractor
Hamby
H. brain retractor
H. clip-applying forceps
H. forceps
H. retractor
H. right-angle clip applier
H. rod
H. twist
H. twist drill
H. wire threader
Hamby-Hibbs retractor
Hamer scalpel
Hamilton
H. bandage
H. deep-surgery forceps
H. forceps
H. pelvic traction screw
tractor
H. tongue depressor
Hamilton-Forewater amniotomy
hook
Hamilton-Steward catheter
Hamis suture
Hamm
H. electrode
H. electrode terminal
adapter
H. fulgurating electrode
H. resectoscope electrode
hammer
Babinski percussion h.
Berliner neurological h.
Berliner percussion h.
Buck h.
Buck neurological h.
Buck percussion h.
Cloward h.
Dejerine h.
Dejerine-Davis percussion h.
Dejerine percussion h.
Epstein h.
h. forceps
fork h.
Gerzog bone h.
Grafco percussion h.
House tapping h.
intranasal h.
Kirk bone h.
Lucae bone h.
Millet test h.

339

hammer *(continued)*
neurological percussion h.
orthopaedic h.
percussion h.
Quisling intranasal h.
Rabiner h.
Rabiner neurological h.
Rica bone h.
slide h.
sliding h.
SMIC bone h.
surgical h.
tapping h.
Taylor percussion h.
Taylor reflex h.
Traube neurological h.
Tromner percussion h.
Wartenberg neurological h.
Williger h.
Hammer mini-fixator
Hammersmith
H. heart valve
H. mitral valve prosthesis
hammock
h. bandage
h. dressing
Hammond
H. alloy
H. argentum mercury
H. blade
H. orthodontic splint
H. winged retractor blade
Hamou
H. endoscope
H. hysteroscope
Hampton
H. electrosurgical unit
H. needle holder
Hamrick
H. elevator
H. suction dissector
H. suction elevator
Hanafee catheter
Hanau face bowe
Hancock
H. aortic valve prosthesis
H. bioprosthetic heart valve
H. bipolar balloon pacing
H. coronary perfusion
catheter
H. embolectomy catheter
H. fiberoptic catheter
H. heterograft heart valve

H. hydrogen detection
catheter
H. luminal
electrophysiologic recording
catheter
H. modified orifice heart
valve
H. temporary cardiac pacing
wire
H. thermodilution catheter
H. wedge-pressure catheter
hand
h. brace
Brueckmann lead h.
h. cock-up snare
h. cock-up splint
Denis Browne retractor
malleable wire h.
h. drill
lead h.
h. nylon scrub brush
pediatric retractor malleable
wire h.
h. retractor
retractor malleable wire h.
h. scrub brush
h. splint
h. surgery rasp
h. trephine
hand-held
h.-h. drill guide
h.-h. exploring electrode
probe
h.-h. nebulizer
h.-h. retractor
handle
Acufex h.
autopsy h.
Bard-Parker h.
Bard-Parker laboratory h.
Bard-Parker surgical h.
Barton traction h.
Bill traction h.
biopsy forceps h.
blade h.
B-P surgical h.
Bruening esophagoscopy
forceps h.
Charnley brace h.
Cloward cross-bar h.
Cloward dowel h.
Corwin knife h.
Cottle modified knife h.

Cottle protected knife h.
ear knife h.
Elliot trephine h.
endoscopic electrode h.
Gigli-saw h.
Hardy knife h.
hexagonal h.
House myringotomy
  knife h.
insulated knife h.
knife h.
laboratory h.
laryngeal h.
laryngeal knife h.
laryngeal mirror h.
lifting h.
Luikart-Bill traction h.
Lynch laryngeal knife h.
Marino rotatable
  transsphenoidal knife h.
Morse instrument h.
myringotomy knife h.
Parker-Bard h.
protected knife h.
rotatable transsphenoidal
  knife h.
Rusch laryngoscope h.
safety h.
saw h.
scalpel h.
Smith endoscopic
  electrode h.
Stiwer scalpel h.
stone basket screw
  mounted h.
Storz ear knife h.
Strully Gigli-saw h.
surgical h.
Tip-Trol h.
T-pin h.
traction h.
tray h.
tympanum perforator h.
Universal h.
Universal chuck h.
V. Mueller Tip-Trol h.
V. Mueller Universal h.
handleless clamp
handpiece
  A-Dec h.
  Cavitron I&A h.
  Chayes h.
  Densco dental h.

Dermacerator h.
Doriot h.
Emesco h.
Imperator h.
infusion h.
Kaessman h.
Kurtin h.
Lares dental h.
Litton dental h.
McIntyre infusion h.
Neuroguide optical h.
phacoemulsification h.
Revelation h.
rotosteotome rotary h.
Sonop h.
Wullstein h.
Wullstein contra-angle h.
Handy-Buck extension tractor
Handy II articulator
hanger
  Adjusta-Rak h.
Hanger prosthesis
hanging cast sling
Hank-Bradley uterine dilator
Hank-Dennen obstretical forceps
Hankins lucite ovoid
Hank uterine dilator
Hanley-McDermott pelvimeter
Hannahan
  H. bur
  H. forceps
Hanna trephine
Hannon
  H. curette
  H. endometrial biopsy
    curette
  H. endometrial curette
Hannover needle holder
Hansen
  H. grasper
  H. keratome guard
Hansen-Street
  H.-S. anchor plate
  H.-S. pin
  H.-S. self-broaching nail
  H.-S. solid intramedullary
    nail
Hanslik patellar prosthesis
haptic
  h. area implant
  h. area lens
  Coburn h.
  modified C-loop h.

haptic *(continued)*
    modified J loop h.
    PMMA h.
haptic-fixated intraocular lens
haptic-sec lens
Hardesty tenotomy hook
hard palate retractor
Hardy
    H. bayonet curette
    H. bayonet enucleator
    H. Bayonet neurosurgical bipolar forceps
    H. bipolar forceps
    H. bivalve speculum
    H. curette
    H. dissector
    H. dressing forceps
    H. enucleator
    H. fork
    H. implant fork
    H. knife handle
    H. lip retractor
    H. microbipolar forceps
    H. microdissector
    H. modification of Bronson-Ray curette
    H. nasal bivalve speculum
    H. pituitary dissector
    H. pituitary spoon
    H. retractor
    H. sellar punch
    H. suction tube
    H. transsphenoidal mirror
Hardy-Duddy
    H.-D. retractor
    H.-D. speculum
    H.-D. vaginal retractor
Hare
    H. compact traction splint
    H. lip traction bow
    H. splint device
    H. traction device
harelip
    h. forceps
    h. needle
    h. suture
Hargin antral trocar
Hargis periosteal elevator
Harken
    H. auricular clamp
    H. ball heart valve
    H. ball valve
    H. cardiovascular forceps

    H. clamp
    H. erysiphake
    H. forceps
    H. heart needle
    H. needle
    H. prosthesis
    H. retractor
    H. rib retractor
    H. rib spreader
    H. valvulotome
Harken-Cooley forceps
Harken-Starr valve
Harlow plate
Harman
    H. eye dressing
    H. fixation forceps
    H. forceps
harmonic suture
Harms
    H. forceps
    H. microtying forceps
    H. probe
    H. suture-tying forceps
    H. trabeculotome
    H. trabeculotomy probe
    H. tying forceps
    H. utility forceps
    H. vessel forceps
Harms-Tubingen
    H.-T. forceps
    H.-T. tying forceps
harness
    Pavlik h.
Harold
    H. Crowe drill
    H. Hayes eustachian bougie
Harpenden
    H. handgrip dynamometer
    H. skinfold calipers
Harper
    H. cervical laminectomy punch
    H. periosteal elevator
Harrah lung clamp
Harrington
    H. bladder retractor
    H. Britetrac retractor
    H. clamp
    H. clamp forceps
    H. deep surgical scissors
    H. erysiphake
    H. forceps
    H. hook clamp

H. hook driver
H. lung-grasping forceps
H. protractor
H. retractor
H. rod
H. scissors
H. spinal elevator
H. splanchnic retractor
H. strut
H. suture
H. sympathectomy retractor
H. thoracic clamp forceps
H. thoracic forceps
H. vulsellum forceps
Harrington-Carmalt clamp
Harrington-Mayo
H.-M. forceps
H.-M. scissors
H.-M. tissue forceps
Harrington-Mixter
H.-M. clamp
H.-M. clamp forceps
H.-M. forceps
H.-M. thoracic clamp
H.-M. thoracic forceps
Harrington-Pemberton
H.-P. retractor
H.-P. sympathectomy
    retractor
Harris
H. angled suture-carrying
    forceps
H. band
H. brace-type reamer
H. catheter
H. dissector
H. femoral head gauge
H. forceps
H. implant
H. leg length calipers set
H. modified J-loop
    intraocular lens
H. precoat neck osteotomy
    guide
H. precoat prosthesis
H. prosthesis
H. protrusio shell
H. rigid quadriped
    intraocular lens
H. separator
H. snare
H. splint sling
H. suture

H. suture-carrying forceps
H. tonsillar knife
H. trephine
H. uterine injector
H. uterine injector catheter
H. wire tightener
Harris-Galante
H.-G. cup
H.-G. porous acetabular
    component
H.-G. porous hip prosthesis
H.-G. prosthesis
Harris-Kronner uterine
manipulator/injector
Harrison
H. capsular knife
H. chalazion retractor
H. curette
H. forked-type strut guide
H. implant
H. interlocked mesh
    dressing
H. interlocked mesh
    prosthesis
H. knife
H. myringoplasty knife
H. retractor
H. scarifying curette
H. suture-removing scissors
H. tucker
Harrison-Shea
H.-S. curette
H.-S. knife curette
Harris-Sinskey microlens hook
Harris-Smith anterior interbody
drill
Harris uterine injection (HUI)
Harshill rectangle
Hart
H. extension finger splint
H. pediatric 3-mirror lens
Hartley
H. implant
H. mammary prosthesis
Hartmann
H. adenoidal curette
H. alligator forceps
H. biopsy punch
H. bone rongeur
H. catheter
H. clamp
H. curette
H. dewaxer speculum

Hartmann *(continued)*
- H. ear-dressing forceps
- H. ear forceps
- H. ear polyp forceps
- H. ear punch
- H. ear rongeur
- H. ear speculum
- H. eustachian catheter
- H. forceps
- H. hemostatic forceps
- H. mosquito forceps
- H. mosquito hemostatic forceps
- H. nasal conchotome
- H. nasal-cutting forceps
- H. nasal-dressing forceps
- H. nasal polyp forceps
- H. nasal punch
- H. nasal speculum
- H. rongeur
- H. speculum
- H. tonsillar dissector
- H. tonsillar punch
- H. tonsillar punch forceps
- H. tuning fork
- H. tuning fork set
- H. uterine biopsy forceps

Hartmann-Citelli
- H.-C. alligator forceps
- H.-C. ear punch
- H.-C. ear punch forceps
- H.-C. forceps

Hartmann-Corgill ear forceps
Hartmann-Gruenwald
- H.-G. nasal-cutting forceps
- H.-G. nasal forceps

Hartmann-Herzfeld
- H.-H. ear forceps
- H.-H. ear rongeur
- H.-H. forceps

Hartmann-Noyes nasal-dressing forceps
Hartmann-Proctor ear forceps
Hartmann-Weingärtner ear forceps
Hartmann-Wullstein
- H.-W. ear forceps
- H.-W. forceps

Hartstein
- H. iris cryoretractor
- H. iris retractor
- H. irrigating iris retractor
- H. retractor

Hartzler
- H. ACS coronary dilation catheter
- H. ACX balloon catheter
- H. angioplasty balloon
- H. balloon catheter
- H. catheter
- H. dilatation catheter
- H. Micro catheter
- H. Micro II catheter
- H. Micro XT catheter
- H. rib retractor
- H. Ultra-Lo-Profile catheter

Harvard
- H. cannula
- H. microbore intravenous extension set
- H. needle

Harvey
- H. Stone clamp
- H. wire scissors

Haslinger
- H. bronchoscope
- H. endoscope
- H. esophagoscope
- H. head holder
- H. headrest
- H. laryngoscope
- H. palate retractor
- H. retractor
- H. tip forceps
- H. tracheobronchoesophagoscope
- H. tracheoscope
- H. uvula retractor

Hasner valve
Hasseltine
Hasson
- H. balloon uterine elevator cannula
- H. cannula
- H. grasper
- H. laparoscope
- H. retractor

Hasson-Eder laparoscope cannula
Hasund appliance
Hatch
- H. catheter
- H. chisel

Hatcher pin
hatchet
- Nordent h.

Hatfield bone curette
Hatt
    H. golf-stick elevator
    H. spoon
Hausmann vascular clamp
Haven skin graft hook
Haverfield
    H. brain cannula
    H. cannula
    H. hemilaminectomy
      retractor
    H. retractor
Haverfield-Scoville
    H.-S. hemilaminectomy
      retractor
    H.-S. retractor
Haverhill
    H. clamp
    H. dermal abrader
    H. needle
Haverhill-Mack clamp
Havlicek
    H. cannula
    H. spiral cannula
    H. trocar
Hawk-Dennen forceps
Hawkins
    H. cervical biopsy forceps
    H. forceps
    H. needle
    H. transhepatic
      cholangiography needle set
Hawks-Dennen
    H.-D. forceps
    H.-D. obstetrical forceps
Hawley
    H. appliance
    H. retainer
Hayden
    H. curette
    H. footplate pick
    H. palate elevator
    H. probe
    H. tonsillar curette
Hayes
    H. anterior resection clamp
    H. anterior resection forceps
    H. anterior resection
      intestinal clamp
    H. anterior resection
      intestinal forceps
    H. clamp
    H. colon clamp

    H. intestinal clamp
    H. Martin forceps
    H. retractor
    H. vaginal speculum
Hayes-Olivecrona
    H.-O. clip forceps
    H.-O. forceps
Hayman dilator
Haynes
    H. brain cannula
    H. cannula
    H. pin
    H. retractor
    H. scissors
Haynes-Griffin mandibular splint
Hays
    H. finger retractor
    H. hand retractor
    H. pharyngoscope
Hayton-Williams
    H.-W. forceps
    H.-W. mouth gag
H-1 catheter
HDL
    high-density lipoprotein
head
    Austin Moore h.
    h. of bed
    h. brace
    Bruening-Storz diagnostic h.
    Bruening-Work diagnostic h.
    coupling h.
    diameter h.
    h. drape
    h. extractor
    h. frame
    h. halter
    h. lamp
    h. mirror
    Morse h.
    Omniflex h.
    Rhoton-Merz rotatable
      coupling h.
    rotatable coupling h.
    Storz-Bruening diagnostic h.
    Work-Bruening diagnostic h.
    Zirconia orthopaedic
      prosthetic h.
headband
    Bosworth h.
    face shield h.
    Gleason h.
    Goot-Lite h.

headband *(continued)*
    Pynchol h.
    Sluder h.
    Storz face shield h.
    Worrall h.
header
    cup pusher h.
headgear
    adaptable class III mask h.
    Kurz pulsation
      orthodontic h.
head holder
    AMSCO h. h.
    Bayless neurosurgical h. h.
    Derlacki-Juers h. h.
    Haslinger h. h.
    Mayfield tic h. h.
    Methodist Hospital h. h.
    Parkinson h. h.
    Shampaine h. h.
headhunter
    h. catheter
    h. visceral angiography
      catheter
headlight
    Goodlite super h.
    Klaar h.
headrest
    adjustable h.
    Adson h.
    Brown-Roberts-Wells h.
    Craig h.
    doughnut h.
    Gardner h.
    Gardner-Wells h.
    Haslinger h.
    horseshoe h.
    Lempert h.
    Light h.
    Light-Veley h.
    Mayfield-Kees h.
    Mayfield pediatric
      horseshoe h.
    Mayfield swivel
      horseshoe h.
    McConnell orthopaedic h.
    Multipoise h.
    neurosurgical h.
    pin h.
    pinion h.
    Richards h.
    Sam Roberts h.
    Shea h.

    Storz adjustable h.
    Veley h.
head/stem spoon separator
healing nut
Healon injection cannula
Healy
    H. forceps
    H. gastrointestinal forceps
    H. intestinal forceps
    H. suture-removing forceps
    H. uterine biopsy forceps
Healy-Jako pediatric subglottiscope
Heaney
    H. clamp
    H. curette
    H. endometrial biopsy
      curette
    H. forceps
    H. hysterectomy forceps
    H. hysterectomy retractor
    H. needle holder
    H. retractor
    H. suture
    H. tissue forceps
    H. uterine curette
    H. vaginal retractor
    H. Vital needle holder
Heaney-Kantor
    H.-K. forceps
    H.-K. hysterectomy forceps
Heaney-Rezek
    H.-R. forceps
Heaney-Simon
    H.-S. forceps
    H.-S. hysterectomy forceps
    H.-S. hysterectomy retractor
    H.-S. retractor
    H.-S. vaginal retractor
Heaney-Stumf forceps
hearing aid *(See* aid)
Hearn needle
Hearst dilator
heart
    h. needle
    h. pacemaker
    Symbion total artificial h.
    h. valve
heater probe
heat exchanger
Heath
    H. chalazion curette
    H. chalazion forceps
    H. clip

H. clip-removing forceps
H. clip-removing scissors
H. curette
H. dilator
H. dissector
H. expressor
H. follicle lid expressor
H. forceps
H. lid expressor
H. mallet
H. mules
H. nasal forceps
H. punctum dilator
H. suture-cutting scissors
H. suture scissors
H. trephine flap dissector
H. wire cutter
H. wire-cutting scissors
heavy
h. cross-slot screwdriver
h. gauge suture
h. retention suture
h. septal scissors
h. silk retention suture
h. silk suture
h. wire suture
heavy-duty pliers with side-cutter
Hebra
H. blade
H. chalazion curette
H. corneal curette
H. curette
Hecht fascia lata forceps
Heck screw
Hedblom
H. costal elevator
H. elevator
H. retractor
H. rib retractor
Hedbloom
H. rib raspatory
Hedstrom file
Hedwig
H. introducer
H. lumen finder
Heermann
H. alligator ear forceps
H. alligator forceps
H. chisel
H. ear forceps
H. forceps
Heffernan nasal speculum

Heffington
H. lumbar seat
H. lumbar seat spinal surgery frame
Hefty bite pin cutter
Hegar
H. dilator
H. needle
H. needle holder
H. rectal dilator
H. uterine dilator
Hegar-Baumgartner
H.-B. needle
H.-B. needle holder
Hegar-Goodell dilator
Hegar-Mayo-Seeley needle holder
Hegar-Olsen needle holder
Hegemann scissors
Hegenbarth
H. clip
H. clip-applying forceps
H. clip forceps
H. forceps
H. wound clip-applying forceps
Hegenbarth-Adams clip
Hegenbarth-Michel clip-applying forceps
Hegge pin
Heidbrink expiratory spill valve
Heidelberg
H. fixation forceps
H. forceps
Heidelberg-R table
Heifitz
H. aneurysm clip
H. bayonet clip applier
H. cerebral aneurysm clamp
H. clip
H. clip applier
H. microclip
H. retractor
H. spatula
Heiming kidney stone forceps
Heimlich
H. chest drain valve
H. heart valve
H. Vygon pneumothorax valve
Heimlich-Gavrilu gastric tube
Hein
H. raspatory
H. rongeur**

Heine gonioscope
Heinkel sigmoidoscope
Heiss
  H. arterial forceps
  H. forceps
  H. hemostatic forceps
  H. mastoid retractor
  H. retractor
  H. vulsellum forceps
Heister mouth gag
Heitz-Boyer clamp
Heiuss soft tissue retractor
Hejnosz radium colpostat
Helanca seamless tube prosthesis
Helfrick
  H. anal retractor
  H. anal ring retractor
  H. retractor
helical
  h. catheter
  h. PTCA dilatation catheter
  h. suture
  h. tube saw
Heliodent dental x-ray unit
Heliodorus bandage
Helistat collagen hemostatic sponge
helium-cadmium diagnostic laser
helium-neon beam (He-Ne)
helium-neon laser
Heller
  H. biopsy forceps
  H. probe
Helmholtz speculum
Helmont speculum
Helsper
  H. laryngectomy button
  H. tracheostomy vent tube
Hemashield collagen-enhanced graft
hemastatic eraser
hemilaminectomy
  h. blade
  h. retractor
hemisphere eye implant
Hemocal hemoperfusion cartridge
Hemoclear dialyzer
hemoclip
  h. clamp
  Weck h.
hemoclip-applying forceps
HemoCue blood hemoglobin test
hemodialysis concentrate

hemodialyzer
  Biospal h.
  Gambro h.
  Polyflux h.
  Redy h.
Hemofreeze blood bag
hemoheater
  Vickers Treonic h.
Hemokart hemoperfusion cartridge
Hem-o-Lok
Hemopad sterile absorbable collagen hemostat
hemorrhoidal
  h. clamp
  h. forceps
  h. ligator
  h. needle
hemostasis
  h. clip
  h. scalp clip
  h. silver clip
hemostat
  Adson h.
  Avitene collagen h.
  Blohmka tonsillar h.
  Boettcher h.
  broadbill h. with push fork
  Collier-DeBakey h.
  Corboy h.
  Corwin h.
  Corwin tonsillar h.
  Crile h.
  curved h.
  Dandy scalp h.
  Davis h.
  Dean h.
  Gutglass h.
  Halsted h.
  Halsted mosquito h.
  Hemopad sterile absorbable collagen h.
  Instat absorbable h.
  Instat collagen absorbable h.
  Jackson h.
  Jackson tracheal h.
  Kelly h.
  Kocher h.
  Lahey h.
  Lewis h.
  Lothrop h.
  Mathrop h.
  McWhorter h.
  mosquito h.

Nu-Knit absorbable h.
Ormco orthodontic h.
orthopaedic h.
Perdue h.
Providence Hospital h.
Raimondi h.
Rankin h.
Rochester-Ochsner h.
Rochester-Péan h.
Sawtell h.
Sawtell-Davis h.
Schnidt h.
Shallcross h.
straight h.
Surgicel absorbable h.
Surgicel Nu-Knit
   absorbable h.
Thrombogen absorbable h.
hemostatic
   h. bag
   h. catheter
   h. cervical forceps
   h. clamp
   h. clip
   h. clip applier
   h. forceps
   h. neurosurgical forceps
   h. suture
   h. thoracic clamp
   h. tissue forceps
   h. tonsillar forceps
   h. tonsillectome
   h. tracheal forceps
hemostatis clip-applying forceps
Hemovac
   H. drain
   H. suction tube
   H. tube
Henderson
   H. approximator
   H. bone chisel
   H. chisel
   H. clamp approximator
   H. retractor
   H. self-retaining retractor
Hendon venoclysis cannula
Hendren
   H. blade
   H. cardiovascular clamp
   H. cardiovascular forceps
   H. clamp
   H. ductus clamp

H. forceps
H. megaureter clamp
H. pediatric forceps
H. pediatric retractor blade
H. ureteral clamp
Hendrickson
   H. bag
   H. drain
   H. hemostatic bag
   H. lithotrite
   H. supapubic drain
He-Ne
   helium-neon beam
   He-Ne laser
Henke
   H. forceps
   H. punch forceps
   H. punch forceps tip
   H. tonsillar dissector
Henke-Stille conchotome
Henley
   H. carotid retractor
   H. dilator
   H. retractor
   H. retractor center blade
   H. retractor set center
      blade
   H. retractor side blade
   H. subclavian artery clamp
   H. vascular clamp
Henner
   H. elevator
   H. endaural elevator
   H. endaural retractor
   H. retractor
   H. T-model endaural
      retractor
Henning
   H. cardia dilator
   H. cast spreader
   H. dilator
   H. plaster cast spreader
Henning-Keinkel stomach probe
Henny laminectomy rongeur
Henrotin
   H. forceps
   H. retractor
   H. uterine vulsellum forceps
   H. vaginal speculum
   H. vulsellum
   H. vulsellum forceps

Henrotin *(continued)*
H. weighted vaginal
    speculum
Henry
H. ciliary forceps
H. instrument tray
H. Schein excavator
H. Schein filling instrument
H. tray
**Henschke-Mauch SNS lower limb
prosthesis**
Henton
H. needle
H. suture needle
H. tonsillar needle
H. tonsillar suture hook
H. tonsillar suture needle
Hepacon
H. cannula
H. catheter
heparin-bonded
h.-b. Bott-type tube
h.-b. tube
heparin-coated
h.-c. catheter
h.-c. guide wire
heparin-flushing needle
heparin needle
hepatic bed
Herbert
H. Adams clamp
H. Adams coarctation
    clamp
H. knee prosthesis
H. sclerotomy knife
**Herchenson esophageal cytology
collector**
Hercules plaster shears
Herculon suture
Herczel
H. dissector
H. elevator
H. periosteal elevator
H. raspatory elevator
H. rib elevator
H. rib raspatory
Herff
H. clamp
H. clip
H. forceps
H. membrane-puncturing
    forceps

Herget
H. biopsy forceps
H. forceps
Heritiz clamp
Herman forceps
Hermann bone-holding forceps
Herman-Taylor gastroscope
hermetically-sealed pacemaker
Hermitex bandage
hernia retractor
Heros chiropody sponge
Herrick
H. clamp
H. forceps
H. kidney clamp
H. kidney forceps
H. kidney pedicle clamp
H. kidney pedicle forceps
H. pedicle clamp
**Hersbury anterior chamber
intraocular lens**
**Hershey left ventricular assist
device**
Hertel
H. bougie urethrotome
H. exophthalmometer
H. forceps
H. kidney stone forceps
H. nephrostomy speculum
H. rigid dilator stone
    forceps
H. rigid kidney stone
    forceps
H. stone forceps
Hertzler
H. baby retractor
H. rib retractor
H. rib spreader
Herz
H. meniscal forceps
H. tendon forceps
Herzenberg bolt
Herzfeld
H. ear forceps
H. forceps
Herzmark fracture frame
Hess
H. capsular forceps
H. capsular iris forceps
H. expressor
H. forceps
H. iris forceps
H. lens scoop

H. lens spoon
H. nerve root retractor
H. screen
H. serrefine
H. tonsillar expressor
Hess-Barraquer
H.-B. forceps
H.-B. iris forceps
Hessburg
H. intraocular lens glide
H. lacrimal needle
H. lens forceps
H. lens-inserting forceps
H. trephine
H. vacuum trephine
Hessburg-Barron trephine
Hesseltine
H. clamp
H. umbilical cord clamp
H. umbiliclip
Hess-Gill
H.-G. eye forceps
H.-G. forceps
H.-G. iris forceps
Hess-Horwitz
H.-H. forceps
H.-H. iris forceps
Hessing brace
heterograft
h. implant
h. prosthesis
Hetherington circular saw
Hevesy polyp forceps
Hewitt
H. mouth gag
H. mouth prop
Hewson
H. breakaway pin
H. drill
H. ligament drill guide
H. passer
Hewson-Richards reamer
hex
h. bar
h. nut-holder pliers
h. socket wrench
h. wrench
Hexabrix contrast material
Hexa-germ scrub soap
hexagonal
h. handle
h. handle osteotome
h. wrench

hexagon snare
hexapolar catheter
Hexascan
Hexcel
H. cast dressing
H. total condylar prosthesis
Hexcelite
H. sheet splint
H. splint
hex-fix external fixator
hexhead
h. bolt
h. pin
h. screwdriver
Heyer-Robertson suprapubic drain
Heyer-Schulte
H.-S. biopsy clamp
H.-S. brain retractor
H.-S. breast implant
H.-S. breast prosthesis
H.-S. catheter
H.-S. clamp
H.-S. device
H.-S. disposal bag
H.-S. drain
H.-S. hydrocephalus shunt
H.-S. Jackson-Pratt wound-
drainage reservoir
H.-S. lens implant
H.-S. muscle biopsy clamp
H.-S. Pour-Safe exudate bag
H.-S. PVC kit
H.-S. Rayport muscle
biopsy clamp
H.-S. reservoir
H.-S. retractor
H.-S. rhinoplasty implant
H.-S. silicone kit
H.-S. valve
H.-S. wedge-suction reservoir
**Heyer-Schulte-Fischer ventricular
cannula**
**Heyer-Schulte-Ommaya CSF
reservoir**
Heyer-Schulte-Portnoy catheter
**Heyer-Schulte-Pudenz cardiac
catheter**
**Heyer-Schulte-Spetzler lumbar
peritoneal shunt**
Hey-Groves needle
Heyman
H. forceps
H. nasal-cutting forceps

Heyman *(continued)*
    H. nasal forceps
    H. nasal scissors
Heyman-Knight nasal dressing forceps
Heyman-Paparella angular scissors
Heyman-Paparella scissors
Hey skull saw
Heywood-Smith
    H.-S. dressing forceps
    H.-S. gallbladder forceps
    H.-S. sponge-holding forceps
HGM intravitreal laser
HG Multilock hip prosthesis
HGP
    HGP II acetabular component
    HGP II acetabular cup
H-H
    H-H open-end alimentation catheter
    H-H Rickham cerebrospinal fluid reservoir
    H-H shunt introducer
Hibbs
    H. biting forceps
    H. blade
    H. bone chisel
    H. bone curette
    H. bone-cutting forceps
    H. bone gouge
    H. bone-holding forceps
    H. chisel
    H. chisel elevator
    H. clamp
    H. costal elevator
    H. curette
    H. forceps
    H. fracture appliance
    H. fracture frame
    H. gouge
    H. laminectomy retractor
    H. mallet
    H. mouth gag
    H. osteotome
    H. periosteal elevator
    H. retractor
    H. retractor blade
    H. self-retaining retractor
    H. spinal fusion chisel elevator
    H. spinal fusion gouge

    H. spinal retractor blade
    H. sponge
Hibbs-Bruns sterilizing rack
Hibb scoop
Hibbs-Spratt
    H.-S. curette
    H.-S. spinal fusion curette
Hibiclens scrub soap
Hibiscrub scrub soap
Hickman
    H. catheter
    H. indwelling catheter
    H. indwelling right atrial catheter
Hickman-Broviac catheter
Hicks lugged plate
Hidalgo catheter
Hiebert
    H. esophageal suture spoon
    H. vascular dilator
Hieshima coaxial catheter
Higbee vaginal speculum
Higgins
    H. bag
    H. catheter
    H. hemostatic bag
Higginson syringe
high
    h. forceps
    h. minus power optics for low vision aid lens
high-capacity
    h.-c. drain
    h.-c. silicone drain
high-density lipoprotein (HDL)
high-fidelity catheter
high-flow
    h.-f. cannula
    h.-f. catheter
    h.-f. coaxial cannula
high-frequency tweezer-type epilator
high-Knight brace
high-risk (HR)
high-risk needle
high-speed
    h.-s. bur
    h.-s. drill
    h.-s. steel bur
HIHA tendon implant
Hildebrandt
    H. uterine forceps
    H. uterine hemostatic forceps

Hildreth
  H. cautery
  H. coagulator
  H. electrode
  H. ocular cautery
  H. rechargable cautery
  H. transilluminator
Hildyard
  H. forceps
  H. nasal forceps
Hilgenreiner brace
Hilger facial nerve stimulator
Hill
  H. nasal raspatory
  H. rectal retractor
  H. retractor
  H. suture
Hill-Bosworth saw
Hill-Ferguson
  H.-F. rectal retractor
  H.-F. retractor
Hillis
  H. eyelid retractor
  H. fetal stethoscope
  H. lid retractor
  H. perforator
  H. stethoscope
Hi-Lo Jet tracheal tube
Hilsinger tonsillar knife
Himalaya dressing forceps
Himmelstein
  H. pulmonary valvulotome
  H. retractor
  H. sternal retractor
Hinderer
  H. cartilage forceps
  H. cartilage-holding forceps
  H. malar prosthesis
hinge
  Lacey rotating h.
  offset h.
  Weser dental h.
hinged
  h. constrained knee prosthesis
  h. great toe replacement prosthesis
  h. Thomas splint
  h. total knee prosthesis
hinged-leaflet vascular prosthesis
hinge-knee prosthesis
hingeless heart valve prosthesis
Hingson-Edwards needle

Hinkle-James rectal speculum
Hinz tongs
HIP
  homograft incus prosthesis
hip
  h. arthroplasty gouge
  Averett total h.
  Bio-Groove h.
  Biomet h.
  Gemini h.
  Gustilo-Kyle total h.
  Howmedica PCA textured h.
  Leinbach head and neck total h.
  PCA total h.
  Precision Osteolock h.
  h. retractor
  h. skid
  h. spica dressing
Hi-Per
  H.-P. Flex exchange wire
  H.-P. Flex wire
Hippel trephine
Hippocrates bandage
Hipps
  H. osteotome
  H. self-retaining retractor
Hipp & Sohn dental scissors
Hircoe denture base material
Hirschberg electromagnet magnet
Hirschman
  H. anoscope
  H. anoscope rectal speculum
  H. clamp
  H. forceps
  H. hemorrhoidal forceps
  H. hook
  H. hooked cannula
  H. iris hook
  H. iris spatula
  H. jeweler's forceps
  H. lens forceps
  H. lens-inserting forceps
  H. lens manipulator
  H. lens spatula
  H. micro-iris hook
  H. nasendoscope
  H. pile clamp
  H. proctoscope
  H. retractor
  H. spatula

Hirschman-Martin proctoscope
Hirsch mucosal clamp
Hirschowitz
    H. fiberscope
    H. gastroduodenal fiberscope
    H. gastroscope
Hirschtick utility shoulder splint
Hirst
    H. forceps
    H. obstetrical forceps
Hirst-Emmet
    H.-E. obstetrical forceps
    H.-E. placental forceps
His
    H. band
    H. catheter
Hishida pine-needle sound
histofreezer
Hitachi
    H. convex-convex biplane
    probe
    H. convex ultrasound probe
    H. fingertip ultrasound
    probe
    H. linear ultrasound probe
    H. multipurpose fingertip
    ultrasound probe
    H. transrectal ultrasound
    probe
    H. transvaginal ultrasound
    probe
hitch
    ankle h.
    girth h.
Hi-Torque
    H.-T. floppy exchange guide
    wire
    H.-T. floppy guide catheter
    H.-T. floppy guide wire
    H.-T. floppy with Propel
    H.-T. intermediate guide
    wire
Hitselberger-McElveen neural
    dissector
Hi Vac tubing
HJB prosthesis
HJD total hip system
Hobbs
    H. medical dilatation
    balloon catheter
    H. needle
    H. polypectomy snare
    H. sheath brush

    H. stent set
    H. stone basket
Hockin lucite ovoid
Hodge
    H. forceps
    H. obstetrical forceps
    H. pessary
Hodgen
    H. apparatus
    H. hip splint
    H. leg splint
Hodlick needle holder
hoe
    Hough h.
    Hough-Saunders stapes h.
    Nordent h.
    stapes h.
Hoen
    H. alligator forceps
    H. bayonet forceps
    H. cannula
    H. dressing forceps
    H. dural separator
    H. forceps
    H. grasping forceps
    H. hemilaminectomy
    retractor
    H. hemostatic forceps
    H. intervertebral disk
    rongeur
    H. laminar gouge
    H. laminectomy rongeur
    H. laminectomy scissors
    H. needle
    H. nerve hook
    H. periosteal elevator
    H. periosteal raspatory
    H. retractor
    H. rongeur
    H. scalp forceps
    H. scalp hemostatic forceps
    H. scalp retractor
    H. skull plate
    H. tissue forceps
    H. ventricular cannula
    H. ventricular needle
Hoffer
    H. corneal marker
    H. forward-cutting knife
    cannula
    H. optical center corneal
    marker

H. ridged intraocular lens
H. ridged lens implant
Hoffmann
H. apex fixation pin
H. clamp
H. ear forceps
H. ear punch forceps
H. ear rongeur
H. external fixation device
H. external fixator
H. eye implant
H. forceps
H. ligament clamp
H. pin
H. scleral fixation pick
H. traction device
H. transfixion pin
Hoffmann-Osher-Hopkins plaster knife
Hoffmann-Pollock forceps
Hoff towel clamp
Hofmeister
H. drainage bag
H. endometrial biopsy curette
Hohmann
H. bone lever
H. clamp
H. retractor
Hohmann-Aldinger bone lever
Hohn
H. catheter
H. vessel dilator
Hoke
H. chisel
H. osteotome
H. spoon
H. sterilizing rack
Hoke-Martin tractor
Hoke-Roberts spoon
Holcombe
H. gastric tourniquet
H. gastric tourniquet clamp
Holden
H. curette
H. uterine curette
holder
A1-Askari needle h.
Abbey needle h.
Adson dural needle h.
Adson needle h.
Aesculap needle h.

Alabama-Green needle eye h.
Alabama needle h.
Alvarado surgical knee h.
Anchor needle h.
anchor needle h.
Anchor tapered spring-needle h.
Andrews rigid chest support h.
Anis-Barraquer needle h.
Anis needle h.
Anspach leg h.
Arruga eye h.
Arruga needle h.
arthroscopic ankle h.
arthroscopic leg h.
Axhausen needle h.
Azar needle h.
baby Barraquer needle h.
baby Crile needle h.
baby Crile-Wood needle h.
Barraquer baby needle h.
Barraquer curved h.
Barraquer eye needle h.
Barraquer needle h.
Barraquer-Troutman needle h.
Baumgartner h.
Baumgartner needle h.
Baum-Metzenbaum needle h.
Baum-Metzenbaum sternal needle h.
Baum needle h.
Baum tonsillar needle h.
bayonet needle h.
bayonet-shaped needle h.
Bechert-Sinskey needle h.
Belin double-ended needle h.
Belin needle h.
Berry needle h.
Bethea sheet h.
Björk-Shiley heart valve h.
bladebreaker h.
Blair-Brown needle h.
Böhler-Steinmann pin h.
bone-graft h.
boomerang needle h.
Bovie h.
Bovie cautery h.
Boyce h.
Boynton needle h.

holder *(continued)*

Bozeman-Finochietto needle h.
Bozeman needle h.
Bozeman-Wertheim needle h.
Brimfield cannulated blade h.
Brown needle h.
Bumgardner dental h.
Bunt forceps h.
Bunt instrument h.
cannula h.
cannula cradle h.
Carb-Bite needle h.
cardiovascular needle h.
Castroviejo-Barraquer needle h.
Castroviejo blade h.
Castroviejo eye needle h.
Castroviejo-Kalt eye needle h.
Castroviejo needle h.
Castroviejo razor h.
Castroviejo-Troutman eye needle h.
Castroviejo-Troutman needle h.
Catalano needle h.
catheter h.
catheter guide h.
Chaffin-Pratt percolator hanger h.
Circon leg h.
clamp h.
Cohan needle h.
Colles needle h.
Collier needle h.
Collins leg h.
Converse needle h.
Cooley Vital microvascular needle h.
Corboy needle h.
Cottle needle h.
Craig headrest h.
Crile-Murray needle h.
Crile needle h.
Crile-Wood needle h.
Crile-Wood Vital needle h.
Crockard suction tube h.
Dainer-Kaupp needle h.
DeBakey needle h.
Dees h.

delicate needle h.
DeMartel-Wolfson clamp h.
Derf h.
Derf eye needle h.
Derf needle h.
Derf Vital needle h.
Derlacki ossicle h.
diamond grip needle h.
Doyen needle h.
ear speculum h.
Eber h.
Eiselsberg-Mathieu needle h.
Elliot femoral condyle h.
Ellis h.
Ellis eye needle h.
Ellis needle h.
Eriksson-Paparella h.
Ermold needle h.
E-Series needle h.
eye needle h.
Ferris Smith needle h.
Finochietto needle h.
foot h.
French-eye needle h.
French-eye Vital needle h.
Furacin gauze h.
Gambro dialyzer h.
Gardner needle h.
Germain needle h.
GHM KLE II x-ray film h.
Giannini needle h.
Gifford h.
Gillies needle h.
Gillquist-Oretorp-Stille needle h.
Graft Assist graft h.
Grant h.
Grant needle h.
Green h.
Greenberg instrument h.
Green eye needle h.
Green needle h.
Grieshaber h.
Grieshaber eye needle h.
Grieshaber needle h.
Hagfer needle h.
Halsey needle h.
Halsey Vital needle h.
Halsey-Webster needle h.
Hampton needle h.
Hannover needle h.
head h. (*See* head holder)
Heaney needle h.

Heaney Vital needle h.
Hegar-Baumgartner needle h.
Hegar-Mayo-Seeley needle h.
Hegar needle h.
Hegar-Olsen needle h.
Hodlick needle h.
hook h.
hookbar h.
Hosel needle h.
House-Urban h.
House-Urban bone h.
House-Urban temporal
  bone h.
Huang vein h.
Hufnagel-Ryder needle h.
Hyde needle h.
instrument h.
h. instrument
intracardiac needle h.
I-tech cannula h.
I-tech needle h.
Ivy needle h.
Jacobson h.
Jacobson needle h.
Jacobson spring-handled
  needle h.
Jacobson Vital needle h.
Jaffe needle h.
Jako laryngeal needle h.
Jameson needle h.
Jannetta bayonet-shaped
  needle h.
Jarcho tenaculum h.
Jarit forceps h.
Jarit microsurgical needle h.
Jarit sternal needle h.
Jarit wire h.
Johnson needle h.
Johnson prostatic needle h.
Jones IMA needle h.
Jones needle h.
Jordan-Caparosa h.
Juers-Derlacki h.
Juers-Derlacki Universal
  head h.
Julian needle h.
Kalman needle h.
Kalt-Arruga needle h.
Kalt eye needle h.
Kalt needle h.
Kalt Vital needle h.
Kilner needle h.
Knolle needle h.

Langenbeck needle h.
Lapides h.
laryngoscope h.
laryngoscope chest
  support h.
laser Heaney needle h.
laser Julian needle h.
leg h.
Lenny Johnson surgical-
  assist knee h.
Lewy chest h.
Lewy laryngoscope h.
Lichtenberg needle h.
Lindley needle h.
Lundia dialyzer h.
Malis needle h.
Masing needle h.
Mason leg h.
Masson-Luethy needle h.
Masson-Mayo-Hegar
  needle h.
Masson needle h.
Masson Vital needle h.
mat h.
Mathieu h.
Mathieu needle h.
Mathieu-Stille needle h.
Mayfield head h.
Mayo h.
Mayo-Hegar curved-jaw
  needle h.
Mayo-Hegar needle h.
Mayo needle h.
McAllister needle h.
McIntyre fish-hook
  needle h.
McPherson microsurgery eye
  needle h.
McPherson needle h.
Metzenbaum needle h.
MGH needle h.
Micra needle h.
micro-infertility needle h.
microneedle h.
microstaple h.
microsurgical needle h.
microvascular needle h.
Millin boomerang needle h.
Mills microvascular
  needle h.
mirror h.
Murray h.
needle h.

holder *(continued)*
Neivert needle h.
nerve h.
Neumann razor blade
  fragment h.
neurosurgical head h.
neurosurgical needle h.
New Orleans needle h.
Octopus h.
O'Gawa needle h.
Okmian microneedle h.
Olsen-Hegar needle h.
Olympic needle h.
Osher needle h.
Paparella monkey-head h.
Paton eye needle h.
Paton needle h.
Pilling needle h.
pin h.
Pittman needle h.
Posilok instrument h.
Potts-Smith needle h.
press plate needle h.
prostatic needle h.
prosthetic valve h.
Quinn h.
Ravich needle h.
razor blade h.
Reill needle h.
Reverdin h.
Rhoton bayonet needle h.
Rhoton microneedle h.
Rhoton needle h.
Rica forceps h.
Rochester needle h.
rod h.
Rogers needle h.
Rubio needle h.
Ryder needle h.
Sarot needle h.
Sarot Vital needle h.
Scanlan microneedle h.
Shea speculum h.
Sheehan-Gillies needle h.
sheet h.
Silber microneedle h.
Silber needle h.
Sims sponge h.
Sinskey needle h.
speculum h.
Spetzler needle h.
S-P needle h.
spring h.

spring-handled needle h.
spring needle h.
Stangel modified Barraquer
  microsurgical needle h.
Stanzel needle h.
Steinmann h.
Stenstrom nerve h.
Stephenson h.
sterile forceps h.
sternal needle h.
Stevens needle h.
Stevenson needle h.
Stille-French cardiovascular
  needle h.
Storz head h.
Storz needle h.
Stratte needle h.
Surcan knee h.
Surcan leg h.
suture h.
Swan needle eye h.
Swiss blade h.
swivel joint suture h.
tapered-spring h.
tapered-spring needle h.
Taylor catheter h.
temporal bone h.
tenaculum h.
Tennant eye needle h.
Tennant thumb-ring
  needle h.
test tube h.
Toennis needle h.
Tomac vest-style h.
Torres needle h.
Troutman-Barraquer
  needle h.
Troutman needle h.
Tru-Cut biopsy needle h.
Turchik instrument h.
Turner-Warwick needle h.
Universal head h.
Universal speculum h.
Vacutainer h.
valve h.
vascular needle h.
Vital Baumgartner needle h.
Vital Castroviejo eye
  needle h.
Vital Castroviejo needle h.
Vital Cooley French eye
  needle h.

Vital Cooley general
tissue h.
Vital Cooley intracardiac
needle h.
Vital Cooley microsurgery
needle h.
Vital Cooley microvascular
needle h.
Vital Cooley needle h.
Vital Cooley neurosurgical
needle h.
Vital Crile-Wood needle h.
Vital DeBakey
cardiovascular needle h.
Vital Derf eye needle h.
Vital Finochietto needle h.
Vital French-eye needle h.
Vital Halsey eye-needle h.
Vital Heaney needle h.
Vital Jacobson needle h.
Vital Jacobson spring-
handled needle h.
Vital Julian needle h.
Vital Kalt eye needle h.
Vital Masson needle h.
Vital Mayo-Hegar needle h.
Vital microsurgery needle h.
Vital microvascular
needle h.
Vital Mills vascular
needle h.
Vital Neivert needle h.
Vital neurosurgical
needle h.
Vital New Orleans
needle h.
Vital Olsen-Hegar needle h.
Vital Rochester needle h.
Vital Ryder needle h.
Vital Sarot needle h.
Vital Stratte needle h.
Vital Wangensteen needle h.
Vital Webster needle h.
V. Mueller laser Rhoton
microneedle h.
V. Mueller-Vital laser
Heaney needle h.
V. Mueller-Vital laser Julian
needle h.
Wangensteen needle h.
Wangensteen Vital needle h.
washer h.
Watanabe pin h.

Watson heart value h.
Web needle h.
Webster-Halsey needle h.
Webster-Kleinert needle h.
Webster needle h.
Webster Vital needle h.
Weck instrument h.
Weck-Rack instrument h.
Weisenbach sterile
forceps h.
well-leg h.
Wertheim needle h.
Wister forceps h.
Worcester instrument h.
Yasargil bayonet needle h.
Yasargil microneedle h.
Yasargil needle h.
Young boomerang needle h.
Young-Hryntschak
boomerang needle h.
Young-Millin h.
Young-Millin boomerang
needle h.
Young needle h.
Zweifel needle h.

holding forceps
hole
guiding catheter with
side h.
Holinger
H. anterior commissure
laryngoscope
H. applicator
H. bronchoscope
H. bronchoscopic magnet
H. bronchoscopic telescope
H. cannula
H. child esophagoscope
H. curved scissors
H. endoscopic magnet
H. esophagoscope
H. forceps
H. hook-on folding
laryngoscope
H. hourglass anterior
commissure laryngoscope
H. hourglass laryngoscope
H. infant bougie
H. infant bronchoscope
H. infant esophageal
speculum
H. infant esophagoscope
H. infant laryngoscope

Holinger *(continued)*
- H. laryngeal dissector
- H. laryngoscope
- H. magnet
- H. modified Jackson laryngoscope
- H. needle
- H. open-end aspirating tube
- H. slotted laryngoscope
- H. specimen forceps
- H. telescope
- H. ventilating fiberoptic bronchoscope

Holinger-Benjamin laser diverticuloscope
Holinger-Garfield laryngoscope
Holinger-Hurst bougie
Holinger-Jackson bronchoscope
Holladay posterior capsular polisher
Hollister
- H. bag
- H. catheter
- H. circumcision device
- H. clamp
- H. colostomy bag
- H. colostomy irrigator
- H. drain
- H. drainage bag
- H. external catheter
- H. First Choice pouch
- H. laryngoscope
- H. self-adhesive catheter

hollow
- h. cannula
- h. chisel
- h. fiber capillary dialyzer
- h. lucite pessary
- h. mill
- h. Silastic disk heart valve
- h. sphere eye implant
- h. sphere orbital implant
- h. sphere prosthesis

hollow-object forceps
Holman
- H. flushing apparatus
- H. lung retractor
- H. retractor

Holman-Mathieu
- H.-M. cannula
- H.-M. salpingography cannula

Holmes
- H. cartilage gouge
- H. chisel
- H. fixation forceps
- H. forceps
- H. nasopharyngoscope
- H. scissors

holmium laser
holmium:YAG laser
Holscher
- H. nerve retractor
- H. nerve root retractor

Holter
- H. catheter
- H. connector
- H. distal atrial catheter
- H. distal catheter passer
- H. distal peritoneal catheter
- H. elliptical valve
- H. external drainage system
- H. hydrocephalus shunt system
- H. in-line shunt filter
- H. introducer
- H. lumboperitoneal catheter
- H. mini-elliptical valve
- H. pump clamp
- H. reservoir
- H. shunt
- H. straight valve
- H. valve
- H. ventricular catheter
- H. ventriculostomy reservoir

Holter-Hausner catheter
Holter-Rickham ventriculostomy reservoir
Holter-Salmon-Rickham ventriculostomy reservoir
Holter-Selker ventriculostomy reservoir
Holth
- H. corneoscleral punch
- H. cystitome
- H. forceps
- H. punch
- H. punch forceps

Holth-Rubin punch
Holt self-retaining catheter
Holtz
- H. curette
- H. ear curette
- H. endometrial curette

Holzbach
    H. abdominal retractor
    H. forceps
    H. hysterectomy forceps
    H. retractor
Holzheimer
    H. mastoid retractor
    H. retractor
    H. skin retractor
Homer
    H. localizaton needle
    H. needle
Homerlok needle
Homiak radium colpostat
homograft
    h. implant
    h. implant material
    h. incus prosthesis (HIP)
    h. prosthesis
Honan
    H. balloon
    H. cuff
    H. pressure cuff
    H. single-use balloon
hone
    Rosen h.
Honeywell recorder
Hood
    H. dermatome
    H. dissector
    H. electrodermatome
    H. manual dermatome
    H. truss
hood
    surgical h.
hooded transilluminator
Hood-Graves vaginal speculum
hook (*See also* buttonhook)
    Abramson h.
    Adson blunt dissecting h.
    Adson brain h.
    Adson dissecting h.
    Adson dural h.
    Adson knot tier h.
    Allport h.
    Andre h.
    h. approximator
    Arruga extraction h.
    Ashbell h.
    attic h.
    Aufranc h.
    Azar lens h.
    Azar lens-manipulating h.

ball nerve h.
Bane h.
Barr crypt h.
Barr fistular h.
Barr rectal h.
Barton double h.
Bellucci h.
Benger probe h.
Berens scleral h.
Bethune nerve h.
biangled h.
Billeau ear h.
Blair palate h.
h. blocker
blunt h.
blunt dissecting h.
blunt iris h.
Boettcher tonsillar h.
bone h.
Bonn iris h.
Bonn micro-iris h.
Bose tracheostomy h.
Boyes-Goodfellow h.
Braun decapitation h.
Braun obstetrical h.
Brimfield cannulated
  grasping h.
Brown h.
Bryant mitral h.
Burch h.
Carroll bone h.
Carroll skin h.
Caspar h.
Catalano muscle h.
Chavasse squint h.
Chernov tracheostomy h.
Clayman iris h.
cleft palate sharp h.
closed h.
Cloward cautery h.
Cloward dural h.
coarctation h.
Collier-Martin h.
Colver examining h.
Colver retractor h.
compression h.
Converse h.
Converse hinged skin h.
Converse skin h.
corkscrew h.
corkscrew dural h.
corneal h.
Cottle h.

hook *(continued)*
    Cottle double h.
    Cottle-Joseph h.
    Cottle nasal h.
    Cottle skin h.
    Crawford h.
    Crile h.
    Crile nerve h.
    Crile single h.
    crural h.
    crypt h.
    Culler rectus muscle h.
    Cushing dural h.
    Cushing gasserian
     ganglion h.
    Cushing nerve h.
    cystic h.
    Dailey fixation h.
    Dandy nerve h.
    Davis h.
    Day ear h.
    destructive obstetrical h.
    Dingman zygomatic h.
    dissecting h.
    distraction h.
    h. distractor
    Dohlman incus h.
    double h.
    double-pronged h.
    double-pronged Cottle h.
    double-pronged Fomon h.
    double-tenaculum h.
    down-angle h.
    Dudley rectal h.
    Dudley tenaculum h.
    dural h.
    ear h.
    Edwards rectal h.
    Emmet tenaculum h.
    Emmet uterine
     tenaculum h.
    extraction h.
    Feaster lens h.
    fenestration h.
    Ferszt dissecting h.
    fibroid h.
    Fink muscle h.
    Fink-Scobie h.
    Finsen tracheal h.
    Finsen wound h.
    Fisch dural h.
    fistular h.
    fixation h.

    fixation twist h.
    flat tenotomy h.
    Fomon h.
    Fomon nasal h.
    footplate h.
    h. forceps
    Frazier cordotomy h.
    Frazier dural h.
    Frazier nerve h.
    Frazier skin h.
    Freer skin h.
    Gam-Mer nerve h.
    Gass retinal detachment h.
    Gillies bone h.
    Gillies-Converse skin h.
    Gillies-Dingman h.
    Gillies dural h.
    Gillies nasal h.
    Gillies skin h.
    Gillies zygoma h.
    goiter h.
    Goldman Universal
     nerve h.
    Goodhill h.
    Graefe h.
    Graefe iris h.
    Graefe strabismus h.
    Graether mushroom h.
    Graham blunt h.
    Graham dural h.
    Graham nerve h.
    Green muscle h.
    Green strabismus h.
    Gross ear h.
    Guthrie h.
    Guthrie eye-fixation h.
    Guthrie fixation h.
    Guthrie iris h.
    Guthrie skin h.
    Gwathmey h.
    Hall modified Moe h.
    Hamilton-Forewater
     amniotomy h.
    Hardesty tenotomy h.
    Harris-Sinskey microlens h.
    Haven skin graft h.
    Henton tonsillar suture h.
    Hirschman h.
    Hirschman iris h.
    Hirschman micro-iris h.
    Hoen nerve h.
    h. holder
    Hough h.

House crural h.
House footplate h.
House incus h.
House oval-window h.
House plate h.
House strut h.
House tragus h.
h. impactor
instant skin h.
intracapsular lens
  expressor h.
intraocular h.
iris h.
irrigating iris h.
irrigation h.
IUD remover h.
Jackson tracheal h.
Jacobson blunt h.
Jaffe iris h.
Jaffe lens-manipulating h.
Jaffe-Maltzman h.
Jaffe micro-iris h.
Jaffe microlens h.
Jako fine ball-tip h.
Jako-Kleinsasser ball-tip h.
Jameson h.
Jameson muscle h.
Jameson strabismus h.
Jannetta h.
Jannetta right-angle h.
Jardine h.
Jarit bone h.
Jarit palate h.
jaw h.
Jeager strabismus h.
Johnson h.
Johnson skin h.
Jordan h.
Joseph h.
Joseph nasal h.
Joseph sharp skin h.
Joseph skin h.
Joseph tenaculum h.
Juers h.
Kelly uterine tenaculum h.
Kelman h.
Kelman irrigation h.
Kelman manipulator h.
Kennerdell-Maroon h.
Kennerdell-Maroon-
  Jameson h.
Kennerdell muscle h.
Kennerdell nerve h.

Kilner goiter h.
Kilner sharp h.
Kilner skin h.
Kimball nephrostomy h.
Kincaid right-angle h.
Kirby double-fixation h.
Kirby intracapsular lens
  expressor h.
Kirby muscle h.
Klapp tendon h.
Kleinert-Kutz h.
Kleinert-Kutz skin h.
Kleinsasser h.
Klemme dural h.
Klintskog amniotomy h.
Knapp h.
Knapp iris h.
Knolle micro-iris h.
Kratz iris push-pull h.
Krayenbuehl h.
Krayenbuehl dural h.
Krayenbuehl nerve h.
Krayenbuehl twist h.
Krayenbuhl h.
Kuglen h.
Kuglen iris h.
Kuglen manipulating h.
Lahey Clinic dural h.
Lahey dural h.
Lange fistular h.
Lange plastic surgery h.
Leader iris h.
Leader vas h.
Leatherman alar h.
Leatherman compression h.
Leinbach olecranon h.
lens h.
Levy-Kuglen iris h.
Lewicky h.
Lewicky microlens h.
Lillie attic h.
Lillie ear h.
Linton vein h.
Loughnane prostatic h.
Lucae h.
Madden sympathectomy h.
Magielski h.
Malgaigne patellar h.
Malis nerve h.
h. manipulator
Manson double-ended
  strabismus h.

hook *(continued)*
 Marino rotatable
  transsphenoidal right-
  angle h.
 Martin h.
 Martin rectal h.
 Maumenee blunt iris h.
 Maumenee iris h.
 Maumenee sharp iris h.
 Mayo fibroid h.
 McIntyre irrigating h.
 McIntyre irrigating iris h.
 McMahon nephrostomy h.
 McReynolds lid-retracting h.
 Meyerding skin h.
 micro-iris h.
 microlens h.
 micronerve h.
 microscopic h.
 microsurgical ear h.
 microvessel h.
 Millard thimble h.
 mitral h.
 Miya h.
 Moe h.
 Morgenstein h.
 Morrison skin h.
 Muelly h.
 Murphy ball-end h.
 muscle h.
 nasal polyp h.
 Neivert nasal h.
 Neivert nasal polyp h.
 nerve h.
 nerve pull h.
 neutral h.
 Newell nucleus h.
 Newhart h.
 New tracheostomy h.
 New tracheotomy h.
 Nova jaw h.
 Nugent iris h.
 oblique h.
 O'Brien rib h.
 obstetrical h.
 obstetrical decapitating h.
 O'Connor h.
 O'Connor flat tenotomy h.
 O'Connor sharp h.
 O'Connor tenotomy h.
 open h.
 ophthalmic h.
 Osher irrigating implant h.
 oval-window h.
 Pajot decapitating h.
 palate h.
 Paul tendon h.
 pedicle h.
 Penn swivel h.
 Pickrell h.
 plain ear h.
 Praeger iris h.
 Pratt crypt h.
 Pratt cystic h.
 Pratt rectal h.
 h. pusher
 Rainen iris h.
 Rainen lens h.
 Rainin iris h.
 Rainin lens h.
 Ramsbotham decapitating h.
 Rappazzo iris h.
 rectal h.
 retractor h.
 h. retractor
 Rhoton h.
 Rhoton nerve h.
 Rica h.
 Rica cerumen h.
 Richards bone h.
 right-angle h.
 Rogozinski h.
 Rolf muscle h.
 Rollet strabismus h.
 Rosser crypt h.
 h. rotary scissors
 rotatable transsphenoidal
  right-angle h.
 Russian fixation h.
 Russian four-pronged
  fixation h.
 Sachs dural h.
 Sadler bone h.
 Saunders-Paparella stapes h.
 Scanlan micronerve h.
 Scanlan microvessel h.
 Scheer h.
 Schnitman skin h.
 Schuknecht footplate h.
 Schuknecht stapes h.
 Schwartz cervical
  tenaculum h.
 h. scissors
 scleral twist fixation h.
 Scobee muscle h.
 Scobee oblique muscle h.

Scoville blunt h.
Scoville curved nerve h.
Scoville dural h.
Scoville retractor h.
Searcy fixation h.
Selverstone cordotomy h.
Shambaugh h.
Shambaugh endaural h.
Shambaugh fistula h.
Shambaugh microscopic h.
sharp h.
Sharpley h.
Shea h.
Shea fenestration h.
Shea fistular h.
Shea oblique h.
Shea stapes h.
Sheets iris h.
Sheets micro-iris h.
Shepard h.
Shepard iris h.
Shepard micro-iris h.
Simon fistula h.
single h.
Sinskey h.
Sinskey iris h.
Sinskey lens h.
Sinskey lens-manipulating h.
Sinskey micro-iris h.
Sinskey microlens h.
Sisson spring h.
skin h.
Sluder sphenoidal h.
Smellie obstetrical h.
SMIC h.
SMIC cerumen h.
Smith expressor h.
Smith lid h.
Smith lid-retracting h.
Smithwick button h.
Smithwick nerve h.
Smithwick
  sympathectomy h.
Speare dural h.
Speer suture h.
spring h.
squint h.
Stallard scleral h.
stapes h.
Stevens muscle h.
Stevens tenotomy h.
Stewart crypt h.
Stewart rectal h.

Stille coarctation h.
St. Martin-Franceschetti
  cataract h.
Storz double-fixation h.
Storz iris h.
Storz twist h.
strabismus h.
Strandell-Stille tendon h.
Strully dural twist h.
strut h.
strut bar h.
Suraci elevator h.
sympathectomy h.
Tauber ligature h.
tenaculum h.
tendon h.
Tennant h.
Tennant anchor lens-
  insertion h.
Tennant iris h.
Tennant lens-
  manipulating h.
tenotomy h.
Toennis dural h.
Tomas iris h.
tonsillar h.
tonsil-suturing h.
Torchia-Kuglen h.
Torchia lens h.
tracheal h.
tracheostomy h.
tracheotomy h.
tragus House h.
triple h.
tubal h.
two-pronged dural h.
Tyrrell h.
Tyrrell iris h.
Tyrrell skin h.
University of Kansas h.
up-angle h.
vas h.
V. Mueller blunt h.
Volkmann bone h.
Volkmann vas h.
von Szulec h.
Wagener h.
Walsh h.
Weary nerve h.
Welch Allyn h.
Wiener h.
Wiener corneal h.
Wiener scleral h.

hook *(continued)*
Wiener suture h.
Wilder foreign body h.
Y-h.
Yankauer h.
Yasargil spring h.
Zaufel-Jansen ear h.
Zoellner h.
zygoma h.
Zylik-Joseph h.
hookbar
h. holder
hooked intramedullary nail
hook-on
h.-o. bronchoscope
h.-o. folding laryngoscope
hook-type
h.-t. dermal curette
h.-t. eye implant
Hooper pediatric scissors
Hope bag
Hopener clamp
Hopkins
H. aortic clamp
H. aortic forceps
H. aortic occlusion clamp
H. arthroscope
H. clamp
H. direct-vision telescope
H. endoscopy telescope
H. fiber-shaft telescope
H. forceps
H. forward-oblique telescope
H. Hospital periosteal
raspatory
H. hysterectomy clamp
H. II optical system
H. lateral telescope
H. nasal endoscopy
telescope
H. pediatric telescope
H. Percuflex drainage
catheter
H. retrospective telescope
H. rigid telescope
H. rod-lens esophagoscope
H. rod-lens telescope
H. sigmoidoscope
H. telescope
H. tympanoscope
**Hopkins-Cushing periosteal
elevator**

Hopp
H. anterior commissure
laryngoscope blade
H. blade
H. laryngoscope
H. laryngoscope blade
Hopp-Morrison laryngoscope
hordeolum eye implant
Horgan
H. blade
H. center blade
H. retractor
Horgan-Coryllos-Moure rib shears
Horgan-Wells rib shears
Horico
H. diamond instrument
H. disk
**Horizon surgical ligating and
marking clip**
horizontal
h. flexible bar retractor
h. mattress suture
h. retractor
h. ring curette
h. suture
Horn endo-otoprobe
horseshoe
h. headrest
h. magnet
h. suture
h. tourniquet
Horsley
H. bone-cutting forceps
H. bone rongeur
H. dural knife
H. dural separator
H. forceps
H. guard
H. suture
H. trephine
Horsley-Stille bone-cutting forceps
hose
Juzo h.
Hosel
H. needle holder
H. retractor
Hosemann
H. choledochus forceps
H. choledochus knife
H. forceps
Hosford
H. dilator

H. double-ended lacrimal
dilator
H. eye dilator
H. foreign body spud
H. lacrimal dilator
H. meibomian gland
expressor
Hosford-Hicks
H.-H. needle
H.-H. transfer forceps
Hoskin forceps
hospital arterial forceps
Hossli suction tube
hot
h. biopsy forceps
h. flexible forceps
Hotchkiss ear suction tube
Hot Ice System III
hot-tipped
h.-t. catheter
h.-t. laser probe
Hotz
H. curette
H. ear curette
H. ear probe
H. probe
Hough
H. alligator forceps
H. anterior crurotomy
nipper
H. bed
H. bur-crurotomy saw
H. chisel
H. curette
H. drum scraper
H. excavator
H. fascial knife
H. footplate auger
H. forceps
H. gouge
H. hoe
H. hook
H. incision knife
H. knife
H. measuring rod
H. middle ear instrument
H. oval-window excavator
H. pick
H. scissors
H. spatula
H. spatula elevator
H. stapedectomy footplate
pick

H. stapedial footplate auger
H. Teflon cutter
H. whirlybird
H. whirlybird excavator
H. whirlybird knife
Hough-Boucheron ear speculum
Hough-Cadogan
H.-C. footpedal suction
control
H.-C. suction tube
Hough-Derlacki mobilizer
Hough-Rosen knife
Hough-Saunders
H.-S. excavator
H.-S. stapes hoe
Houghton rongeur
Hough-Wullstein
H.-W. bur saw
H.-W. crurotomy saw bur
**hourglass anterior commissure
laryngoscope**
Hourin
H. needle
H. tonsillar needle
House
H. adapter
H. alligator crimper forceps
H. alligator forceps
H. alligator grasping forceps
H. alligator scissors
H. alligator strut forceps
H. blade
H. bur
H. calipers
H. calipers strut
H. chisel
H. crural hook
H. cup forceps
H. curette
H. cutoff adapter
H. cutting block
H. detachable blade
H. dissector
H. ear curette
H. ear elevator
H. ear forceps
H. ear knife
H. ear separator
H. elevator
H. endaural elevator
H. endolymphatic shunt
H. endolymphatic shunt
tube

House *(continued)*
- H. endolymphatic shunt tube introducer
- H. excavator
- H. footplate chisel
- H. footplate hook
- H. forceps
- H. Gelfoam press
- H. Gelfoam pressure forceps
- H. grasping forceps
- H. hand-held retractor
- H. hand retractor
- H. implant
- H. incudostapedial joint knife
- H. incus hook
- H. irrigator
- H. knife
- H. knife blade
- H. lancet knife
- H. malleus nipper
- H. measuring rod
- H. middle ear instrument
- H. middle ear mirror
- H. miniature forceps
- H. myringoplasty knife
- H. myringotomy knife
- H. myringotomy knife handle
- H. needle
- H. neurovascular clip
- H. obtuse pick
- H. ophthalmic blade
- H. oval-cup forceps
- H. oval-window hook
- H. oval-window pick
- H. pick
- H. piston
- H. piston prosthesis
- H. piston wire
- H. plate hook
- H. pressure forceps
- H. retractor
- H. scissors
- H. separator
- H. sickle knife
- H. stapes curette
- H. stapes elevator
- H. stapes needle
- H. stapes speculum
- H. strut calipers
- H. strut forceps
- H. strut guide
- H. strut hook
- H. strut pick
- H. sucker irrigator
- H. suction adapter
- H. suction tube
- H. suction tube adapter
- H. tantalum prosthesis
- H. tapping hammer
- H. Teflon-coated elevator
- H. Teflon cutting block
- H. tragus hook
- H. T-tube irrigator
- H. tympanoplasty curette
- H. tympanoplasty knife
- H. wire-fat prosthesis
- H. wire guide
- H. wire loop
- H. wire prosthesis
- H. wire stapes prosthesis
- H. wire strut guide

House-Barbara
- H.-B. needle
- H.-B. pick
- H.-B. shattering needle

House-Baron
- H.-B. suction tube
- H.-B. tube

House-Bellucci scissors

House-Bellucci-Shambaugh
- H.-B.-S. alligator scissors
- H.-B.-S. scissors

House-Billeau ear loop

House-Buck curette

House-Crabtree
- H.-C. dissector
- H.-C. dissector pick

House-Delrin cutting block

House-Derlacki chisel

House-Dieter
- H.-D. eye forceps
- H.-D. malleus nipper

House-Hough excavator

House-Paparella
- H.-P. curette
- H.-P. stapes curette

Housepian sellar punch

Houser
- H. silicone T-tube tube
- H. tube

House-Radpour
- H.-R. irrigator
- H.-R. suction irrigator
- H.-R. suction tube

House-Rosen
    H.-R. knife
    H.-R. needle
House-Saunders middle ear curette
House-Sheehy knife curette
House-Stevenson
    H.-S. irrigator
    H.-S. suction irrigator
    H.-S. suction tube
House-Urban
    H.-U. bone holder
    H.-U. dissector
    H.-U. holder
    H.-U. marker
    H.-U. microsurgery
      cinecamera
    H.-U. middle fossa retractor
    H.-U. Pentax camera
    H.-U. retractor
    H.-U. rotary dissector
    H.-U. taste tester
    H.-U. temporal bone holder
    H.-U. tube
    H.-U. UEM-100 cinecamera
    H.-U. vacuum rotary
      dissector
House-Urban-Stille camera
House-Wullstein
    H.-W. cup forceps
    H.-W. ear forceps
    H.-W. forceps
    H.-W. oval-cup forceps
    H.-W. perforating bur
Houspian clip-applying forceps
Housset-Debray gastroscope
Houston nasal osteotome
Houtz endometrial curette
Hoverbed
HOW
    hypothermia oxygen warmer
Howard
    H. basket
    H. closing forceps
    H. corneal abrader
    H. forceps
    H. Jones needle
    H. spinal curette
    H. spiral dislodger
    H. spiral stone dislodger
    H. stone basket
    H. stone dislodger
    H. tonsillar forceps
    H. tonsil-ligating forceps

Howard-DeBakey aortic aneurysm
  clamp
Howard-Flaherty
    H.-F. spiral dislodger
    H.-F. spiral stone dislodger
Howard-Schatz laser
Howarth nasal raspatory
Howell
    H. biliary aspiration needle
    H. Rotatable BII
      papillotome
    H. Rotatable BII
      sphincterotome
Howmedica
    H. cement
    H. PCA textured hip
    H. pediatric osteotomy
      system
    H. prosthesis
    H. total ankle system
Howorth
    H. elevator
    H. osteotome
    H. prosthesis
    H. retractor
    H. toothed retractor
Howse-Coventry
    H.-C. hip apparatus
    H.-C. prosthesis
Hoxworth
    H. clip
    H. forceps
Hoyer snare
Hoyt
    H. deep-surgery forceps
    H. forceps
    H. hemostatic forceps
Hoytenberger tissue forceps
Medi-Tech HP Flo-Switch
HP M1350A fetal monitor
HPS II total hip prosthesis
HR
    high-risk
      HR needle
Hruby
    H. contact implant
    H. contact lens
    H. laser
    H. lens
Hryntschak catheter
HS
    hysterosalpingography

HSG
hysterosalpingography
HSG tray
HSS total condylar knee prosthesis
Huang
H. Universal arm retractor
H. Universal flexible arm
H. vein holder
Hubbard
H. airplane vent tube
H. bolt
H. corneoscleral forceps
H. electrode
H. forceps
H. plate
H. retractor
Hubbard-Nylok bolt
Hubell meatoscope
Huber
H. forceps handle
H. needle
Hub saw
Hudgins
H. cannula
H. salpingography cannula
Hudson
H. adapter
H. All-Clear nasal cannula
H. bone drill
H. bone retractor
H. brace
H. brace with bur
H. brain forceps
H. bur
H. cerebellar attachment
H. cerebellar attachment drill
H. cerebellar extension
H. clamp
H. conical bur
H. cranial bur
H. cranial drill
H. cranial forceps
H. cranial rongeur forceps
H. dressing forceps
H. drill
H. forceps
H. retractor
H. rongeur forceps
H. shank
H. tissue-dressing forceps
H. tissue forceps

Hudson-Jones knee cage brace
Huegli
H. meatoscope
H. meatotome
Hueter
H. bandage
H. perineal dressing
Huey scissors
Huffman
H. infant vaginal speculum
H. infant vaginoscope
Huffman-Graves
H.-G. adolescent vaginal speculum
H.-G. vaginal speculum
Huffman-Huber
H.-H. infant vaginoscope
H.-H. vaginoscope
Hufford esophagoscope
Hufnagel
H. aortic clamp
H. ascending aortic clamp
H. clamp
H. commissurotomy knife
H. forceps
H. implant
H. low-profile heart prosthesis
H. mitral valve forceps
H. mitral valve-holding forceps
H. valve-holding clamp
Hufnagel-Kay
H.-K. heart valve
H.-K. valve
Hufnagel-Ryder needle holder
Hu-Friedy
H.-F. dental bur
H.-F. elevator
Huger diamond-back nasal scissors
Hughes
H. eye implant
H. fulguration electrode
H. implant
Hugh Young pedicle clamp
Hugly aspirating tube
HUI
Harris uterine injection
HUI catheter
HUI Mini-Flex uterine injector
Huibregtse biliary stent set

Huibregtse-Katon
   H.-K. ERCP catheter
   H.-K. papillotome
Huibregtse-Kato sphincterotome
Hulka
   H. cannula
   H. clip
   H. clip applier
   H. clip forceps
   H. tenaculum
   H. tenaculum forceps
   H. uterine cannula
   H. uterine manipulator
   H. uterine tenaculum
Hulka-Kenwick
   H.-K. forceps
   H.-K. uterine-elevating
     forceps
   H.-K. uterine elevator
   H.-K. uterine-manipulating
     forceps
Hulten-Stille cannula
Humby knife
Hume
   H. aortic clamp
   H. clamp
humeral
   h. cutting guide
   h. impactor
   h. reamer
   h. retractor
   h. saw
HUMI cannula
hump
   h. forceps
   h. gouge
Humphrey
   H. automatic keratometer
   H. coronary sinus-sucker
     suction tube
   H. retinal imager
Humphries
   H. aortic aneurysm clamp
   H. aortic clamp
   H. clamp
   H. reverse-curve aortic
     clamp
Hundley knee knife
Hunkeler
   H. intraocular lens
   H. lightweight intraocular
     lens implant

Hunt
   H. angiographic trocar
   H. arachnoid dissector
   H. bladder retractor
   H. chalazion forceps
   H. clamp
   H. colostomy clamp
   H. dissector
   H. forceps
   H. metal sound
   H. needle
   H. organizer
   H. retractor
   H. tumor forceps
   H. vessel forceps
Hunter
   H. curette
   H. large uterine curette
   H. one-piece all-PMMA
     intraocular lens
   H. rod
   H. separator
   H. splinter forceps
   H. tendon prosthesis
   H. uterine curette
Hunter-Satinsky clamp
Hunter-Sessions
   H.-S. balloon
   H.-S. vena cava-occluding
     balloon catheter
Hunt-Reich secondary cannula
Hunt-Yasargil pituitary forceps
Hupp
   H. retractor
   H. tracheal retractor
Hurd
   H. angular electrode
   H. bipolar diathermy
     electrode
   H. bone forceps
   H. dissector
   H. electrode
   H. elevator
   H. forceps
   H. needle
   H. pillar retractor
   H. retractor
   H. septal bone-cutting
     forceps
   H. septal elevator
   H. septal forceps
   H. septum-cutting forceps
   H. suture needle

Hurd *(continued)*
   H. tonsillar dissector
   H. tonsillar pillar retractor
   H. tonsillar suturing needle
   H. turbinate electrode
Hurd-Morrison dissector
Hurdner tissue forceps
Hurd-Weder
   H.-W. dissector
   H.-W. tonsillar dissector
Hurricaine gel
Hurson
   H. flexible pressure clamp
   H. flexible retractor
   H. flexible sliding clamp
Hurst
   H. bullet-tip dilator
   H. dilator
   H. esophageal dilator
   H. mercury dilator
   H. mercury-filled dilator
   H. mercury-filled esophageal bougie
Hurst-Maloney dilator
Hurst-Tucker pneumatic dilator
Hurteau forceps
Hurtig dilator
Hurwitt catheter
Hurwitz
   H. clamp
   H. esophageal clamp
   H. intestinal clamp
   H. thoracic trocar
   H. trocar
Huse cannula
Husk
   H. mastoid rongeur
   H. rongeur
Hutch evacuator
Hutchins
   H. biopsy needle
   H. needle
Hutchinson iris retractor
Huxley respirator
Huzly
   H. applicator
   H. aspirator
Hyams
   H. catheter
   H. clamp
   H. double-lumen catheter
   H. meatus clamp

Hyams-Timberlake wire loop for electrode
HybridFit
   H. total hip system
   H. total knee system
Hyde
   H. astigmatism ruler
   H. corneal forceps
   H. forceps
   H. "frog" irrigating cannula
   H. needle holder
hydraclip
Hydracon contact lens
HydraCross TLC PTCA catheter
Hydragrip
   H. clamp
   H. clamp insert
Hydrajaw insert
Hydrasoft contact lens
hydraulic
   h. knee unit prosthesis
   h. vein stripper
Hydro-Cast
Hydroflex
   H. penile implant
   H. penile prosthesis
   H. penile semirigid implant
Hydrogel expansile intraocular lens
Hydrojette aspirator
Hydron Burn Bandage
hydrophilic contact lens
Hydroset root canal sealer
hydrostatic
   h. bag
   h. balloon
   h. balloon catheter
   h. bed
   h. dilator
   h. dissector
hydroxyapatite (HA)
   h. implant material
   h. ossicular prosthesis
hyfrecator
   Bircher h.
   h. coagulator
   Hall-Fish h.
Hyfrecutter
Hylinks clip
hymenal band
Hymes scleral knife
Hymes-Timberlake electrode
hyoid-cutting forceps
Hypaque contrast material

hyperalimentation catheter
hyperbaric bed
hyperextension brace
hyperextension fracture frame
Hyperflex flexible guide wire
Hypertie bandage
hypodermic needle
hypogastric artery forceps
hypophyseal forceps
hypophysectomy forceps
Hypospray jet injection needle
hypothermia oxygen warmer
  (HOW)
hysterectomy
  h. clamp
  h. forceps
  h. kit
  h. retractor
hysterosalpingography (HS, HSG)
  h. catheter

hysteroscope
  ACMI h.
  AMSCO h.
  Baggish h.
  contact h.
  Elmed h.
  examining h.
  fiberoptic h.
  Hamou h.
  Leisegang flexible h.
  Leisegang LM-FLEX 7
    flexible h.
  Scopemaster h.
  h. sheath
  Storz h.
  Van Der Pas h.
Hysterovac drain
Hysto-vac drain
Hy-Tape

I&A
    irrigating-aspirating
    irrigating and aspirating
    irrigation and aspiration
    irrigation-aspiration
        I&A kit
        I&A machine
        McIntyre I&A system
        Simcoe I&A system
IAB
    intra-aortic balloon
        IAB catheter
IABP
    intra-aortic balloon pump
        IABP intra-aortic balloon
          pump
I-beam
        I.-b. cement punch
        I.-b. hemiarthroplasty hip
          prosthesis
        I.-b. press-fit punch
Icarex 25 Med mirror reflex lens
  camera
IC bed
ice
        i. bag
        i. clot evacuator
ice-tong calipers
ICLH
    Imperial College of London
      Hospital
      ICLH apparatus
Icofly infusion needle
ICP
    intracranial pressure
      ICP catheter
ICS
    International compression
      system
Ideal tourniquet
Idecap dialyzer
Iglesias
        I. continuous flow
          resectoscope
        I. dilator
        I. electrode
        I. evacuator
        I. fiberoptic resectoscope
        I. microlens resectoscope
        I. resectoscope

IKI catgut suture
Ikuta clamp approximator
ILA stapling device
ileal reservoir catheter
ileostomy
    i. appliance
    i. bag
Ilex
    I. stomal seal
    I. stoma protective cream
iliac
    i. clamp
    i. forceps
    i. graft separator
iliac-femoral cannula
Iliff
    I. blepharochalasis forceps
    I. clamp
    I. lacrimal trephine
    I. trephine
Iliff-Park speculum
Iliff-Wright needle
Ilizarov limb-lengthening system
Illinois needle
Illouz
    I. cannula
    I. suction cannula
illuminated
    i. probe
    i. speculum
    i. ureter probe
illuminator
    Barkan i.
    Britetrac i.
    fiberoptic surgical field i.
    intramedallary i.
    Novar oral i.
    Pilling fiberoptic i.
    slit i.
    suspended operating i.
Ilopan disposable syringe
ILS
    intraluminal stapler
IM
    intramedullary
      IM nail
      IM tendon stripper
IMA
    inferior mesenteric artery
    internal mammary artery

IMA *(continued)*
  IMA forceps
  IMA graft
  IMA scissors
Image custom external breast prosthesis
imager
  Humphrey retinal i.
Imatron CT bone mineral phantom
Imax periotips
imbricating suture
IMED infusion device
IM/EM
  intramedullary/extramedullary
    IM/EM tibial resection guide
    IM/EM tibial resection stylus
Imexdop CT Doppler
IMMA lens
immediate
  i. postoperative prosthesis (IPOP)
  i. postoperative prosthesis dressing
Immergut
  I. suction-coagulation tube
  I. suction tube
immobilizer
  arm and shoulder i.
  Velpeau-style shoulder i.
  Westfield-style acromioclavicular i.
immobilizing bandage
immovable bandage
impactor
  Bio-Moore II stem i.
  Cloward bone graft i.
  Cloward dowel i.
  Dawson-Yuhl i.
  femoral i.
  glenoid implant base i.
  hook i.
  humeral i.
  Judet i. for acetabular cup
  lateral gutter i.
  Moe i.
  mushroom i.
  orthopaedic i.
  i. plate
  Pollock wimp wire i.
  Raylor bone i.
  spondylophyte i.

impactor-extractor
IMP-Capello arm support
impedance electrode
Imperator handpiece
Imperatori
  I. forceps
  I. laryngeal forceps
Imperial alloy
Imperial College of London Hospital (ICLH)
impermeable dressing
Imperson catheter
Impex aspiration & injection needle
implant
  accessory eye i.
  accordion i.
  acorn-shaped i.
  acorn-shaped eye i.
  acrylic ball eye i.
  acrylic conformer eye i.
  acrylic eye i.
  Acufex-Suretac i.
  Acuflex intraocular lens i.
  adhesive silicone i.
  adjustable breast i.
  adrenal medullary i.
  AGC knee program i.
  alar-columellar i.
  Allen i.
  Allen-Brailey intraocular lens i.
  Allen eye i.
  Allen orbital i.
  Allen Supramid i.
  Alpar i.
  Alpar intraocular lens i.
  AMO intraocular lens i.
  AMO scleral i.
  AO/ASIF orthopaedic i.
  Appolionio eye i.
  Arenberg-Denver inner-ear valve i.
  Arion i.
  Arruga i.
  Arruga eye i.
  Arruga-Moura-Brazil orbital i.
  Arruga movable eye i.
  articulated chin i.
  artificial joint i.
  Ashworth-Blatt i.
  aspheric lens i.

A-type dental i.
Azar Tripod eye i.
Balnetar i.
Bard i.
Barkan i.
Barraquer i.
Bechert intraocular lens i.
Bechtol i.
Beekhuis-Supramid
  mentoplasty
  augmentation i.
Berens i.
Berens conical eye i.
Berens eye i.
Berens orbital i.
Berens pyramidal eye i.
Berens-Rosa eye i.
Berens sphere eye i.
Bietti eye i.
bifocal eye i.
bilumen mammary i.
Binder submalar i.
Binkhorst i.
Binkhorst eye i.
Binkhorst lens i.
Blair-Brown i.
i. blank
Boberg-Ans i.
Bonaccolto eye i.
Branemark
  osseointegration i.
Braun i.
Brawner eye i.
Brawner orbital i.
breast i.
Brown-Dohlman corneal i.
Brown-Dohlman eye i.
build-up eye i.
Bunker i.
candle vaginal cesium i.
cardiovascular i.
carpal lunate i.
Carrion-Small penile i.
cartilage i.
Cartwright i.
Castroviejo i.
Castroviejo acrylic i.
Castroviejo eye i.
Celestin i.
celluloid i.
Chatzidakis i.
chessboard i.
chin i.

Choyce i.
Choyce eye i.
Choyce intraocular eye i.
Choyce-Mark eye i.
Clayman lens i.
Coburn anterior chamber
  intraocular lens i.
Coburn Mark IX eye i.
cochlear i.
Cogan-Boberg-Ans lens i.
collagen i.
i. collar
columellar i.
conical i.
conical eye i.
contact shell i.
conventional reform eye i.
conventional shell-type
  eye i.
Copeland intraocular lens i.
Copeland lens i.
Core-Vent i.
corneal i.
corneal eye i.
Corning i.
corrected cosmetic contact
  shell eye i.
Cox-Uphoff i.
Cronin i.
Cronin mammary i.
CUI columellar i.
CUI dorsal i.
CUI malar i.
CUI rhinoplasty i.
curl-back shell eye i.
curvilinear chin i.
Custodis i.
custom-contoured i.
Cutler i.
Cutler eye i.
3D Accuscan facial i.
Dacron i.
Dannheim eye i.
DCS i.
DeBakey i.
defibrillator i.
dental i.
De Paco i.
DePuy orthopaedic i.
Dermostat i.
Dermostat orbital i.
DeWecker eye i.
Doherty i.

implant *(continued)*
 Doherty eye i.
 Doherty sphere eye i.
 Donnheim i.
 dorsal columella i.
 dorsal column stimulator i.
 double-lumen breast i.
 Dow Corning i.
 Dragstedt i.
 dual-compartment gel-
  inflatable mammary i.
 Duehr-Allen eye i.
 dummy sources in
  cesium i.
 Duracon knee i.
 dural i.
 Edwards i.
 Edwards Teflon
  intracardiac i.
 Ehmke platinum Teflon i.
 electrical i.
 endometrial i.'s
 endometriotic i.
 endo-osseous i.
 endo-osseous dental i.
 Epstein lens i.
 Esser i.
 Ethrone i.
 E-type dental i.
 Ewald-Walker knee i.
 Ewing eye i.
 expandable breast i.
 extended anatomical high-
  profile malar i.
 Extrafil breast i.
 eye i.
 eye sphere i.
 fascia lata i.
 feathered extended malar i.
 fenestra i.
 Ferguson i.
 fetal substantia nigra i.'s
 Fibrel gelatin matrix i.
 finger joint i.
 Finney penile i.
 flexible Dualens i.
 flexible rod penile i.
 Flexi-Flate II penile i.
 Flexi-Flate penile i.
 Flexi-Rod II penile i.
 i. forceps
 Fox i.
 Fox eye i.

Fox eyelid i.
Fox sphere i.
Fox sphere eye i.
free i.
Frey eye i.
Frey tunneled eye i.
front build-up eye i.
full-dimpled lucite eye i.
full-thickness i.
Fyodorov i.
Fyodorov eye i.
Fyodorov lens i.
Fyodorov type II lens i.
Fyodorov type I lens i.
Galin intraocular lens i.
Garcia-Novito eye i.
gel-filled i.
Gelfilm retinal i.
Gelfilm retinal orbital i.
gel-saline mammary i.
Gerow Small-Carrion
 penile i.
Gillies i.
glass sphere i.
glass sphere eye i.
gold i.
gold eye i.
Goldmann multimirrored
 lens i.
Gold-Mules eye i.
gold sphere eye i.
Gore-Tex vascular i.
Gott i.
great toe i.
Guist eye i.
Guist sphere eye i.
Haik i.
Haik eye i.
haptic area i.
Harris i.
Harrison i.
Hartley i.
hemisphere eye i.
heterograft i.
Heyer-Schulte breast i.
Heyer-Schulte lens i.
Heyer-Schulte rhinoplasty i.
HIHA tendon i.
Hoffer ridged lens i.
Hoffmann eye i.
hollow sphere eye i.
hollow sphere orbital i.
homograft i.

hook-type eye i.
hordeolum eye i.
House i.
Hruby contact i.
Hufnagel i.
Hughes i.
Hughes eye i.
Hunkeler lightweight
  intraocular lens i.
Hydroflex penile i.
Hydroflex penile
  semirigid i.
Insall-Burstein intracondylar
  knee i.
Intermedics intraocular
  lens i.
Interpore osteointegrated i.
interstitial i.
intraorbital i.
Iowa i.
Iowa eye i.
Iowa orbital i.
iridium i.
iridium wire i.
Ivalon i.
Ivalon eye i.
Ivalon sponge eye i.
Jardon-Straith chin i.
Jardon-Straith nasal i.
joint i.
Jordan i.
Jordan eye i.
Keragen i.
King i.
King orbital i.
Koeppe gonioscopic lens i.
Koeppe intraocular lens i.
Kratz i.
Kratz-Sinskey intraocular
  lens i.
Krause-Wolfe i.
Kryptok bifocal lens i.
Lacey total knee i.
Landegger orbital i.
Landegger orbital eye i.
LaPorte total toe i.
Lash-Loeffler i.
Lemoine eye i.
Lemoine orbital i.
lens i.
Levitt i.
Levitt eye i.
Lifecath peritoneal i.

Lincoff i.
Lincoff eye i.
Lincoff scleral sponge eye i.
Little intraocular lens i.
Liverpool elbow i.
Loptex laser intraocular
  lens i.
low-implant breast i.
low-profile breast i.
lucite i.
lucite eye i.
lucite sphere i.
lunate i.
Lyda Ivalon-Lucite orbital i.
lymphoma i.
MacIntosh i.
magnetic i.
magnetic eye i.
malar i.
mammary i.
Marlex mesh i.
McGhan i.
McGhan breast i.
McGhan eye i.
Medallion intraocular lens i.
Medical Optics eye i.
Medical Workshop
  intraocular lens i.
Melauskas orbital i.
Meme mammary i.
Mentor malleable semirigid
  penile i.
meridianal eye i.
Mersilene i.
meshed ball i.
metallic i.
metal orthopaedic i.
metastatic i.
metatarsophalangeal i.
  (MTPI)
methyl methacrylate eye i.
middle ear i.
3M mammary i.
modular i.
Molteno drainage eye i.
motility eye i.
Muhlberger i.
Muhlberger orbital i.
Mules i.
Mules eye i.
Mules sphere eye i.
Müller shield eye i.
Naden-Rieth i.

implant *(continued)*
nasal dorsal i.
Neer II total shoulder
system i.
Norplant i.
Novito eye i.
Ollier-Thiersch i.
O'Malley self-adhering
lens i.
orbital i.
orbital eye i.
orbital floor i.
ORC posterior chamber
intraocular lens i.
orthotic attachment i.
Osseodent dental i.
osseous i.
Osteogen resorbable
osteogenic bone-filling i.
Padgett i.
Panje i.
paraffin i.
Pasqualini i.
patch i.
patella-resurfacing i.
peanut eye i.
Pearce vaulted-Y lens i.
pectoralis muscle i.
pedicle i.
penile i.
percutaneous dorsal column
stimulator i.
permanent i.
Phystan i.
pin i.
Pisces i.
planoconvex eye i.
plastic i.
plastic ball i.
plastic sphere eye i.
Platina intraocular lens i.
Plexiglas i.
Plexiglas eye i.
PMI i.
polyethylene eye i.
polyethylene sphere i.
Polystan i.
polyvinyl sponge i.
Porex Medpor i.
Porex PHA i.
Precision-Cosmet intraocular
lens i.
Precision eye i.

press-fit i.
Proplast i.
Proplast facial i.
Proplast preformed i.
pyramidal eye i.
radiocarpal i.
radium i.
Radovan breast i.
Rastelli i.
Rayner-Choyce eye i.
reform i.
reform eye i.
removable i.
retinal Gelfilm i.
Reuter bobbin i.
Reverdin i.
reverse-shaped eye i.
rhinoplasty i.
Ridley anterior chamber i.
Ridley Mark II lens i.
Roberts dental i.
Rodin i.
Rodin orbital i.
Rosa-Berens eye i.
Ruedemann eye i.
Ruiz plano fundus lens i.
SACH i.
Sauerbruch i.
Schepens hollow
hemisphere i.
scleral i.
scleral buckle eye i.
scleral buckler i.
scleral eye i.
seed i.
semishell eye i.
serrefine i.
shell i.
shell eye i.
shell-type eye i.
Shepard intraocular lens i.
Ship arthroplasty i.
Sichel i.
Sichel movable i.
Sichel orbital i.
Silastic i.
Silastic chin i.
Silastic corneal eye i.
Silastic Cronin i.
Silastic eye i.
Silastic finger i.
Silastic penile i.
Silastic rhinoplasty i.

Silastic scleral buckler
  eye i.
Silastic silicone rubber i.
Silastic subdermal i.
Silastic testicular i.
Silastic toe i.
silicone i.
silicone buckling i.
silicone button eye i.
silicone eye i.
silicone-filled breast i.
silicone meshed motility i.
silicone nasal strut i.
silicone pad eye i.
silicone rod i.
silicone sleeve eye i.
silicone sponge i.
silicone strip eye i.
silicone tire eye i.
Siloxane i.
Siltex mammary i.
Simcoe i.
Simcoe-Amo eye i.
Simcoe eye i.
Simcoe intraocular lens i.
Sinskey lens i.
Sled i.
Small-Carrion Silastic rod
  for penile i.
Smith orbital floor i.
Snellen conventional reform
  eye i.
Snellen eye i.
soft silicone sphere i.
solid silicone with Supramid
  mesh i.
spermatocele i.
sphere i.
sphere eye i.
spherical i.
spherical eye i.
split-thickness i.
sponge i.
stainless steel i.
Stone i.
Stone eye i.
Straith chin i.
Straith nasal i.
Strampelli i.
S-type dental i.
subdermal i.
submucosal i.
subperiosteal i.

superficial i.
Supramid i.
surface eye i.
Surgibone i.
Surgicel i.
Surgitek i.
Surgitek Flexi-Flate II
  penile i.
Surgitek mammary i.
Swanson i.
Swanson carpal lunate i.
Swanson carpal scaphoid i.
Swanson finger joint i.
Swanson great toe i.
Swanson hemi-i.
Swanson radial head i.
Swanson radiocarpal i.
Swanson trapezium i.
Swanson ulnar head i.
Swanson wrist joint i.
Swiss MP joint i.
Syed-Neblett i.
Syed template i.
tantalum i.
tantalum eye i.
tantalum mesh eye i.
Teflon i.
Teflon mesh i.
Teflon orbital floor i.
tendon i.
Tennant Anchorflex lens i.
Tensilon i.
Terino anatomical chin i.
testicular i.
Tevdek i.
Thiersch i.
tire eye i.
total top i.
Townley i.
transosteal pin i.
trapezium i.
trial i.
Troncoso i.
Troutman i.
Troutman eye i.
Troutman magnetic i.
T-type dental i.
tunneled eye i.
Ultex i.
Ultrox i.
unicompartmental knee i.
Unilab Surgibone surgical i.
ureteral i.

implant *(continued)*
   Uribe i.
   Uribe orbital i.
   Usher Marlex mesh i.
   U-type dental i.
   VA i.
   VA magnetic i.
   VA magnetic orbital i.
   Varilux i.
   Vitallium i.
   Vitallium eye i.
   Vivosil i.
   Volk conoid i.
   Walter Reed i.
   Weavenit i.
   Weber i.
   Weber hip i.
   Weck-cel i.
   Wheeler i.
   Wheeler eye i.
   Wheeler sphere eye i.
   wire mesh eye i.
   Wolfe i.
   Wölfe-Krause i.
   Zest subperiosteal i.
   Zyderm i.
   Zyderm collagen i.
   Zyplast i.
implantable
   i. clip
   i. neural stimulator
   i. pacemaker
implantation
   i. forceps
   Surgicel i.
implanted
   i. electrode
   i. malleable clip
   i. pacemaker
   i. suture
implanter
   Geuder i.
implant material (*See also* material)
   acrylic i. m.
   allogeneic lyophilized bone grafts i. m.
   bioceramic i. m.
   Bonaccolto monoplex orbital i. m.
   bone i. m.
   celluloid i. m.
   corundum ceramic i. m.

cyanoacrylate fixed orbital silicone sleds i. m.
Dermostat eye i. m.
Edwards Teflon intracardiac patch i. m.
Ethrone i. m.
Expander mammary i. m.
Fletching femoral hernia i. m.
homograft i. m.
hydroxyapatite i. m.
Iowa i. m.
Keolar i. m.
Landegger orbital i. m.
Lash-Loeffler penile i. m.
Lincoff sponge i. m.
Linkow dental i. m.
L-rod i. m.
Malteno tube i. m.
methyl methacrylate i. m.
Ommaya reservoir i. m.
Paladon i. m.
paraffin i. m.
Pearman penile i. m.
polyether i. m.
polyethylene i. m.
polyurethane i. m.
polyvinyl i. m.
Schepens hollow silicone hemisphere i. m.
Scialom dental i. m.
Shearing posterior chamber i. m.
shell i. m.
Small-Carrion penile i. m.
solid buckling i. m.
solid silicone i. m.
solid silicone exoplant i. m.
Spitz-Holter valve i. m.
sponge silicone i. m.
Stimoceiver i. m.
Szulc orbital i. m.
tissue mandrel i. m.
titanium i. m.
transcatheter umbrella i. m.
tunnel-type i. m.
Usher Marlex mesh i. m.
Vitallium i. m.
Implens intraocular lens
Impra
   I. Flex vascular graft
   I. microporous PTFE vascular graft

I. peritoneal catheter
I. vascular graft
impregnated
    i. dressing
    i. electrode
Impregum impression material
impression material syringe
IMSI-Metripond operating room table
inactive electrode
incandescent
    i. endoscope lamp
    i. sheath
InCare brace
incise drape
incision
    i. dilator
    i. knife
    i. retractor
    i. spreader
incisive suture
Inclan graft
Incono bag
incontinence clamp
incudostapedial
    i. joint knife
    i. knife
incus replacement prosthesis
Indiana reamer
Indian club needle
India rubber suture
indicator
    Berens-Tolman i.
    Berens-Tolman ocular hypertension i.
    Neesone root canal depth i.
    Pio root canal depth i.
indifferent electrode
indirect ophthalmoscope
Indong Oh prosthesis
indwelling
    i. catheter
    i. stent
    i. ureteral stent
infant
    i. abdominal retractor
    i. abduction splint
    i. biopsy forceps
    i. bronchoscope
    i. catheter
    i. dilator
    i. esophagoscope
    i. eyelid retractor

i. female catheter
i. male catheter
i. retractor
i. rib retractor
i. rib shears
i. soap
i. telescope
i. urethrotome
i. urethrotome blade
i. vaginoscope
i. vascular clamp
i. ventilation monitor
inferior
    i. mesenteric artery (IMA)
    i. vena cava (IVC)
    i. vena caval clip
inflatable
    i. catheter
    i. cuff
    i. Foley bag catheter
    i. mammary prosthesis
    i. Mentor penile prosthesis
    i. penile prosthesis
    i. splint
    i. tourniquet cuff
    i. tracheal tube cuff
inflated balloon
inflator
    Bonney retrograde i.
    Ogden-Senturia eustachian i.
inflow cannula
infraorbital suture
infrared ray photocoagulator
infundibular
    i. forceps
    i. punch
    i. rongeur forceps
Infusaid
    I. catheter
    I. Infuse-A-Port
    I. needle
    I. pump
Infuse-A-Port
    Infusaid I.-A.-P.
infuser
    Ohio pressure i.
    Parker micropump insulin i.
    pen pump insulin i.
infusion
    i. cannula
    i. catheter
    i. device

infusion *(continued)*
    i. handpiece
    i. tube
Ingals
    I. antral cannula
    I. cannula
    I. flexible silver cannula
    I. nasal speculum
    I. rectal injection cannula
Inge
    I. laminar retractor
    I. laminar spreader
    I. laminectomy retractor
    I. retractor
    I. spreader
Ingersoll
    I. adenoid curette
    I. curette
    I. needle
    I. tonsillar needle
Ingraham-Fowler
    I.-F. clip-applying forceps
    I.-F. cranium clip
    I.-F. tantalum clip
    I.-F. tantalum cranium clip
Ingraham skull punch
Ingram
    I. catheter
    I. trocar
ingress/egress cannula
inguinal truss
inhalation cannula
inhalator
    OIC emergency oxygen i.
    Oxy-Quik Mark IV
      oxygen i.
inhaler
    Schimelbusch i.
    ultrasound i.
inhibitor
    vaporizing rust i.
initial incision retractor
Injectate probe
injection
    i. cannula
    i. needle
Injectoflex respirator jet
injector
    DG77 jet i.
    Harris uterine i.
    HUI Mini-Flex uterine i.
    Lakatos Teflon i.
    Marcon-Haber varices i.

    Medrad contrast medium i.
    Miller ratchet i.
    Robinject needle i.
    uterine i.
inlet
    Berry rotating i.
    i. cannula
    Fish i.
    i. forceps
in-line venous pressure monitor
inner
    i. cannula
    i. coaxial irrigating cannula
Innomed
    I. bone curette
    I. curette
Innsbruck electrode
Inokucki vascular stapler
Inoue balloon catheter
Inpersol peritoneal dialysis set
input device
Inronail finger or toenail
    prosthesis
Insall-Burstein
    I.-B. intracondylar knee
      implant
    I.-B. knee prosthesis
insert
    articular i.
    clamp i.
    Dischler rectoscopic
      suction i.
    Endostat calibration pod i.
    Fogarty i.
    Fogarty-Hydragrip i.
    Fogarty-Softjaw i.
    Hydragrip clamp i.
    Hydrajaw i.
    i. mattress suture
    retainer i.
    Softjaw i.
    tray i.
inserter
    Armstrong "V" tube
      suction i.
    Buck femoral cement
      restrictor i.
    diaphragm i.
    Moon-Robinson prosthesis i.
    Robinson-Moon prosthesis i.
    twist-in drain tube i.
    Tytan tube i.
insertion forceps

insertor
>DDT lock screw i.
>deluxe FIN pin i.
>Storz i.
>subperiosteal glass bead i.

insitu
>i. bypass instrument set
>i. valve-cutter kit
>i. valve scissors

Inspiron device
Instant Fever Tester thermometer
instant skin hook
Instasan scrub soap
Instat
>I. absorbable hemostat
>I. collagen absorbable
> hemostat

Instra-Rack
>I.-R. count bar
>I.-R. security rod
>I.-R. separator clip

Instrument
>Accurate Surgical and
> Scientific I.'s (ASSI)
>I. Makar Switching Stick

instrument
>Abradabloc dermabrasion i.
>accessory i.
>arterial oscillator
> endarterectomy i.
>Atlas orthogonal
> percussion i.
>Austin middle ear i.
>i. basket
>Bellucci middle ear i.
>Biomer microsuturing i.
>bone abduction i.
>Britetrac fiberoptic i.
>Cheshire-Poole-Yankauer
> suction i.
>chiropractic adjusting i.
>circumcision i.
>i. cleaner
>Cobb spinal i.
>i. coding tape
>conization i.
>contour-facilitating i. (CFI)
>cortex extractor i.
>cryosurgical i.
>cutting i.
>Daisy irrigation-aspiration i.
>Delcom filling i.

Diamond-Lite
>cardiovascular i.
Dix double-ended i.
Dreyfus prosthesis
>placement i.
Dyonics arthroscopic i.
Endoloop chromic ligature
>suture i.
Fleming conization i.
G-C filling i.
Graefe i.
graft measuring i.
grasping i.
Guilford-Wright middle
>ear i.
Halifax fine adjustment i.
Henry Schein filling i.
i. holder
holder i.
Horico diamond i.
Hough middle ear i.
House middle ear i.
irrigating-aspirating i.
ITD-FG dental diamond i.
Jordan middle ear i.
Jordan strut-measuring i.
Keeler cryosurgical i.
Kimberley diamond i.
Kitner blunt dissecting i.
knot-tying i.
Kos middle ear i.
Krwawicz cataract
>cryosurgical i.
ligature-passing i.
i. lubricant
lumbar accessory i.
lung i.
Matsuda titanium surgical i.
McCabe measuring i.
McGee middle ear i.
measuring i.
3M filling i.
Micromedics surgical i.
microneurosurgical i.
middle ear i.
Millet neurological test i.
Miracompo filling i.
Monarch II bleaching i.
Nordent filling i.
orthopaedic cutting i.
Paparella middle ear i.
Plastibell compression i.
reduction i.

instrument *(continued)*
    Rosen middle ear i.
    Safco diamond i.
    Salinger reduction i.
    Schafer cortical hearing i.
    Scheer middle ear i.
    Schuknecht middle ear i.
    Seiffert suturing i.
    i. set for angled blade
    Shea middle ear i.
    Shea prosthesis placement i.
    SITE I&A i.
    Smillie cartilage i.
    Smith-Miller-Patch
      cryosurgical i.
    Snowden-Pencer laparoscopic
      cholecystectomy i.
    i. stabilizer pad
    Steele filling i.
    stereotaxic i.
    i. stringer
    strut measuring i.
    suturing i.
    Todd-Wells human
      stereotaxic i.
    i. tray
    tray i.
    Ultra-Cut Cobb spinal i.
    ultrasonic bone-cutting i.
    Universal nasal i. handle
    ureteral visualization i.
    Valleylab laparoscopic i.
    vertebral body biopsy i.
    Vibrasonic hearing i.
    vitrectomy i.
    Wallach mini-freezer
      cryosurgical i.
    Wiet graft-measuring i.
    Wigand endoscopic i.
    Wright-Guilford middle
      ear i.

instrumentation
    Accu-Line knee i.
    Bio-Moore II i.
    compression i.
    Cooley i.
    Cotrel-Dubousset i.
    DeBakey i.
    L-rod i.
    Russell-Taylor interlocking
      nail i.
    TAG i.

    Texas Scottish Rite
      Hospital i.
    TSRH i.
    Zielke i.

instrument-grasping forceps
instrument-handling forceps
insufflation device
insufflator
    Bonney i.
    Buckstein colonic i.
    colonic i.
    Eder i.
    gas i.
    Kelly i.
    Kidde tubal i.
    KLI i.
    laparoscopic i.
    Milex vaginal i.
    Pneumomat laparoscopic i.
    Sieger i.
    Stille i.
    variable flow i.
    Weber colonic i.

insulated
    i. bayonet forceps
    i. forceps
    i. knife handle
    i. monopolar forceps
    i. tissue forceps

Intact
    I. catheter
    I. xenograft valve

Integral
    I. distal centralizer
    I. hip system
    I. Interlok femoral
      prosthesis

Integrity
    I. acetabular cup screw
    I. neutral liner
    I. shell

InteguDerm dressing
Interad whole body CT scanner
interbody
    i. fusion rasp
    i. graft tamp
    i. rasp

intercardiac sucker
Interceed
    I. absorbable adhesion
      barrier
    I. adhesion barrier

intercerebral electrode

Interpore

interchangeable | in-the-ear

interchangeable
    i. vein stripper
    i. vein stripper olive
intercostal
    i. catheter
    i. drain
    i. trocar
interdental splint
interdermal buried suture
Interface arterial blood filter
interference
    i. fit
    i. screw
Interfit-Pharmacea Intermedic
    intraocular lens
Interflux intraocular lens
interlocking
    i. sound
    i. suture
Interlok primary femoral
    component
intermaxillary
    i. suture
    i. wire
Intermedics
    I. Cyberlith X
      multiprogrammable
      pacemaker
    I. intraocular lens implant
    I. lithium-powered
      pacemaker
    I. pacemaker
    I. Quantum pacemaker
    I. Quantum unipolar
      pacemaker
    I. Thinlith II pacemaker
intermittent
    i. positive pressure
      breathing (IPPB)
    i. suture
internal
    i. ear prosthesis
    i. fixation device
    i. mammary artery (IMA)
    i. mammary artery catheter
internasal suture
International compression system
    (ICS)
International standard goniometer
interosseous wire
interpalpebral suture
Interpore osteointegrated implant

interrupted
    i. black silk suture
    i. chromic catgut suture
    i. chromic suture
    i. cotton suture
    i. far-near suture
    i. fine silk suture
    i. Lembert suture
    i. mattress suture
    i. near-far suture
    i. nylon suture
    i. plain catgut suture
    i. silk suture
    i. suture
    i. vertical mattress suture
Intersept cardiotomy reservoir
Interson biopsy needle guide
interspace
    i. shaper
    i. width marker
Interstate spatula
interstitial implant
Intertach pacemaker
intervener
    Love-Gruenwald i.
interventional catheter
intervertebral
    i. curette
    i. disk forceps
    i. disk rongeur
    i. disk rongeur forceps
    i. spreader
intestinal
    i. anastomosis clamp
    i. anastomosis forceps
    i. bag
    i. clamp
    i. closing forceps
    i. decompression trocar
    i. forceps
    i. holding forceps
    i. needle
    i. occlusion clamp
    i. occlusion retractor
    i. plication needle
    i. resection clamp
    i. ring clamp
    i. suture
    i. tissue forceps
    i. tissue-holding forceps
in-the-bag lens
in-the-ear (ITE)
    i.-t.-e. hearing aid

Intimax
- I. biliary catheter
- I. cholangiography catheter
- I. occlusion catheter
- I. vascular catheter

intra-aortic
- i.-a. balloon (IAB)
- i.-a. balloon assist device
- i.-a. balloon catheter
- i.-a. balloon pump (IABP)

IntraArc 9963 arthroscopic power system

intra-arterial
- i.-a. cannula
- i.-a. chemotherapy catheter

intracapsular
- i. lens expressor
- i. lens expressor hook
- i. lens forceps
- i. lens loop

intracardiac
- i. cannula
- i. catheter
- i. needle holder
- i. retractor
- i. sucker
- i. sucker connector
- i. sucker guard
- i. suction tube
- i. sump tube

Intracath catheter
intracervical bag
intracoronary
- i. guiding catheter
- i. perfusion catheter

intracranial
- i. pressure catheter
- i. pressure monitoring device
- i. pressure monitor screw

intracranial pressure (ICP)
intracuticular
- i. nylon suture
- i. suture

intradermal
- i. mattress suture
- i. suture

IntraDop intraoperative Doppler
Intraflex intramedullary pin extractor
intragastric balloon
intraligamentary syringe
intraluminal stapler (ILS)

intramedallary illuminator
intramedullary (IM)
- i. alignment rod
- i. bar
- i. broach
- i. brush
- i. canal plug
- i. device
- i. drill
- i. fixation device
- i. guide
- i. pin
- i. reamer
- i. Rush rod

intramedullary/extramedullary (IM/EM)
intranasal
- i. bivalve splint
- i. hammer

Intran disposable intrauterine pressure measurement catheter
intraocular
- i. balloon
- i. cannula
- i. forceps
- i. hook
- i. irrigating forceps
- i. lens (IOL)
- i. lens cannula
- i. lens forceps
- i. lens glide

Intraoptics intraocular lens
intraoral stent
intraorbital implant
intrascapular roll
Intrasil catheter
IntraSite gel wound dressing
intrathoracic forceps
intrauterine
- i. cannula
- i. catheter
- i. contraceptive device (IUCD)
- i. device (IUD)
- i. insemination catheter (IUI)
- i. pessary
- i. pressure catheter

intravascular ultrasound (IVUS)
intravenous (IV)
- i. accurate control (IVAC)
- i. catheter

i. needle
i. pacing catheter
intraventricular pressure monitoring catheter
intravitreal
i. cryoprobe
i. laser
Intrepid
I. balloon catheter
I. percutaneous transluminal coronary angioplasty catheter
I. PTCA catheter
introducer
ACS percutaneous i.
Allen eye i.
Allen sphere i.
Angestat hemostasis i.
Angetear tear-away i.
Cardak percutaneous catheter i.
Carter eye sphere i.
Carter sphere i.
i. catheter
catheter i.
Cook micropuncture i.
Desilets-Hoffman i.
Desilets-Hoffman micropunch i.
Desilets-Hoffman pacemaker i.
Dumon-Gilliard prosthesis i.
Encapsulon sheath i.
endolymphatic shunt tube i.
Eric Lloyd i.
Goodhill strut i.
Hall self-holding i.
Hedwig i.
H-H shunt i.
Holter i.
House endolymphatic shunt tube i.
Maryfield i.
Morgan vent tube i.
Neuroguide peel-away catheter i.
peel-away i.
Pennine-O'Neil urinary catheter i.
Ramses diaphragm i.
Razi cannula i.
Richardson polyethylene tube i.

Speck i.
sphere i.
Storz vent tube i.
Tuohy-Borst side-arm i.
UMI transseptal Cath-Seal catheter i.
Uni-Shunt with reservoir i.
USCI i.
ventricular catheter i.
Wellwood-Ferguson i.
introducing forceps
intubation laryngoscope
invaginator
Lempert i.
inverted
i. cone bur
i. knot suture
i. suture
inverter
Barrett appendix i.
Damian i.
Mayo-Boldt i.
Wangensteen tissue i.
inverting suture
Ioban
I. antimicrobial incise drape
I. drape
I. Steri-drape
iodine
i. catgut suture
i. cup
iodized surgical gut suture
iodochromic catgut suture
iodophor Steri-drape
Iogel intraocular lens
iohexol contrast material
IOL
intraocular lens
IOL dialer
IOLAB
I. Azar intraocular lens
I. intraocular lens
I. lens
Ionescu-Shiley
I.-S. aortic valve prosthesis
I.-S. heart valve
I.-S. pericardial patch
I.-S. pericardial valve graft
I.-S. pericardial xenograft
Ionguard titanium modular head component
ion laser
Iopamidol contrast material

Ioprep scrub soap
Ioptex intraocular lens
Iowa
    I. eye implant
    I. forceps
    I. implant
    I. implant material
    I. membrane forceps
    I. membrane-puncturing
      forceps
    I. orbital implant
    I. pudendal needle guide
    I. State fixation forceps
    I. State forceps
    I. total hip prosthesis
    I. trumpet
    I. trumpet needle guide
    I. trumpet pudendal needle
      guide
    I. University elevator
    I. University periosteal
      elevator
Iowa-Mengert membrane forceps
IPAS
    IPAS flexible cannula
    IPAS syringe
IPOP
  immediate postoperative
    prosthesis
    IPOP cast dressing
IPPB
  intermittent positive pressure
    breathing
Irby head frame
Irene lens
iridium
    i. implant
    i. prosthesis
    i. wire implant
iridium-192 loaded stent
iridocapsular intraocular lens
iridocapsulotomy scissors
iris
    i. bipolar forceps
    i. claw lens
    i. clip intraocular lens
    i. disposable retractor
    i. expressor
    i. forceps
    i. hook
    i. knife
    i. knife-needle
    i. lens manipulator

    i. microforceps
    i. repositor
    i. retractor
    i. scissors
    i. spatula
    i. supported intraocular lens
    i. supported lens
    i. suture microforceps
    i. tissue forceps
    i. with Barraquer handle
      scissors
iron
  Lusskin subungual
    hematoma i.
Iron interne retractor
irrigating
    i. and aspirating (I&A)
    i. and aspirating coaxial
      cannula
    i. cannula
    i. catheter
    i. curette
    i. cystitome
    i. dialer
    i. Dilaprobe
    i. iris hook
    i. lens loupe
    i. lens manipulator
    i. mushroom retractor
    i. notched spatula
    i. probe
    i. sheath
    i. short sharp cystitome
    i. spatula
    i. tip
    i. uterine curette
    i. vectis
    i. vectis loop
irrigating-aspirating (I&A)
    i.-a. instrument
irrigating-positioning needle
irrigation
    i. and aspiration (I&A)
    i. catheter
  Colon-A-Sun colonic i.
    i. hook
irrigation-aspiration (I&A)
    i.-a. kit
    i.-a. system
irrigator
  anterior chamber i.
  antral i.
  Barraquer i.

Baumrucker clamp i.
Bishop-Harman anterior
  chamber i.
Carabelli i.
Dento-Spray oral i.
DeVilbiss eye i.
Doss automatic percolator i.
Dougherty anterior
  chamber i.
endoscopic i.
Fink i.
Fisch bone drill i.
Fluvog i.
Fox hydrostatic i.
Gibson anterior chamber i.
Goldstein anterior
  chamber i.
Gum Machine oral i.
Hollister colostomy i.
House i.
House-Radpour i.
House-Radpour suction i.
House-Stevenson i.
House-Stevenson suction i.
House sucker i.
House T-tube i.
Kelman i.
Kemp i.
Lukens double-channel i.
McKenna Tide-Ur-Ator i.
Moncrieff anterior
  chamber i.
nasal i.
Perio Pik i.
Perry ostomy i.
Pro Pulse i.
Radpour i.
Radpour-House i.
Radpour-House suction i.
Rollett anterior chamber i.
Shambaugh i.
Shea i.
sinus i.
Sterling-Sylva i.
suction i.
Sylva anterior chamber i.
Thornwald i.
Thornwald antral i.
Water Pik i.
Wells i.
Younge i.
irrigator-aspirator
  Fluvog i.-a.

Irrigo syringe
Irvine scissors
Isaacs endometrial cell sampler
Isberg scleral plug
ischial
  i. brace
  i. weightbearing brace
  i. weightbearing leg brace
Ishihara color test
isoelastic pelvic prosthesis
isolation
  i. face mask
  i. forceps
isolator
  Vickers i.
Isosal syringe
Isotac pilot wire
isotopic pulse generator pacemaker
Israel
  I. blunt rake retractor
  I. dissector
  I. nasal rasp
  I. rake retractor
  I. rasp
  I. retractor
  I. suction suction tube
  I. tongue depressor
  I. tonsillar dissector
Itard
  I. catheter
  I. eustachian catheter
ITD-FG dental diamond
  instrument
ITE
  in-the-ear
I-tech
  I.-t. cannula
  I.-t. cannula holder
  I.-t. cannula tray
  I.-t. intraocular foreign body
    forceps
  I.-t. needle holder
  I.-t. splinter forceps
  I.-t. tying forceps
I-tech-Castroviejo bladebreaker
IUCD
  intrauterine contraceptive device
IUD
  intrauterine device
    IUD remover hook
IUI
  intrauterine insemination
  catheter

IV
    intravenous
      IV catheter
      IV needle
IVAC
    intravenous accurate control
      IVAC ventilator
Ivalon
      I. dressing
      I. eye implant
      I. graft
      I. implant
      I. prosthesis
      I. sponge
      I. sponge eye implant
      I. suture
Ivan
      I. laryngeal applicator
      I. nasopharyngeal applicator

IVC
    inferior vena cava
Medi-Tech IVC filter
IVD rongeur
Iverson dermabrader
Ives
      I. anoscope
      I. rectal speculum
Ives-Fansler anoscope
Ivinsco cervical dilator
Ivocryl resin
IVT percutaneous catheter introducer sheath
IVUS
    intravascular ultrasound
Ivy
      I. mastoid rongeur
      I. needle holder
Iwashi clamp approximator

Jabaley scissors
Jaboulay button
jacket
    body j.
    Bonchek-Shiley cardiac j.
    Calot j.
    cuirass j.
    Kydex body j.
    Minerva back j.
    Minerva plastic j.
    Orthoplast j.
    plaster-of-Paris j.
    radix Raney j.
    Raney j.
    Risser wedging j.
    Royalite body j.
    Sayre j.
    Von Lackum transection
      shift j.
    Willock j.
    Willock respiratory j.
    Wilmington j.
jacket-type chest dressing
Jackson
    J. alligator forceps
    J. alligator grasping forceps
    J. anterior commissure
      laryngoscope
    J. approximation forceps
    J. aspirating tube
    J. biopsy forceps
    J. bite block
    J. bone-extension clamp
    J. bone-holding clamp
    J. bougie
    J. broad-blade staple forceps
    J. bronchial dilator
    J. button forceps
    J. clamp
    J. cone-shaped tracheal tube
    J. costophrenic
      bronchoscope
    J. cross-action forceps
    J. cup round-punch forceps
    J. cylindrical-object forceps
    J. dilator
    J. double-concave rat-tooth
      forceps
    J. double-ended retractor
    J. double-prong forceps

    J. down-jaw forceps
    J. dull-pointed forceps
    J. endoscopic forceps
    J. esophageal dilator
    J. esophageal scissors
    J. esophageal shears
    J. esophagoscope
    J. fenestrated meat forceps
    J. fenestrated peanut-
      grasping forceps
    J. fiberoptic slide
      laryngoscope
    J. filiform bougie
    J. forceps
    J. forward-grasping forceps
    J. full-lumen bronchoscope
    J. full-lumen esophagoscope
    J. goiter retractor
    J. head-holding forceps
    J. hemostat
    J. hemostatic forceps
    J. hollow-object forceps
    J. infant biopsy forceps
    J. infant forceps
    J. lacrimal intubation set
    J. laryngeal applicator
    J. laryngeal applicator
      forceps
    J. laryngeal atomizer
    J. laryngeal basket forceps
    J. laryngeal-dressing forceps
    J. laryngeal forceps
    J. laryngeal-grasping forceps
    J. laryngeal punch forceps
    J. laryngeal ring-rotation
      forceps
    J. laryngeal scissors
    J. laryngectomy tube
    J. laryngofissure forceps
    J. laryngoscope
    J. laryngostat
    J. magnification ruler set
    J. open-end aspirating tube
    J. papilloma forceps
    J. perichondrial elevator
    J. probe
    J. punch
    J. punch forceps
    J. radiopaque bougie
    J. retractor

Jackson *(continued)*
  J. right-angle retractor
  J. ring-jaw forceps
  J. ring-rotation forceps
  J. rongeur
  J. rotation forceps
  J. scalpel
  J. self-retaining goiter
    retractor
  J. sharp-pointed forceps
  J. side-curved forceps
  J. silver tracheostomy tube
  J. sister-hook forceps
  J. sliding laryngoscope
  J. spinal surgery table
  J. sponge carrier
  J. square punch tip
  J. square-specimen forceps
  J. standard bronchoscope
  J. standard laryngoscope
  J. staple bronchoscope
  J. tenaculum
  J. tendon forceps
  J. tracheal bistoury
  J. tracheal bistoury knife
  J. tracheal bougie
  J. tracheal dilator
  J. tracheal forceps
  J. tracheal hemostat
  J. tracheal hemostatic
    forceps
  J. tracheal hook
  J. tracheal retractor
  J. tracheal scalpel
  J. tracheal tenaculum
  J. tracheal tube
  J. tracheoscope
  J. tracheotomic bistoury
  J. triangular-punch forceps
  J. tunneler
  J. turbinate scissors
  J. vaginal retractor
  J. vaginal speculum
  J. velvet-eye aspirating tube
  J. velvet-eye tube
  J. warning stop tube
Jackson-Moore shears
Jackson-Mosher
  J.-M. cardiospasm dilator
  J.-M. dilator
Jackson-Plummer dilator

Jackson-Pratt
  J.-P. bifurcated drain
    extension
  J.-P. catheter
  J.-P. dissector
  J.-P. drain
  J.-P. flat drain kit
  J.-P. hysterectomy kit
  J.-P. large-volume round
    silicone drain kit
  J.-P. large-volume suction
    reservoir
  J.-P. PVC kit
  J.-P. round PVC drain
  J.-P. silicone flat drain
  J.-P. silicone hubless flat
    drain
  J.-P. silicone round drain
  J.-P. suction drain
  J.-P. suction tube
  J.-P. T-tube drain
Jackson-Rees endotracheal tube
Jackson-Trousseau dilator
Jacob
  J. clamp
  J. forceps
  J. tenaculum
  J. uterine tenaculum
  J. uterine vulsellum forceps
  J. vulsellum
  J. vulsellum forceps
  J. vulsellum uterine
    tenaculum
Jacobaeus thoracoscope
Jacobaeus-Unverricht thoracoscope
Jacobs
  J. biopsy forceps
  J. chuck adapter
  J. chuck drill
  J. clamp
  J. snap-lock chuck
  J. tenaculum
  J. vulsellum
Jacobson
  J. bayonet-shaped scissors
  J. bipolar forceps
  J. bladder retractor
  J. blood vessel probe
  J. blunt hook
  J. bulldog clamp
  J. clamp
  J. counter-pressure elevator
  J. curette

J. dressing forceps
J. endarterectomy spatula
J. forceps
J. fork
J. goiter retractor
J. hemostatic forceps
J. holder
J. microbulldog clamp
J. microdressing forceps
J. microscissors
J. modified vessel clamp
J. mosquito forceps
J. needle holder
J. probe
J. retractor
J. scissors
J. spring-handled needle holder
J. spring-handled scissors
J. suture pusher
J. vas deferens probe
J. vessel clamp
J. vessel knife
J. vessel punch
J. Vital needle holder

Jacobson-Potts
    J.-P. clamp
    J.-P. vessel clamp
Jacobs-Palmer laparoscope
Jacob-Swan gonioscopic prism
Jacobus mammotone
Jacques gastric tube
Jade Audio-Starr hearing aid
Jaeger
    J. keratome
    J. keratome knife
    J. lid plate
    J. lid plate retractor
    J. lid retractor
    J. retractor
Jaeger-Whiteley catheter
Jaffe
    J. eyelid speculum
    J. iris hook
    J. lens-manipulating hook
    J. lens spatula
    J. lid retractor
    J. lid speculum
    J. micro-iris hook
    J. microlens hook
    J. needle holder
    J. one-piece all-PMMA intraocular lens

J. spatula
J. suturing forceps
J. wire lid retractor
Jaffe-Bechert nucleus rotator
Jaffe-Givner lid retractor
Jaffe-Maltzman
    J.-M. hook
    J.-M. lens manipulator
Jager meniscal forceps
Jahnke anastomosis clamp
Jahnke-Cook-Seeley clamp
Jako
    J. clamp
    J. facial nerve monitor
    J. fine ball-tip hook
    J. forceps
    J. knot pusher
    J. laryngeal forceps
    J. laryngeal knife
    J. laryngeal mirror
    J. laryngeal needle holder
    J. laryngeal probe
    J. laryngeal suction tube
    J. laryngoscope
    J. laser aspirating tube
    J. laser retractor
    J. laser trocar
    J. microlaryngeal cup forceps
    J. microlaryngeal forceps
    J. microlaryngeal grasping forceps
    J. microlaryngeal scissors
    J. microlaryngoscope
    J. probe
    J. suction-irrigator
    J. suction tube
    J. transilluminator
Jako-Cherry laryngoscope
Jako-Kleinsasser
    J.-K. ball-tip hook
    J.-K. knife
    J.-K. microforceps
    J.-K. microscissors
Jako-Pilling laryngoscope
Jalaguier-Reverdin needle
Jamar dynamometer
James
    J. lumbar peritoneal catheter
    J. wound approximation forceps

Jameson
J. calipers
J. eye calipers
J. forceps
J. hook
J. muscle clamp
J. muscle forceps
J. muscle hook
J. muscle recession forceps
J. needle
J. needle holder
J. recession forceps
J. scissors
J. strabismus forceps
J. strabismus hook
J. strabismus needle
J. tracheal muscle forceps
Jameson-Metzenbaum scissors
Jameson-Werber scissors
Jamshidi
J. biopsy needle
J. liver biopsy needle
J. needle
Jamshidi-Kormed bone marrow biopsy needle
Janes
J. fracture appliance
J. fracture frame
Janet bladder swab
Janeway gastroscope
Janko clamp
Jannetta
J. alligator grasping forceps
J. aneurysm neck dissector
J. angular elevator
J. angular knife
J. bayonet forceps
J. bayonet-shaped needle holder
J. bayonet-shaped scissors
J. dissector
J. double-pronged fork
J. duckbill elevator
J. forceps
J. hook
J. knife
J. microbayonet forceps
J. posterior fossa retractor
J. probe
J. retractor
J. right-angle hook
J. scissors

Jannetta-Kurze
J.-K. dissecting scissors
J.-K. scissors
Jansen
J. bayonet dressing forceps
J. bayonet ear forceps
J. bayonet forceps
J. bayonet nasal forceps
J. bayonet rongeur
J. bone curette
J. bone rongeur
J. clamp
J. curette
J. dissecting forceps
J. dressing forceps
J. ear forceps
J. forceps
J. mastoid raspatory
J. mastoid retractor
J. monopolar forceps
J. mouth gag
J. nasal-dressing forceps
J. periosteotome
J. retractor
J. scalp retractor
J. thumb forceps
Jansen-Cottle rongeur
Jansen-Gifford
J.-G. mastoid retractor
J.-G. retractor
Jansen-Gruenwald forceps
Jansen-Middleton
J.-M. forceps
J.-M. nasal-cutting forceps
J.-M. rongeur
J.-M. septal forceps
J.-M. septal punch
J.-M. septotomy forceps
J.-M. septum-cutting forceps
Jansen-Mueller forceps
Jansen-Newhart
J.-N. mastoid probe
J.-N. probe
Jansen-Sluder mouth gag
Jansen-Struyken
J.-S. forceps
J.-S. septal forceps
Jansen-Wagner
J.-W. mastoid retractor
J.-W. retractor
Jansen-Zaufel rongeur

Japanese
- J. Bruening anastigmatic aural magnifier
- J. Bruening magnifier

Japonicum laminaria

Jaquet apparatus

Jarcho
- J. cannula
- J. forceps
- J. self-retaining uterine cannula
- J. tenaculum
- J. tenaculum forceps
- J. tenaculum holder
- J. uterine cannula
- J. uterine tenaculum
- J. uterine tenaculum forceps

Jardine hook

Jardon eye shield

Jardon-Straith
- J.-S. chin implant
- J.-S. nasal implant

Jarit
- J. air injection cannula
- J. anterior resection clamp
- J. bipolar coagulator
- J. bladebreaker
- J. bone hook
- J. brain forceps
- J. cartilage clamp
- J. comedo extractor
- J. cross-action retractor
- J. dissecting scissors
- J. endarterectomy scissors
- J. finger goniometer
- J. flat-tip scissors
- J. forceps
- J. forceps holder
- J. hand surgery osteotome
- J. intestinal clamp
- J. lacrimal cannula
- J. lower lateral scissors
- J. mallet
- J. meniscal clamp
- J. microstitch scissors
- J. microsurgery scissors
- J. microsurgical needle holder
- J. microsuture tying forceps
- J. mosquito forceps
- J. palate hook
- J. periosteal elevator
- J. peripheral vascular scissors
- J. pin cutter
- J. plaster knife
- J. plaster shears
- J. renal sinus retractor
- J. reverse adenoid curette
- J. small bone-holding clamp
- J. spring wire retractor
- J. sterilizer forceps
- J. sternal needle holder
- J. stitch scissors
- J. tendon-pulling forceps
- J. three-prong cast spreader
- J. tube-occluding forceps
- J. tuning fork
- J. utility shears
- J. wire holder
- J. wire-pulling forceps

Jarit-Allis tissue forceps

Jarit-Crafoord forceps

Jarit-Dandy forceps

Jarit-Deaver retractor

Jarit-Graves vaginal speculum

Jarit-Kerrison rongeur

Jarit-Liston bone-cutting forceps

Jarit-Mason
- J.-M. cast breaker
- J.-M. pediatric cast breaker

Jarit-Pederson vaginal speculum

Jarit-Poole abdominal suction tube

Jarit-Ruskin rongeur

Jarit-Yankauer suction tube

Jarvis
- J. clamp
- J. forceps
- J. hemorrhoidal forceps
- J. pile clamp
- J. snare

Jasbee esophagoscope

Javal ophthalmometer

Javerts
- J. placental forceps
- J. polyp forceps

Javid
- J. bypass clamp
- J. bypass tube
- J. carotid artery bypass clamp
- J. carotid artery clamp
- J. carotid clamp
- J. carotid shunt
- J. catheter

Javid *(continued)*
  J. clamp
  J. shunt
jaw
  j. hook
  j. rongeur
  j. spreader
  j. spring clip
Jayles forceps
Jazbi
  J. dissector
  J. suction tonsillar dissector
  J. tonsillar dissector
JB-1 catheter
JB catheter
Jeager strabismus hook
Jeb graft
Jefferson
  J. retractor
  J. self-retaining retractor
Jehle coronary perfusion catheter
jejunostomy
  percutaneous endoscopic j.
    (PEJ)
Jelco
  J. catheter
  J. intravenous stylet
  J. needle
Jelenko
  J. arch bar
  J. bar
  J. facial fracture appliance
  J. pliers
  J. splint
jelly
  Argyle lubricating j.
  j. dressing
  electrode j.
  K-Y lubricating j.
  Lubrajel lubricating j.
Jelm
  J. catheter
  J. two-way catheter
Jena colposcope
Jena-Schiotz tonometer
Jenkins chisel
Jennings
  J. Loktite mouth gag
  J. mouth gag
Jennings-Skillern mouth gag
Jenning-Streifeneder gastroscope
Jenny mammary prosthesis

Jensen
  J. capsular polisher
  J. forceps
  J. intraocular lens forceps
  J. lens forceps
  J. lens-inserting forceps
Jensen-Thomas irrigating-aspirating cannula
Jentzer trephine
Jergensen reamer
Jergensen-Trinkle reamer
Jervey
  J. forceps
  J. iris forceps
Jesberg
  J. aspirating tube
  J. bronchoscope
  J. clamp
  J. esophagoscope
  J. forceps
  J. grasping forceps
  J. infant bronchoscope
  J. laryngectomy clamp
  J. oval esophagoscope
  J. upper esophagoscope
Jesco scissors
J.E. Sheehan chisel
Jet
  J. shield
  J. Vac cement dispenser
jet
  Injectoflex respirator j.
  Riwomat respirator j.
jeweler's
  j. bipolar forceps
  j. forceps
  j. pickup forceps
Jewett
  J. bar
  J. bone chip packer
  J. bone extractor
  J. brace
  J. double-angled osteotomy plate
  J. driver
  J. electrode
  J. fracture appliance
  J. frame
  J. hyperextension brace
  J. nail
  J. pick-up screw
  J. prosthesis
  J. slotted plate

J. socket reamer
J. urethral sound
J. uterine dilator
J. uterine sound
JFB III endoscope
J-guide wire
jig
    chamfer j.
Jimmy
    J. dislodger
    J. dissector
    J. John colonic irrigation
      system
Jinotti dual-purpose catheter
JL-4 catheter
JL-5 catheter
J-loop
    J-l. electrode
    J-l. intraocular lens
    J-l. posterior chamber
      intraocular lens
JMS injection needle
Joal lens
Jobert
    J. de Lamballe suture
    J. suture
Jobson-Horne
    J.-H. cotton applicator
    J.-H. probe
Jobson-Pynchon tongue depressor
Jobst
    J. dressing
    J. mammary support
      dressing
    J. postoperative air-boot
    J. prosthesis
Jobstens neurostimulator
Joe's hoe retractor
Johannsen lag screw
Johannsen-Stille lag screw
Johanson-Stille cystotomy trocar
John
    J. A. Tucker
      mediastinoscope
    J. Green calipers
    J. Green pendulum scalpel
Johns Hopkins
    J. H. bulldog clamp
    J. H. clamp
    J. H. coarctation clamp
    J. H. forceps
    J. H. gallbladder forceps

J. H. gallbladder retractor
J. H. gall duct forceps
J. H. hemostatic forceps
J. H. modified Potts clamp
J. H. occluding forceps
J. H. retractor
J. H. serrefine forceps
J. H. stone basket
Johnson
    J. basket
    J. brain tumor forceps
    J. canaliculus wire
    J. cheek retractor
    J. coagulation suction tube
    J. dental band
    J. erysiphake
    J. evisceration knife
    J. forceps
    J. gauze sponge
    J. hook
    J. hook retractor
    J. intestinal tube
    J. needle holder
    J. prostatic needle holder
    J. ptosis forceps
    J. ptosis knife
    J. retractor
    J. screwdriver
    J. skin hook
    J. spatula
    J. stone basket
    J. stone dislodger
    J. swab sampler
    J. thoracic forceps
    J. twin-wire appliance
    J. ureteral basket
    J. ureteral stone basket
    J. ventriculogram retractor
Johnson-Bell erysiphake
Johnson & Johnson
    J & J Band-Aid sterile
      drape
    J & J dressing
    J & J saliva ejector
    J & J tourniquet
Johnson-Kerrison punch
Johnson-Tooke corneal knife
Johnston
    J. clamp
    J. dilator
    J. gastrostomy plug
    J. infant dilator

joint
  CUI j.
  j. implant
Jo-Kath catheter
joker dissector
Jolly
  J. dilator
  J. uterine dilator
Jonas-Graves vaginal speculum
Jonas prosthesis
Jonathan Livingston Seagull patella prosthesis
Jonell
  J. countertraction finger splint
  J. thumb splint
Jones
  J. adenoid curette
  J. arm splint
  J. brace
  J. canaliculus dilator
  J. cervical knife
  J. clamp
  J. curette
  J. dilator
  J. dissecting scissors
  J. dressing
  J. forceps
  J. forearm splint
  J. hemostatic forceps
  J. IMA diamond knife
  J. IMA epicardial retractor
  J. IMA forceps
  J. IMA kit
  J. IMA needle holder
  J. IMA scissors
  J. lacrimal canaliculus dilator
  J. metacarpal splint
  J. nasal splint
  J. needle holder
  J. pin
  J. punctum dilator
  J. retractor
  J. suture
  J. tear duct tube
  J. thoracic clamp
  J. towel clamp
  J. towel forceps
Jonesco
  J. bone wire guide
  J. wire suture needle

Joplin
  J. bone-holding forceps
  J. forceps
  J. tendon passer
  J. tendon stripper
  J. toe prosthesis
Jordan
  J. bur
  J. canal elevator
  J. canal incision knife
  J. capsular knife
  J. dilator
  J. elevator
  J. eye implant
  J. hook
  J. implant
  J. middle ear instrument
  J. needle
  J. perforating bur
  J. stapedectomy knife
  J. strut forceps
  J. strut-measuring instrument
  J. wire loop dilator
Jordan-Caparosa holder
Jordan-Day
  J.-D. bur
  J.-D. cutting bur
  J.-D. dermatome
  J.-D. drill
  J.-D. fenestration bur
  J.-D. polishing bur
Jordan-Hermann chisel
Jordan-Rosen
  J.-R. curette
  J.-R. elevator
Jorgenson
  J. dissecting scissors
  J. gallbladder scissors
  J. retractor
  J. scissors
Joseph
  J. angular knife
  J. antral perforator
  J. bayonet saw
  J. bistoury knife
  J. button-end knife
  J. cervical knife
  J. chisel
  J. clamp
  J. double-edged knife
  J. guard
  J. hook

J. hook retractor
J. knife
J. measuring ruler
J. nasal brace
J. nasal elevator
J. nasal hook
J. nasal knife
J. nasal rasp
J. nasal saw
J. nasal splint
J. periosteal elevator
J. periosteal raspatory
J. periosteotome
J. punch
J. rasp
J. raspatory
J. saw
J. saw protector
J. scissors
J. septal bar
J. septal clamp
J. septal clamp facial
   fracture appliance
J. septal fracture appliance
J. septal frame
J. septal splint
J. sharp skin hook
J. skin hook
J. skin hook retractor
J. skin retractor
J. tenaculum hook
J. wound retractor
Joseph-Farrior saw
Joseph-Killian septal elevator
Joseph-Maltz
   J.-M. angular saw
   J.-M. knife
   J.-M. nasal saw
   J.-M. scissors
Josephson
   J. catheter
   J. quadpolar catheter
Joseph-Stille saw
Joseph-Verner
   J.-V. raspatory
   J.-V. saw
Jostra
   J. arterial blood filter
   J. cardiotomy reservoir
   J. catheter
Jousto dropfoot splint, skid
   orthosis
JR-4 catheter

JR-5 catheter
J-scope esophagoscope
J-shaped I&A cannula
Judd
   J. cannula
   J. clamp
   J. cystoscope
   J. forceps
   J. strabismus forceps
   J. suture forceps
   J. trocar
   J. urethroscope
Judd-Allis
   J.-A. clamp
   J.-A. forceps
   J.-A. intestinal forceps
   J.-A. intestinal retractor
   J.-A. tissue forceps
Judd-DeMartel
   J.-D. forceps
   J.-D. gallbladder forceps
Judd-Mason
   J.-M. bladder retractor
   J.-M. prostatic retractor
   J.-M. retractor
Judet
   J. dissector
   J. impactor for acetabular
      component
   J. impactor for acetabular
      cup
   J. prosthesis
   J. strut
Judkins
   J. catheter
   J. coronary catheter
   J. guiding catheter
   J. left coronary catheter
   J. right coronary catheter
   J. torque-control catheter
   J. USCI catheter
Judkins-4 guiding catheter
Juers
   J. crimper forceps
   J. curette
   J. ear curette
   J. forceps
   J. hook
   J. lingual forceps
   J. wire crimper
Juers-Derlacki
   J.-D. holder
   J.-D. Universal head holder

Juers-Lempert
  J.-L. endaural rongeur
  J.-L. forceps
  J.-L. rongeur
  J.-L. rongeur forceps
Juevenelle clamp
jugal suture
jugum forceps
Julian
  J. cystoresectoscope
  J. forceps
  J. needle holder
  J. splenorenal forceps
  J. thoracic artery forceps
  J. thoracic forceps
  J. thoracic hemostatic
    forceps
Julian-Damian
  J.-D. clamp
  J.-D. thoracic forceps

Julian-Fildes clamp
jumbo biopsy forceps
junctional pacemaker
Jung microtome knife
Junior Tompkins portable aspirator
Jurasz
  J. forceps
  J. laryngeal forceps
Jurgan pin
Jutte tube
Juzo hose
J-Vac
  J-V. bulb suction reservoir
  J-V. catheter
  J-V. closed wound drainage
    system
  J-V. drain

Kader
- K. fishhook needle
- K. gastrostomy
- K. intestinal spatula
- K. needle

Kadesky forceps
Kadir Hi-Torque guide wire
Kaessman handpiece
Kahler
- K. biopsy forceps
- K. bronchial biopsy forceps
- K. bronchial forceps
- K. bronchoscopic forceps
- K. bronchus-grasping forceps
- K. double-action tip
- K. laryngeal biopsy forceps
- K. laryngeal forceps
- K. polyp forceps

Kahn
- K. cannula
- K. dilator
- K. forceps
- K. scissors
- K. tenaculum forceps
- K. traction tenaculum
- K. trigger cannula
- K. uterine cannula
- K. uterine dilator
- K. uterine trigger cannula
- K. uterine trigger cannula extension tip

Kahn-Graves vaginal speculum
Kahostat wound dressing
Kalamarides dural retractor
Kal-Dermic suture
Kalinowski
- K. ear speculum
- K. perforator
- K. rasp

Kalinowski-Verner
- K.-V. ear speculum
- K.-V. rasp

Kalk
- K. electrode
- K. esophagoscope
- K. palpitation probe

Kall modification of Silverman needle
Kallmorgen vaginal spatula

Kalman
- K. forceps
- K. needle holder
- K. occluding forceps
- K. tube-occluding forceps

Kalos pacemaker
Kalt
- K. capsule forceps
- K. corneal needle
- K. eye needle
- K. eye needle holder
- K. eye spoon
- K. forceps
- K. needle
- K. needle holder
- K. suture
- K. vein needle
- K. Vital needle holder

Kalt-Arruga needle holder
Kamerling one-piece all-PMMA intraocular lens
Kaminsky
- K. catheter
- K. stent

Kanavel
- K. brain-exploring cannula
- K. cannula
- K. cock-up splint
- K. conductor
- K. exploring cannula

Kanavel-Senn retractor
Kane
- K. clamp
- K. obstetrical clamp
- K. umbilical clamp
- K. umbilical cord clamp

kangaroo tendon suture
Kansas
- K. City band truss
- K. University corneal forceps

Kantor
- K. circumcision clamp
- K. clamp
- K. forceps

Kantor-Berci laryngoscope
Kantrowitz
- K. clamp
- K. dressing forceps
- K. forceps

Kantrowitz *(continued)*
   K. hemostatic clamp
   K. pacemaker
   K. thoracic clamp
   K. thoracic forceps
   K. tissue forceps
Kaplan
   K. needle
   K. resectoscope
   K. tracheostomy needle
Kapp
   K. applying forceps
   K. clamp
   K. clip
   K. forceps
   K. micro-arterial clamp
   K. microclamp
Kapp-Beck
   K.-B. bronchial clamp
   K.-B. clamp
   K.-B. coarctation clamp
   K.-B. colon clamp
   K.-B. forceps
Kapp-Beck-Thomson clamp
Kaps operating microscope
Kara
   K. cataract-aspirating
      cannula
   K. cataract needle
   K. erysiphake
   K. needle
Karamar-Mailatt tarsorrhaphy
   clamp
Karaya
   K. adhesive appliance
   K. dressing
   K. electrode
   K. ring ileostomy appliance
   K. seal ileostomy appliance
   K. seal ileostomy stomal
      bag
Karickhoff
   K. keratoscope
   K. laser lens
Karl
   K. Storz Calcutript
   K. Storz coagulator
   K. Storz flexible
      ureteropyeloscope
Karmen catheter
Karmody vascular spring retractor
Karolinska-Stille punch

Karp
   K. aortic punch
   K. aortic punch forceps
Karras
   K. angiography needle
   K. needle
Kartchner carotid artery clamp
Kartchner carotid clamp
Kartch pigtail probe
Karwetsky U-bow activator
Kashiwabara laryngeal mirror
Kaslow
   K. gastrointestinal tube
   K. tube
Katena
   K. blade
   K. ring
   K. spatula
Katon catheter
Katsch chisel
Katzeff cartilage scissors
Katzen
   K. balloon catheter
   K. wire
Katzenstein rectal cannula
Katzin-Barraquer
   K.-B. Colibri forceps
   K.-B. corneal forceps
   K.-B. forceps
Katzin corneal transplant scissors
Katzin-Long balloon
Katzin-Troutman scissors
Kaufer type II retractor
Kaufman
   K. adapter
   K. catheter
   K. clamp
   K. ENT forceps
   K. eye vitrector
   K. forceps
   K. hemostat clip applier
   K. III anti-incontinence
      prosthesis
   K. II vitrector
   K. incontinence device
   K. insulated forceps
   K. insulated monopolar
      forceps
   K. kidney clamp
   K. male urinary
      incontinence prosthesis
Kay
   K. aortic anastomosis clamp

K. aortic clamp
K. balloon
K. clamp
Kay-Cross suction tip suction tube
Kaye
K. fine-dissecting scissors
K. scissors
Kay-Lambert clamp
Kay-Shiley
K.-S. disk valve prosthesis
K.-S. heart valve
Kay-Suzuki
K.-S. heart valve
K.-S. prosthesis
Kazanjian
K. action-type osteotome
K. bar
K. bone-cutting forceps
K. button
K. cutting forceps
K. forceps
K. guide
K. nasal-cutting forceps
K. nasal forceps
K. nasal hump-cutting
forceps
K. nasal hump forceps
K. nasal splint
K. T-bar
K. tooth button
Kazanjian-Cottle forceps
Kazanjian-Goldman rongeur
KBM
KBM absorbent gauze
KBM cotton ball
KBM gauze swab
**KDF-2.3 intrauterine insemination
catheter**
K dissector sponge
Kean-M-4 occluder
Kearns
K. bag catheter
K. bladder dilator
K. dilator
Kebab graft
KED
Kendrick extrication device
Keeler
K. camera
K. cryophake
K. cryosurgical instrument
K. lamp
K. microscissors

K. ophthalmoscope
K. panoramic surgical
telescope
K. pantoscope
K. prosthesis
K. Pulsair noncontact
tonometer
K. spotlight lens loupe
K. wide-angle lens loupe
Keeley vein stripper
keel stent
keeper
line k.
Nelson line k.
Keer aneurysm clip
Kees clip applier
Kehr
K. gallbladder tube
K. T-tube
Keisler lacrimal cannula
Keisley suture
Keith
K. abdominal needle
K. drain
K. needle
Keithley clamp kit
Keitzer infant urethrotome
Keizer
K. eye retractor
K. lid retractor
K. retractor
Keizer-Lancaster eye speculum
Keller-Blake leg splint
Keller cephalometric device
Kelling gastroscope
Kellman-Elschnig spatula
Kellogg tongue depressor
Kelly
K. abdominal retractor
K. adenotome
K. arterial forceps
K. clamp
K. curette
K. cystoscope
K. dilator
K. direct vision adenotome
K. dressing forceps
K. endoscope
K. fistular scissors
K. forceps
K. hemostat
K. hemostatic forceps
K. hose clamp

Kelly *(continued)*
- K. inflatable T-tube
- K. insufflator
- K. intestinal needle
- K. needle
- K. orifice dilator
- K. ovum forceps
- K. placental forceps
- K. plication suture
- K. polypus forceps
- K. proctoscope
- K. punch
- K. rectal speculum
- K. retractor
- K. scissors
- K. sigmoidoscope
- K. sphincter dilator
- K. sphincteroscope
- K. suture
- K. tissue forceps
- K. tube
- K. urethral forceps
- K. uterine dilator
- K. uterine scissors
- K. uterine tenaculum hook
- K. vulsellum

Kelly-Descemet membrane punch
Kelly-Gray
- K.-G. curette
- K.-G. uterine curette
- K.-G. uterine forceps

Kelly-Kennedy suture
Kelly-Murphy
- K.-M. forceps
- K.-M. hemostatic forceps
- K.-M. hemostatic uterine vulsellum forceps

Kelly-Rankin forceps
Kelly-Sims
- K.-S. retractor
- K.-S. vaginal retractor

Kelly-Wick vascular tunneler
Kelman
- K. air cystotome
- K. aspirator
- K. cannula
- K. Cry-O-Cadet
- K. cyclodialysis cannula
- K. cystotome
- K. cystotome knife
- K. dipstick
- K. double-bladed cystotome
- K. forceps

- K. hook
- K. II three-point fixation rigid tripod intraocular lens
- K. implantation forceps
- K. intraocular forceps
- K. iris retractor
- K. irrigation hook
- K. irrigator
- K. irrigator forceps
- K. knife cannula cystotome
- K. knife cystotome
- K. manipulator hook
- K. modern flexible tripod intraocular lens
- K. Multiflex intraocular lens
- K. needle
- K. Omnifit intraocular lens
- K. Omnifit lens
- K. phacoemulsifier
- K. Quadraflex intraocular lens
- K. retractor
- K. S-flex intraocular lens

Kelman-McPherson
- K.-M. corneal forceps
- K.-M. forceps
- K.-M. microtying forceps
- K.-M. suture forceps
- K.-M. tissue forceps
- K.-M. tying forceps

Kel retractor
Kelsey
- K. clamp
- K. pile clamp

Kelsey-Fry bone awl
Kelvin pacemaker
Kemp irrigator
Ken
- K. driver
- K. Drive sleeve
- K. nail
- K. screwdriver
- K. sliding nail

Kendrick extrication device (KED)
Kennedy
- K. bar
- K. forceps
- K. ligament augmentation device
- K. uterine vulsellum forceps
- K. vulsellum forceps

**Kennedy-Cornwell bladder
  evacuator**
Kennerdell
  K. bayonet forceps
  K. medial orbital retractor
  K. muscle hook
  K. nerve hook
  K. spatula
Kennerdell-Maroon
  K.-M. dissector
  K.-M. duckbill elevator
  K.-M. elevator
  K.-M. hook
  K.-M. orbital retractor
  K.-M. probe
Kennerdell-Maroon-Jameson hook
Kensey atherectomy catheter
Kent forceps
Kenwood
  K. finger cot
  K. laparotomy sponge
Keolar implant material
Keragen implant
keratome
  Agnew k.
  Atkinson k.
  Beaver k.
  Berens k.
  k. blade
  Castro-Martinez k.
  Castroviejo k.
  Castroviejo angled k.
  Czermak k.
  Daily k.
  Fink-Rowland k.
  Fuchs k.
  Grieshaber k.
  Jaeger k.
  Kirby k.
  Kirby-Duredge k.
  Lancaster k.
  Landolt k.
  Lichtenberg k.
  Martinez-Castro k.
  McCaslin wave-edge k.
  McReynolds-Castroviejo k.
  McReynolds pterygium k.
  Rowland k.
  Storz-Duredge k.
  Thomas k.
  Wiener k.
keratometer
  Autoref k.

Canon automatic k.
Humphrey automatic k.
k. lens
Marco k.
Storz k.
surgical k.
Terry k.
keratoplasty scissors
keratoprosthesis
keratoscope
  Karickhoff k.
  Klein self-luminous k.
keratotomy forceps
Kerlix
  K. bandage
  K. conforming bandage
    dressing
  K. dressing
  K. laparotomy sponge
Kern
  K. bone clamp
  K. bone-holding clamp
  K. bone-holding forceps
  K. clamp
  K. forceps
  K. miniforceps
**Kernan-Jackson coagluating
  bronchoscope**
Kerner dental mirror
Kern-Lane bone-holding forceps
Kerpel bone curette
Kerr
  K. abduction splint
  K. clip
  K. clip applier
  K. drill
  K. electro-torque drill
  K. hand drill
Kerrison
  K. cervical rongeur
  K. forceps
  K. laminectomy punch
  K. lumbar rongeur
  K. mastoid rongeur
  K. punch
  K. retractor
  K. rongeur
  K. rongeur forceps
Kerrison-Costen rongeur
Kerrison-Ferris Smith rongeur
Kerrison-Jacoby punch
Kerrison-Morgenstein rongeur
Kerrison-Rhoton sellar punch

Kerrison-Schwartz rongeur
Kerrison-Spurling rongeur
Kersting colostomy clamp
Kesilar cannula
Kesling tooth-spacing spring
Kessel osteotomy plate
Kessler
    K. podiatry rasp
    K. prosthesis
    K. suture
Kestler ambulatory head tractor
Kestrel disinfector
Ketac liner
Kevorkian
    K. biopsy forceps
    K. curette
    K. endocervical curette
    K. endometrial curette
    K. endometrial uterine
    curette
    K. forceps
    K. uterine biopsy forceps
Kevorkian-Younge
    K.-Y. biopsy curette
    K.-Y. biopsy forceps
    K.-Y. cervical biopsy
    forceps
    K.-Y. curette
    K.-Y. endocervical biopsy
    curette
    K.-Y. forceps
    K.-Y. uterine applicator
    K.-Y. uterine biopsy forceps
    K.-Y. uterine curette
Key
    K. elevator
    K. periosteal elevator
key
    Allen-type hex k.
keyed supracondylar plate
Keyes
    K. biopsy punch
    K. bone-splitting chisel
    K. chisel
    K. cutaneous biopsy punch
    K. cutaneous punch
    K. cutaneous trephine
    K. dermal punch
    K. lithotrite
    K. punch
    K. skin punch
    K. splitting chisel
Keyes-Ultzmann-Luer cannula

Keymed
    K. dilator
    K. esophageal tube
    K. fiberoptic scope
Keys-Briston type spline
Keys-Kirschner traction bow
Keystone splint
keyway
    OEC lag screw component
    with k.
Kezerian
    K. chisel
    K. curette
    K. gouge
    K. osteotome
K-Gar
    K-G. clamp
    K-G. umbilical clamp
Khodadad
    K. clamp
    K. clip
    K. forceps
    K. microclamp
    K. microclip
    K. microclip forceps
Khosia cautery
Kidd
    K. cystoscope
    K. instrument rack
    K. trocar
    K. U-tube
Kidde
    K. nebulizer
    K. tourniquet
    K. tourniquet cuff
    K. tubal insufflator
    K. uterine cannula
Kidde-Robbins tourniquet
kidney
    k. clamp
    Duo-Klex artificial k.
    Elmar artificial k.
    k. forceps
    k. internal splint catheter
    k. internal stent catheter
    k. needle
    k. pedicle clamp
    k. pedicle forceps
    k. retractor
    k. stone forceps
    k. suturing needle
kidney-elevating forceps
kidney internal splint/stent (KISS)

Kido suprapubic trocar
Kiefer clamp
Kiel graft
Kielland (*var. of* Kjelland)
Kiene bone tamp
Kifa
  K. catheter
  K. clip
  K. green, grey, red, yellow
    catheter
Killearn rongeur
Killey molar retractor
Killian
  K. antral cannula
  K. apparatus
  K. cannula
  K. chisel
  K. cutting forceps tip
  K. dissector
  K. double-articulated forceps
    tip
  K. forceps
  K. frontal sinus chisel
  K. gouge
  K. laryngeal spatula
  K. nasal cannula
  K. nasal speculum
  K. probe
  K. rectal speculum
  K. septal compression
    forceps
  K. septal elevator
  K. septal forceps
  K. septal speculum
  K. suspension apparatus
  K. suspension gallows
  K. suspension gallows
    apparatus
  K. tonsillar knife
  K. tube
Killian-Claus chisel
Killian-Eichen cannula
Killian-Halle nasal speculum
Killian-Jameson forceps
Killian-King
  K.-K. goiter retractor
  K.-K. retractor
Killian-Lynch
Killian-Reinhard chisel
Kilner
  K. chisel
  K. elevator
  K. goiter hook

  K. malar lever
  K. mouth gag
  K. nasal retractor
  K. needle holder
  K. retractor
  K. retrograde chisel
  K. sharp hook
  K. skin hook
  K. skin hook retractor
  K. skin wound retractor
  K. suture carrier
Kilner-Dott mouth gag
Kilpatrick retractor
Kimball
  K. catheter
  K. nephrostomy hook
Kimberley diamond instrument
Kimpton vein spreader
**Kim-Ray Greenfield vena cava
  filter**
Kimura platinum spatula
KinAir bed
Kincaid right-angle hook
Kindt
  K. arterial clamp
  K. carotid artery clamp
  K. carotid clamp
  K. clamp
Kinematic
  K. facebow
  K. II condylar and
    stabilizer total knee system
  K. II rotating-hinge knee
    system
  K. II total knee prosthesis
  K. rotating-hinge total knee
**Kinemax modular condylar and
  stabilizer total knee system**
Kinemetric guide system
kinetic
  k. continuous passive
    motion device
  k. CPM device
King
  K. adenoidal punch
  K. brace
  K. cardiac bioptome
  K. catheter
  K. cervical brace
  K. connector adapter
  K. corneal trephine
  K. goiter retractor

409

King *(continued)*
  K. goiter self-retaining
    retractor
  K. guiding catheter
  K. implant
  K. multipurpose catheter
  K. multipurpose coronary
    graft catheter
  K. needle
  K. orbital implant
  K. retractor
  K. suture needle
  K. tissue forceps
King-Hurd
  K.-H. dissector
  K.-H. retractor
  K.-H. tonsillar dissector
King-Prince
  K.-P. forceps
  K.-P. recession forceps
Kingsley
  K. forceps
  K. grasping forceps
  K. orthodontic plate
kink-resistant
  k.-r. catheter
  k.-r. peritoneal catheter
Kinsella
  K. elevator
  K. periosteal elevator
Kinsella-Buie
  K.-B. clamp
  K.-B. lung clamp
KIP laser
Kirby
  K. cataract knife
  K. corneoscleral forceps
  K. curved zonular separator
  K. cylindrical zonular
    separator
  K. double-ball separator
  K. double-curve lens loupe
  K. double-fixation hook
  K. expressor
  K. eye tissue forceps
  K. fixation forceps
  K. flat zonular separator
  K. forceps
  K. hook expressor
  K. intracapsular lens
    expressor
  K. intracapsular lens
    expressor hook

  K. intracapsular lens
    expressor with cylindrical
    separator
  K. intracapsular lens
    expressor with double-ball
    separator
  K. intracapsular lens
    expressor with flat
    separator
  K. intracapsular lens forceps
  K. intracapsular lens loop
  K. intracapsular lens loupe
  K. intracapsular separator
    lens expressor with curved
    zonular separator
  K. iris forceps
  K. iris spatula
  K. keratome
  K. lens expressor
  K. lens forceps
  K. lens spoon
  K. lid retractor
  K. muscle hook
  K. retractor
  K. separator
  K. suture
  K. tissue forceps
Kirby-Arthus fixation forceps
Kirby-Bracken iris forceps
Kirby-Duredge
  K.-D. keratome
  K.-D. knife
Kirchner
  K. retractor
  K. wire
Kirk
  K. bone hammer
  K. mallet
  K. orthopaedic mallet
Kirkheim-Storz urethrotome
Kirkland
  K. curette
  K. periodontal pack
  K. retractor
Kirklin
  K. atrial retractor
  K. sternal awl
Kirkpatrick
  K. forceps
  K. tonsillar forceps
Kirmisson
  K. elevator
  K. periosteal elevator

K. periosteal raspatory
K. raspatory
K. respirator
Kirschner
K. abdominal retractor
K. apparatus
K. bone drill
K. boring wire
K. extension bow
K. femoral canal plug
K. guiding probe
K. II-C shoulder system
K. suture
K. total shoulder prosthesis
K. traction apparatus
K. Universal self-centering
captive-head bipolar
component
K. wire
K. wire cutter
K. wire drill
K. wire pin
K. wire traction bow
K. wire tractor
**Kirschner-Balfour abdominal
retractor**
Kirschner-Ullrich forceps
Kirwan
K. bipolar coagulator
K. coaptation ophthalmic
bipolar forceps
K. cranioblade
K. iris curved ophthalmic
bipolar forceps
K. iris straight ophthalmic
bipolar forceps
K. jeweler's curved
ophthalmic bipolar forceps
K. jeweler's insulated
straight ophthalmic bipolar
forceps
K. Nadler-style coaptation
ophthalmic bipolar forceps
**Kirwan-Adson ophthalmic bipolar
forceps**
**Kirwan-Tenzel ophthalmic bipolar
forceps**
Kishi lens
Kish urethral catheter
KISS
kidney internal splint/stent
KISS catheter
kissing balloon

Kistner
K. button
K. dissector
K. plastic tracheostomy
tube
K. probe

kit
Adjust-A-Flow colostomy
irrigation k.
aneuroplastic k.
ankle traction k.
Arrow pneumothorax k.
biopsy k.
Biosearch jejunostomy k.
Bookwalter rectal k.
Bookwalter small incision k.
Brimms Quik-Fix denture
repair k.
brush biopsy k.
Budde halo blade k.
Burnett Pap smear k.
CAPIS k.
Cartmill feeding tube k.
Castaneda k.
Ceramco porcelain k.
cervical traction k.
clip gun tray k.
Cloward anterior fusion k.
Cloward PLIF II k.
Cloward posterior lumbar
interbody fusion k.
Codman disposable ICP k.
Codman IMA k.
contour defect molding k.
corner k.
cranioplastic k.
Crystar porcelain k.
CTS Relief k.
Dentifix denture repair k.
Diethrich k.
Diethrich coronary artery
bypass k.
Dover midstream urine
collection k.
drain flat k.
Dynacor enema cleansing k.
Enemette enema
cleansing k.
E-Series micro-infertility k.
Etch-Master k.
Fresenius Euro-Collins k.

kit *(continued)*

Gill ureteral brush biopsy k.
Glove-n-Gel amniotomy k.
Halifax interlaminar clamp k.
Heyer-Schulte PVC k.
Heyer-Schulte silicone k.
hysterectomy k.
I&A k.
insitu valve-cutter k.
irrigation-aspiration k.
Jackson-Pratt flat drain k.
Jackson-Pratt hysterectomy k.
Jackson-Pratt large-volume round silicone drain k.
Jackson-Pratt PVC k.
Jones IMA k.
Keithley clamp k.
Ko-Lec-Pac urinary collection k.
Leather in-situ valve-cutter k.
Lister suture removal k.
Malis brain retractor k.
Marlen biliary drainage k.
microvascular STA-MCA k.
neonatal internal jugular puncture k.
neurological k.
Osteoloc endodontic stabilization k.
Pap smear k.
parallel pin k.
percutaneous catheter introducer k.
Perry Noz-Stop k.
Preci-Vertix k.
Rosenberg meniscal repair k.
Shofu porcelain stain k.
shunt k.
Starlite endodontic implant starter k.
Straith nasal splint k.
support k.
thermodilution catheter introducer k.
tuboplasty surgical k.
UMI amniocentesis k.
ureteral brush biopsy k.
Wood colonic k.
Wound-Evac k.
Xomed sinus irrigation k.

Kitchen

K. postpartum gauze packer
K. postpartum packer

Kitner

K. blunt dissecting instrument
K. blunt dissector
K. clamp
K. dissecting scissors
K. dissector
K. forceps
K. goiter forceps
K. retractor
K. thyroid-packing forceps

Kiwisch bandage

Kjelland, Kielland

K. blade
K. forceps
K. obstetrical forceps

Kjelland-Barton forceps

Kjelland-Luikart

K.-L. forceps
K.-L. obstetrical forceps

Klaar headlight

Klaff septal speculum

Klammt elastic open activator

Klapp tendon hook

Klatskin

K. biopsy needle
K. liver biopsy needle
K. needle

Klauber

K. band setter
K. pusher-burnisher

Klause antral punch

Klause-Carmody antral punch

Klebanoff

K. bougie
K. common duct sound
K. gallstone scoop

Kleegman

K. cannula
K. dilator

KleenSpec

K. disposable anoscope
K. disposable laryngoscope
K. disposable speculum
K. disposable vaginal speculum
K. fiberoptic disposable sigmoidoscope

K. forceps
K. laryngoscope
K. otoscope adapter
K. sigmoidoscope
Kleer base plate
Kleesattel
K. elevator
K. raspatory
Klein
K. self-luminous keratoscope
K. ventilation tube
Kleinert-Kutz
K.-K. bone-cutting forceps
K.-K. bone file
K.-K. bone rongeur
K.-K. clamp
K.-K. clamp approximator
K.-K. cutter
K.-K. dissector
K.-K. elevator
K.-K. hook
K.-K. hook retractor
K.-K. microclip
K.-K. rongeur
K.-K. rongeur forceps
K.-K. skin hook
K.-K. tendon-passing forceps
K.-K. tendon retriever
K.-K. tendon retriever
  forceps
Kleinert-Ragnell retractor
Kleinert suture
Kleinsasser
K. anterior commissure
  laryngoscope
K. hook
K. knife
K. laryngoscope
K. lens loupe
K. microlaryngeal scissors
K. operating laryngoscope
K. probe
K. retractor
Kleinsasser-Riecker laryngoscope
Kleinschmidt appendectomy clamp
Klemme
K. appendectomy retractor
K. dural hook
K. gasserian ganglion
  retractor
K. laminectomy retractor
K. retractor

Klenzak
K. brace
K. double-upright splint
Kleppinger
K. bipolar forceps
K. forceps
Klevas clamp
KLI
KLI bipolar forceps
KLI forceps
KLI insufflator
KLI laprocator laparoscope
KLI monopolar forceps
Klima-Rosegger sternal needle
Kliners alar retractor
Kling
K. adhesive dressing
K. bandage
K. cervical brace
K. conform dressing
K. dressing
K. gauze bandage
K. gauze dressing
Klinikum-Berlin tubing clamp
Klinkenbergh-Loth scissors
Klintskog amniotomy hook
Klondike bed
Kloti cutter
Klutch denture adhesive
Klute clamp
KM-1 breast pump
KM-3A
KM-3A liner
KM-3A shell
KM-4
KM-4 liner
KM-4 shell
KMC hip system
KMP fenestrated femoral stem
KMW hip system
Knapp
K. blade
K. cataract knife
K. cataract spoon
K. cyclodialysis spatula
K. cystitome
K. eye speculum
K. forceps
K. hook
K. iris hook
K. iris knife
K. iris knife-needle
K. iris probe

Knapp *(continued)*
K. iris repositor
K. iris scissors
K. iris spatula
K. knife-needle
K. lacrimal retractor
K. lacrimal sac retractor
K. lens scoop
K. lens spoon
K. needle
K. probe
K. retractor
K. speculum
K. strabismus scissors
K. trachoma forceps
Knapp-Culler speculum
Knapp-Luer trachoma forceps
knee
k. brace splint
k. immobilizer splint
Kinematic rotating-hinge
total k.
Miller-Galante
unicompartmental k.
PCA modular total k.
PCA revision total k.
PCA unicompartmental k.
k. retractor
k. splint
Stanmore total k.
variable axis k.
knife
Abraham tonsillar k.
Adson dural k.
Adson sharp k.
Agnew canaliculus k.
Alcon ophthalmic k.
Aleman meniscotomy k.
Alexander otoplasty k.
Allen-Barkan k.
Allen-Hanbury k.
amputation k.
angular k.
A-OK crescent k.
A-OK ophthalmic k.
A-OK phacoemulsification
slit k.
arachnoid k.
Arenberg endolymphatic
sac k.
Arthro-Lok k.
arthroscopy k.
Atkins tonsillar k.

Austin dental k.
Austin dissection k.
Austin sickle k.
Auth k.
Ayre cone k.
Ayre-Scott cervical cone k.
Backhaus cervical k.
Bailey-Glover-O'Neil
commissurotomy k.
Bailey-Morse mitral k.
Bailey round k.
Ballenger cartilage k.
Ballenger mucosal k.
Ballenger nasal k.
Ballenger septal k.
Ballenger swivel k.
Bard-Parker k.
Barkan goniotomy k.
Barker Vacu-tome
suction k.
Baron k.
Baron ear k.
Barraquer corneal k.
Barrett uterine k.
bayonet k.
Beard lid k.
Beaver ear k.
Beaver goniotomy needle k.
Beaver tonsillar k.
Beck tonsillar k.
Beer cataract k.
Bellucci k.
Bellucci lancet k.
Berens iris k.
Berens sclerotomy k.
Bickle microsurgical k.
bistoury k.
k. blade
Blair-Brown skin graft k.
Blair cleft palate k.
Blake gingivectomy k.
Bock k.
Bodenham-Blair skin
graft k.
Bodenham-Humby skin
graft k.
Bodian discission k.
Bonta mastectomy k.
Bosher commissurotomy k.
Braithwaite skin graft k.
Brock mitral valve k.
Brock pulmonary valve k.
Brophy bistoury k.

Brophy cleft palate k.
Brown-Blair skin graft k.
Brown cleft palate k.
Buck ear k.
Buck myringotomy k.
Bucy cordotomy k.
Burford-Lebsche sternal k.
button-end k.
Caltagirone skin graft k.
Canad meniscal k.
canal k.
canaliculus k.
Canfield tonsillar k.
k. cannula cystitome
capsule k.
Carter septal k.
cartilage k.
Castroviejo ophthalmic k.
Castroviejo-Wheeler
  discission k.
cataract k.
Catlin amputing k.
Cave cartilage k.
cervical cone k.
circle k.
Cobbett skin graft k.
cold k.
cold coning k.
Collings k.
Collins k.
Colver tonsillar k.
Concept arthroscopic k.
Converse k.
Converse nasal k.
cordotomy k.
corneal k.
cornea-splitting k.
Cornman dissecting k.
Cottle k.
Cottle double-edged k.
Cottle nasal k.
Crescent plaster k.
Crile k.
Crile cleft palate k.
Crile ganglion k.
Crile gasserian ganglion k.
Cronin palate k.
Crosby k.
Culbertson canal k.
Curdy schlerotome k.
Cushing dural hook k.
k. cystotome
Davidoff cordotomy k.

Daviel chalazion k.
Davis k.
Day tonsillar k.
Dean capsulotomy k.
Dean tonsillar k.
DeLee laparotrachelotomy k.
Dench ear k.
DePalma k.
Derlacki capsular k.
Dermot-Pierce ball-tipped k.
Derra commissurotomy k.
Derra guillotine k.
D'Errico laminar k.
Desmarres iris k.
Desmarres paracentesis k.
Deutschman cataract k.
Devonshire k.
diamond k.
Dintenfass-Chapman k.
Dintenfass ear k.
discission k.
dissection k.
k. dissector
double-edged k.
double-edged sickle k.
double-ended flap k.
Douglas tonsillar k.
Downing cartilage k.
drum elevator k.
Dupuytren k.
Duredge Paufique k.
ear k.
ear furuncle k.
k. electrode
Elschnig cataract k.
Elschnig pterygium k.
Equen-Neuffer laryngeal k.
Esmarch plaster k.
eye k.
facial nerve k.
Farrior-McHugh ear k.
Farrior otoplasty k.
Farrior septal cartilage
  stripper k.
Farrior sickle k.
Farrior triangular k.
feather k.
Ferris Robb tonsillar k.
Fine-Gill corneal k.
Fisher k.
Fisher tonsillar k.
flap k.
Fletcher tonsillar k.

knife *(continued)*
Foerster capsulotomy k.
Fomon k.
Fomon double-edge k.
Fowler-Zollner k.
Frazier cordotomy k.
Frazier pituitary
  capsulectomy k.
Freer-Ingal nasal k.
Freer-Ingal submucous k.
Freer nasal k.
Freer septal k.
Freer submucous k.
Frieberg cartilage k.
Friesner ear k.
Gandhi k.
Gerzog ear k.
Gerzog-Ralks k.
Gill corneal k.
Gill iris k.
Gillquist-Oretorp-Stille k.
gingivectomy k.
Glasscock-House k.
Goldman guillotine nerve k.
goniotomy k.
Goodhill k.
Goodhill-Down k.
Goodyear tonsillar k.
Graefe cataract k.
Graefe cystitome k.
Graefe iris k.
Graf cervical cordotomy k.
Green cataract k.
Grieshaber k.
Groff electrosurgical k.
Guilford-Wright
  crurotomy k.
Guilford-Wright double-
  edged k.
Guilford-Wright elevator k.
Guilford-Wright elevator
  flap k.
Guilford-Wright flap k.
Guilford-Wright
  incudostapedial k.
Guilford-Wright roller k.
Guy tenotomy k.
Haab after-cataract k.
Haab needle k.
Halle dural k.
Halle trigeminus k.
k. handle
Harrison k.

Harrison capsular k.
Harrison myringoplasty k.
Harris tonsillar k.
Herbert sclerotomy k.
Hilsinger tonsillar k.
Hoffmann-Osher-Hopkins
  plaster k.
Horsley dural k.
Hosemann choledochus k.
Hough k.
Hough fascial k.
Hough incision k.
Hough-Rosen k.
Hough whirlybird k.
House k.
House ear k.
House incudostapedial
  joint k.
House lancet k.
House myringoplasty k.
House myringotomy k.
House-Rosen k.
House sickle k.
House tympanoplasty k.
Hufnagel
  commissurotomy k.
Humby k.
Hundley knee k.
Hymes scleral k.
incision k.
incudostapedial k.
incudostapedial joint k.
iris k.
Jackson tracheal bistoury k.
Jacobson vessel k.
Jaeger keratome k.
Jako-Kleinsasser k.
Jako laryngeal k.
Jannetta k.
Jannetta angular k.
Jarit plaster k.
Johnson evisceration k.
Johnson ptosis k.
Johnson-Tooke corneal k.
Jones cervical k.
Jones IMA diamond k.
Jordan canal incision k.
Jordan capsular k.
Jordan stapedectomy k.
Joseph k.
Joseph angular k.
Joseph bistoury k.
Joseph button-end k.

Joseph cervical k.
Joseph double-edged k.
Joseph-Maltz k.
Joseph nasal k.
Jung microtome k.
Kelman cystotome k.
Killian tonsillar k.
Kirby cataract k.
Kirby-Duredge k.
Kleinsasser k.
Knapp cataract k.
Knapp iris k.
Korte plaster k.
Kreissl meatotomy k.
Krull acetabular k.
Kyle crypt k.
Ladd k.
Lancaster k.
Lance k.
lancet k.
Lange blade k.
Lange cartilage k.
Langenbeck flap k.
Lang eye k.
Lanigan cartilage k.
laryngeal k.
Lebsche sternal k.
Lee cartilage k.
Lee Cohen k.
Leksell gamma k.
Leland-Jones tonsillar k.
Leland tonsillar k.
Lempert k.
ligamentum teres k.
Lillie tonsillar k.
Lindvall meniscectomy k.
Lindvall-Stille meniscal k.
Lipschiff k.
Liston amputating k.
Lothrop tonsillar k.
Lowe-Breck cartilage k.
Lowell glaucoma k.
Lowe microtome k.
Lucae ear perforation k.
Lundsgaard-Burch k.
Lynch k.
Lynch obtuse-angle
  laryngeal k.
Lynch right-angle k.
Lynch straight k.
Lynch tonsillar k.
MacCallum k.
Machemer scleral k.

MacKenty cleft palate k.
Magielski bayonet canal k.
Maltz button-end k.
Maltz cartilage k.
Mandelbaum ear k.
Marcks k.
margin-finishing k.
Martinez corneal
  dissector k.
Maumenee k.
Maumenee goniotomy k.
Mayo k.
McCabe canal k.
McGee tympanoplasty k.
McHugh facial nerve k.
McHugh-Farrior canal k.
McHugh flap k.
McKeever cartilage k.
McMurray tenotomy k.
McPherson-Wheeler eye k.
McPherson-Ziegler micro-
  iris k.
McReynolds-Castroviejo
  pterygium k.
McReynolds pterygium k.
Mead lancet k.
meniscal k.
meniscectomy k.
Mercer cartilage k.
Metzenbaum septal k.
Meyer k.
Meyhöffer k.
Meyhöffer eye k.
Micra k.
micro-iris k.
micrometer k.
microsurgical k.
Millette tonsillar k.
Millette-Tyding k.
Miltex ligature k.
Mitchell cartilage k.
Moncorps k.
Moorehead ear k.
Morgenstein periosteal k.
Moritz-Schmidt k.
Murphy plaster k.
myringoplasty k.
myringotomy k.
nasal k.
Neff meniscal k.
Neivert tonsillar k.
Newman uterine k.
Niche k.

knife *(continued)*
Niedner commissurotomy k.
Nordent periodontic k.
Nunez-Nunez mitral
   stenosis k.
Olivecrona trigeminal k.
Olk membrane peeler k.
Oretorp retractable k.
orthopaedic k.
Osher diamond k.
Osher micrometer
   cataract k.
Pace hysterectomy k.
Page tonsillar k.
Paparella canal k.
Paparella elevator k.
Paparella-House k.
Paparella incudostapedial k.
Paparella incudostapedial
   joint k.
Paparella sickle k.
paracentesis k.
Parker serrated discission k.
Parker tenotomy k.
Paton corneal k.
Paufique corneal k.
Paufique Duredge k.
Paufique graft k.
pick k.
plaster k.
Politzer angular ear k.
Politzer ear k.
Politzer-Ralks k.
Pope rectal k.
Potter modified k.
Potter sickle k.
Potts expansile k.
pterygium k.
pull knife k.
radial keratotomy k.
Ralks reversible k.
Rayport dural k.
Reese ptosis k.
Rehne skin graft k.
Reiner k.
Reiner plaster k.
retrograde k.
Rica trigeminal k.
Ridlon plaster k.
right-angle k.
Rish cartilage k.
Rizzuti-Spizziri k.
Rizzuti-Spizziri cannula k.

Rizzuti stitch-removal k.
Robb tonsillar k.
Robertson tonsillar k.
Robinson flap k.
Rochester mitral stenosis k.
Roger septal k.
roller k.
Rosen cartilage k.
Rosen ear incision k.
Rosen incision k.
round k.
round ruby k.
Royce bayonet ear k.
Royce ear k.
ruby k.
Ryerson tenotome k.
Salenius meniscal k.
sapphire k.
Sarot k.
Sato corneal k.
scarifier k.
Scheer elevator k.
Scheie goniopuncture k.
Scheie goniotomy k.
Scholl meniscal k.
Schuknecht roller k.
Schuknecht sickle k.
Schultze ambryotomy k.
Schwartz cordotomy k.
Seiler tonsillar k.
Sellor mitral valve k.
semilunar cartilage k.
septal k.
serrated fine-cutting k.
Sexton ear k.
Shaffer modification of
   Barkan k.
Shambaugh k.
Shambaugh-Lempert k.
sharp k.
Shea k.
Shea incision k.
Sheehy canal k.
Sheehy-House k.
Sheehy myringotomy k.
Sheehy round k.
Sichel iris k.
sickle k.
Silver k.
Silverstein micro-utility k.
Silverstein round k.
Silverstein sickle k.
Simon fistula k.

Simons cleft palate k.
Sluder k.
SMIC sternal k.
Smillie k.
Smillie cartilage k.
Smillie meniscal k.
Smith cataract k.
Smith cordotomy k.
Smith-Fisher cataract k.
Smith-Green cataract k.
Smith-Green eye k.
Speed-Sprague k.
Spizziri k.
Spizziri cannula k.
k. spud
stapedectomy k.
Stecher arachnoid k.
sternal k.
Stewart cartilage k.
stiletto k.
Stiwer furuncle k.
Storz k.
Storz-Duredge cataract k.
Storz folding-handle ear k.
Storz sheath-handle ear k.
straight k.
Strayer meniscal k.
Stryker-School meniscal k.
Suker spatula k.
Swan k.
Swan spade-type needle k.
swivel k.
Sword k.
Tabb double-ended flap k.
Tabb ear k.
Tabb flap k.
Tabb myringoplasty k.
Tabb pick k.
Taylor k.
tendon k.
terres k.
testing drum k.
thermal k.
Thiersch skin graft k.
Thornton T-incision
  diamond k.
Tobold laryngeal k.
Toennis dural k.
tonsillar k.
Tooke k.
Tooke angled k.
Tooke corneal k.
Tooke cornea-splitting k.

Tooke iris k.
Torchia corneal k.
trifacet k.
trigeminal k.
triple-edge diamond-blade k.
Troutman corneal k.
Troutman-Tooke corneal k.
Tubby tenotomy k.
Tweedy canaliculus k.
twin k.
Tydings tonsillar k.
Ullrich fistular k.
Ullrich uterine k.
unitome k.
Vacu-tome k.
Vannas abscess k.
Vaughan abscess k.
vessel k.
Vic hair transplant k.
Vic Vallis running hair k.
Virchow brain k.
Virchow cartilage k.
Virchow skin graft k.
V-lance eye k.
Wagner k.
Walb k.
Walton ear k.
Watson skin graft k.
Weber k.
Weber canaliculus k.
Weber iris k.
Webster skin graft k.
Weck k.
Weiss-pattern k.
Wheeler k.
Wheeler discission k.
Wheeler iris k.
Wilder cystitome k.
Williams cartilage k.
Woodruff spatula k.
Wright-Guilford double-
  edged k.
Wright-Guilford elevator k.
Wright-Guilford elevator-
  flap k.
Wright-Guilford flap k.
Wright-Guilford
  incudostapedial k.
Wright-Guilford roller k.
Wullstein double-edged k.
X-Acto utility k.
Yamanda k.
Yasargil arachnoid k.

knife *(continued)*
    Yund k.
    Yund ligamentum teres k.
    Ziegler iris k.
knife-needle
    Girard-Swan knife-needle
    Knapp iris knife-needle
    McCaslin knife-needle
    Ziegler knife-needle
    Ziegler iris knife-needle
knife-pick
    Tabb k.-p.
Knight
    K. biopsy needle
    K. brace
    K. forceps
    K. nasal-cutting forceps
    K. nasal forceps
    K. nasal scissors
    K. nasal septum-cutting forceps
    K. needle
    K. polyp forceps
    K. septal forceps
    K. septum-cutting forceps
    K. Sluder nasal forceps
    K. turbinate forceps
Knighton
    K. hemilaminectomy self-retaining retractor
    K. retractor
Knighton-Crawford forceps
Knighton-Kerrison punch
Knight-Sluder forceps
knitted
    k. graft
    k. prosthesis
    k. Teflon prosthesis
    k. vascular prosthesis
Knoche tube
Knodt distraction rod
Knolle
    K. anterior chamber irrigating cannula
    K. cannula
    K. capsular polisher
    K. capsular scraper
    K. capsular scratcher
    K. dipstick
    K. lens cortex spatula
    K. lens gauge
    K. lens implantation forceps
    K. lens nucleus spatula
    K. lens spatula
    K. micro-iris hook
    K. needle holder
    K. polisher
    K. scraper
Knolle-Kelman
    K.-K. cannulated cystitome
    K.-K. sharp cystitome
Knolle-Pearce
    K.-P. cannula
    K.-P. irrigating lens loop
    K.-P. lens loop
    K.-P. vectis
Knolle-Shepard lens forceps
Knolle-Volker lens-holding forceps
Knolls irrigating cannula
knot-holding forceps
knot tier
knot-tying instrument
Knowles
    K. bandage scissors
    K. hip pin
    K. pin
    K. pin nail
knuckle-bender splint
Knutsson
    K. penile clamp
    K. urethrography clamp
Koagamin dressing
Kobak needle
Kobayashi vacuum extractor
Kocher
    K. arterial forceps
    K. bladder retractor
    K. bladder spatula
    K. blade retractor
    K. bone retractor
    K. brain spoon
    K. bronchocele sound
    K. clamp
    K. depressor
    K. dissector
    K. elevator
    K. forceps
    K. gallbladder retractor
    K. goiter director
    K. goiter dissector
    K. goiter self-retaining retractor
    K. grooved director
    K. hemostat
    K. hemostatic forceps
    K. intestinal clamp

K. intestinal forceps
K. kidney-elevating forceps
K. Micro-Line intestinal forceps
K. needle
K. periosteal dissector
K. periosteal elevator
K. probe
K. raspatory
K. retractor
K. spatula
Kocher-Crotti
K.-C. goiter retractor
K.-C. goiter self-retaining retractor
K.-C. retractor
Kocher-Langenbeck retractor
Kocher-Ochsner
K.-O. forceps
K.-O. hemostatic forceps
Kocher-Wagner retractor
Koch-Julian sphincterotome
Koch-Mason dressing
Kodel sling
Kodex drill
Koeberlé forceps
Koenig
K. elevator
K. graft
K. grooved director
K. probe
K. raspatory
K. retractor
K. tonsillar swab
K. vascular forceps
K. vein retractor
Koenig-Stille scissors
Koeppe
K. diagnostic lens
K. gonioscopic lens
K. gonioscopic lens implant
K. intraocular lens implant
K. lamp
Koerte
K. gallstone forceps
K. retractor
Koffler
K. forceps
K. septal bone forceps
K. septal forceps
Koffler-Hajek
K.-H. laminectomy rongeur
K.-H. sphenoidal punch

Koffler-Lillie
K.-L. forceps
K.-L. septal forceps
Kogan
K. endocervical speculum
K. endospeculum
K. endospeculum forceps
K. endospeculum speculum
K. speculum
K. urethra speculum
Kohlman
K. dilator
K. urethral dilator
Kohn needle
Kokowicz raspatory
Kolb
K. bronchial forceps
K. forceps
K. trocar
Ko-Lec-Pac urinary collection kit
Koln clip
Kolobow membrane lung
Kolodny
K. clamp
K. forceps
Konan microscope
Koneg retractor
Kontack temporary crown
Kontron
K. balloon
K. intra-aortic balloon
K. intra-aortic balloon pump
Koontz
K. hernia needle
K. needle
Kopan needle
Kopetzky
K. bur
K. sinus bur
Kormed
K. disposable liver biopsy needle
K. needle
K. peritoneal lavage tray
Korotkoff
K. sound
K. soundgraph
Korte
K. abdominal spatula
K. gallstone forceps
K. plaster knife
K. retractor

Korte-Wagner retractor
Korth ureterotome
Kos
- K. attic cannula
- K. cannula
- K. chisel
- K. crimper forceps
- K. curette
- K. ear suction tube
- K. elevator
- K. middle ear instrument
- K. pick

Koslowski
- K. hip nail
- K. microforceps

Kowa
- K. angiographic camera
- K. camera
- K. fundus camera
- K. hand camera
- K. Optimed camera
- K. portable slit lamp
- K. retinal camera

Koylon foam rubber dressing
Kozlinski retractor
Kozlowski tube
K-37 pediatric arterial blood filter
K-Pratt dilator
Krackow HTO blade staple
Kraff
- K. capsular polisher
- K. intraocular utility forceps
- K. lens-inserting forceps
- K. nucleus lens loop
- K. suturing forceps
- K. tying forceps

Kraff-Osher lens forceps
Kraff-Utrata intraocular utility forceps
Kramer
- K. direct-vision telescope
- K. ear speculum
- K. forceps
- K. operating laryngoscope
- K. telescope

Krasky retractor
Kratz
- K. angled cystitome
- K. capsular scraper
- K. capsular scratcher
- K. cystitome
- K. implant

- K. iris push-pull hook
- K. lens
- K. lens-inserting forceps
- K. modified J-loop intraocular lens
- K. polisher
- K. posterior chamber intraocular lens
- K. scraper
- K. scratcher

Kratz-Barraquer
- K.-B. speculum
- K.-B. wire eye speculum

Kratz-Johnson modified J-loop intraocular lens
Kratz-Sinskey intraocular lens implant
Krause
- K. angular oval punch
- K. antral trocar
- K. biopsy forceps
- K. cannula
- K. ear polyp snare
- K. ear snare
- K. esophagoscopy forceps
- K. forceps
- K. laryngeal snare
- K. nasal polyp snare
- K. nasal snare
- K. nasal snare cannula
- K. nasal snare wire carrier
- K. oval punch tip
- K. punch forceps
- K. punch forceps tip
- K. square-basket tip
- K. through-cutting forceps tip
- K. transverse suture
- K. Universal forceps

Krause-Davis spatula
Krause-Wolfe
- K.-W. graft
- K.-W. implant
- K.-W. prosthesis

Krayenbuehl
- K. dural hook
- K. hook
- K. nerve hook
- K. twist hook

Krayenbuhl hook
K reamer
Krego elevator

Kreischer
    K. bone chisel
    K. chisel
Kreissl meatotomy knife
Kremer
    K. fixation forceps
    K. triple-optical zone
       corneal marker
Krentz
    K. gastroscope
    K. photogastroscope h
Kretschmer retractor
Kreuscher
    K. scissors
    K. semilunar cartilage
       scissors
Kreutzmann
    K. cannula
    K. trocar
Krieger wide-field fundus lens
Krinsky-Prince accommodation
   ruler
Kristeller
    K. retractor
    K. vaginal retractor
    K. vaginal speculum
Kristiansen eyelet lag screw
Krol esophageal dilator
Krol-Koski tracheal dilator
Kron
    K. bile duct dilator
    K. dilator
    K. gallbladder dilator
    K. gall duct dilator
    K. gall duct probe
    K. probe
Kronecker
    K. aneurysm needle
    K. needle
Kronendonk pin
Kroner apparatus
Kronfeld
    K. electrode
    K. eyelid retractor
    K. forceps
    K. micropin forceps
    K. pin
    K. retractor
    K. surface electrode
    K. suturing forceps
Krönlein
Krönlein-Berke retractor
Krönlein hemostatic forceps

K root canal file
Krosnick vesicourethral suspension
   clamp
Krull acetabular knife
Krumeich steriscope
Krwawicz cataract cryosurgical
   instrument
Kry-Med 300 probe
Kryptok
    K. bifocal lens implant
    K. bifocals lens
krypton laser
K/S-Allis forceps
KSK articulator
KSO brace
KTK laminaria tent
KTP
    KTP argon video laser
    KTP laser
    KTP 532 laser
KTP/532 surgical laser system
KTP/YAG surgical laser system
Kudo elbow component
Kuglen
    K. angled lens manipulator
    K. hook
    K. iris hook
    K. lens manipulator
    K. manipulating hook
    K. retractor
    K. straight lens manipulator
Kuhlman
    K. brace
    K. cervical brace
Kuhne coverglass forceps
Kuhn endotracheal tube
Kuhnt
    K. capsular forceps
    K. fixation forceps
    K. forceps
    K. gouge
Kulvin-Kalt
    K.-K. forceps
    K.-K. iris forceps
    K.-K. mules
Kummel intestinal spatula
Küntscher
    K. cloverleaf nail
    K. driver
    K. extractor
    K. intramedullary nail
    K. nail
    K. nail driver

Küntscher *(continued)*
- K. pin
- K. reamer
- K. rod
- K. traction apparatus

Küntscher-Hudson brace

Kurlander orthopaedic wrench

Kurosaka screw

Kurtin
- K. handpiece
- K. planing dermabrasion brush
- K. vein stripper
- K. wire brush

Kurze
- K. dissecting scissors
- K. dissector
- K. forceps
- K. microbiopsy forceps
- K. micrograsping forceps
- K. micro-instrument with scissors tip
- K. microscissors
- K. pickup forceps
- K. suction-irrigator
- K. suction tube

Kurz pulsation orthodontic headgear

Kushner-Tandatnick
- K.-T. curette
- K.-T. endometrial biopsy curette

Küstner
- K. suture
- K. tenaculum
- K. uterine tenaculum forceps

Kuttner
- K. dissector
- K. wound stretcher

Kutzmann clamp

Kwapis
- K. interdental forceps
- K. ligature carrier
- K. subcondylar retractor

Kwik wax

K-wire driver

Kwitko
- K. conjunctival spreader
- K. lens spatula

K-Y
- K-Y lubricating jelly
- K-Y pliers

Kydex
- K. body jacket
- K. brace

Kyle
- K. applicator
- K. crypt knife
- K. nasal speculum

Kypher suture

labial bar
laboratory handle
Laborde
    L. dilator
    L. forceps
    L. tracheal dilator
labyrinth curette
LaCarrere
    L. electrode
    L. electrodiaphake
lace suture
Lacey
    L. prosthesis
    L. rotating hinge
    L. total knee implant
lachrymal (*var. of* lacrimal)
lacidem suture
Lack tongue retractor
Lacor tube
lacrimal, lachrymal
    l. apparatus
    l. canaliculus dilator
    l. cannula
    l. chisel
    l. dilator
    l. duct probe
    l. needle
    l. probe
    l. retractor
    l. sac retractor
    l. sound
    l. stent
lacrimoconchal suture
lacrimoethmoidal suture
lacrimomaxillary suture
lacrimoturbinal suture
Lactina breast pump
Lactomer copolymer absorbable
  stapler
LAD
    ligament augmentation device
Ladd
    L. band
    L. calipers
    L. clamp
    L. elevator
    L. intracranial pressure
    monitor
    L. knife

    L. lid clamp
    L. raspatory
LaForce
    L. adenotome
    L. adenotome blade
    L. golf-club knife spud
    L. hemostatic tonsillectome
    L. knife "golf-club" spud
    L. spud
LaForce-Grieshaber adenotome
LaForce-Stevenson adenotome
LaForce-Storz adenotome
Lagleyze needle
Lagrange
    L. scissors
    L. sclerectomy scissors
Lagrange-Letoumel hip prosthesis
lag screw
Lahey
    L. arterial forceps
    L. bag
    L. bronchus clamp
    L. Carb-Edge scissors
    L. carrier
    L. catheter
    L. clamp
    L. Clinic dural hook
    L. Clinic nerve root
    retractor
    L. Clinic retractor
    L. Clinic skull trephine
    L. Clinic spinal fusion
    gouge
    L. Clinic thin osteotome
    L. delicate scissors
    L. dissecting forceps
    L. drain
    L. dural hook
    L. forceps
    L. gall duct forceps
    L. goiter retractor
    L. goiter-seizing forceps
    L. goiter tenaculum
    L. goiter vulsellum forceps
    L. hemostat
    L. hemostatic forceps
    L. ligature carrier
    L. ligature passer
    L. lock arterial forceps
    L. needle

Lahey *(continued)*
- L. operating scissors
- L. retractor
- L. scissors
- L. suture
- L. tenaculum forceps
- L. thoracic
- L. thoracic clamp
- L. thoracic forceps
- L. thyroid retractor
- L. thyroid tenaculum forceps
- L. thyroid tissue traction forceps
- L. thyroid traction forceps
- L. thyroid traction vulsellum forceps
- L. traction forceps
- L. Y-tube tube

Lahey-Babcock forceps
Lahey-Péan forceps
Lahey-Sweet dissecting forceps
Laidley double-catheterizing cystoscope
Laing
- L. concentric hip cup
- L. cup
- L. hip cup prosthesis
- L. osteotomy plate

Laird spatula
Lajeune hemostatic forceps
Lakatos Teflon injector
Lakeside
- L. cotton roll
- L. nasal scissors

Lalonde tendon approximator
Lamb cannula
Lambda
- L. Omni Stanicor pacemaker
- L. pacemaker

lambdoid suture
Lambert
- L. aortic clamp
- L. chalazion forceps
- L. forceps

Lambert-Berry rib raspatory
Lambert-Kay
- L.-K. anastomosis forceps
- L.-K. aortic clamp
- L.-K. clamp
- L.-K. vascular clamp

Lambert-Lowman
- L.-L. bone clamp
- L.-L. clamp

Lambotte
- L. bone chisel
- L. bone-holding clamp
- L. bone-holding forceps
- L. chisel
- L. fibular forceps
- L. forceps
- L. osteotome
- L. raspatory
- L. rib raspatory
- L. splitting chisel

Lambotte-Henderson osteotome
Lambrinudi splint
lamellar blade
laminar
- l. dissector
- l. elevator
- l. spreader

laminaria
- l. cervical dilator
- l. cervical tent
- Japonicum l.
- l. seaweed obstetrical dilator
- l. tent

laminectomy
- l. blade
- l. chisel
- l. raspatory
- l. retractor
- l. rongeur
- l. rongeur forceps
- l. self-retaining retractor
- l. wedge sponge

Laminex needle
Lamis
- L. infusion system
- L. patellar clamp

Lamont
- L. elevator
- L. nasal rasp
- L. nasal saw

lamp
- Bausch-Lomb Thorpe slit l.
- Binner head l.
- Buie sigmoidoscope replacement l.
- l. bulb
- Campbell slit l.
- Davis l.
- Eldridge-Green l.

examining l.
Faro coolbeam l.
Grafco perineal l.
Haag-Streit slit l.
head l.
incandescent endoscope l.
Keeler l.
Koeppe l.
Kowa portable slit l.
Nikon slit l.
Quick-Lite l.
Reichert slit l.
Rusch laryngoscope l.
Rycroft l.
sigmoidoscope
  replacement l.
slit l.
slit illuminator slit l.
Thorpe slit l.
Topcon slit l.
Universal l.
Universal Mack l.
Uviolite l.
xenon l.

Lancaster
  L. eye speculum
  L. keratome
  L. knife
  L. magnet
  L. ocular transilluminator
  L. sclerotome
  L. speculum
Lancaster-O'Connor
  L.-O. forceps
  L.-O. speculum
Lanceford prosthesis
Lance knife
lancet
  l. knife
  Microlance blood l.
lancet-shaped
  l.-s. biopsy forceps
  l.-s. electrode
Landau
  L. dilator
  L. speculum
  L. trocar
  L. vaginal retractor
Landegger
  L. orbital eye implant
  L. orbital implant
  L. orbital implant material
Landers-Foulks prosthesis

Lane's sail [handwritten annotation]

Landers vitrectomy lens forceps
Landolt
  L. cannula
  L. keratome
  L. spreader
Landon
  L. colpostat
  L. forceps
  L. narrow-bladed retractor
Lane
  L. band
  L. bone forceps
  L. bone-holding clamp
  L. bone-holding forceps
  L. catheter
  L. clamp
  L. cleft palate needle
  L. dissector
  L. elevator
  L. fasciatome
  L. forceps
  L. fracture plate
  L. gastroenterostomy clamp
  L. gastrointestinal forceps
  L. intestinal clamp
  L. intestinal forceps
  L. lever
  L. mouth gag
  L. needle
  L. periosteal elevator
  L. periosteal raspatory
  L. rectal catheter
  L. retractor
  L. screwdriver
  L. suturing needle
  L. tissue forceps
  L. towel clamp
  L. ureteral meatotomy
    electrode
Lang
  L. dissector
  L. eye knife
  L. eye scoop
  L. iris forceps
  L. suture
Lange
  L. antral punch
  L. approximation forceps
  L. blade
  L. blade knife
  L. bone elevator
  L. cartilage knife
  L. eye speculum

Lange *(continued)*
- L. fistular hook
- L. mouth gag
- L. plastic surgery hook
- L. retractor
- L. skinfold calipers

Lange-Converse nasal root rongeur
Lange-Hohmann bone lever
Langenbeck
- L. amputation saw
- L. bone-holding forceps
- L. elevator
- L. flap knife
- L. forceps
- L. metacarpal saw
- L. needle holder
- L. periosteal elevator
- L. periosteal raspatory
- L. periosteal retractor
- L. raspatory
- L. retractor

Langenbeck-Cushing vein retractor
Langenbeck-Green retractor
Langenbeck-Mannerfelt retractor
Langenbeck-O'Brien raspatory
Langinate impression material
Lanigan cartilage knife
LAP-13 Ranfac cholangiographic catheter
Lapadis ileostomy bag
Laparocam
- Storz L.

Laparomed
- L. cholangiogram device
- L. cholangiogram vacuum system
- L. suture-applier device

laparoscope
- ACMI l.
- Cabot Medical Corporation diagnostic l.
- Cabot Medical Corporation operating l.
- Circon-ACMI diagnostic l.
- Daniel double-punch laser l.
- Dyonics rod lens l.
- Eder l.
- Elmed diagnostic l.
- Elmed operating l.
- Frangenheim l.
- Fujinon diagnostic l.
- Fujinon operating l.
- Hasson l.
- Jacobs-Palmer l.
- KLI laprocator l.
- Lent l.
- Marlow Surgical Technologies, Inc. diagnostic l.
- Marlow Surgical Technologies, Inc. operating l.
- Menghini-Wildhirt l.
- offset operating l.
- Olympus diagnostic l.
- Olympus operating l.
- Richard Wolf l.
- Richard Wolf Medical Instruments diagnostic l.
- Richard Wolf Medical Instruments operating l.
- Ruddock l.
- Sharplav l.
- Solos Endoscopy diagnostic l.
- Stoltz l.
- Storz l.
- Storz diagnostic l.
- Storz operating l.
- Wildhirt l.
- Wisap/USA diagnostic l.
- Wisap/USA operating l.
- Wolf l.
- Wolf insufflation l.
- zero-degree l.
- Ziskie operating l.

laparoscopic
- l. cannula
- l. forceps
- l. insufflator
- l. scissors
- l. sleeve

Laparostat
- Olsen self-retaining L.
- L. with fiber diversion
- L. with irrigation and aspiration

laparotomy
- l. ring
- l. sponge
- l. sponge ring
- l. sponge ring

Laparo Vac irrigation and aspiration system
Lapides
- L. catheter

L. collecting bag
L. holder
L. needle
Lapidus bed
Laplace
L. forceps
L. liver retractor
L. retractor
LaPorte total toe implant
Lar-A-Jext laryngectomy tube
Lardennois button
Lares dental handpiece
Large
L. clamp
L. vena caval clamp (Alfred M. Large)
large
l. antral cannula
l. bowel curette
l. physiological cup
l. tray
l. uterine curette
large-bore
l.-b. cannula
l.-b. catheter
l.-b. needle
large-diameter
l.-d. optics intraocular lens
l.-d. optics lens
large-loop electrode
large-lumen catheter
large-volume
l.-b. round silicone drain
l.-b. suction reservoir
LaRocca nasolacrimal tube
LaRoque suture
Larrey
L. bandage
L. dressing
Larry
L. probe
L. rectal director
L. rectal probe
Larsen tendon forceps
laryngeal
l. applicator
l. applicator forceps
l. atomizer
l. basket forceps
l. biopsy forceps
l. bronchial grasping forceps
l. cannula
l. curette forceps

l. dilator
l. dissector
l. forceps
l. grasping forceps
l. handle
l. knife
l. knife handle
l. mirror
l. mirror handle
l. probe
l. punch forceps
l. retractor
l. rotation forceps
l. saw
l. scissors
l. snare
l. sponge carrier
l. sponging forceps
l. suction tube
l. trocar
laryngeal-bronchial telescope
laryngectomy
l. clamp
l. tube
laryngofissure
l. forceps
l. retractor
laryngonasopharyngoscope
Berci-Ward l.
laryngopharyngoscope
Berci-Ward l.
Proctor l.
Stuckrad magnifying l.
laryngoscope
adult l.
adult reverse-bevel l.
Albert-Andrews l.
Andrews l.
Andrews infant l.
anterior commissure l.
Atkins-Tucker l.
Atkins-Tucker shadow-free l.
baby Miller l.
Belscope l.
Benjamin binocular slimline l.
Benjamin pediatric l.
Bizzarri-Guiffrida l.
l. blade
Briggs l.
Broyles l.
Broyles anterior commissure l.

laryngoscope *(continued)*
Broyles optical l.
Broyles wasp-waist l.
Burton l.
l. chest support holder
Chevalier Jackson l.
Clerf l.
commissure l.
Dedo l.
Dedo-Jako l.
Dedo laser l.
Dedo-Pilling l.
direct l.
disposable l.
dual distal-lighted l.
ESI l.
fiberoptic l.
fiberoptic slide l.
Fink l.
Finnoff l.
Flagg l.
folding l.
l. folding blade
Foregger l.
Fragen l.
Garfield-Holinger l.
Guedel l.
Guedel-Negus l.
Haslinger l.
l. holder
Holinger l.
Holinger anterior
  commissure l.
Holinger-Garfield l.
Holinger hook-on folding l.
Holinger hourglass l.
Holinger hourglass anterior
  commissure l.
Holinger infant l.
Holinger modified
  Jackson l.
Holinger slotted l.
Hollister l.
hook-on folding l.
Hopp l.
Hopp-Morrison l.
hourglass anterior
  commissure l.
intubation l.
Jackson l.
Jackson anterior
  commissure l.
Jackson fiberoptic slide l.

Jackson sliding l.
Jackson standard l.
Jako l.
Jako-Cherry l.
Jako-Pilling l.
Kantor-Berci l.
KleenSpec l.
KleenSpec disposable l.
Kleinsasser l.
Kleinsasser anterior
  commissure l.
Kleinsasser operating l.
Kleinsasser-Riecker l.
Kramer operating l.
laser l.
Lewy l.
Lewy multipurpose anterior
  commissure l.
Lindholm operating l.
Lundy l.
Lynch l.
Lynch suspension l.
Machida l.
Machida fiberoptic l.
MacIntosh l.
Magill l.
Mantel l.
McIntosh l.
Miller l.
mirror l.
multipurpose l.
multipurpose anterior
  commissure l.
Negus l.
Olympus ENF-P2 flexible l.
optical l.
Ossoff-Karlan l.
Ossoff-Karlan-Dedo l.
Ossoff-Karlan-Jako l.
Ossoff-Karlan laser l.
polio l.
l. profilometer
reverse-bevel l.
Rica l.
Rica anesthetic l.
Rica anterior commissure l.
Rica infant l.
Riecker-Kleinsasser l.
Roberts l.
Roberts self-retaining l.
rotating l.
Rusch l.
Sam Roberts l.

Sam Roberts self-retaining l.
Sanders l.
Sanders intubation l.
self-retaining l.
shadow-free l.
Shapshay-Healy l.
Siker mirror l.
sliding l.
slotted l.
SMIC l.
SMIC anterior commisure l.
standard l.
standard Jackson l.
Stange l.
Storz anterior commissure l.
Storz-Hopkins l.
Storz infection ventilation l.
Storz-Riecker l.
straight-blade l.
suspension l.
Tucker l.
Tucker anterior
  commissure l.
Tucker-Holinger l.
Tucker-Jako l.
Tucker mid-lighted optic
  slide l.
Tucker slotted l.
wasp-waist l.
Weerda l.
Welch Allyn l.
Welch Allyn disposable l.
Welch Allyn KleenSpec
  disposable l.
Wisconsin l.
Wis-Foregger l.
Wis-Hipple l.
Yankauer l.

laryngostat
Jackson l.
Lewy l.
Priest wasp-waist l.
Proctor l.
Proctor-Hellens l.
Roman l.

laryngostroboscope
Nagashima LS-3 l.

larynx
American artificial l.
Electronic Artificial l.
external auditory l.
Xomed intraoral artificial l.

Lasag contact lens

Laser
L. Fiber Director
L. ovary forceps

laser
Albarran l.
AMO l.
argon l.
argon-krypton l.
atheroblation l.
l. balloon
balloon-centered argon l.
Biophysic Medical l.
Britt argon l.
carbon dioxide l.
l. catheter
Chromaser dermatology l.
Chrys surgical CO_2 l.
Cilco l.
CO_2 l.
Coherent argon l.
Coherent radiation argon l.
Coherent system of CO_2
  surgical l.
Cooper argon l.
CooperVision l.
CooperVision argon l.
dye l.
Endo-Lase CO_2 l.
erbium-YAG l.
Excimer l.
Excimer cool l.
l. fiber
fluorescence-guided
  "smart" l.
l. fume absorber
gas l.
green l.
l. Heaney needle holder
helium-cadmium
  diagnostic l.
helium-neon l.
He-Ne l.
HGM intravitreal l.
holmium l.
holmium:YAG l.
Howard-Schatzl.
Hruby l.
intravitreal l.
ion l.
l. Julian needle holder
KIP l.
krypton l.
KTP l.

laser *(continued)*
    KTP 532 l.
    KTP argon video l.
    l. laryngeal suction tube
    l. laryngoscope
    Lasertek l.
    Lasertek YAG l.
    Lassag Micropter II l.
    MCM smart l.
    Medilas Nd:YAG surgical l.
    l. microlaryngeal cup forceps
    l. microlaryngeal grasping forceps
    l. micromanipulator for surgical microscope
    l. microsurgery set
    Mira l.
    l. mirror
    Moeller l.
    Multilase Nd:YAG surgical l.
    Nd:YAG l.
      neodymium-doped yttrium-aluminum-garnet laser
    neodymium l.
    neodymium-doped yttrium-aluminum-garnet l. (Nd:YAG laser)
    Neurolase microsurgical CO_2 l.
    Ophthalas l.
    potassium titanyl phosphate (KTP) l.
    l. probe
    red l.
    l. ridge lens
    l. rod
    rotational ablation l.
    ruby l.
    l. scalpel
    Sharplan l.
    Sharplan CO_2 l.
    Sharplan Medilas Nd:YAG surgical l.
    Sharplan surgical l.
    SharpLase Nd:YAG l.
    SITE l.
    SITE argon l.
    SLT CL100 Contact l.
    SLT CL MD/110 Contact l.
    SLT CL MD/Dual contact l.
    SLT Contact l.
    smart l.
    Spectra-Physics argon l.
    Spectra-Physics microsurgical l.
    spectroscopy-directed l.
    stereotaxic l.
    Storz l.
    l. surgery set
    surgical l.
    l. taper
    thulium holmium:YAG l.
    l. tubal scissors
    tunable dye l.
    Visulas Nd:YAG l.
    Wild l.
    Xanar 20 Amulase CO_2 l.
    YAG l.
    Zeiss l.
    Zeiss H l.
    Zeiss MD l.

laser-bronchoscope
    Dumon l.-b.

Laserscope disposable Endostat fiber

LaserSonics Nd:YAG LaserBlade scalpel

Lasertek
    L. laser
    L. YAG laser

Lash-Loeffler
    L.-L. implant
    L.-L. penile implant material
    L.-L. penile prosthesis

Lassag Micropter II laser

latent pacemaker

lateral
    l. band
    l. guide pin
    l. gutter impactor
    l. microlens telescope
    l. osteotome
    l. positioner
    l. retractor

latex
    l. bag
    l. band
    l. catheter
    l. drain
    l. O band

l. rubber tourniquet strap
l. sponge graft

Lathbury
L. applicator
L. cotton applicator

lathe-cut polymethyl methacrylate intraocular lens

Latrobe
L. retractor
L. soft palate retractor

Lattimer Silastic testicular prosthesis

Lauer forceps

Laufe
L. aspirating curette
L. cervical dilator
L. divergent outlet forceps
L. forceps
L. obstetrical forceps
L. polyp forceps
L. portable uterine evacuator
L. retractor
L. uterine polyp forceps

Laufe-Barton-Kjelland obstetrical forceps

Laufe-Barton-Kjelland-Piper obstetrical forceps

Laufe-Barton obstetrical forceps

Laufe-Novak
L.-N. diagnostic curette
L.-N. gynecologic curette

Laufe-Piper
L.-P. forceps
L.-P. obstetrical forceps
L.-P. uterine polyp forceps

Laufe-Randall
L.-R. curette
L.-R. gynecologic curette

Laufman forceps

Laurens-Alcatel nuclear powered pacemaker

lavage
Easi-Lav gastric l.
pulse l.
Tum-E-Vac gastric l.

lavaging catheter

Laval advancement forceps

LaVeen helical stripper

Lawford speculum

Lawrence
L. deep forceps
L. deep-surgery forceps

L. forceps
L. hemostatic forceps

Lawrie
L. modified circumflex scissors
L. scissors

Lawton
L. corneal scissors
L. forceps

Lawton-Balfour self-retaining retractor

Lawton-Schubert biopsy forceps

Lawton-Wittner cervical biopsy forceps

Layden infant lens

Layman tongue depressor

Lazar microsuction forceps

L-buttress plate

LDL
low-density lipoprotein

LDS
LDS clip
LDS disposable unit

lead
CCS endocardial pacing l.
endocardial balloon l.
endocardial cardiac l.
epicardial l.
l. hand
myocardial l.
permanent cardiac pacing l.
permanent pacing l.
l. plate
l. suture
temporary pervenous l.

Leadbetter-Politano ureteral implant prosthesis

Leader
L. forceps
L. iris hook
L. vas hook
L. vas isolation forceps

Leader-Kohlman dilator

lead-filled mallet

lead-shot tie suture

leaflet retractor

Leahey
L. clamp
L. marginal chalazion forceps
L. suture forceps

Leake Dacron mandible prosthesis

Leasure
- L. aspirator
- L. nasal forceps
- L. round punch tip
- L. tracheal retractor
- L. tuning fork

Leather
- L. antegrade valvulotome
- L. in-situ bypass instrument set
- L. in-situ valve-cutter kit
- L. retrograde valvulotome

Leather-Karmody in-situ valve scissors

Leatherman
- L. alar hook
- L. compression hook
- L. trochanteric retractor

leather valve cutter

Leaver sclerotomy forceps

Le Blond R diamond dental bur

Lebsche
- L. chisel
- L. forceps
- L. raspatory
- L. rongeur
- L. saw
- L. sternal chisel
- L. sternal knife
- L. sternal punch
- L. sternal punch forceps
- L. sternal shears

LeCocq brace

Lectrosonic gel

LeDentu suture

Ledor pigtail catheter

LeDran suture

Lee
- L. bracket
- L. bronchial clamp
- L. cartilage knife
- L. Cohen knife
- L. cryoprobe
- L. delicate hemostatic forceps
- L. diamond bur
- L. double-ended retractor
- L. graft
- L. lingual button
- L. microvascular clamp
- L. needle
- L. orthodontic resin
- L. right-angle clamp

Lee-Cohen septal elevator

Leeds-Northrup Speedomax recorder

Lee-Fischer plastic bracket

Lees
- L. arterial forceps
- L. clamp
- L. nontraumatic forceps
- L. right-angle clamp
- L. vascular clamp
- L. wedge resection clamp

Leff
- L. alloy
- L. stethoscope

Lefferts
- L. bone-cutting forceps
- L. forceps
- L. rib shears
- L. rib spreader

LeFort
- L. catheter
- L. dilator
- L. filiform
- L. filiform bougie
- L. filiform guide
- L. male catheter
- L. sound
- L. suture
- L. urethral catheter
- L. urethral sound
- L. uterine sound

left
- l. uterine displacement device (LUD)
- l. ventricular (LV)
- l. ventricular assist device (LVAD)
- l. ventricular clamp catheter

leg
- l. and ankle traction
- l. brace
- l. holder
- l. sling

Legend pacemaker

Legen self-retaining retractor

legging
- traction l.

Legg osteotome

leg-holding device

Legueu
- L. bladder retractor
- L. kidney retractor

L. retractor
L. spatula
Lehman
  L. aortographic catheter
  L. catheter
  L. pancreatic manometry catheter
  L. ventriculography catheter
  L. wire-guided biliary manometry catheter set
Lehnhardt Universal cap
Leicaflex camera
Leigh
  L. capsular forceps
  L. forceps
  L. right-handed forceps
Leighton needle
Leinbach
  L. head and neck endoprosthesis
  L. head and neck total hip
  L. hip prosthesis
  L. olecranon hook
  L. olecranon screw
  L. osteotome
  L. prosthesis
Leios pacemaker
Leisegang
  L. flexible hysteroscope
  L. LM-FLEX 7 flexible hysteroscope
Leiske style intraocular lens
Leiter tube
Leivers
  L. blade
  L. formed-type bite
  L. mouth gag
  L. mouth gag frame
  L. swivel-type bite
Lejeune
  L. applicator
  L. cotton applicator
  L. forceps
  L. thoracic forceps
Leksell
  L. bone rongeur
  L. forceps
  L. frame
  L. gamma knife
  L. grooved director
  L. laminectomy rongeur
  L. rongeur
  L. rongeur forceps

L. stereotaxic frame
L. sternal approximator
L. trephine
Leksell-Stille rongeur
Leland-Jones
  L.-J. clamp
  L.-J. forceps
  L.-J. peripheral vascular clamp
  L.-J. tonsillar knife
  L.-J. vascular clamp
Leland tonsillar knife
Lell
  L. esophagoscope
  L. laryngofissure saw
  L. tracheal tube
Lembert suture
Lem-Blay
  L.-B. circumcision clamp
  L.-B. clamp
Lemmon
  L. blade
  L. contractor
  L. intimal dissector
  L. rib approximator
  L. self-retaining sternal retractor
  L. sternal approximator
  L. sternal retractor
  L. sternal spreader
Lemmon-Russian forceps
Lemoine
  L. eye implant
  L. forceps
  L. orbital implant
  L. serrefine
Lemoine-Searcy anchor
Lemole
  L. atrial valve self-retaining retractor
  L. mitral valve retractor
Lempert
  L. bone curette
  L. bone rongeur
  L. bur
  L. curette
  L. diamond-dust polishing bur
  L. elevator
  L. endaural curette
  L. endaural rongeur
  L. excavator
  L. fenestration bur

Lempert *(continued)*
- L. fine curette
- L. forceps
- L. headrest
- L. heavy elevator
- L. invaginator
- L. knife
- L. malleus cutter
- L. malleus nipper
- L. malleus punch
- L. narrow elevator
- L. perforator
- L. retractor
- L. rongeur
- L. rongeur forceps

Lempert-Beckman-Colver endaural speculum

Lempert-Colver
- L.-C. endaural speculum
- L.-C. retractor

Lempert-Juers rongeur

Lempert-Storz lens loupe

Lempka vein stripper

length
- neck l.

Lenny Johnson surgical-assist knee holder

Lenox
- L. Hill brace
- L. Hill knee brace
- L. Hill Spectralite knee brace

lens
- Abraham contact l.
- Abraham iridectomy laser l.
- Abraham YAG laser l.
- AC l.
- acrylic l.
- Advent Flurofocon contact l.
- Albarran l.
- Alcon intraocular l.
- Allergan Advent contact l.
- Allergan Medical Optics l.
- Allergan-Simcoe C-loop intraocular l.
- all-in-the-bag intraocular l.
- all-PMMA intraocular l.
- all-PMMA one-piece C-loop intraocular l.
- Amercal intraocular l.
- Amercal-Shepard intraocular l.
- American Medical Optics l.
- AMO l.
- Anis two flexible closed loops intraocular l.
- anterior chamber intraocular l.
- AO l.
- Aquaflex contact l.
- Arnott one-piece all-PMMA intraocular l.
- aspheric l.
- Azar intraocular l.
- Azar Mark II intraocular l.
- bag-fixated intraocular l.
- Barkan infant l.
- Barkan operating l.
- Baron intraocular l.
- Barraquer l.
- Barraquer J-loops intraocular l.
- Barrett hydrogel intraocular l.
- Bechert l.
- Bechert one-piece all-PMMA intraocular l.
- biconvex intraocular l.
- bifocal l.
- Binkhorst collar stud intraocular l.
- Binkhorst intraocular l.
- Binkhorst mustache lens intraocular l.
- Binkhorst two modified J-loops intraocular l.
- Blumenthal intraocular l.
- Boberg l.
- Boberg-Ans intraocular l.
- l. cannula
- capsular style l.
- Capsulform l.
- Cardona focalizing fundus l.
- cast-molded PMMA intraocular l.
- CGI-1 contact l.
- Charles intraocular l.
- Charles irrigating l.
- Charles irrigating contact l.
- Choyce l.
- Choyce intraocular l.
- Choyce Mark intraocular l.
- Choyce-Tennant l.
- Cilco intraocular l.
- Cilco MonoFlex PMMA l.

Cilco Optiflex intraocular l.
Cilco posterior chamber
 intraocular l.
Clayman l.
l. clip
C-loop intraocular l.
closed-loop intraocular l.
Coburn l.
Coburn intraocular l.
Coburn Optical Industries-
 Feaster intraocular l.
Coburn-Storz intraocular l.
Cogan-Boberg-Ans l.
compressible acrylic
 intraocular l.
compression-molded PMMA
 intraocular l.
contact l.
CooperVision-Cilco
 intraocular l.
CooperVision-Cilco Kelman
 multiflex all-PMMA
 intraocular l.
CooperVision-Cilco Novaflex
 anterior chamber
 intraocular l.
Copeland l.
Copeland anterior chamber
 intraocular l.
Copeland radial loop
 intraocular l.
diopter l.
disk lens intraocular l.
Donnheim l.
Dubroff radial loop
 intraocular l.
Duragel l.
endocapsular artificial lens
 intraocular l.
l. enucleation scoop
Epstein collar stud acrylic l.
Epstein-Copeland l.
Epstein intraocular l.
Epstein posterior chamber l.
European in-the-bag l.
l. expressor
extended wear soft
 contact l. (EWSCL)
Feaster Dualens
 intraocular l.
Feaster dual-placement
 intraocular l.
Fechner intraocular l.

Flexcon l.
flexible fluoropolymer
 contact l.
flexible-loop anterior
 chamber intraocular l.
flexible-loop posterior
 chamber intraocular l.
folding l.
l. forceps
FormFlex formocresal l.
FormFlex intraocular l.
Foroblique l.
four-footed lens l.
four-piece intraocular l.
four-point fixation
 intraocular l.
Fresnel l.
Friedman-Hruby l.
fundal laser l.
Fyodorov four-loop iris clip
 intraocular l.
Fyodorov intraocular l.
Fyodorov-Sputnik FFP
 contact intraocular l.
Fyodorov type II
 intraocular l.
Fyodorov type I
 intraocular l.
Galand in-the-bag l.
Galand-Knolle modified J-
 loop intraocular l.
l. glide cutter
Goldmann contact l.
Goldmann three-mirror
 gonioscopy l.
gradient index l.
GRIN l.
haptic area l.
haptic-fixated intraocular l.
haptic-sec l.
Harris modified J-loop
 intraocular l.
Harris rigid quadriped
 intraocular l.
Hart pediatric 3-mirror l.
Hersbury anterior chamber
 intraocular l.
high minus power optics
 for low vision aid l.
Hoffer ridged intraocular l.
l. hook
Hruby l.
Hruby contact l.

lens *(continued)*
Hunkeler intraocular l.
Hunter one-piece all-PMMA intraocular l.
Hydracon contact l.
Hydrasoft contact l.
Hydrogel expansile intraocular l.
hydrophilic contact l.
IMMA l.
l. implant
l. implantation forceps
Implens intraocular l.
Interfit-Pharmacea Intermedic intraocular l.
Interflux intraocular l.
in-the-bag l.
intraocular l. (IOL)
Intraoptics intraocular l.
Iogel intraocular l.
IOLAb l.
IOLAB Azar intraocular l.
IOLAB intraocular l.
Ioptex intraocular l.
Irene l.
iridocapsular intraocular l.
iris claw l.
iris clip intraocular l.
iris supported l.
iris supported intraocular l.
Jaffe one-piece all-PMMA intraocular l.
J-loop intraocular l.
J-loop posterior chamber intraocular l.
Joal l.
Kamerling one-piece all-PMMA intraocular l.
Karickhoff laser l.
Kelman II three-point fixation rigid tripod intraocular l.
Kelman modern flexible tripod intraocular l.
Kelman Multiflex intraocular l.
Kelman Omnifit l.
Kelman Omnifit intraocular l.
Kelman Quadraflex intraocular l.
Kelman S-flex intraocular l.
keratometer l.

Kishi l.
Koeppe diagnostic l.
Koeppe gonioscopic l.
Kratz l.
Kratz-Johnson modified J-loop intraocular l.
Kratz modified J-loop intraocular l.
Kratz posterior chamber intraocular l.
Krieger wide-field fundus l.
Kryptok bifocals l.
large-diameter optics l.
large-diameter optics intraocular l.
Lasag contact l.
laser ridge l.
lathe-cut polymethyl methacrylate intraocular l.
Layden infant l.
Leiske style intraocular l.
Lester notch intraocular l.
Levick one-piece all-PMMA intraocular l.
Lewicky intraocular l.
Lindstrom modified J-loop, three-piece reverse PMMA optic intraocular l.
Little-Arnott tripod intraocular l.
l. loop
loop l.
loop-fixated intraocular l.
l. loop forceps
l. loupe
Lovac fundus contact l.
Lovac six-mirror gonioscopic l.
low-power optics for myopic correction l.
Lynell intraocular l.
Machemer magnifying vitrectomy l.
Maltese cross l.
l. manipulator
Mazzocco compressible silicone l.
Mazzocco silicone intraocular l.
McLean prismatic fundus laser l.
Mehta intraocular l.
meniscal l.

meniscal posterior concave
  intraocular l.
3M intraocular l.
l. mitral heart valve
modified C-loops
  intraocular l.
modified J-loop, posterior
  chamber intraocular l.
Momosi spider lens
  intraocular l.
multiple-piece intraocular l.
Novaflex intraocular l.
NuVue l.
Omnifit intraocular l.
one-piece intraocular l.
open l.
open-loop intraocular l.
optical radiation
  intraocular l.
Optiflex intraocular l.
ORC intraocular l.
Osher-Fresnel intraocular l.
Packard intraocular l.
Palmer l.
Palmer-Buono contact l.
Pannu II intraocular l.
Pannu intraocular l.
Pearce-Keates bifocal l.
Pearce-Keates bifocal
  intraocular l.
Pearce posterior chamber
  intraocular l.
Pearce Tripod intraocular l.
Perspex CQ intraocular l.
Peyman-Green vitrectomy l.
Peyman special optics for
  low vision l.
Phaco-flex l.
Pharmacia Intermedics
  ophthalmics intraocular l.
Pharmacia intraocular l.
plano l.
planoconcave l.
planoconvex l.
plus power l.
PMMA intraocular l.
Pointer one-piece all-PMMA
  intraocular l.
polypropylene intraocular l.
posterior chamber
  intraocular l.
posterior convex
  intraocular l.

l. pusher
Rapazzo intraocular l.
Rayner-Choyce intraocular l.
reverse intraocular l.
ridged lenses l.
ridged lenses intraocular l.
ridged posterior chamber
  intraocular l.
rigid intraocular l.
Ritch contact l.
Ritch trabeculoplasty laser l.
Rodenstock l.
Rohm and Haas PMMA
  intraocular l.
Roussel-Fankhauser
  contact l.
Ruiz fundus contact l.
Ruiz fundus laser l.
Ruiz plano fundus l.
Sableflex anterior chamber
  intraocular l.
sapphire l.
l. scoop
semiflexible intraocular l.
semirigid intraocular l.
Severin multiple closed-loop
  intraocular l.
Shah-Shah intraocular l.
Shearing intraocular l.
Shearing J-Loop
  intraocular l.
Shearing posterior chamber
  intraocular l.
Shearing S-style anterior
  chamber intraocular l.
Sheets closed-loop posterior
  chamber intraocular l.
Sheets two flexible closed
  loops intraocular l.
Shepard flexible anterior
  chamber intraocular l.
Shepard Universal
  intraocular l.
short C-loop intraocular l.
Siepser intraocular l.
silica contact l.
silvered contact l.
Simcoe C-loop intraocular l.
Sinskey l.
Sinskey intraocular l.
Sinskey-style J-loop
  intraocular l.
Slimfit l.

lens *(continued)*
 soft intraocular l.
 SOLA VIP l.
 l. spatula
 l. spoon
 Stankiewicz iris clip
  intraocular l.
 Starr Surgical polyimide
  loop intraocular l.
 Strampelli l.
 Supramid l.
 Surefit l.
 Surefit intraocular l.
 Surgidev intraocular l.
 Surgidev Leiske anterior
  chamber intraocular l.
 Tennant Anchorflex
  intraocular l.
 Thorpe gonioprism l.
 Thorpe 4-mirror
  goniolaser l.
 Thorpe 4-mirror vitreous
  fundus laser l.
 three-footed lens
  intraocular l.
 three-mirror intraocular l.
 three-piece modified J-loop
  intraocular l.
 three-point fixation
  intraocular l.
 Tolentino vitrectomy l.
 toric l.
 tripod intraocular l.
 Troncoso tubular l.
 Truvision Omni l.
 Ultex l.
 ultraviolet-blocking
  intraocular l.
 uniplanar intraocular l.
 uvea-fixated intraocular l.
 uvea-supported l.
 uvea-supported intraocular l.
 UVR-absorbing l.
 UVR-absorbing intraocular l.
 Varigray l.
 Varilux infinity l.
 Varilux Plus l.
 Volk conoid l.
 Wang l.
 Worst l.
 Worst lobster-claw l.
 Worst Medallion l.
 Yalon intraocular l.

 Zeiss aspheric l.
 Ziski iris clip intraocular l.
 Zoeffle soft intraocular l.
lensometer
Lent
 L. laparoscope
 L. photolaparoscope
Lente
 L. probe
 L. silver nitrate probe
Lentulo
 L. drill
 L. spiral drill
Leo
 L. Schwartz multipurpose
  forceps
 L. Schwartz sponge-holding
  forceps
Leonard
 L. deep forceps
 L. deep-surgery forceps
 L. forceps
Leone expansion screw
Lepley-Ernst tube
Leptos pacemaker
Leriche
 L. forceps
 L. hemostatic forceps
 L. spatula
 L. tissue forceps
Lerman hinge brace
Lermoyez nasal punch
LeRoy
 L. catheter
 L. clip
 L. clip-applying forceps
 L. disposable scalp clip
 L. infant clip-applying
  forceps
 L. infant scalp clip
 L. scalp clip
LeRoy-Raney scalp clip
L'Esperance
 L. erysiphake
 L. needle
 L. right-angle erysiphake
Lespinasse suture
Lester
 L. A. Dine camera
 L. fixation forceps
 L. forceps
 L. lens manipulator
 L. notch intraocular lens

Lester-Burch eye speculum
Letournel acetabular fracture bone
  plate
Leukos pacemaker
leukotome
    Bailey l.
    Dorsey transorbital l.
    Freeman transorbital l.
    Lewis l.
    Lours l.
    Love l.
    McKenzie l.
    Nosik transorbital l.
    Tworek transorbital l.
Leukotrap red cell storage system
Leung endoscopic nasal biliary
  drainage set
Leurs nasal rasp
Leusch atraumatic obturator
Levant
    L. dislodger
    L. stone dislodger
    L. stone dislodger basket
levator snare
LeVeen
    L. ascites shunt
    L. catheter
    L. peritoneal shunt
    L. shunt
Levenson tissue forceps
lever
    Alexander bone l.
    Bennett bone l.
    bone l.
    Bristow l.
    Buck-Gramcko bone l.
    Charnley femoral l.
    Cottle bone l.
    Hohmann-Aldinger bone l.
    Hohmann bone l.
    Kilner malar l.
    Lane l.
    Lange-Hohmann bone l.
    Murphy-Lane l.
    Norrbacka-Stille l.
    l. pessary
    Sellheim obstetrical l.
    Tager l.
    Torpin obstetrical l.
    Verbrugge-Müller bone l.
    Wagner bone l.
Lever-Mini chisel

Levick one-piece all-PMMA
  intraocular lens
Levin
    L. duodenal tube
    L. electrode
    L. tube catheter
Levin-Davol tube
Levine
    L. curetting spud
    L. foreign body spud
Levinthal surgery retractor
Levis
    L. arm splint
Levitt
    L. eye implant
    L. implant
Levora fixation forceps
Levret forceps
Levy-Kuglen
    L.-K. iris hook
    L.-K. lens manipulator
Levy-Okun stripper
Levy perineal retractor
Lewicky
    L. capsular scraper
    L. cortex extractor
    L. cystitome
    L. hook
    L. intraocular lens
    L. IOL spatula
    L. maintainer
    L. microlens hook
    L. needle
    L. threaded infusion
      cannula
Lewin
    L. baseball finger splint
    L. bone clamp
    L. bone-holding clamp
    L. bone-holding forceps
    L. bunion dissector
    L. clamp
    L. dissector
    L. finger splint
    L. forceps
    L. sesamoidectomy dissector
    L. spinal-perforating forceps
Lewin-Stern
    L.-S. finger splint
    L.-S. thumb splint
Lewis
    L. dental mirror
    L. forceps

Lewis *(continued)*
- L. hemostat
- L. intramedullary device
- L. laryngectomy tube
- L. lens loop
- L. lens loupe
- L. lens scoop
- L. leukotome
- L. mouth gag
- L. nasal rasp
- L. periosteal elevator
- L. periosteal raspatory
- L. rasp
- L. recording cystometer
- L. retractor
- L. septal forceps
- L. suspension device
- L. tongue depressor
- L. tonsillar hemostatic forceps
- L. tonsillar screw
- L. tonsillar snare
- L. ureteral stone isolation forceps

Lewis-Leigh positive-pressure nonrebreathing valve

Lewkowitz
- L. forceps
- L. lithotomy forceps
- L. ovum forceps
- L. placental forceps

Lewy
- L. chest holder
- L. laryngoscope
- L. laryngoscope holder
- L. laryngostat
- L. multipurpose anterior commissure laryngoscope
- L. suspension apparatus
- L. Teflon glycerine-mixture injection needle
- L. Teflon glycerine-mixture syringe

Lewy-Holinger
- L.-H. needle
- L.-H. Teflon injection needle

Lewy-Rubin
- L.-R. needle
- L.-R. Teflon glycerine-mixture injection needle

Lexer
- L. chisel
- L. dissecting scissors
- L. gouge
- L. mini gouge
- L. osteotome
- L. scissors
- L. tissue forceps

Lexer-Durotip dissecting scissors

Lex-Ton lumbar laminectomy frame

Leydig drain

Leyla
- L. brain retractor
- L. flexible arm
- L. retractor
- L. self-retaining brain retractor

Leyla-Yasargil
- L.-Y. retractor
- L.-Y. self-retaining retractor

Leyro-Diaz
- L.-D. forceps
- L.-D. thoracic forceps

Lezius suction tube

L-F Uniflex diathermy electrosurgical unit

Lichtenberg
- L. corneal trephine
- L. keratome
- L. needle holder

Lichtwicz
- L. abdominal trocar
- L. antral cannula
- L. antral needle
- L. antral trocar
- L. needle

Lichtwicz-Bier antral needle

lid
- l. clamp
- l. everter
- l. expressor
- l. forceps
- l. plate
- l. retractor
- l. scalpel
- l. speculum

Liddicoat aortic valve retractor

Liddle
- L. aortic clamp
- L. clamp

Lieberman
- L. abrader
- L. forceps
- L. proctoscope

L. sigmoidoscope
L. sigmoidoscope with
  swinging window
L. suturing forceps
L. tying forceps
Lieberman-Pollock
  L.-P. double corneal forceps
  L.-P. forceps
Lieb-Guerry forceps
Liebreich probe
Lieppman
  L. cystitome
  L. microcystitome
  L. sharp cystitome
  L. spatula
Lifecath
  L. catheter
  L. peritoneal implant
Lifeline electrode
Life-Lok clamp
Lifemed
  L. blood tubing
  L. cannula
  L. heterologous heart valve
life-saving tube
lift
  Wigmore plaster saw
    with l.
lifter
  tissue l.
  waltzing areolar l.
  Yasargil tissue l.
lifting handle
Ligaclip
ligament
  l. augmentation device
    (LAD)
  l. clamp
ligamenta flava forceps
ligament-grasping forceps
ligamentum teres knife
Ligapak suture
Lig-A-Ring separator
Liga surgical clip
ligation suture
ligator
  Barron l.
  Barron hemorrhoidal l.
  Centrix PDQ l.
  Clarke-Reich l.
  Gigator hemorehoidal l.
  hemorrhoidal l.
  Lurz-Goltner l.

McGivney hemorrhoidal l.
Preston-Hopkins l.
Rudd l.
Salvatore umbilical cord l.
Sanford l.
Scanlan l.
Tucker hemorrhoidal l.
Twist-Mate l.
ligature
  l. cannula
  l. carrier
  l. director
  l. forceps
  l. guide
  l. needle
  l. passer
  l. scissors
  l. suture
  l. tucker
ligature-carrying
  l.-c. aneurysm forceps
  l.-c. forceps
ligature-passing instrument
light
  AMSCO l.
  l. carrier
  Castle surgical l.
  Chick surgical l.
  Clar head l.
  Co-Axa l.
  l. cross-slot screwdriver
  dermatologic ultraviolet l.
  floor-standing surgical l.
  Fotofil activator l.
  Fragen laryngoscope
    fiberoptic l.
  Gass neurosurgical l.
  overhead l.
  l. pipe
  ultraviolet l.
  Witt dental l.
lighted
  l. retractor
  l. speculum
Light headrest
Light-Veley
  L.-V. apparatus
  L.-V. automatic cranial drill
  L.-V. bur
  L.-V. cranial drill
  L.-V. drill
  L.-V. headrest

Liguory endoscopic nasal biliary drainage set
Liks Russian disk rotation heart valve
Lilienthal
    L. probe
    L. rib guillotine
    L. rib spreader
Lilienthal-Sauerbruch
    L.-S. retractor
    L.-S. rib spreader
Lillehei
    L. forceps
    L. pacemaker
    L. retractor
    L. valve forceps
    L. valve-grasping forceps
    L. valve prosthesis
Lillehei-Kaster
    L.-K. cardiac valve prosthesis
    L.-K. heart valve
Lillehei-Warden catheter
Lillie
    L. antral trocar
    L. attic cannula
    L. attic hook
    L. cannula
    L. ear hook
    L. forceps
    L. frontal sinus probe
    L. gouge
    L. intestinal forceps
    L. intestinal tissue forceps
    L. nasal speculum
    L. pillar retractor
    L. probe
    L. rectus tendon clamp
    L. retractor
    L. rongeur
    L. scissors
    L. tissue-holding forceps
    L. tonsillar knife
    L. tonsillar scissors
Lillie-Killian
    L.-K. forceps
    L.-K. septal bone forceps
    L.-K. septal forceps
Lillie-Koffler tool
limbal suture
limbic suture
Lin clamp

Lincoff
    L. catheter
    L. design of Storz scleral buckling balloon catheter
    L. eye implant
    L. implant
    L. scleral sponge eye implant
    L. sponge
    L. sponge implant material
    L. sponge rod
Lincoln
    L. pediatric scissors
    L. scissors
Lincoln-Metzenbaum scissors
Linde
    L. cryogenic probe
    L. cryoprobe
Lindeman
    L. bur
    L. cannula
    L. needle
    L. self-retaining uterine vacuum cannula
    L. transfusion needle
Lindeman-Silverstein
    L.-S. Arrow tube
    L.-S. ventilation tube
Lindholm
    L. microlaryngoscope
    L. operating laryngoscope
Lindholm-Stille elevator
Lindley
    L. needle holder
    L. scissors
Lindner
    L. anastomosis clamp
    L. comeoscleral suture
    L. cyclodialysis spatula
Lindsay-Rea forceps
Lindstrom modified J-loop, three-piece reverse PMMA optic intraocular lens
Lindvall meniscectomy knife
Lindvall-Stille meniscal knife
line
    Codman ICP monitoring l.
    l. keeper
linear
    l. polyethylene suture
    l. scissor punch
    l. stapler
    l. stapling device

Lineback adenoidal punch
linen
    l. suture
    l. thread suture
liner
    Ardee denture l.
    Calcipulpe cavity l.
    Cavitec cavity l.
    Cavoline cavity l.
    Enduron acetabular l.
    Integrity neutral l.
    Ketac l.
    KM-4 l.
    KM-3A l.
    polyethylene l.
    provisional l.
    Pulpdent cavity l.
    rubber bite l.
    splint l.
    Tempo denture l.
    Tubulitec cavity l.
liners
lingual
    l. arch
    l. bar
    l. forceps
    l. spatula
Link approximator
Linkow dental implant material
Linnartz
    L. clamp
    L. forceps
    L. intestinal clamp
    L. stomach clamp
Linn-Graefe iris forceps
Linton
    L. clamp
    L. esophageal tube
    L. retractor
    L. splanchnic retractor
    L. tourniquet
    L. tourniquet clamp
    L. vein hook
    L. vein stripper
Linton-Blakemore needle
Linton-Nachlas tube
Linx
    L. extension wire
    L. guide wire extension
Lion hearing aid
lion-jaw
    l.-j. bone-holding forceps
    l.-j. clamp
    l.-j. forceps
lip
    l. clamp
    l. retractor
    l. suture
    l. traction bow
lipodissector
Lippes loop intrauterine device
Lippman hip prosthesis
Lipschiff knife
Lipschwitz needle
Lipscomb-Anderson drill guide
Liqui-Cor gel
liquid
    l. conductor Bovie
    Touchup acrylic coating l.
Listening Glass hearing aid
Lister
    L. bandage
    L. bandage scissors
    L. conjunctival forceps
    L. dressing
    L. forceps
    L. mules
    L. scissors
    L. suture removal kit
Lister-Burch eye speculum
List needle
Liston
    L. amputating knife
    L. bone-cutting forceps
    L. forceps
    L. plaster-of-Paris scissors
    L. shears
    L. splint
Liston-Key-Horsley forceps
Liston-Littauer bone-cutting forceps
Liston-Luer-Whiting rongeur
Liston-Ruskin shears
Liston-Stille
    L.-S. bone-cutting forceps
    L.-S. double-action bone-
      cutting forceps
    L.-S. forceps
lith II pacemaker
lithium pacemaker
lithium-powered pacemaker
Lithostar lithotripsy unit
lithotomy forceps
lithotriptor
    Dornier l.
    manual l.

lithotriptor *(continued)*
Pentax l.
l. probe
lithotriptoscope
Ravich l. with Luer lock
lithotrite
Alcock l.
Bigelow l.
Hendrickson l.
Keyes l.
Löwenstein l.
Ravich l.
Reliquet l.
Teale gorget l.
Littauer
L. bone-cutting forceps
L. ciliary forceps
L. ear-dressing forceps
L. ear forceps
L. ear polyp forceps
L. forceps
L. nasal-dressing forceps
L. rongeur
L. scissors
L. stitch scissors
L. suture scissors
Littauer-Liston
L.-L. bone-cutting forceps
L.-L. forceps
Littauer-West cutting forceps
Littell cannula
Litt forceps
Little
L. intraocular lens implant
L. retractor
L. suture scissors
Little-Arnott tripod intraocular lens
Littler
L. scissors
L. suture-carrying scissors
Littlewood
L. forceps
L. tissue forceps
Littmann defibrillation pad
Litton dental handpiece
Littre suture
Litvak-Pereyra ligature needle
Litwak
L. cannula
L. clamp
L. general utility scissors
L. mitral valve scissors

Litwin
L. angled scissors
L. scissors
liver
l. bed
l. biopsy needle
l. biopsy set
l. needle
l. retractor
liver-holding clamp
Livermore trocar
Liverpool elbow implant
live splint
Livingston
L. bar
L. forceps
L. intramedullary bar
living suture
Ljunggren-Stille tenotome
Llobera
L. fixation forceps
L. forceps
Lloyd
L. adapter counterbore
L. bronchial catheter
L. catheter
L. double catheter
L. esophagoscopic catheter
L. nail extractor
Lloyd-Davis
L.-D. clamp
L.-D. occlusion forceps
L.-D. rectal scissors
L.-D. sigmoidoscope
lobectomy
l. forceps
l. scissors
lobe forceps
lobe-grasping forceps
lobe-holding forceps
Lobell
L. forceps
L. splinter forceps
Lobenstein-Tarnier forceps
lobotomy
l. electrode
l. needle
lobster-tail catheter
localizer
Urrets-Zavalia l.
localizing electrode
locator, locater
ASIS femoral head l.

Berman l.
Bronson-Turner foreign
  body l.
Porex nerve l.
saddle l.
lock
Codman disposable ICP
  Luer l.
English l.
French l.
German l.
Luer l.
l. needle
pivot l.
sliding l.
l. suture
Locke bone clamp
locked suture
Lockhart-Mummery
L.-M. probe
L.-M. retractor
locking
anatomic medullary l.
  (AML)
l. clamp
l. nut
l. peg
l. running suture
l. screw
l. suture
lock-stitch suture
Lockwood
L. clamp
L. forceps
L. intestinal forceps
L. tissue forceps
Lockwood-Allis
L.-A. forceps
L.-A. intestinal forceps
L.-A. tissue forceps
Loeffler suture
Loewi suspension device
Lofberg
L. thyroid retractor
L. vaginal speculum
Lofric disposable urethral catheter
Lofstrand brace
Logan
L. bow with teeth
L. dissector
L. lacrimal sac self-retaining
  retractor

L. lip traction bow
L. periosteal elevator
L. retractor
L. traction bow with teeth
Lok-it screwdriver
Lok-Mesh bonding base
Lok-screw
L.-s. double-slot screwdriver
L.-s. screwdriver
Lollipop Stick
Lombard-Beyer
L.-B. forceps
L.-B. rongeur
L.-B. rongeur forceps
Lombard-Boies mastoid rongeur
Lombard rongeur
London
L. College foil carrier
L. forceps
L. narrow-bladed retractor
L. retractor
L. tissue forceps
Long
L. forceps
L. forceps with teeth
L. hysterectomy forceps
L. Island College Hospital
  forceps
L. Island College Hospital
  placental forceps
L. Island forceps
L. needle
long
l. back-handed elevator
l. needle
l. scalpel
l. tissue forceps
Longdwel
L. catheter
L. catheter needle
L. needle
L. Teflon catheter
long-handle curette
long-handle offset gouge
longitudinal suture
long-jaw basket forceps
long-leg brace
Longmire-Mueller curved
  valvulotome
Longmire-Storm clamp
Longmire valvulotome
Lonnecken tube

Look
 L. coaxial flexible
  disposable cannula
 L. single-use cannula
loop (*See also* loupe)
 Adler l.
 Adler tripronged lens
  error l.
 Amenabar l.
 Arlt lens l.
 Axenfeld nerve l.
 l. ball electrode
 Beck-Schenck
  tonsillectome l.
 Beck twisted wire l.
 Beck twisted wire snare l.
 Billeau l.
 Billeau ear l.
 Billeau-House ear l.
 Cannon endarterectomy l.
 Clayman-Knolle irrigating
  lens l.
 l. curette
 cutting l.
 Diaflex retrieval l.
 ear l.
 l. electrode
 foreign body l.
 Gobin-Weiss l.
 House-Billeau ear l.
 House wire l.
 intracapsular lens l.
 irrigating vectis l.
 Kirby intracapsular lens l.
 Knolle-Pearce irrigating
  lens l.
 Knolle-Pearce lens l.
 Kraff nucleus lens l.
 l. lens
 lens l.
 Lewis lens l.
 McKenzie leukotomy l.
 New Orleans lens l.
 nucleus l.
 nucleus removal l.
 nylon l.
 l. retractor
 retrieval l.
 l. scaler
 l. shunt
 Simcoe l.
 Simcoe double-end lens l.
 Simcoe nucleus l.

 Simcoe nucleus delivery l.
 Simcoe nucleus lens l.
 Snellen lens l.
 soft wire l.
 spring wire l.
 Sur-Fit l.
 Surgitie ligating l.'s
 l. suture
 tonsillar l.
 tonsillectome l.
 Torchia vectis l.
 tri-pronged l.
 Troutman lens l.
 twisted wire snare l.
 Uresil radiopaque silicone-
  band vessel l.'s
 vascular l.
 vectis l.
 Vedder l.
 vessel l.
 V. Mueller vascular l.
 Weber-Elschnig l.
 Wilder lens l.
 wire l.
loop-fixated intraocular lens
loop-type
 l.-t. snare forceps
 l.-t. stone-crushing forceps
Loopuyt needle
loose
 l. body forceps
 l. body grasper
 l. body suction forceps
Lopez-Reinke tonsillar dissector
Lo-Por
 L.-P. prosthesis
 L.-P. vascular graft
LoPresti
 L. fiberoptic esophagoscope
 L. panendoscope
Lo-Profile
 L.-P. balloon
 L.-P. balloon catheter
 L.-P. II balloon catheter
 L.-P. steerable dilatation
  catheter
**Loptex laser intraocular lens
 implant**
Lordan chalazion forceps
Lord-Blakemore tube
Lore
 L. forceps
 L. subglottic forceps

L. suction tip-holding
forceps
L. suction tube
L. suction tube-holding
forceps
L. tendon grip forceps
Lore-Lawrence tracheotomy tube
Lorenz brace
Lorenzo
L. reamer
L. screw
L. SMO prosthesis
Lorie
L. antral trephine
L. cheek retractor
L. retractor
Lorna
L. nonperforating towel
clamp
L. nonperforating towel
forceps
Loth-Kirschner drill
Lothrop
L. dissector
L. forceps
L. hemostat
L. ligature forceps
L. retractor
L. tonsillar knife
L. tonsillar retractor
L. uvula retractor
Lottes
L. nail
L. pin
L. reamer
L. triflange intramedullary
nail
Loughnane prostatic hook
Louisville elevator
Lounsbury
L. curette
L. placental curette
loupe (*See also* loop)
Amenabar lens l.
Arlt lens l.
Atwood l.
Aus-Jena-Gullstrand lens l.
Bausch and Lomb
Duoloupe lens l.
Beck l.
Beebe lens l.
Berens lens l.
Berger l.

Berget lens l.
binocular l.
Callahan lens l.
Clayman-Knolle lens l.
Codman lens l.
Codman magnifying l.
corneal monocular l.
Daviel lens l.
Denlan magnifying l.
Duoloupe lens l.
fiberoptic l.
Gill-Welsh lens l.
Gill-Welsh-Morrison lens l.
Gullstrand lens l.
Gullstrand-Zeiss lens l.
irrigating lens l.
Keeler spotlight lens l.
Keeler wide-angle lens l.
Kirby double-curve lens l.
Kirby intracapsular lens l.
Kleinsasser lens l.
Lempert-Storz lens l.
lens l.
Lewis lens l.
Magill magnifying l.
l. magnification
Magni focuser lens l.
Mark II lens l.
May hook-on lens l.
New Orleans lens l.
Oculus lens l.
Opticaid lens l.
Optivisor lens l.
prism l.
Simcoe nucleus lens l.
Stierlen lens l.
Storz Universal lens l.
surgical l.
Troutman lens l.
Ward-Lempert lens l.
Weber-Elschnig lens l.
Wilder lens l.
Zein l.
Zeiss lens l.
Lours leukotome
Loute wire tightener
Lovac
L. fundus contact lens
L. six-mirror gonioscopic
lens
Love
L. leukotome
L. nasal splint

Love *(continued)*
    L. nasopharyngeal retractor
    L. nerve retractor
    L. nerve root retractor
    L. retractor
    L. uvula retractor
Love-Adson
    L.-A. elevator
    L.-A. periosteal elevator
Love-Gruenwald
    L.-G. alligator forceps
    L.-G. forceps
    L.-G. intervener
    L.-G. intervertebral disk
      rongeur
    L.-G. laminectomy rongeur
    L.-G. pituitary forceps
    L.-G. pituitary rongeur
    L.-G. rongeur
Lovejoy retractor
Love-Kerrison
    L.-K. forceps
    L.-K. rongeur
    L.-K. rongeur forceps
Lovelace
    L. bladder forceps
    L. forceps
    L. gallbladder traction
      forceps
    L. hemostatic forceps
    L. hemostatic tissue forceps
    L. lung forceps
    L. lung-grasping forceps
    L. thyroid-traction forceps
    L. thyroid-traction vulsellum
      forceps
    L. tissue forceps
    L. traction lung forceps
    L. traction tissue forceps
Loversan infusion set
Löw-Beer forceps
low-contact stress plate
low-density lipoprotein (LDL)
Lowe-Breck cartilage knife
Lowell
    L. glaucoma knife
    L. needle
    L. pleural needle
Lowe microtome knife
Löwenberg forceps
Löwenstein lithotrite
lower
    l. forceps

l. gall duct forceps
l. lateral forceps
l. occlusive clamp
Lowette needle
Lowette-Verner needle
Lowis
    L. intervertebral disk
      forceps
    L. IV disk rongeur forceps
    L. periosteal elevator
Lowman
    L. bone clamp
    L. bone-holding clamp
    L. bone-holding forceps
    L. clamp
    L. forceps
    L. hand retractor
    L. retractor
Lowman-Gerster bone clamp
Lowman-Hoglund clamp
low-power optics for myopic
  correction lens
low-profile
    l.-p. breast implant
    l.-p. mitral heart valve
    l.-p. prosthesis
    l.-p. valve
    l.-p. with antisiphon valve
Lowsley
    L. forceps
    L. grasping forceps
    L. needle
    L. prostate retractor
    L. prostatic forceps
    L. prostatic lobe-holding
      forceps
    L. prostatic tractor
    L. retractor
    L. ribbon-gut needle
Lowsley-Luc forceps
Lowsley-Peterson
    L.-P. cystoscope
    L.-P. endoscope
low-viscosity bone cement
low-viscosity cement (LVC)
L-plate plate
LPS
    LPS balloon
    LPS catheter
L-resection guide
L-rod
    L-r. implant material
    L-r. instrumentation

L-shaped elevator
LSU reciprocation-gait orthosis brace
Luango curette
Lubafax dressing
Lubke-Berci Versa-lite
Lubrajel lubricating jelly
lubricant
    instrument l.
    Weck-Kare instrument l.
    Weck-Lube instrument l.
    Wec-Kreem instrument l.
Luc
    L. ethmoidal forceps
    L. forceps
    L. nasal-cutting forceps
    L. septal forceps
    L. septum-cutting forceps
Lucae
    L. bayonet
    L. bayonet dressing forceps
    L. bayonet ear forceps
    L. bayonet tissue forceps
    L. bone hammer
    L. bone mallet
    L. dissecting forceps
    L. dressing forceps
    L. ear forceps
    L. ear perforation knife
    L. ear probe
    L. ear speculum
    L. eustachian catheter
    L. forceps
    L. hook
    L. mallet
    L. mastoid mallet
    L. probe
Lucas
    L. chisel
    L. curette
    L. gouge
Lucchese mitral valve dilator
lucite
    l. eye implant
    l. implant
    l. sphere implant
Luck
    L. bone drill
    L. bone saw
    L. drill
    L. fasciatome
Luck-Bishop saw

LUD
    left uterine displacement device
        LUD device
Ludwig middle ear applicator
Luedde exophthalmometer
Luer
    L. adapter
    L. bone curette
    L. bone rongeur
    L. connector
    L. curette
    L. eye speculum
    L. fenestrated lens scoop
    L. forceps
    L. hemorrhoidal forceps
    L. lock
    L. lock adapter
    L. lock connector
    L. lock needle
    L. mallet
    L. needle
    L. reconstruction plate
    L. retractor
    L. rongeur
    L. rongeur forceps
    L. speaking tube
    L. "S" retractor
    L. suction cannula adapter
    L. thoracic rongeur
    L. tracheal cannula
    L. tracheal double-ended retractor
    L. tracheal retractor
    L. tracheal tube
    L. tube
Luer-Friedmann rongeur
Luer-Hartmann rongeur
Luer-Koerte gallstone scoop
Luer-Liston-Wheeling rongeur
Luer-Stille rongeur
Luer-Whiting
    L.-W. forceps
    L.-W. rongeur forceps
Luhr
    L. fixation system
    L. implant screw
    L. mandibular plate
    L. MCS bone plate
    L. microbone plate
    L. mini fixation bone plate
    L. MRS system
    L. screw

Luikart
    L. forceps
Luikart-Bill
    L.-B. forceps
    L.-B. traction handle
Luikart-Kjelland
    L.-K. forceps
    L.-K. obstetrical forceps
Luikart-McLane forceps
Luikart-Simpson
    L.-S. forceps
    L.-S. obstetrical forceps
Lukens
    L. aspirator
    L. bone wax dressing
    L. cannula
    L. catgut suture
    L. collector
    L. double-channel irrigator
    L. epiglottic retractor
    L. orthodontic band
    L. retractor
    L. thymus retractor
    L. tracheal double-ended
      retractor
    L. tracheal retractor
Lulu clamp
Lumaguide infusion catheter
lumbar
    l. accessory instrument
    l. accessory set
    l. aortography needle
    l. peritoneal catheter
    l. puncture needle
    l. retractor
    l. subarachnoid catheter
    l. suture
Lumbard airway
lumbosacral support pelvic traction
lumbotomy retractor
lumbrical bar
Lumelec catheter
lumen
    l. cannula
    l. finder
Lumi alloy
LUMINA
    L. operating telescope
    L. rod lens arthroscope
    L.-SL telescope
Lumix dental x-ray unit
lunate implant
Lunderquist guide wire

Lunderquist-Ring torque guide
Lundholm
    L. plate
    L. screw
Lundia dialyzer holder
Lundsgaard
    L. blade
    L. sclerotome
Lundsgaard-Burch
    L.-B. corneal rasp
    L.-B. knife
    L.-B. sclerotome
Lundy
    L. fascial needle
    L. laryngoscope
    L. needle
    L. tubing hand roller
Lundy-Irving
    L.-I. caudal needle
    L.-I. needle
Lundy tubing hand-roller
lung
    l. clamp
    l. dissecting scissors
    l. exclusion clamp
    l. forceps
    l. instrument
    Kolobow membrane l.
    membrane artificial l.
    l. retractor
    Sci-Med Life Systems, Inc.
      membrane artificial l.
    l. tissue forceps
lung-grasping forceps
Luongo
    L. cannula
    L. curette
    L. hand retractor
    L. needle
    L. retractor
    L. septal elevator
    L. sphenoid irrigating
      cannula
Lurz-Goltner ligator
Lusskin
    L. bone drill
    L. drill
    L. subungual hematoma
      iron
Luster investment material
Luther-Peter
    L.-P. lid everter
    L.-P. retractor

Lutz
- L. forceps
- L. septal forceps
- L. septal ridge-cutting forceps
- L. septal ridge forceps

Luxo illuminated magnifier
Luys separator
LV
- left ventricular
- LV apex cannula

LVAD
- left ventricular assist device

LVC
- low-viscosity cement

Lyda Ivalon-Lucite orbital implant
Lyman-Smith
- L.-S. brace
- L.-S. toe drop brace
- L.-S. tractor

lymphoma implant
Lynch
- L. blunt dissector
- L. cup-shaped curette forceps
- L. curette
- L. dissector
- L. electrode
- L. forceps
- L. knife

- L. laryngeal dissector
- L. laryngeal forceps
- L. laryngeal knife handle
- L. laryngoscope
- L. mucosa separator plate
- L. obtuse-angle laryngeal knife
- L. right-angle knife
- L. scissors
- L. septal splint
- L. spatula
- L. straight knife
- L. suspension apparatus
- L. suspension laryngoscope
- L. tonsillar dissector
- L. tonsillar knife

Lynell intraocular lens
LYOfoam
- L. C dressing
- L. dressing
- L. wound dressing

Lyon
- L. forceps
- L. tube

lyophilized graft
Lyster water bag
Lytle
- L. metacarpal splint
- L. suture

M

M Beaver blade
M bur (M-1, M-2, etc.)

3M

3M drape
3M dressing
3M filling instrument
3M intraocular lens
3M limb isolation bag
3M mammary implant
3M matrix tape
3M Vi-drape

MacAusland

M. bone mallet
M. chisel
M. dissector
M. finishing-ball reamer
M. finishing-cup reamer
M. hip skid
M. muscle retractor
M. reamer
M. retractor
M. skid

MacAusland-Kelly retractor
MacCallum knife
MacDonald

M. clamp
M. dissector
M. gastric clamp
M. periosteal elevator

Macewen

M. drill
M. saw

Macey tendon carrier
MacGregor

M. conjunctival forceps
M. forceps
M. mules

Machemer

M. calipers
M. diamond-dusted forceps
M. magnifying vitrectomy
lens
M. scleral knife
M. VISC vitrector

Machida

M. fiber-duodenoscope
M. fiberoptic laryngoscope
M. flexible endoscope
M. laryngoscope

machine

AK-10 dialysis m.
Cavitron m.
Cavitron-Kelman
phacoemulsification m.
CooperVision I&A m.
Drake-Willard
hemodialysis m.
Drake-Willock dialysis m.
Epilatron hair-removal m.
Fresenius dialysis m.
I&A m.
Narkomed anesthesia m.
Narkomed subcompact
anesthesia m.
Portadial kidney m.

MacIntosh

M. blade
M. fiberoptic laryngoscope
blade
M. implant
M. laryngoscope
M. stainless steel
laryngoscope blade
M. tibial plateau prosthesis

Mack

M. ear plug
M. lingual tonsillar
tonsillectome
M. serrefine
M. tonometer

MacKay

M. contour retractor
M. contour self-retaining
retractor
M. nasal splint
M. retractor

Mackay-Marg tonometer
MacKenty

M. cleft palate knife
M. forceps
M. laryngectomy tube
M. periosteal elevator
M. scissors
M. septal elevator
M. sphenoidal punch
M. tissue forceps

**MacKenty-Converse periosteal
elevator**

Mackler
    M. intraluminal tube
    M. intraluminal tube
      prosthesis
MacKool capsule retractor
Maclay tonsillar scissors
Mac-Lee enema bag
MacNab-English shoulder
    prosthesis
MacNamara cataract spoon
Macon Hospital speculum
MacQuigg-Mixter forceps
Macrofit hip prosthesis
macromanipulators
    Microbeam I, II, III, IV m.
MacroVac
Macula retinoscope
Madayag needle
Madden
    M. clamp
    M. dissector
    M. forceps
    M. intestinal clamp
    M. ligature carrier
    M. sympathectomy hook
Madden-Potts
    M.-P. forceps
    M.-P. intestinal forceps
    M.-P. tissue forceps
Maddox
    M. caudal needle
    M. needle
    M. rod
Madoff suction tube
Maestro
    M. implantable cardiac
      pacemaker
    M. pacemaker
magazine clip
Magicap
    Coltene M.
Magielski
    M. bayonet canal knife
    M. chisel
    M. coagulating forceps
    M. coagulation cautery
    M. coagulator
    M. curette
    M. elevator
    M. forceps
    M. hook
    M. needle
    M. stapes chisel

    M. tonsillar forceps
    M. tonsil-seizing forceps
Magielski-Heermann
    M.-H. forceps
    M.-H. strut forceps
Magill
    M. band
    M. catheter forceps
    M. catheter-introducing
      forceps
    M. endotracheal catheter
    M. endotracheal cathether-
      introducing forceps
    M. endotracheal forceps
    M. forceps
    M. laryngoscope
    M. magnifying loupe
    M. orthodontic band
    M. tube
Maglinte catheter
Magnatone hearing aid
magnesium tuning fork
Magneson strut
magnet
    Alnico Magneprobe m.
    Atlas-Storz eye m.
    Berman m.
    Bonaccolto m.
    Bronson m.
    Bronson-Magnion m.
    Coronet m.
    Equen stomach m.
    eye m.
    Firlene eye m.
    Grafco m.
    Gruening eye m.
    Haab eye m.
    Hirschberg electromagnet m.
    Holinger m.
    Holinger bronchoscopic m.
    Holinger endoscopic m.
    horseshoe m.
    Lancaster m..
    Mellinger m.
    Mueller giant eye m.
    Norris tip m.
    Patel intraocular m.
    Ralks m.
    Ralks eye m.
    Schumann giant eye m.
    Scientronics m.
    Storz-Atlas eye m.
    suction m.

surgical power m.
Sweet eye m.
Szulc eye m.
Thomas m.
Trowbridge-Campau eye m.
Wildgen-Reck metal
  locator m.
magnetic
  m. cup
  m. extractor
  m. eye implant
  m. eye probe
  m. implant
  m. retriever
Magnevist contrast material
magnifier
  anastigmatic aural m.
  aural m.
  Bruening aural m.
  Bruening Japanese
    anastigmatic aural m.
  Bruening-Storz anastigmatic
    aural m.
  ear speculum with m.
  Japanese Bruening m.
  Japanese Bruening
    anastigmatic aural m.
  Luxo illuminated m.
  Storz-Bruening m.
  Storz-Bruening anastigmatic
    aural m.
Magni focuser lens loupe
magnifying glasses
Magnuson
  M. abduction humeral
    splint
  M. circular twin saw
  M. double counter-rotating
    saw
  M. single circular saw
  M. twist drill
  M. valve prosthesis
Magnuson-Cromie prosthesis
Magovern
  4-A M. heart valve
  M. heart valve
Magovern-Cromie
  M.-C. heart valve
  M.-C. prosthesis
Magrina-Bookwalter
  M.-B. vaginal Deaver blade
  M.-B. vaginal lateral blade

M.-B. vaginal posterior
  blade
M.-B. vaginal retractor
M.-B. vaginal retractor ring
Maguire-Harvey cutter
Mahoney
  M. dilator
  M. intranasal antral
    speculum
Mahorner
  M. dilator
  M. retractor
  M. thyroid retractor
Mahurkar
  M. catheter
  M. dual-lumen dialysis
    catheter
  M. dual-lumen femoral
    catheter
  M. fistular needle
Maier
  M. dressing forceps
  M. forceps
  M. polyp forceps
  M. sponge forceps
  M. uterine-dressing forceps
  M. uterine forceps
Mailler
  M. colon forceps
  M. cut-off forceps
  M. intestinal forceps
  M. rectal forceps
Maine gonioscope
Maingot
  M. clamp
  M. gallbladder tube
  M. hysterectomy forceps
maintainer
  anterior chamber m.
  filter m.
  Gerber space m.
  Lewicky m.
  self-retaining chamber m.
Maisonneuve
  M. bandage
  M. urethrotome
Maison retractor
Majewski nasal curette
Major
major
  m. airway
  m. connector bar
Major amblyoscope

Maki scissors
Maklakoff tonometer
Mala-paedic shoe
malar implant
Malcolm-Rand cranial x-ray frame
male catheter
Malecot
    M. catheter
    M. drain
    M. four-wing drain
    M. nephrostomy catheter
    M. self-retaining urethral
      catheter
    M. Silastic catheter
    M. suprapubic catheter
    M. suprapubic cystostomy
      catheter
    M. two-wing drain
    M. urethral catheter
    M. 2-wing catheter
    M. 4-wing catheter
    M. 2-wing drain
    M. 4-wing drain
male/female washer
Malette-Spencer coronary cannula
Malgaigne
    M. apparatus
    M. clamp
    M. patellar hook
Maliniac
    M. nasal brace
    M. nasal rasp
    M. nasal retractor
    M. retractor
Malis
    M. angled-up bipolar
      forceps
    M. bipolar coagulation
      forceps
    M. bipolar coagulator
    M. bipolar cutting forceps
    M. bipolar irrigating forceps
    M. brain retractor kit
    M. cerebellar retractor
    M. cerebral retractor
    M. clip applier
    M. CMC-II PC bipolar
      coagulator
    M. coagulator
    M. cup forceps
    M. curette
    M. dissector
    M. elevator

    M. forceps
    M. hinge clamp
    M. irrigating forceps stylet
    M. irrigation tubing set
    M. ligature passer
    M. needle holder
    M. nerve hook
    M. neurosurgical scissors
    M. retractor
    M. scissors
    M. titanium microsurgical
      forceps
    M. vessel supporter
Malis-Frazier suction tube
Malis-Jensen
    M.-J. bipolar forceps
    M.-J. forceps
Malith pacemaker
malleable
    m. blade
    m. blade retractor
    m. copper retractor
    m. passing needle
    m. probe
    m. retractor
    m. ribbon retractor
    m. spatula
    m. stainless steel retractor
    m. stylet
mallet
    Bakelite m.
    Bergman m.
    Blount nylon m.
    bone m.
    Boxwood m.
    brass m.
    Brown m.
    Carroll aluminum m.
    cervical m.
    Chandler m.
    Children's Hospital m.
    copper m.
    Cottle m.
    Crane m.
    fiber m.
    Gerzog m.
    Hajek m.
    Heath m.
    Hibbs m.
    Jarit m.
    Kirk m.
    Kirk orthopaedic m.
    lead-filled m.

Lucae m.
Lucae bone m.
Lucae mastoid m.
Luer m.
MacAusland bone m.
Mead m.
Meyerding m.
nasal m.
nylon face m.
nylon head m.
Ombrédanne m.
Ralks m.
Rica bone m.
Richards combination m.
Rissler m.
Rush m.
slotted m.
SMIC surgical m.
Smith-Petersen m.
solid copper head m.
standard pattern m.
Stille m.
surgical m.
White m.
malleus
m. cutter
m. forceps
m. nipper
malleus-incus prosthesis
Mallinckrodt
M. angiographic catheter
M. catheter
M. Laser-Flex tube
Mallor pacemaker
Mallory-Head
M.-H. hip prosthesis
M.-H. Interlok calcar
trimmer
M.-H. Interlok primary
femoral component
M.-H. Interlok rasp
M.-H. Interlok reamer
M.-H. modular acetabular
template
M.-H. porous primary
femoral prosthesis
Malm-Himmelstein pulmonary
valvulotome
malomaxillary suture
Maloney
M. catheter
M. dilator
M. endo-otoprobe

M. esophageal dilator
M. mercury-filled dilator
M. mercury-filled esophageal
dilator
M. no-hole lens manipulator
M. tapered bougie
M. tapered mercury-filled
esophageal bougie
M. tapered-tip dilator
malsensing pacemaker
Malström vacuum extractor
Malström-Westman cannula
Malteno tube implant material
Maltese cross lens
Maltz
M. bayonet saw
M. button-end knife
M. cartilage knife
M. nasal rasp
M. needle
M. rasp
M. retractor
Maltz-Anderson
M.-A. nasal rasp
M.-A. rasp
Maltz-Lipsett
M.-L. nasal rasp
M.-L. rasp
Maltzman needle
mamillary suture
Mammalok
M. localization needle
M. needle
mammary
m. implant
m. prosthesis
m. support dressing
mammary-coronary tissue forceps
Mammatech breast prosthesis
mammometer
mammotone
Jacobus m.
Rogers m.
Manan needle
Manchester
M. knee replacement
M. nasal osteotome
M. ovoid
Manchu cotton dressing
Mancke flex-rigid gastroscope
Mancusi-Ungaro scissors
Mandelbaum
M. cannula

Mandelbaum *(continued)*
    M. catheter
    M. ear knife
mandibular
    m. arch bar
    m. mesh
mandrel
mandril graft
mandrin
    m. dilator
    wire m.
Mangoldt epithelial graft
Manhattan
    M. Eye and Ear corneal
      dissector
    M. Eye and Ear probe
    M. Eye and Ear spatula
    M. Eye and Ear suturing
      forceps
Mani
    M. catheter
    M. cerebral catheter
manifold
manipulator
    Barrett flange lens m.
    Barrett irrigating lens m.
    button lip lens m.
    Feaster lens m.
    Gall-Addison uterine m.
    Hirschman lens m.
    hook m.
    Hulka uterine m.
    iris lens m.
    irrigating lens m.
    Jaffe-Maltzman lens m.
    Kuglen angled lens m.
    Kuglen lens m.
    Kuglen straight lens m.
    lens m.
    Lester lens m.
    Levy-Kuglen lens m.
    Maloney no-hole lens m.
    McIntyre irrigating iris m.
    Osher nucleus lens m.
    Sinskey lens m.
    Smith-Leiske lens m.
    uterine m.
manipulator/injector
    Harris-Kronner uterine m./i.
Mannerfelt
    M. chisel
    M. gouge

    M. raspatory
    M. retractor
Mann forceps
Manning
    M. forceps
    M. retractor
Mannis suture probe
manometer-tipped catheter
Mansfield
    M. balloon
    M. balloon catheter
    M. balloon dilatation
      catheter
    M. dilatation balloon
      catheter
    M. forceps
Manson-Aebli corneal scissors
Manson double-ended strabismus
    hook
Mantel laryngoscope
Mantisol drain
Mantoux needle
Mantz
    M. dilator
    M. rectal dilator
manual
    m. dermatome
    m. dermatome adapter
    m. dermatome brush
    m. dermatome thickness
      gauge
    m. esthesiometer
    m. lithotriptor
    m. osteotome
    m. resuscitation bag
    m. retractor
    m. surgical chisel
many-tailed
    m.-t. bandage
    m.-t. dressing
MAPF (textured surface) femoral
    stem
Maquet
    M. operating table
    M. velox table
Marax dilator
Marbach episiotomy scissors
Marble bone pin
March-Barton forceps
March laser sclerostomy needle
Marcks knife

Marco
    M. ARK-2000 refractor
    M. keratometer
Marcon Colon Decompression set
Marcon-Haber varices injector
Marcuse
    M. forceps
    M. tube clamp
Mardis-Dangler ureteral stent set
marginal
    m. chalazion forceps
    m. clamp
margin-finishing knife
Margolis appliance
Margulies intrauterine device
Marici bronchoscope
Marin
    M. bur
    M. reamer
Marino
    M. rotatable transsphenoidal enucleator
    M. rotatable transsphenoidal horizontal-ring curette
    M. rotatable transsphenoidal instrument set
    M. rotatable transsphenoidal knife handle
    M. rotatable transsphenoidal right-angle hook
    M. rotatable transsphenoidal round dissector
    M. rotatable transsphenoidal spatula dissector
    M. rotatable transsphenoidal vertical-ring curette
Marion
    M. drain
    M. oxygen resuscitation system
    M. screw
Marion-Reverdin needle
Mark
    M. II Chandler retractor
    M. II lens loupe
    M. III halo system
Mark-7 intrauterine sound
marker
    Accu-Line surgical m.
    CA 125 serum tumor m.
    Castroviejo scleral m.
    Codman m.
    corneal m.
    Donahoo m.
    face-lift m.
    Feldman radial keratotomy m.
    fine-line tissue m.
    Gass scleral m.
    Glomark fluorescent skin m.
    gold ear m.
    Gonin-Amsler m.
    Gonnin-Amsler scleral m.
    Green corneal m.
    Green-Kenyon m.
    Green-Kenyon corneal m.
    Green optical crater m.
    Hoffer corneal m.
    Hoffer optical center corneal m.
    House-Urban m.
    interspace width m.
    Kremer triple-optical zone corneal m.
    Mickey and Minnie surgical m.
    Neumann double m.
    Neumann double-corneal m.
    Neumann-Shepard corneal m.
    Neumann-Shepard optical center m.
    Neumann-Shepard optical center corneal m.
    Neumann-Shepard oval optical center m.
    O'Connor scleral m.
    ocular m.
    Oshar-Newmann 8-line corneal m.
    Osher-Neumann m.
    Osher-Neumann corneal m.
    oval optical zone m.
    radial keratotomy m.
    RK m.
    round optical zone m.
    Ruiz adjustable m.
    Ruiz-Shepard m.
    Saunders-Paparella m.
    scleral m.
    Shepard optical center m.
    Simcoe corneal m.
    skin m.
    Sklar scribe skin m.
    Thornton corneal m.
    Thornton low-profile m.

marker *(continued)*
    Thornton optical center m.
    T-incision m.
    TLS surgical m.
    trephine m.
    vein graft ring m.
    Vismark surgical skin m.
    window rasp m.
marker-calipers
Markham biopsy needle
Markham-Meyerding
    M.-M. hemilaminectomy
      retractor
    M.-M. retractor
marking
    m. calipers
    m. pen
    m. scissors
Markley
    M. orthodontic wire
    M. retention pin
    M. retractor
Markwalder
    M. forceps
    M. rib rongeur
Marlen
    M. biliary drainage kit
    M. colostomy appliance
    M. ileostomy bag
    M. leg bag
    M. weightless bag
Marlex
    M. band
    M. bandage
    M. mesh graft
    M. mesh implant
    M. mesh prosthesis
    M. mesh snare
    M. methyl methacrylate
      prosthesis
    M. suture
Marlin thoracic catheter
Marlow
    M. Surgical Technologies,
      Inc. diagnostic laparoscope
    M. Surgical Technologies,
      Inc. operating laparoscope
Marmor modular knee prosthesis
Maroon-Jannetta dissector
Maroon lip curette
Marquardt bone rongeur
Marquez-Gomez conjunctival graft
Marshall V-suture

Marshik
    M. forceps
    M. tonsillar forceps
    M. tonsil-seizing forceps
Marstock apparatus
Martel
    M. clamp
    M. conductor
    M. intestinal clamp
Marten hair eye brush
Martin
    M. abdominal retractor
    M. ballpoint scissors
    M. bandage
    M. bipolar coagulation
      forceps
    M. blade
    M. bur
    M. cartilage clamp
    M. cartilage forceps
    M. cartilage scissors
    M. cheek retractor
    M. clamp
    M. dermal curette
    M. diamond wire cutter
    M. endarterectomy stripper
    M. forceps
    M. hip gouge
    M. hook
    M. laryngectomy tube
    M. lip retractor
    M. meniscal forceps
    M. muscle clamp
    M. nasopharyngeal biopsy
      forceps
    M. nasopharyngeal forceps
    M. needle
    M. nerve root retractor
    M. palate retractor
    M. pelvimeter
    M. probe
    M. rectal hook
    M. rectal hook retractor
    M. rectal speculum
    M. retractor
    M. rubber dressing
    M. snare
    M. tenaculum
    M. throat scissors
    M. thumb forceps
    M. tissue forceps
    M. tracheostomy tube
    M. uterine fistula probe

M. uterine needle
M. uterine sound
M. uterine tenaculum
   forceps
M. vaginal retractor
M. vaginal speculum
Martinex knife-dissector
Martinez
M. corneal dissector knife
M. corneal trephine
M. disposable trephine
M. double-ended corneal
   dissector
M. scleral centering ring
Martinez-Castro keratome
Martini bone curette
Marx needle
Maryan
M. biopsy punch forceps
M. forceps
Maryfield
M. introducer
M. introducer catheter
Mary Jane breast pump
Masciuli silicone sponge
Mashemer cutter
Masing needle holder
mask
isolation face m.
Rudolph m.
surgical m. *bag valve mask*

Mason
M. clamp
M. leg holder
M. splint
M. suction tube
M. tonsil suction dissector
M. vascular clamp
Mason-Allen
M.-A. hand splint
M.-A. snare
M.-A. Universal hand splint
**Mason-Auvard weighted vaginal
speculum**
Mason-Judd
M.-J. bladder retractor
M.-J. retractor
M.-J. self-retaining retractor
Mason-School aspirating needle
**Massachusetts General Hospital
(MGH)**
Massie
M. driver

M. extractor
M. II nail
M. II plate
M. screwdriver
M. sliding nail
M. sliding nail tube
Masson
M. fascial needle
M. fascial stripper
M. fasciatome
M. needle
M. needle holder
M. Vital needle holder
Masson-Luethy needle holder
Masson-Mayo-Hegar needle holder
mastectomy skin flap retractor
Master
M. Flow Pumpette
M. screwdriver
MasterCraft hearing aid
Masters intestinal clamp
Masterson
M. clamp
M. curved clamp
M. hysterectomy forceps
M. pelvic clamp
M. straight clamp
Masters-Schwartz
M.-S. intesstinal clamp
M.-S. liver clamp
Mastin
M. clamp
M. goiter forceps
M. muscle clamp
M. muscle forceps
M. muscle tissue forceps
mastoid
m. bone bur
m. bur
m. catheter
m. chisel
m. curette
m. dressing
m. gouge
m. probe
m. retractor
m. rongeur
m. rongeur forceps
m. searcher
m. self-retaining retractor
m. suction tube
m. suture
mastoid-retaining retractor

Masy angioscope
mat
    m. holder
    silicone-spiked m.
Matas
    M. band
    M. vessel band
Matchett-Brown
    M.-B. hip endoprosthesis
    M.-B. prosthesis
    M.-B. stem rasp
material (*See also* implant material)
    ACCO impression m.
    Accuflex impression m.
    Accu-Gel impression m.
    Accu-Mix impression m.
    Adaptic II dental
      restorative m.
    Agarloid impression m.
    Algee impression m.
    Alginate impression m.
    Algitec impression m.
    Aneuroplast acrylic m.
    Angiovist contrast m.
    Astron investment m.
    Audisil silicone ear
      mold m.
    Augmen bone-grafting m.
    Aurovest investment m.
    barium contrast m.
    Castorit investment m.
    Celestin graft m.
    Coe impression m.
    Coe investment m.
    Coltene impression m.
    Coltex impression m.
    Compafill MH dental
      restorative m.
    Compalay dental
      restorative m.
    Compamolar dental
      restorative m.
    Conray contrast m.
    cranioplastic acrylic
      cranioplasty m.
    Cristobalite investment m.
    Cystografin contrast m.
    Dentemp filling m.
    Dentloid impression m.
    Derma-Sil impression m.
    diatrizoate contrast m.
    Diviplast impression m.

    Durafill dental
      restorative m.
    Endur bonding m.
    Estilux dental restorative m.
    E-Z M barium contrast m.
    Fastcure denture repair m.
    Flexistone impression m.
    Fotofil dental restorative m.
    Gastrografin contrast m.
    G-C Vest investment m.
    gold weight and wire spring
      implant m.
    Hexabrix contrast m.
    Hircoe denture base m.
    Hypaque contrast m.
    implant m.
    Impregum impression m.
    iohexol contrast m.
    Iopamidol contrast m.
    Langinate impression m.
    Luster investment m.
    Magnevist contrast m.
    Omniflex impression m.
    Omnipaque contrast m.
    Opotow filling m.
    Optiray contrast m.
    Ortho-Jel impression m.
    Palfique Estelite tooth
      shade resin m.
    Paradentine dental
      restorative m.
    Pearlon impression m.
    Perma-Cryl denture base m.
    Permatone denture m.
    Platorit investment m.
    Polybar contrast m.
    Porocoat m.
    Proplast II porous
      implant m.
    Proplast I porous
      implant m.
    Provit filling m.
    Pyrost bone replacement m.
    Ramitec bite m.
    Raybar 75 contrast m.
    Rayvist contrast m.
    Rema-Exakt investment m.
    Renografin contrast m.
    Scutan temporary splint m.
    Septosil impression m.
    Sili-Gel impression m.
    SMS investment m.

SR-Isosit dental
restorative m.
SR-Ivocap denture m.
SR-Ivolen impression m.
SR-Ivoseal impression m.
^{99m}Tc Cardiolyte
contrast m.
^{99m}Tc Cardiotech
contrast m.
^{99m}Tc disofenin contrast m.
^{99m}Tc DTPA contrast m.
^{99m}Tc MDP contrast m.
^{99m}Tc sulfur colloid
contrast m.
Tru-Chrome band m.
twisted cotton
nonabsorbable surgical
suture m.
Wirosol investment m.
Wirovest investment m.
Mathews
M. drill
M. drill point
M. hand drill
M. load drill
M. osteotome
M. rectal speculum
Mathieu
M. double-ended retractor
M. foreign body forceps
M. holder
M. needle
M. needle holder
M. pliers
M. raspatory
M. retractor
M. tongue forceps
M. tongue-seizing forceps
M. urethral forceps
Mathieu-Stille needle holder
Mathrop hemostat
matrix
ACCOR dental m.
m. band
Walser m.
Matson
M. raspatory
M. rib elevator
M. rib stripper
Matson-Alexander
M.-A. elevator
M.-A. raspatory
M.-A. rib stripper

Matson-Mead
M.-M. apicolysis retractor
M.-M. periosteum stripper
Matson-Plenk raspatory
**Matsuda titanium surgical
instruments**
Mattis
M. corneal scissors
M. scissors
Mattison-Upshaw retractor
Mattox aortic clamp
Mattox-Potts scissors
mattress suture
Matzenauer
M. speculum
M. vaginal speculum
Mauermayer
M. resectoscope
M. stone punch
Maumenee
M. blunt iris hook
M. corneal forceps
M. cross-action capsular
forceps
M. erysiphake
M. forceps
M. goniotomy knife
M. iris hook
M. knife
M. needle
M. sharp iris hook
M. straight-action capsule
forceps
M. tissue forceps
M. vitreous-aspirating needle
M. vitreous needle
**Maumenee-Barraquer vitreous
sweep spatula**
Maumenee-Colibri
M.-C. corneal forceps
M.-C. forceps
Maumenee-Park
M.-P. erysiphake
M.-P. eye speculum
Maunder oral screw mouth gag
Maunoir scissors
Maunsell suture
Max
M. Fine forceps
M. Fine tying forceps
M. Force biliary balloon
dilatation catheter
M. forceps

Maxam suture
Maxi-Driver driver
Maxilith
  M. pacemaker
  M. pacemaker pulse
  generator
maxillary
  m. arch bar
  m. disimpaction forceps
  m. fracture forceps
  m. sinus cannula
maxillofacial
  m. bone screw
  m. osteotome
Maxi-Myst nebulizer system
Max-I-Probe irrigation probe
Maxon
  M. absorbable suture
  M. suture
May
  M. hook-on lens loupe
  M. kidney clamp
  M. ophthalmoscope
Mayer
  M. forceps
  M. nasal splint
  M. pessary
Mayfield
  M. aneurysm clamp
  M. aneurysm forceps
  M. applying forceps
  M. bayonet osteotome
  M. CIS-RE aneurysm clip
  M. clip
  M. clip applicator
  M. clip applier
  M. curette
  M. forceps
  M. head holder
  M. instrument table
  M. malleable brain spatula
  M. pediatric horseshoe
  headrest
  M. pediatric horseshoe pad
  M. retractor
  M. skull clamp
  M. skull clamp adapter
  M. skull clamp pin
  M. skull pin
  M. spinal curette
  M. swivel horseshoe
  headrest
  M. tic head holder

Mayfield-Kees
  M.-K. clip
  M.-K. headrest
Mayo
  M. abdominal retractor
  M. bone-cutting forceps
  M. cannula
  M. carrier
  M. catgut needle
  M. clamp
  M. common duct probe
  M. common duct scoop
  M. coronary perfusion
  cannula
  M. coronary perfusion tip
  M. curved scissors
  M. cystic duct scoop
  M. dissecting scissors
  M. elbow prosthesis
  M. external vein stripper
  M. fibroid hook
  M. forceps
  M. gallbladder scoop
  M. gall duct scoop
  M. gallstone scoop
  M. goiter ligature carrier
  M. holder
  M. instrument table
  M. instrument tray
  M. intestinal needle
  M. kidney clamp
  M. kidney forceps
  M. kidney pedicle forceps
  M. kidney stone probe
  M. knife
  M. linen suture
  M. long dissecting scissors
  M. needle
  M. needle holder
  M. operating scissors
  M. perfusing "O" ring
  M. probe
  M. retractor
  M. round blade scissors
  M. scissors
  M. scoop
  M. stand
  M. straight scissors
  M. suture
  M. table
  M. tissue forceps
  M. total ankle prosthesis
  M. tray

M. trocar needle
M. trocar-point needle
M. ureter isolation forceps
M. uterine probe
M. uterine scissors
M. vein stripper
M. vessel clamp

Mayo-Adams
M.-A. appendectomy retractor
M.-A. retractor
M.-A. self-retaining retractor

Mayo-Blake
M.-B. gallstone forceps
M.-B. stone forceps

Mayo-Boldt inverter
Mayo-Collins
M.-C. appendectomy retractor
M.-C. double-ended retractor
M.-C. mastoid retractor
M.-C. retractor

Mayo-Guyon
M.-G. clamp
M.-G. kidney clamp
M.-G. vessel clamp

Mayo-Harrington
M.-H. dissecting scissors
M.-H. forceps
M.-H. scissors

Mayo-Hegar
M.-H. curved-jaw needle holder
M.-H. needle holder

Mayo-Lexer scissors
Mayo-Lovelace
M.-L. abdominal retractor
M.-L. clamp
M.-L. retractor
M.-L. spur crusher
M.-L. spur crushing clamp

Mayo-Myers
M.-M. external vein stripper
M.-M. stripper

Mayo-New scissors
Mayo-Noble
M.-N. dissecting scissors
M.-N. scissors

Mayo-Ochsner
M.-O. cannula
M.-O. forceps

M.-O. suction trocar cannula
M.-O. trocar

Mayo-Péan
M.-P. forceps
M.-P. hemostatic forceps

Mayo-Potts dissecting scissors
Mayo-Robson
M.-R. clamp
M.-R. forceps
M.-R. gallstone scoop
M.-R. gastrointestinal forceps
M.-R. intestinal clamp
M.-R. intestinal forceps

Mayo-Russian
M.-R. forceps
M.-R. gastrointestinal forceps
M.-R. tissue forceps

Mayo-Simpson retractor
Mayo-Sims
M.-S. dissecting scissors
M.-S. scissors

Mayo-Stille
M.-S. operating scissors
M.-S. scissors

Mazlin intrauterine device
Mazzacco flexible lens forceps
Mazzariello-Caprini
M.-C. stone forceps
M.-C. stone forceps sterilizing case

Mazzocco
M. compressible silicone lens
M. silicone intraocular lens

MB
MB band
MB fraction

McAllister
M. needle holder
M. scissors

McAtee
M. apparatus
M. compression screw device
M. olecranon device

McBratney aspirating speculum
McBride
M. cup
M. plate
M. prosthesis

McBride-Moore prosthesis
McBurney
 M. fenestrated retractor
 M. retractor
 M. thyroid retractor
McCabe
 M. antral retractor
 M. canal knife
 M. crurotomy saw
 M. crus guide fork
 M. facial nerve dissector
 M. flap knife dissector
 M. measuring instrument
 M. parotidectomy retractor
 M. perforation rasp
 M. posterior fossa retractor
McCabe-Farrior rasp
McCaffrey positioner
McCannel suture
McCarey-Kaufman solution
McCarthy
 M. bladder evacuator
 M. catheter
 M. coagulation electrode
 M. continuous-flow
 resectoscope
 M. diathermic knife
 electrode
 M. electrode
 M. endoscope
 M. fiberoptic Foroblique
 telescope
 M. forceps
 M. Foroblique operating
 telescope
 M. Foroblique panendoscope
 cystoscope
 M. fulgurating electrode
 M. infant electrotome
 M. loop operating electrode
 M. microlens resectoscope
 M. miniature electrotome
 M. miniature loop electrode
 M. miniature resectoscope
 M. miniature telescope
 M. multiple resectoscope
 M. punctate electrotome
 M. telescope
 M. visual forceps
 M. visual hemostatic
 forceps

McCarthy-Alcock
 M.-A. forceps
 M.-A. hemostatic forceps
McCarthy-Campbell miniature
 cystoscope
McCaskey
 M. antral catheter
 M. antral curette
 M. catheter
 M. curette
 M. sphenoid cannula
McCaslin
 M. knife-needle
 M. needle-knife
 M. wave-edge keratome
McCleery-Miller
 M.-M. clamp
 M.-M. intestinal anastomosis
 clamp
 M.-M. intestinal clamp
 M.-M. locking device
McClintock
 M. placental forceps
 M. uterine forceps
McClure iris scissors
McCollough
 M. elevator
 M. osteotome
 M. rasp
McConnell orthopaedic headrest
McCoy
 M. forceps
 M. septal forceps
 M. septum-cutting forceps
McCrae dilator
McCravey forceps
McCrea
 M. cystoscope
 M. infant sound
 M. sound
McCullough
 M. externofrontal retractor
 M. forceps
 M. hysterectomy clamp
 M. retractor
 M. strabismus forceps
 M. suture forceps
 M. suture-tying forceps
 M. suturing forceps
 M. utility forceps
McCurdy
 M. needle
 M. staphylorrhaphy needle

McDavid knee brace
McDermott
  M. clip
  M. extractor
  M. Surgiclip
McDonald clamp
McDowell
  M. mouth gag
  M. needle
McElroy curette
**McElveen-Hitselberger neural
  dissector**
McFadden
  M. aneurysm clip
  M. clip
  M. Surgiclip
  M. Vari-Angle aneurysm
  clip
  M. Vari-Angle clip applier
McFarland tibial graft
McGannon
  M. eye retractor
  M. forceps
  M. iris retractor
  M. lens forceps
  M. retractor
McGaw
  M. skinfold calipers
  M. tape measure
McGee
  M. canal elevator
  M. ear piston prosthesis
  M. footplate pick
  M. middle ear instrument
  M. needle perforating
  M. oval-window rasp
  M. piston
  M. prosthesis needle
  M. raspatory
  M. splint
  M. tympanoplasty knife
  M. wire-closure forceps
  M. wire crimper
  M. wire-crimping forceps
McGee-Caparosa wire crimper
McGee-Paparella
  M.-P. forceps
  M.-P. wire-crimping forceps
McGee-Priest
  M.-P. forceps
  M.-P. wire-closure forceps
  M.-P. wire crimper
  M.-P. wire-crimping forceps

McGee-Priest-Paparella
  M.-P.-P. closure forceps
  M.-P.-P. crimper-forceps
  M.-P.-P. forceps
McGhan
  M. breast implant
  M. breast prosthesis
  M. eye implant
  M. implant
  M. plastic surgical needle
McGill
  M. forceps
  M. neurological percussor
  M. retractor
McGivney
  M. hemorrhoidal forceps
  M. hemorrhoidal ligator
McGoey-Evans
  M.-E. acetabular cup
  M.-E. cup
McGoey Vitallium punch
**McGood coronary perfusion
  catheter**
McGoon
  M. cannula
  M. coronary perfusion
  catheter
McGowan-Keeley tube
McGowan needle
McGravey
  M. forceps
  M. tissue forceps
McGraw suture
McGregor
  M. conjunctival forceps
  M. forceps
  M. needle
McGuire
  M. clamp
  M. corneal scissors
  M. forceps
  M. marginal chalazion
  forceps
  M. rib spreader
  M. tendon tucker
McHenry
  M. forceps
  M. tonsillar artery forceps
  M. tonsillar forceps
McHugh
  M. facial nerve knife
  M. flap knife
  M. oval speculum

McHugh-Farrior canal knife
McIndoe
  M. bone-cutting forceps
  M. chisel
  M. dissecting forceps
  M. dressing forceps
  M. forceps
  M. nasal chisel
  M. rasp
  M. raspatory
  M. retractor
  M. rongeur forceps
  M. scissors
McIntire
  M. aspiration-irrigation
  system
  M. needle
  M. splint
McIntosh
  M. double-lumen catheter
  M. forceps
  M. hemodialysis catheter
  M. laryngoscope
  M. laryngoscope blade
  M. suture-holding forceps
McIntyre
  M. angled cannula
  M. anterior chamber
  cannula
  M. aspiration needle
  M. cannula
  M. coaxial cannula
  M. coaxial irrigating-
  aspirating system
  M. cystitome
  M. fish-hook needle holder
  M. guarded cystitome
  M. guarded irrigating
  cystitome set
  M. I&A system
  M. infusion handpiece
  M. infusion set
  M. irrigating hook
  M. irrigating iris hook
  M. irrigating iris
  manipulator
  M. irrigating spatula
  M. irrigation-aspiration
  system
  M. irrigation needle
  M. lacrimal cannula
  M. microhook
  M. nylon cannula connector

  M. reverse cystotome
  M. spatula
  M. staight ant. chamber
  cannula
  M. suture tamper
  M. truncated cone
McIntyre-Binkhorst irrigating
  cannula
McIver
  M. catheter
  M. nephrostomy catheter
McIvor
  M. mouth gag
  M. mouth gag tongue blade
McKay
  M. ear forceps
  M. forceps
McKee
  M. brace
  M. femoral prosthesis
  M. prosthesis
  M. speculum
  M. trifin nail
McKee-Farrar
  M.-F. acetabular cup
  M.-F. cup
  M.-F. hip prosthesis
McKeever
  M. cartilage knife
  M. patellar cap prosthesis
McKenna
  M. Tide-Ur-Ator evacuator
  M. Tide-Ur-Ator irrigator
McKenzie
  M. bone drill
  M. brain clip
  M. brain clip-applying
  forceps
  M. brain clip-cutting forceps
  M. bur
  M. clamp
  M. clip
  M. clip-applying forceps
  M. clip-holding rack
  M. clip-introducing forceps
  M. clip rack
  M. cranial drill
  M. drill
  M. enlarging bur
  M. forceps
  M. grasping forceps
  M. hemostasis clip
  M. leukotome

M. leukotomy loop
M. perforating twist drill
M. perforator drill
M. silver brain clip
M. silver clip
M. V-clip

McKesson
M. mouth gag
M. mouth probe
M. pneumothroax apparatus
M. suction bottle unit

McKinney
M. eye speculum
M. fixation ring
M. speculum

McKissock
M. areolar template
M. suture

McLane
M. obstetrical forceps
M. pile forceps

McLane-Luikart obstetrical forceps
McLane-Tucker-Kjelland forceps
McLane-Tucker-Luikart forceps
McLane-Tucker obstetrical forceps
McLaughlin
M. carpal scaphoid screw
M. hip plate
M. laser mirror
M. laser rod
M. laser vaginal measuring rod
M. nail
M. plate
M. quartz rod
M. speculum

McLean
M. capsular forceps
M. capsulotomy scissors
M. clamp
M. corneoscleral suture
M. ophthalmological forceps
M. prismatic fundus laser lens
M. tonometer

McLearie bone forceps
McLeod padded clavicular splint
McLight PCL brace
McMahon nephrostomy hook
McMaster bone graft
MCM smart laser
McMurray tenotomy knife
McMurtry-Schlesinger shunt tube

McNaught prosthesis
McNealey-Glassman
M.-G clamp
M.-G visceral retainer

McNealey-Glassman-Babcock forceps
McNealey-Glassman-Mixter
M.-G.-M. clamp
M.-G.-M. forceps
M.-G.-M. ligature-carrying aneurysm forceps

McNealey visceral retractor

McNeil-Goldman
M.-G blepharostat
M.-G blepharostat ring
M.-G scleral ring

McNutt
M. driver
M. extractor

MCP
metacarpophalangeal

McPherson
M. angled bipolar forceps
M. angled forceps
M. corneal forceps
M. corneal section scissors
M. curved bipolar iris forceps
M. eye speculum
M. forceps
M. iris spatula
M. irrigating forceps
M. lens forceps
M. microbipolar forceps
M. microconjunctival scissors
M. microcorneal forceps
M. micro-iris forceps
M. micropin forceps
M. microsurgery eye needle holder
M. microsuture forceps
M. microtenotomy scissors
M. micro-utility suture scissors
M. needle holder
M. rack
M. speculum
M. straight bipolar forceps
M. straight bipolar iris forceps
M. suture-tying forceps
M. suturing forceps

McPherson *(continued)*
  M. trabeculotome
  M. tying forceps
McPherson-Castroviejo
  M.-C. corneal scissors
  M.-C. forceps
  M.-C. microcorneal scissors
McPherson-Pierse
  M.-P. forceps
  M.-P. microcorneal forceps
  M.-P. microsuturing forceps
McPherson-Vannas
  M.-V. micro-iris scissors
  M.-V. scissors
McPherson-Westcott
  M.-W. conjunctival scissors
  M.-W. scissors
  M.-W. stitch scissors
McPherson-Wheeler
  M.-W. blade
  M.-W. eye knife
McPherson-Ziegler micro-iris knife
McQuigg
  M. clamp
  M. forceps
  M. right-angle clamp
McQuigg-Mixter
  M.-M. bronchial forceps
  M.-M. forceps
McReynolds
  M. driver
  M. driver-extractor
  M. extractor
  M. eye spatula
  M. lid-retracting hook
  M. pterygium keratome
  M. pterygium knife
  M. pterygium scissors
McReynolds-Castroviejo
  M.-C. keratome
  M.-C. pterygium knife
McShirley amalgamator
McWhinnie
  M. dissector
  M. electrode
  M. tonsillar dissector
McWhorter
  M. hemostat
  M. tonsillar forceps
MD brace
MDP
  methylene diphosphonate

MDS
  MDS adhesive
  MDS Truspot articulating film
Meacham-Scoville forceps
Mead
  M. bone rongeur
  M. bridge remover
  M. crown remover
  M. dental rongeur
  M. lancet knife
  M. mallet
Meadox
  M. dacron mesh
  M. Dardik biograft
  M. graft sizer
  M. ICP monitor
  M. Microvel double-velour Dacron graft
  M. Microvel graft
  M. Surgimed cathether
  M. Teflon felt pledget
  M. vascular graft
measure
  McGaw tape m.
  special distance m.
measuring
  m. gauge
  m. guide
  m. instrument
  m. rod
Measuroll suture
meat
  m. forceps
  m. hook retractor
meatal
  m. clamp
  m. dilator
  m. sound
meat-grasping forceps
meatoscope
  Hubell m.
  Huegli m.
meatotome
  Bunge ureteral m.
  Ellik m.
  Huegli m.
  Riba electrical ureteral m.
meatotomy electrode
mechanical
  m. device
  m. finger
  m. finger forceps

m. forceps
m. respirator
m. ventilator
mechanic's
m. pin
m. waste dressing
Meckel
M. band
M. rod
M. scan
Mecon-I hearing aid
meconium aspirator
Medallion
M. intraocular lens implant
M. lens expressor
Meda 2500 TENS unit
Med-Co flexible catheter
Medcor pacemaker
Medela
M. Apgar timer
M. breast pump
Medelec-Van Gogh electroencephalographic recording system
Medena continent ileostomy catheter
median palatine suture
mediastinal
m. cannula
m. catheter
m. drain
mediastinoscope
Carlens m.
Freiburg m.
Goldberg MPC m.
John A. Tucker m.
mediastinoscopy aspirating needle
Medi-Breather IPPB device
Medical
M. Design brace
M. Optics eye implant
M. Workshop intraocular lens implant
Medicam
Medici aerosol adhesive tape remover dressing
medicinal nebulizer
Medicon
M. contractor
M. forceps
M. rib retractor
M. wire-twister forceps

Medicon-Jackson
M.-J. forceps
M.-J. rectal forceps
Medicon-Packer mosquito forceps
Medicus bed
Medicut
M. cannula
M. catheter
M. intravenous needle
M. needle
Mediform dural graft
Medi-graft vascular prosthesis
Medi-Laser
Mochida CO2 M.-L.
Medilas Nd:YAG surgical laser
Medina
M. catheter
M. ileostomy catheter
Meding
M. tonsil enucleator tonometer
M. tonsil enucleator tonsillectome
Medinvent vascular stent
MediPort-DL double-lumen catheter
MediPort implanted vascular device
Mediscus low-air-loss bed
Mediskin hemostatic sponge
Medisystems fistular needle
Meditape
Medi-Tech
M.-T. arterial dilatation catheter
M.-T. balloon catheter
M.-T. bipolar probe
M.-T. catheter
M.-T. catheter system
M.-T. fascial dilator
M.-T. flexible stiffening cannula
M.-T. guide wire
M.-T. HP Flo-Switch
M.-T. IVC filter
M.-T. Mansfield dilating catheter
M.-T. sheath
M.-T. steerable catheter
M.-T. stone basket
medium
m. chromic suture

medium *(continued)*
> m. forceps
> Gastrovist contrast m.

Med-Neb respirator

Medoc-Celestin endoprosthesis prosthesis

Medrad
> M. angiographic catheter
> M. catheter
> M. contrast medium injector

Medrafil
> M. suture
> M. wire suture

Medscand Cytobrush Plus

Medtel pacemaker

Medtronic
> M. Activitrax pacemaker
> M. balloon catheter
> M. Byrel-SX pacemaker
> M. corkscrew electrode pacemaker
> M. Cyberlith pacemaker
> M. demand pacemaker
> M. external/internal pacemaker
> M. Hall prosthetic heart valve
> M. pacemaker
> M. Pacette pacemaker
> M. pulse generator
> M. Symbios pacemaker

Medtronic-Alcatel pacemaker

Medtronic-Laurens-Alcatel pacemaker

Medtronic-Zyrel pacemaker

medullary
> m. canal reamer
> m. nail
> m. pin

Medwatch telemetry system

Medx camera

Meeker
> M. artery forceps
> M. clamp
> M. deep-surgery forceps
> M. forceps
> M. gallbladder forceps
> M. gallstone clamp
> M. hemostatic forceps
> M. intestinal forceps

Meek snare

Meek-style clavicular strap

Meek-Wall
> M.-W. dermatome
> M.-W. microdermatome

Meerschaum probe

Mefix adhesive tape

Megadyne Fann E-Z Clean laparoscopic electrode

megaureter clamp

Mehta intraocular lens

meibomian
> m. expressor forceps
> m. forceps

Meigs
> M. curette
> M. endometrial curette
> M. retractor
> M. suture
> M. uterine curette

Melauskas orbital implant

Meller
> M. cyclodialysis spatula
> M. lacrimal sac retractor
> M. retractor

Mellinger
> M. eye speculum
> M. fenestrated blades speculum
> M. magnet

Mellinger-Axenfeld eye speculum

Melt elevator

Meltzer
> M. adenoid punch
> M. nasopharyngoscope
> M. tonsillar punch

membrane
> m. artificial lung
> m. forceps
> Gore-Tex surgical m.
> m. perforator

membrane-puncturing forceps

Meme
> M. breast prosthesis
> M. mammary implant

Mendel ligature forceps

Mendez
> M. degree calipers
> M. degree gauge
> M. ultrasonic cystotome

Mendez-Schubert aortic punch

Menge
> M. pessary
> M. stem pessary

Mengert membrane-puncturing forceps
Menghini
- M. biopsy needle
- M. cannula
- M. liver biopsy needle
- M. needle
- M. set

Menghini-Wildhirt
- M.-W. laparoscope
- M.-W. peritoneoscope

meniscal
- m. clamp
- m. curette
- m. cutter
- m. hook scissors
- m. knife
- m. lens
- m. mirror
- m. repair needle
- m. retractor
- m. spoon
- m. suture grabber

meniscectomy
- m. blade
- m. knife
- m. probe
- m. scissors

meniscotome
- Bowen-Grover m.
- Drompp m.
- Dyonics m.
- Ruuska m.
- Smillie m.

Meniscus Mender II system
Mentanium vitreoretinal instrument set
Mentor
- M. biliary stent
- M. bladder pacemaker
- M. breast prosthesis
- M. coudé catheter
- M. fine-focus microscope
- M. Foley catheter
- M. Foley catheter with comfort sleeve
- M. inflatable penile prosthesis
- M. injector gun
- M. malleable semirigid penile implant
- M. microscope

- M. penile prosthesis
- M. prostate biopsy needle
- M. Self-Cath penile prosthesis
- M. Tele-Cath ileal conduit sampling catheter
- M. wet-field coagulator
- M. wet-field cordless coagulator

Mentor-Urosan external catheter
Mercedes tip cannula
Mercer cartilage knife
Mercier catheter
Merck respirator
mercury
- m. cell-powered pacemaker
- Hammond argentum m.
- SS white m.

mercury-containing balloon
mercury-filled
- m.-f. dilator
- m.-f. esophageal bougie

mercury-weighted dilator
meridianal eye implant
Merlin stone forceps
Merlis obstetrical excavator
Merocel sponge
Merriam forceps
Merrill-Levassier retractor
Merrimack laser adapter
Mershon
- M. band pusher
- M. spring

Mersilene
- M. band
- M. dressing
- M. graft
- M. implant
- M. mesh dressing
- M. sling
- M. suture

Mers suture
Merthiolate
- M. dressing
- M. swab

Mertz keratoscopy ring
Merz
- M. aortic punch
- M. hysterectomy forceps

Merz-Vienna
- M.-V. nasal speculum
- M.-V. speculum

Mesalt
    M. dressing
    M. sterile dressing
mesh
    Auto Suture surgical m.
    Dacron m.
    Dexon polyglycolic acid m.
    m. graft
    mandibular m.
    Meadox dacron m.
    m. myringotomy tube
    PGA m.
    skin graft expander m.
    stainless steel m.
    Supramid m.
    surgical metallic m.
    m. suture
    titanium m.
meshed ball implant
mesher
    skin graft m.
    Zimmer skin graft m.
mesocaval H-graft shunt
mesocolic band
mesonephric drain
metacarpal
    m. broach
    m. double-ended retractor
    m. saw
metacarpophalangeal (MCP)
metal
    m. adapter
    m. ball-tip catheter
    m. band
    m. band suture
    m. cannula
    m. catheter
    m. clamp
    m. clip
    m. dead-ender
    m. electrode
    m. Fox shield
    m. needle
    m. orthopaedic implant
    m. pin
    m. ruler
    m. splint
    m. tongue depressor
Metaline dressing
metallic
    m. clamp
    m. fixation device
    m. implant

metallic-tip cannula
Meta MV cardiac pacemaker
Metaport catheter
metastatic implant
metatarsal stem broach
metatarsophalangeal
    m. endoprosthesis
    m. implant (MTPI)
Metavox hearing aid
Metcalf spring drop brace
Metcher eye speculum
Metcoff pediatric biopsy needle
meter
    Cybex finger-clip pulse m.
    Peakometer urinary flow
      rate m.
    Wright peak-flow m.
Metermatic nasal nebulizer
methacrylate
    polymethyl m. (PMMA)
Methodist
    M. Hospital head holder
    M. vascular suction tube
methyl
    m. methacrylate eye implant
    m. methacrylate graft
    m. methacrylate implant
      material
methylene diphosphonate (MDP)
metopic suture
Metras
    M. bronchial catheter
    M. catheter
Mettler Dia-Sonic electrosurgical
    unit
Metz
    Metzenbaum
Metzelder modification activator
Metzel-Wittmoser forceps
Metzenbaum (Metz)
    M. chisel
    M. delicate scissors
    M. dissecting scissors
    M. forceps
    M. long scissors
    M. needle holder
    M. operating scissors
    M. scissors
    M. septal knife
    M. tonsillar forceps
Metzenbaum-Lipsett scissors
Metzenbaum-Tydings forceps

Meurig Williams spinal fusion
plate
Mewissen infusion catheter
Mexican bat
Meyer
    M. biliary retractor
    M. cyclodiathermy needle
    M. knife
    M. needle
    M. olive-tipped vein
      stripper
    M. spiral vein stripper
    M. vein stripper
Meyerding
    M. bone graft
    M. bone skid
    M. chisel
    M. curette
    M. curved gouge
    M. finger retractor
    M. gouge
    M. hip skid
    M. laminectomy blade
    M. laminectomy retractor
    M. laminectomy self-
      retaining retractor
    M. mallet
    M. osteotome
    M. prosthesis
    M. retractor
    M. retractor blade
    M. saw-toothed curette
    M. self-retaining retractor
    M. shoulder skid
    M. skid
    M. skin hook
Meyerding-Deaver retractor
Meyhöffer, Meyhoeffer
    M. chalazion curette
    M. curette
    M. eye knife
    M. knife
MGH
    Massachusetts General Hospital
    MGH forceps
    MGH knee prosthesis
    MGH needle holder
    MGH osteotome
    MGH periosteal elevator
    MGH uterine vulsellum
      forceps
    MGH vulsellum
    MGH vulsellum forceps

MG II total knee system
MGM glenoidal punch
Miami fracture brace
MIC gastrostomy tube
Michael Reese prosthesis
Michel
    M. aortic clamp
    M. clamp
    M. clip
    M. clip-applying forceps
    M. clip-removing forceps
    M. forceps
    M. rhinoscopic mirror
    M. scalp clip
    M. skin clip
    M. suture clip
    M. suture clip-applying
      forceps
    M. tissue forceps
    M. wound clip
    M. wound clip-applying
      forceps
    M. wound clip forceps
    M. wound clip-removing
      forceps
Michele trephine
Michelson infant bronchoscope
Michelson-Sequoia air drill
Michels pick
Michel-Wachtenfeldt clip
Michigan
    M. forceps
    M. intestinal forceps
    M. University intestinal
      forceps
Mickey and Minnie surgical
  marker
Micra
    M. knife
    M. needle holder
Micrins forceps
micro
    m. cross-action bulldog
      clamp
    m.-infertility dissecting
      scissors
    m.-infertility needle holder
    m.-infertility scissors
    m.-oscillating saw
    m. "penny" sucker suction
      tube
Micro-Aire
    M.-A. bone saw

Micro-Aire *(continued)*
    M.-A. bur
    M.-A. drill
    M.-A. osteotome
    M.-A. pulse lavage system
    M.-A. surgical instrument
      system
micro-Allis forceps
micro-anastomosis
    m.-a. approximator
    m.-a. clip
    m.-a. clip approximator
micro-arterial
    m.-a. clamp
    m.-a. forceps
micro-aspirator
    Ergo m.-a.
microballoon
    m. probe
    Rand m.
microbayonet
    m. forceps
    m. rasp
    m. scoop
Microbeam I, II, III, IV
    macromanipulators
microbiopsy forceps
microbipolar forceps
microblade
    Beaver m.
microbone curette
microbronchoscopic
    m. grasping forceps
    m. tissue forceps
microbrush
microbulldog
    m. clamp
    m. clip
microcalipers
    Storz m.
microcautery unit
microclamp
    m. clip
    m. forceps
    Kapp m.
    Khodadad m.
Microclens wipes
microclip
    m. forceps
    Heifitz m.
    Khodadad m.
    Kleinert-Kutz m.
    Williams m.

    Yasargil m.
    Zylik m.
microconjunctival scissors
microcorneal
    m. forceps
    m. scissors
microcrimped prosthesis
microcup
    m. forceps
    m. pituitary forceps
microcurette
    Rhoton m.
    Ruggles m.
microcut bandsaw
microcystitome
    Lieppman m.
microdermatome
    Meek-Wall m.
microdissecting forceps
microdissector
    Crockard m.
    Hardy m.
    Yasargil m.
Microdon dressing
microdressing forceps
microdrill
    Shea m.
micro-electrode
micro-extractor forceps
Microfoam
    M. dressing
    M. surgical tape
microforceps
    Adson m.
    Anis m.
    Collis m.
    iris m.
    iris suture m.
    Jako-Kleinsasser m.
    Koslowski m.
    Nicola m.
    Pierse-type m.
    Rhoton m.
    Scanlan m.
    Sparta m.
    V. Mueller laser Rhoton m.
    Yasargil m.
Micro-Guide catheter
micro-Halstead arterial forceps
microhemostat
    O'Brien-Storz m.
microhook
    Bonn m.

McIntyre m.
Shambaugh-Derlacki m.
Simcoe m.
microhysteroscope
micro-impactor
Codman m.-i.
micro-instrument tray
micro-invasive catheter
micro-iris
m.-i. hook
m.-i. knife
m.-i. scissors
micro-irrigator
Stryker m.-i.
microkeratome
Microknit
M. arterial prosthesis
M. patch graft
M. vascular graft
Microlance blood lancet
microlaryngeal
m. cup-shaped forceps
m. grasping forceps
m. laser operating platform
m. laser probe
m. scissors
m. suction laser operating
platform
microlaryngoscope
Abramson-Dedo m.
anterior commissure m.
Fragen anterior
commissure m.
Jako m.
Lindholm m.
microlens
m. cystourethroscope
m. direct-vision telescope
m. Foroblique telescope
m. hook
m. urethroscope
Microlet electrode needle
Micro-Line arterial forceps
Microlith
M. pacemaker pulse
generator
M. P pacemaker
Microloc knee system
microloupe
microlumbar
m. diskectomy retractor
m. retractor
micromanometer-tip catheter

micromeasurer
Micromedics surgical instrument
micrometer
m. knife
Tolman m.
micromirror
Apfelbaum micromirror
Silverstein micromirror
Micron
microneedle
m. holder
m. holder forceps
micronerve
m. hook
microneurosurgical
m. forceps
m. instrument
micropin
m. forceps
Pischel m.
micropituitary scissors
micropoint needle
Micropore surgical tape dressing
microprobe
Micro-Pulsar TENS unit
microrasp
Scanlan m.
microraspatory
Yasargil m.
microreciprocating saw
microrongeur
Davol m.
microruler
Stecher m.
microsagittal saw
microscissors
Collis m.
Gill-Welsh Vannas
angled m.
Jacobson m.
Jako-Kleinsasser m.
Keeler m.
Kurze m.
Rhoton m.
round-tip m.
Scanlan m.
Shutt m.
V. Mueller laser Rhoton m.
Yasargil m.
microscope
CooperVision m.
corneal m.
fiberoptic m.

microscope *(continued)*
  Hallpike-Blackmore ear m.
  Kaps operating m.
  Konan m.
  laser micromanipulator for
    surgical m.
  Mentor m.
  Mentor fine-focus m.
  surgical m.
  Topcon m.
  Zeiss operating m.
microscopic
  m. hook
  m. scissors
Microseal nebulizer
microserrefine
  Storz m.
Micro-Sharp blade
Microsnap hemostatic forceps
Microson hearing aid
microspatula
  Osher malleable m.
Microspike approximator
microsponge
  Weck-cel m.
Micross
  M. catheter
  M. dilatation catheter
microstaple holder
Microstar dialysis system
Microstat
microstimulator
microstomia prevention appliance
  (MPA)
microsurgical
  m. biopsy forceps
  m. dissector
  m. ear hook
  m. ear pick
  m. forceps
  m. grasping forceps
  m. knife
  m. needle holder
  m. retractor
  m. scissors
  m. tying forceps
microsuture-tying forceps
Microtek
  M. cupped forceps
  M. scissors
microtenotomy scissors
Microthin P2 pacemaker

microtip
  m. bipolar jeweler's forceps
  m. forceps
microtissue forceps
microtying
  m. eye forceps
  m. forceps
MicroTymp tympanometric device
micro-utility
  m.-u. forceps
  m.-u. scissors
microvascular
  m. clamp
  m. clamp-applying forceps
  m. forceps
  m. modified Alm retractor
  m. needle holder
  m. scissors
  m. STA-MCA kit
  m. tying forceps
Microvasic Rigiflex balloon
Microvasive
  M. biliary device
  M. sclerotherapy needle
Microvel
  M. graft
  M. prosthesis
Microvena Amplatz snare
microvessel hook
microvitrector
microvitreoretinal (MVR)
  m. blade
  m. spatula
Microvit scissors
Microwec scissors
micturition bag
Midas Rex drill
middle
  m. ear aspirator
  m. ear calipers
  m. ear chisel
  m. ear curette
  m. ear excavator
  m. ear forceps
  m. ear implant
  m. ear instrument
  m. ear ring curette
  m. ear strut forceps
  m. ear suction cannula
  m. palatine suture
Middledorpf retractor
Middlesex-Pointe retractor

480

Middleton
    M. adenoid curette
    M. curette
midforceps
midoccipital electrode
midstream aortogram catheter
Mignon cataract extractor
Mija ligature carrier
Mikaelsson catheter
Mikros pacemaker
Mikro-tip
    M.-t. angiocatheter
    M.-t. catheter
    M.-t. transducer
Mikulicz
    M. abdominal retractor
    M. clamp
    M. drain
    M. forceps
    M. liver retractor
    M. peritoneal clamp
    M. peritoneal forceps
    M. retractor
    M. spatula
    M. spur-crusher
    M. tonsillar forceps
Mikulicz-Radecki
    M.-R. clamp
    M.-R. drain
Mikulicz spur-crusher
Milan uterine curette
Milch resection plate
Miles
    M. antral curette
    M. clamp
    M. clip
    M. rectal clamp
    M. retractor
    M. skin clip
    M. Teflon clip
    M. vena caval clip
Milette-Tyding dissector
Milewski driver
Milex
    M. forceps
    M. Jel-Jector vaginal
      applicator
    M. pessary
    M. retractor
    M. spatula
    M. vaginal insufflator
mill
    hollow m.

    OrthoBlend powered
      bone m.
Millar
    M. micromonometer
      catheter
    M. Mikro-Tip catheter
      pressure transducer
    M. pigtail angiographic
      catheter
    M. transducer
Millard thimble hook
Miller
    M. articulating forceps
    M. bayonet forceps
    M. bone file
    M. bougie
    M. bracket positioner
    M. curette
    M. cystoscope
    M. dental elevator
    M. dilator
    M. dissecting scissors
    M. endotracheal tube
    M. fiberoptic laryngoscope
      blade
    M. forceps
    M. injector bezel
    M. laryngoscope
    M. operating scissors
    M. rasp
    M. ratchet injector
    M. rectal forceps
    M. rectal scissors
    M. retractor
    M. stainless steel
      laryngoscope blade
    M. tonsillar dissector
    M. tube
    M. vaginal speculum
Miller-Abbott
    M.-A. catheter
    M.-A. double-lumen
      intestinal tube
    M.-A. intestinal tube
Miller-Apexo elevator
Miller-Galante
    M.-G. hip prosthesis
    M.-G. revision knee system
    M.-G. total knee system
    M.-G. unicompartmental
      knee

Miller-Senn
    M.-S. double-ended retractor
    M.-S. retractor
Miller-vac drain
Millesi
    M. interfascicular graft
    M. scissors
Millet
    M. needle
    M. neurological test
      instrument
    M. test hammer
Millette tonsillar knife
Millette-Tyding knife
Millex filter
Milligan
    M. dissector
    M. double-ended dissector
    M. self-retaining retractor
    M. speculum
Milliknit
    M. arterial prosthesis
    M. graft
millimeter ruler
Millin
    M. bladder neck spreader
    M. bladder retractor
    M. bladder spatula
    M. boomerang needle
      holder
    M. capsular forceps
    M. capsule-grasping forceps
    M. clamp
    M. forceps
    M. ligature-guiding forceps
    M. lobe-grasping forceps
    M. prostatectomy forceps
    M. retractor
    M. retropublic bladder
      retractor
    M. self-retaining retractor
    M. side blade
    M. solid malleable center
      blade
    M. suction tube
    M. T-shaped forceps
Millin-Bacon
    M.-B. bladder neck spreader
    M.-B. bladder retractor
    M.-B. bladder self-retaining
      retractor
    M.-B. retractor

    M.-B. retropubic
      prostatectomy retractor
milliner's needle
millinery bag
Millipore
    M. filter
    M. suture
Mill-Rose
    M.-R. biopsy forceps
    M.-R. cytology brush
    M.-R. spiral stone basket
    M.-R. stone basket
    M.-R. tube
Mills
    M. circumflex scissors
    M. coronary endarterectomy
      set
    M. coronary endarterectomy
      spatula
    M. mammary-coronary
      tissue forceps
    M. microvascular needle
      holder
    M. operative peripheral
      angioplasty catheter
    M. saphenous-aortic tissue
      forceps
    M. scissors
    M. tissue forceps
    M. valvulotome
Milroy-Piper suction tube
Milteck scissors
Miltex
    M. gun
    M. ligature knife
    M. retractor
    M. rib spreader
Milwaukee
    M. brace
    M. scoliosis brace
    M. snare
Miner osteotome
Minerva
    M. back jacket
    M. plastic jacket
Mingograf electroencephalograph
miniapplier
miniature
    m. bulldog clamp
    m. intestinal forceps
    m. loop electrode
    m. multipurpose clamp
    m. sound

minibasket
    Shutt m.
    Wilson-Cook m.
miniblade
minibladebreaker
    Troutman-Barraquer
      minibladebreaker
miniclip
    Stangel fallopian tube m.
minicurette
minicut bandsaw
mini-echo sounder
mini-fixator
    Hammer M.-F.
miniforceps
    Kern m.
mini-Hohmann retractor
minilaparotomy Falope-ring
  applicator
Minilith
    M. pacemaker
    M. pacemaker pulse
      generator
minimagnet
    Hamblin m.
minimallet
    Gam-Mer m.
mini-micro forceps
miniosteotome
    Gam-Mer m.
Mini-Profile dilatation catheter
minirazor bladebreaker
Minispace IUI catheter
ministaple
    Richards m.
Ministem TENS unit
mini-Stryker power drill
mini-Ullrich bone clamp
minivise
    Budde halo flex arm m.
mini-Wright peak flowmeter
Minix pacemaker
Minneapolis hip prosthesis
Minnesota
    M. impedance cardiograph
    M. retractor
    M. tube
minor connector bar
Minos air drill
Mira
    M. coagulator
    M. drill

    M. female trochanteric
      reamer
    M. femoral head reamer
    M. laser
    M. photocoagulator
Mira-Charnley reamer
Miracompo filling instrument
Miratract
mirror
    bayonet transsphenoidal m.
    Buckingham m.
    m. cannula
    Everclear laryngeal m.
    Grafco head m.
    Grafco laryngeal m.
    Hardy transsphenoidal m.
    head m.
    m. holder
    House middle ear m.
    Jako laryngeal m.
    Kashiwabara laryngeal m.
    Kerner dental m.
    laryngeal m.
    m. laryngoscope
    laser m.
    Lewis dental m.
    McLaughlin laser m.
    meniscal m.
    Michel rhinoscopic m.
    Oliair mouth m.
    Olyco mouth m.
    Olympia mouth m.
    Poh mouth m.
    rhinoscopic m.
    SMIC mouth m.
    Stiwer laryngeal m.
Mirrorreflex camera
Mischer-Pudenz shunt
Mischler shunt
Misdome-Frank curette
Mishima-Hedbys attachment
  pacemeter
Mishler
    M. dual-chamber valve
    M. flushing valve
Miskimon
    M. cerebellar retractor
    M. cerebellar self-retaining
      retractor
Mistette nasal spray pump
Mitamura fine ceramic heart valve

Mitchel-Adam
  M.-A. clamp
  M.-A. multipurpose clamp
Mitchel aortotomy clamp
Mitchell
  M. basket
  M. cartilage knife
  M. stone basket
  M. ureteral stone dislodger
Mitchell-Diamond
  M.-D. biopsy forceps
  M.-D. forceps
Mitek
  M. anchor
  M. anchor system
  M. quick anchor appliance
Mithoefer-Jansen mouth gag
Mitraflex
  M. multilayer wound
    dressing
  M. wound dressing
mitral
  m. forceps
  m. hook
  m. valve dilator
  m. valve-holding forceps
  m. valve retractor
  m. valve scissors
Mitrathane wound dressing
Mitrothin P2 pacemaker
Mitsubishi
  M. angioscope
  M. angioscopic catheter
Mittlemeir ceramic hip prosthesis
Mityvac
  M. extractor
  M. vacuum delivery system
  M. vacuum extraction
    system
  M. vacuum extractor
Mixter
  M. arterial forceps
  M. baby hemostatic forceps
  M. brain biopsy punch
  M. clamp
  M. common duct Dilaprobe
  M. common duct Dilaprobe
    dilator
  M. common duct probe
  M. Dilaprobe probe
  M. dilating probe
  M. dilator
  M. forceps

  M. full-curve forceps
  M. gallbladder forceps
  M. gall duct forceps
  M. gall duct probe
  M. gallstone forceps
  M. hemostatic forceps
  M. irrigating Dilaprobe
    dilator
  M. irrigating probe
  M. ligature-carrier clamp
  M. mosquito forceps
  M. needle
  M. operating scissors
  M. pediatric forceps
  M. pediatric hemostatic
    forceps
  M. probe
  M. right-angle clamp
  M. thoracic clamp
  M. thoracic clamp forceps
  M. thoracic forceps
  M. tube
  M. ventricular needle
Mixter-McQuigg forceps
Mixter-O'Shaughnessy
  M.-O. dissecting forceps
  M.-O. forceps
  M.-O. hemostatic forceps
  M.-O. ligature forceps
Mixter-Paul
  M.-P. arterial forceps
  M.-P. hemostatic forceps
Mixtner catheter
Miya hook
Mizutani laminaria tent
Mizzy needle
MM band
MMS low-profile acetabular cup
Moberg
  M. bone plate
  M. chisel
  M. forceps
  M. retractor
Moberg-Stille
  M.-S. forceps
  M.-S. retractor
mobilizer
  Derlacki m.
  Derlacki ear m.
  Derlacki-Hough m.
  Hough-Derlacki m.
Mobin-Uddin vena cava filter
Mochida CO2 Medi-Laser

MOD
>MOD femoral drill guide
>MOD unicompartmental
>knee system

modelling carver

modified
>m. CIF needle
>m. C-loop haptic
>m. C-loops intraocular lens
>m. J loop haptic
>m. J-loop, posterior
>chamber intraocular lens
>m. Moore hip locking
>prosthesis
>m. sclerectomy punch
>m. spatula needle
>m. suction tube
>m. Younge forceps

Modny
>M. drill
>M. guide
>M. pin

modular
>m. Austin-Moore hip
>prosthesis
>m. calcar replacement stem
>m. head remover
>m. implant
>m. Iowa Precoat total hip
>prosthesis
>m. Lenbach hip system
>m. prosthesis

module
>dialysate preparation m.

Moe
>M. bone curette
>M. gouge
>M. hook
>M. impactor
>M. intertrochanteric plate
>M. osteotome
>M. subcutaneous rod

Moehle
>M. corneal forceps
>M. forceps

Moeller laser

Moersch
>M. bronchoscope
>M. bronchoscopic forceps
>M. bronchoscopic specimen
>forceps
>M. cardiospasm dilator
>M. electrode

>M. esophagoscope
>M. forceps

Moffat-Robinson bone pate
collector

Mogen circumcision clamp

Mohr
>M. clamp
>M. finger splint
>M. pinchcock clamp

moist dressing

mold
>acrylic m.
>Altchek vaginal m.
>Counsellor vaginal m.
>flavine wool m.
>Silastic m.
>silicone m.
>sodium alginate wool m.

moleskin
>m. bandage
>m. traction hitch dressing

Mollison
>M. mastoid rongeur
>M. retractor
>M. self-retaining retractor

Molt
>M. curette
>M. dissector
>M. elevator
>M. forceps
>M. mouth gag
>M. pedicle forceps
>M. periosteal elevator

Molteno drainage eye implant

Moltz-Storz tonsillectome

Mo-Mark curette

Momberg
>M. tourniquet
>M. tube

Momosi spider lens intraocular
lens

Monaco broach

Monaghan
>M. respirator
>M. ventilator

Monaldi drain

Monarch II bleaching instrument

Moncorps knife

Moncrieff
>M. anterior chamber
>cannula
>M. anterior chamber
>irrigating cannula

Moncrieff *(continued)*
  M. anterior chamber
    irrigator
  M. cannula
monitor
  ASN m.
  automatic single-needle m.
    (ASN)
  Biocon impedance
    plethysmography cardiac
    output m.
  blood perfusion m. (BPM)
  cardiac m.
  Cardiotach fetal m.
  Codman intracranial
    pressure m.
  DeVilbiss Mini-Dop
    fetal m.
  DeVilbiss OB-Dop fetal m.
  Eucotone m.
  Fetalert fetal heart m.
  HP M1350A fetal m.
  infant ventilation m.
  in-line venous pressure m.
  Jako facial nerve m.
  Ladd intracranial
    pressure m.
  Meadox ICP m.
  Myotone EMG m.
  Neuroguide m.
  nocturnal penile
    tumescence m. (NPT
    monitor)
  noninvasive continuous
    cardiac output m.
  Pocket-Dop II fetal heart
    rate m.
  respiratory function m.
  Sonicaid SYSTEM 8000
    fetal m.
  Terumo Doppler fetal heart
    rate m.
  Thermograph
    temperature m.
  ultrasound m.
  Verner-Smith m.
  Wakeling fetal heart m.
monitored bed
monitoring cannula
Monk prosthesis
Monks malar elevator
monocular
  m. bandage

  m. dressing
  m. eye dressing
  m. indirect ophthalmoscope
Monod punch forceps
monofilament
  m. clear suture
  m. green suture
  m. nylon suture
  m. steel suture
  m. suture
  m. wire suture
Monoject
  M. bone marrow aspirator
  M. laceration irrigation tray
Monomer filter
monopolar
  m. coagulating forceps
  m. electrocautery
  m. forceps
  m. insulated forceps
  m. temporary electrode
Monorail angioplasty catheter
monostrut heart valve
Montague
  M. abrader
  M. proctoscope
  M. sigmoidoscope
Montefiore tracheal tube
Montenovesi
  M. cranial forceps
  M. cranial rongeur
  M. cranial rongeur forceps
Montgomery
  M. esophageal tube
  M. laryngeal stent
  M. strap dressing
  M. tracheal cannula
  M. tracheal fenestrator
  M. tracheal T-tube
  M. tracheal tube
  M. vaginal speculum
Montgomery-Bernstine speculum
**Montgomery-Lofgren tapered Safe-
  T-Tube**
**Monticelli-Spinelli circular external
  fixation system**
Montrose dressing applicator
Moody
  M. fixation forceps
  M. forceps
Moon rectal retractor

Moon-Robinson
    M.-R. prosthesis inserter
    M.-R. stapes prosthesis
Moore
    M. adjustable nail
    M. blade plate
    M. bone drill
    M. bone elevator
    M. bone reamer
    M. bone retractor
    M. button
    M. chisel
    M. disk
    M. drill
    M. driver
    M. elevator retractor
    M. fixation pin
    M. forceps
    M. gallbladder spoon
    M. gall duct scoop
    M. gallstone scoop
    M. gouge
    M. hip endoprosthesis
    system
    M. hip prosthesis
    M. hollow chisel
    M. hook drive-extractor
    M. hooked extractor
    M. lens forceps
    M. lens-implanting forceps
    M. lens-inserting forceps
    M. nail extractor
    M. nail set
    M. osteotome
    M. prosthesis-mortising
    chisel
    M. rasp
    M. retractor
    M. spinal fusion gouge
    M. stem rasp
    M. thoracoscope
    M. tracheostomy button
Moore-Blount
    M.-B. driver
    M.-B. extractor
    M.-B. plate
    M.-B. screwdriver
Moorehead
    M. cheek retractor
    M. clamp
    M. dental retractor
    M. dissector
    M. ear knife

    M. elevator
    M. lid clamp
    M. periosteotome
    M. retractor
Moore-Troutman corneal scissors
Moran-Karaya
    M.-K. disk
    M.-K. ring
    M.-K. sheet
morcellizer
    Rubin m.
    Rubin septal m.
    Yarmo m.
Morch
    M. respirator
    M. swivel adapter
    M. swivel tracheostomy
    tube
    M. ventilator
Moren-Moretz vena caval clip
Moreno
    M. clamp
    M. gastroenterostomy clamp
Moretz
    M. clip
    M. prosthesis
    M. Tiny Tytan ventilation
    tube
    M. Tytan ventilation tube
Morgan
    M. proctoscope
    M. vent tube introducer
Morgan-Boehm proctoscope
Morgenstein
    M. blunt forceps
    M. gouge
    M. hook
    M. periosteal knife
    M. pick
    M. pick
    M. spatula
Morgenstein-Kerrison rongeur
Moritz-Schmidt
    M.-S. forceps
    M.-S. knife
    M.-S. laryngeal forceps
Morris
    M. aortic clamp
    M. biphase screw
    M. cannula
    M. catheter
    M. drain
    M. forceps

Morris *(continued)*
  M. mitral valve spreader
  M. retractor
  M. Silastic thoracic drain
  M. thoracic catheter
Morrison-Hurd
  M.-H. dissector
  M.-H. pillar retractor
  M.-H. retractor
  M.-H. tonsillar dissector
Morrison skin hook
Morrissey Gigli-saw guide
Morsch-Retec respirator
Morse
  M. backward-cutting aortic
    scissors
  M. blade
  M. head
  M. instrument handle
  M. modified Finochietto
    retractor
  M. retractor
  M. scissors
  M. sternal retractor
  M. sternal spreader
  M. stopcock
  M. suction tube
  M. taper
  M. taper cone provisional
  M. taper stem
  M. towel clip
  M. valve retractor
Morse-Andrews suction tube
Morse-Ferguson suction tube
Morson
  M. forceps
  M. retractor
  M. trocar
mortising chisel
Morton
  M. bandage
  M. dislodger
  M. stone dislodger
Mortson
  M. clip
  M. V-shaped clip
Morwel
  M. cannula
  M. silhouette suction
    apparatus
Moseley
  M. fasciatome
  M. glenoid rim prosthesis

Mosher
  M. bag
  M. curette
  M. drain
  M. esophagoscope
  M. ethmoid curette
  M. ethmoid punch forceps
  M. forceps
  M. intubation tube
  M. Life Saver antichoke
    suction device
  M. lifesaver retractor
  M. life-saving suction tube
  M. life-saving tube
  M. nasal speculum
  M. retractor
  M. strip
  M. urethral speculum
mosquito
  m. clamp
  m. forceps
  m. hemostat
  m. hemostatic forceps
  m. lid clamp
Moss gastric decompression tube
mother-daughter endoscope
motility eye implant
motion
  continuous passive m.
    (CPM)
Mott
  M. double-ended retractor
  M. raspatory
  M. retractor
Mottgen goniometer
Moule screw pin
Moult curette
Moulton lacrimal tube
Mount
  M. forceps
  M. intervertebral disk
    forceps
  M. intervertebral disk
    rongeur forceps
Mount-Mayfield
  M.-M. aneurysm forceps
  M.-M. forceps
Mount-Olivecrona
  M.-O. clip applier
  M.-O. forceps
Mouradian
  M. humeral fixation system
  M. humeral rod

Moure-Coryllos rib shears
Moure esophagoscope
mouse-tooth
  m.-t. clamp
  m.-t. forceps
Mousseau-Barbin esophageal tube
mouth
  m. gag (*See* gag)
  m. gag frame
  m. gag set
  m. gag tongue blade
  m. gag tongue depressor
    blade
  m. gag tooth plate
Moynihan
  M. bile duct probe
  M. clamp
  M. clip
  M. forceps
  M. gall duct forceps
  M. gallstone probe
  M. gallstone scoop
  M. intestinal forceps
  M. kidney pedicle forceps
  M. probe
  M. respirator
  M. towel clamp
  M. towel forceps
Moynihan-Navratil forceps
MPA
  microstomia prevention
    appliance
MP-A-1 catheter
MP-A-2 catheter
MPC coagulation forceps
MPF catheter
MPL
  MPL aspirating syringe
  MPL dental needle
  MPL Hypo intraosseous
    needle
MPR drain catheter
Mr. PainAway Health-Up TENS
  unit
Mt. Clemens Hospital clip applier
MTPI
  metatarsophalangeal implant
Mt. Sinai skull clamp pin
Muck
  M. forceps
  M. tonsillar forceps
mucosal
  m. cuff

  m. elevator
  m. separator plate
mucotome
  Castroviejo-Steinhauser m.
  Norelco m.
mucous forceps
Mueller (*See also* Müller, V.
  Mueller)
  M. alkaline battery cautery
  M. aortic clamp
  M. bronchial clamp
  M. bur
  M. catheter
  M. clamp
  M. curette
  M. Currentrol cautery
  M. electric corneal trephine
  M. electronic tonometer
  M. eye speculum
  M. forceps
  M. giant eye magnet
  M. lacrimal sac retractor
  M. needle
  M. pediatric clamp
  M. retractor
  M. saw
  M. shield
  M. speculum
  M. suction tube
  M. telescope
  M. tongue blade
  M. total hip prosthesis
  M. vena caval clamp
Mueller-Balfour
  M.-B. retractor
  M.-B. self-retaining retractor
Mueller-Charnley hip prosthesis
Mueller-Frazier suction tube
Mueller-LaForce adenotome
Mueller-Markham patent ductus
  forceps
Mueller-Pool suction tube
Mueller-Pynchon suction tube
Mueller-Yankauer suction tube
Muelly hook
Muer anoscope
Mufson-Cushing retractor
Muhlberger
  M. implant
  M. orbital implant
  M. orbital prosthesis
Muir
  M. cautery clamp

Muir *(continued)*
M. clamp
M. hemorrhoidal forceps
M. rectal cautery clamp
M. rectal speculum
Muirhead-Little pelvic rest tractor
Muirhead pelvic rest
Muldoon
M. dilator
M. lacrimal dilator
M. lacrimal probe
M. lid retractor
M. meibomian forceps
M. tube
Mules
M. eye implant
M. graft
M. implant
M. prosthesis
M. scoop
M. sphere eye implant
mules
Bishop-Harman m.
Colibri m.
Gill-Hess m.
Graefe m.
Halsted m.
Heath m.
Kulvin-Kalt m.
Lister m.
MacGregor m.
Paton-Berens m.
Müller (*See also* Mueller, V. Mueller)
M. coronary perfusion cannula
M. shield eye implant
Müller-type
M.-t. acetabular cup
M.-t. femoral head replacement
Mulligan
M. anastomosis clamp
M. cervical biopsy punch
M. dissector
M. Silastic prosthesis
Mullins
M. blade
M. catheter
M. tongue depressor
M. transseptal catheter
multiaction pin cutter

Multiclip disposable ligating clip device
Multicor
M. cardiac pacemaker
M. Gamma pacemaker
M. II pacemaker
multielectrode impedance catheter
multifilament
m. steel suture
m. suture
Multifire
M. GIA 50 stapler
M. GIA 60 stapler
M. TA 30 stapler
M. TA 50 stapler
M. TA 60 stapler
M. TA stapler
Multi-Fit Luer-Lok control tonsillar syringe
Multilase Nd:YAG surgical laser
multilead electrode
Multilith pacemaker
Multi-Lock knee brace
multilumen
m. catheter
m. probe
Multi-Med triple-lumen infusion catheter
multiple-piece intraocular lens
multiple-pin hole occluder
multiple-point electrode
Multipoise headrest
MultiPolar bipolar cup
multipolar impedance catheter
multiprogrammable
m. pacemaker
m. pulse generator
multipurpose
m. angled clamp
m. anterior commissure laryngoscope
m. ball electrode
m. catheter
m. clamp
m. curved clamp
m. forceps
m. laryngoscope
m. retractor
m. valve
Multistim electrode catheter
multistrand suture
multitoothed cartilage forceps
Mumford Gigli-saw guide

Munchen
    M. curette
    M. endometrial biopsy
      curette
Mundie
    M. forceps
    M. placental forceps
Munich-Crosstreet anoscope
Munro
    M. brain scissors
    M. retractor
    M. self-retaining retractor
Murdock eye speculum
Murdock-Wiener eye speculum
Murdoon eye speculum
Murless
    M. fetal head extractor
    M. head extractor
    M. head extractor forceps
    M. head retractor
Murphy
    M. ball-end hook
    M. ball reamer
    M. bone skid
    M. brace
    M. button
    M. chisel
    M. common duct dilator
    M. dilator
    M. forceps
    M. gallbladder retractor
    M. gouge
    M. intestinal needle
    M. needle
    M. plaster knife
    M. punch
    M. rake retractor
    M. retractor
    M. splint
    M. tonsillar forceps
Murphy-Balfour
    M.-B. center blade
    M.-B. retractor
**Murphy-Johnson anastomosis
button**
Murphy-Lane
    M.-L. bone elevator
    M.-L. bone skid
    M.-L. lever
    M.-L. skid
Murphy-Péan hemostatic forceps
Murray
    M. forceps

    M. holder
    M. knee prosthesis
Murray-Jones arm splint
Murray-Thomas arm splint
**Murtagh self-retaining infant scalp
retractor**
muscle
    m. biopsy clamp
    m. clamp
    m. forceps
    m. hook
musculotendinous cuff
Museholdt
    M. forceps
    M. nasal-dressing forceps
Museux
    M. forceps
    M. tenaculum
    M. tenaculum forceps
    M. uterine forceps
    M. uterine vulsellum
      forceps
    M. vulsellum forceps
**Museux-Collins uterine vulsellum
forceps**
mush clamp
mushroom
    m. catheter
    m. impactor
Musial tissue forceps
Musken tonometer
muslin dressing
mustache dressing
Mustarde
    M. awl
    M. forceps
    M. suture
**MVE-50 implantable myocardial
electrode**
MVR
    microvitreoretinal
    MVR blade
MVS
    MVS cannula
    MVS phacoemulsifier
myelography needle
Myers
    M. interchangeable vein
      stripper
    M. knee retractor
    M. retractor
    M. spiral vein stripper
    M. vein stripper

Myerson
- M. antral trocar
- M. biting punch
- M. biting tip
- M. bronchial forceps
- M. electrode
- M. forceps
- M. laryngeal forceps
- M. laryngectomy saw
- M. miniature laryngeal
  biopsy forceps
- M. resin
- M. wash tube

Myerson-Moncrieff cannula
Mylar catheter
Myles
- M. adenotome
- M. antral curette
- M. cannula
- M. clamp
- M. curette
- M. forceps
- M. forceps punch
- M. guillotine
- M. guillotine adenotome
- M. guillotine tonsillectome
- M. hemorrhoidal clamp
- M. hemorrhoidal forceps
- M. nasal-cutting forceps
- M. nasal forceps
- M. nasal punch
- M. nasal speculum
- M. punch
- M. sinus antral cannula
- M. sinus cannula
- M. tonsillectome snare

Myles-Ray speculum
Mynol endodontic cement
myocardial
- m. clamp
- m. dilator
- m. electrode
- m. lead

Myocure blade
myoma screw
myomatome
- Segond m.

Myopulse muscle stimulator
Myosynchron muscle stimulator
Myotone EMG monitor
Myowire
- M. cardiac electrode
- M. II cardiac electrode

myringoplasty knife
myringotome
- barbed m.
- Buck m.
- Rica m.
- SMIC m.

myringotomy
- m. drain tube
- m. ear blade
- m. knife
- m. knife blade
- m. knife handle
- m. knife ophthalmic blade

Myrtle leaf probe

N

Nabatoff vein stripper
Nachlas gastrointestinal tube
Nachlas-Linton tube
Naclerio diaphragm retractor
Naden-Rieth
    N.-R. implant
    N.-R. prosthesis
Nadler
    N. bipolar coaptation
      forceps
    N. scissors
Naegele
    N. forceps
    N. obstetrical forceps
Nagaraja endoscopic nasal biliary
  drainage set
Nagashima
    N. antroscope trocar
    N. electrogustometer
    N. electronystagmograph
    N. LS-3 laryngostroboscope
    N. right-angle antroscope
Nagel anomaloscope
Nager
    N. palatal needle
    N. tonsillar needle
Nagielski needle
nail
    Augustine boat n.
    Barr bolt n.
    n. bed
    boat n.
    Böhler hip n.
    Brooker-Wills n.
    cannulated n.
    Capener n.
    closed n.
    cloverleaf n.
    Curry hip n.
    Delitala T-nail n.
    Delta Recon n.
    diamond n.
    Dooley n.
    n. drill
    Ender n.
    Engel-May n.
    fluted n.
    four-flanged n.
    Gissane spike n.
    Grosse & Kempf femoral n.

Grosse & Kempf tibial n.
Hansen-Street self-
  broaching n.
Hansen-Street solid
  intramedullary n.
hooked intramedullary n.
IM n.
Jewett n.
Ken n.
Ken sliding n.
Knowles pin n.
Koslowski hip n.
Küntscher n.
Küntscher cloverleaf n.
Küntscher intramedullary n.
Lottes n.
Lottes triflange
  intramedullary n.
Massie II n.
Massie sliding n.
McKee trifin n.
McLaughlin n.
medullary n.
Moore adjustable n.
Neufeld n.
n. nipper
noncannulated n.
Nylok self-locking n.
Nystroem hip n.
Nystroem-Stille hip n.
OEC/Kuntscher Interlocking
  Pathfinder n.
Pidcock n.
n. plate
Pugh self-adjusting n.
Recon n.
Rush n.
Russell-Taylor n.
Schneider intramedullary n.
n. scissors
n. set
Slocum-Smith-Petersen n.
slotted n.
Smillie n.
Smith-Petersen
  cannulated n.
Staples osteotomy n.
Steinmann n.
supracondylar n.
Sven Johansson hip n.

nail *(continued)*
    Temple University n.
    Thatcher n.
    Thornton n.
    Tiemann n.
    Venable-Stuck n.
    Vesely n.
    Vesely-Street n.
    Vitallium n.
    V-medullary n.
    Watson-Jones n.
    Webb bolt n.
    Z-fixation n.
    Zickel n.
    Zimmer telescoping n.
nail-cutting forceps
nail-extracting forceps
nail nipper
    English n. n.
    Turnbull n. n.
nail-nipper scissors
Nakayama
    N. anastomosis apparatus
    N. clamp
    N. microvascular stapler
    N. ring
    N. staple
Nalebuff-Goldman strut
Nalzene filter
Namic
    N. angiographic syringe
    N. catheter
    N. localization needle
Narkomed
    N. anesthesia machine
    N. subcompact anesthesia
    machine
narrow
    n. elevator
    n. retractor
    n. washer
nasal
    n. airway
    n. alligator forceps
    n. aspirator
    n. bivalve speculum
    n. bone forceps
    n. cannula
    n. cartilage-holding forceps
    n. catheter
    n. chisel
    n. curette

    n. dilator
    n. dissector
    n. dorsal implant
    n. endoscopic telescope
    n. forceps
    n. gouge
    n. hump-cutting forceps
    n. insertion forceps
    n. irrigator
    n. knife
    n. knife blade
    n. lower lateral forceps
    n. mallet
    n. needle
    n. needle holder forceps
    n. osteotome
    n. pack
    n. polyp forceps
    n. polyp hook
    n. probe
    n. punch
    n. rasp
    n. retractor
    n. saw
    n. saw blade
    n. scissors
    n. septal forceps
    n. snare
    n. snare cannula
    n. snare wire
    n. snare wire carrier
    n. speculum
    n. splint
    n. suction cup
    n. suction tube
    n. suture
    n. suture needle
    n. tampon
    n. tampon sponge
    n. tenaculum
    n. tenaculum set
nasal-cutting forceps
nasal-dressing forceps
nasal-grasping forceps
nasal-packing forceps
nasal-tip dressing
Nasa-Spec nasal speculum
nasendoscope
    Hirschman n.
Nash needle
Nashold electrode
nasobiliary catheter

nasofrontal
    n. osteotome
    n. suture
nasolacrimal duct probe
nasomaxillary suture
nasopharyngeal
    n. biopsy forceps
    n. retractor
    n. speculum
nasopharyngolaryngofiberscope
    Pentax n.
nasopharyngoscope
    Broyles n.
    flexible n.
    Holmes n.
    Meltzer n.
    National n.
nasostat
    Gottschalk n.
Naso-Tamp nasal packing sponge
nasotrachael catheter
Nathan pacemaker
National
    N. all-metric
      transilluminator
    N. cautery
    N. cautery electrode
    N. coagulator
    N. ear speculum
    N. electricator
    N. general purpose
      cystoscope
    N. Graves vaginal speculum
    N. nasopharyngoscope
    N. opal-glass
      transilluminator
    N. proctoscope
natural
    n. pacemaker
    n. suture
Natural-Lok acetabular cup
Natural-Lok acetabular cup
  prosthesis
Natvig wire-twister forceps
Naugh os calcis apparatus tractor
NBIH catheter
NCT
    Non-Contact tonometer
Nd:YAG laser
Neal
    N. cannula
    N. catheter

    N. catheter trocar
    N. fallopian cannula
near-and-far suture
near-far suture
Nebauer
    N. ophthalmoendoscope
    N. ophthalmoscope
NEB total hip prosthesis
nebulizer
    bulb-operated n.
    DeVilbiss n.
    Emerson-Segal Medimizer
      demand n.
    hand-held n.
    Kidde n.
    medicinal n.
    Metermatic nasal n.
    Microseal n.
    Omron compressor n.
    penicillin n.
    Raindrop medication n.
    Selrodo n.
    ultrasonic n.
neck
    n. length
    n. rest
neck-wrap halter
needle
    abdominal n.
    Abrams n.
    Abrams pleural n.
    abscission n.
    Accucore II biopsy n.
    Ackerman n.
    Acland n.
    ACS n.
    active length n.
    Addix n.
    Adson n.
    Adson aneurysm n.
    Adson-Murphy n.
    Adson-Murphy trocar
      point n.
    Adson scalp n.
    Adson suture n.
    advancement n.
    Agnew n.
    Agnew tattooing n.
    air aspirator n.
    Albarran-Reverdin n.
    Alexander n.
    Alexander tonsillar n.
    Altmann n.

needle *(continued)*
    AMC n.
    Amplatz n.
    Amplatz angiography n.
    Amsler n.
    Amsler aqueous transplant n.
    Anchor surgical n.
    anesthesia n.
    anesthesia block n.
    aneurysm n.
    angiography n.
    angular n.
    anterior chamber receiving n.
    antral n.
    antral trocar n.
    antrum-exploring n.
    aortic root perfusion n.
    aortic vent n.
    aortic vent n.
    aortogram n.
    aortography n.
    Arkan sharpening-stone n.
    arterial n.
    arterial blood n.
    arteriography n.
    aspirating n.
    aspiration biopsy n.
    Atkinson n.
    Atkinson retrobulbar n.
    Atraloc n.
    atraumatic n.
    atraumatic suture n.
    Austin n.
    AV fistula n.
    Babcock n.
    Ballade n.
    Barbara n.
    Bard biopsy n.
    Barker n.
    Barraquer n.
    Barraquer-Vogt n.
    Barrett n.
    Barrett hebosteotomy n.
    B-D n.
    B-D bone marrow biopsy n.
    B-D spinal n.
    Beath n.
    Becton-Dickinson Teflon-sheathed n.
    Beeth n.
    Bengash n.

    bent n.
    Berbecker n.
    Bergeret-Reverdin n.
    Berges-Reverdin n.
    Beyer n.
    Beyer paracentesis n.
    Biegelseisen n.
    Bierman n.
    biopsy n.
    Biosearch n.
    bipolar n.
    Birtcher electrosurgical n.
    Black-Decker n.
    Blackmon n.
    Blair-Brown n.
    block anesthesia n.
    blunt n.
    blunt-point n.
    bone marrow biopsy n.
    Bonney n.
    Bonney curved n.
    Bonney suture n.
    boomerang n.
    boomerang bladder n.
    Bovie n.
    Bowman n.
    Bowman cataract n.
    Bowman eye n.
    Bowman iris n.
    brain biopsy n.
    Braun n.
    breast localization n.
    Brockenbrough n.
    Brockenbrough curved n.
    Brockenbrough transseptal n.
    Brophy n.
    Brophy-Deschamps n.
    Brown n.
    Brown cleft palate n.
    Brown-Sanders fascial n.
    Brown staphylorrhaphy n.
    Brughleman n.
    Brunner n.
    Brunner ligature n.
    Buerger n.
    Buerger prostatic n.
    Buncke quartz n.
    Bunnell n.
    Bunnell tendon n.
    butterfly n.
    butterfly IV n.
    BV-2 n.
    BV100 n.

Calhoun n.
Calhoun-Hagerless n.
Calhoun-Merz n.
Campbell n.
Campbell ventricular n.
cardioplegic n.
Carlens n.
carotid angiogram n.
Carpule n.
Carroll n.
Castroviejo n.
cataract n.
cataract-aspirating n.
catgut n.
catheter n.
caudal n.
cerebral angiography n.
cerebral angiography
  puncture n.
cervical n.
cervical suture n.
Charles n.
Charles fluted n.
Charleston antral n.
Charles vacuuming n.
Charlton n.
Charlton antral n.
Chiba n.
Chiba biopsy n.
Chiba eye n.
Chiba transhepatic
  cholangiography n.
Childs-Phillips n.
Childs-Phillips intestinal
  plication n.
Cibis n.
Cibis ski n.
CIF n.
Clagett n.
Clas von Eichen n.
cleft palate n.
Cloquet n.
Cobb-Ragde n.
Cobe AV fistular n.
Colts cutting n.
Colver n.
Colver tonsillar n.
Concept Multi-Liner
  lining n.
Concept suturing n.
Cone n.
cone biopsy n.
Cone ventricular n.

Conrad-Crosby n.
Conrad-Crosby bone marrow
  biopsy n.
Continental n.
control-release n.
conventional n.
Cook-Longdwel n.
Cook percutaneous entry n.
Cooley aortic vent n.
Cooley ventricular n.
Cooper n.
Cooper
  chemopallidectomy n.
Cooper ligature n.
Cooper pallidectomy n.
Cope n.
Cope biopsy n.
Cope pleural biopsy n.
Cope thoracentesis n.
copper-clad steel n.
corneal n.
corneal suture n.
Coston iris n.
couching n.
Cournand n.
Cournand arterial n.
Cournand arteriography n.
Cournand-Grino n.
Cournand-Grino
  angiography n.
Craig n.
Craig biopsy n.
Crawford n.
Crawford fascial n.
Crosby biopsy n.
CTX n.
CU-8 n.
Culp biopsy n.
Curry n.
Curry cerebral n.
curved n.
curved suture n.
Cushing n.
Cushing ventricular n.
cutting n.
cyclodiathermy n.
dacryocystorhinostomy n.
Daily cataract n.
Daiwa dental n.
Daiwa disposable n.
Damshek n.
Dandy n.
Dandy-Cairns brain n.

needle *(continued)*
Dandy-Cairns ventricular n.
Dandy ventricular n.
Dattner n.
Davis n.
Davis knife-n.
Davis tonsillar n.
Dean n.
Dean antral n.
Dean iris knife-n.
Dean-Senturia n.
DeBakey n.
debridement n.
Dees n.
Dees renal n.
Dees suture n.
Deknatel n.
Deknatel K-n.
Delbet-Reverdin n.
Denis Browne n.
Denis Browne cleft
 palate n.
DePuy-Weiss tonsillar n.
D'Errico ventricular n.
Deschamps n.
Deschamps ligature n.
Deschamps-Navratil n.
Deschamps-Navratil
 ligature n.
desiccation n.
desiccation-fulguration n.
Desmarres n.
Desmarres eye n.
Desmarres paracentesis n.
Devonshire n.
diamond-point suture n.
diathermic n.
Dingman n.
Dingman malleable
 passing n.
Dingman passing n.
discission n.
diskographic n.
disposable aspiration n.
disposable biopsy n.
disposable injection n.
disposable suturing n.
Dispos-A-Ture single-use
 surgical n.
Dix n.
DLP cardioplegic n.
docking n.
Docktor n.

Dorsey n.
Dos Santos aortography n.
Dos Santos lumbar
 aortography n.
double-barreled n.
double-lumen n.
double-tipped center-
 threading n.
Douglas suture n.
Doyen n.
Drapier n.
Drews lavage n.
D-Tach n.
Duff debridement n.
Dupuy-Dutemps n.
Dupuy-Weiss n.
Dupuy-Weiss tonsillar n.
dural n.
Durham n.
DuVries n.
Dyonics n.
East Grinstead n.
egress n.
n. electrode
Emmet n.
Emmet-Murphy n.
epilation n.
Epstein n.
Erosa disposable
 hypodermic n.
Estridge ventricular n.
Ethicon TG Plus n.
Ethicon TGW n.
exploring n.
extrusion n.
eyed n.
eyed suture n.
eyeless n.
eyeless atraumatic suture n.
eyeless suture n.
E-Z-EM biopsy n.
E-Z-EM cut biopsy n.
Falk n.
Farah cystoscopic n.
fascial n.
Federspiel n.
Feild-Lee biopsy n.
Fein n.
Fein antral trocar n.
Ferguson n.
Ferguson round-body n.
Ferguson suture n.

Ferris disposable bone
    marrow aspiration n.
filter n.
fine n.
Finochietto n.
Fischer n.
Fischer pneumothoracic n.
Fisher n.
Fisher eye n.
fishhook n.
fistular n.
flat spatula n.
flexible injection n.
Floyd n.
Floyd pneumothorax
    injection n.
flute n.
Flynt n.
Flynt aortography n.
Foltz n.
n. forceps
foreign body n.
Frackelton n.
Frackelton fascial n.
Framer tendon-passing n.
Francke n.
Frankfeldt n.
Frankfeldt hemorrhoidal n.
Franklin liver puncture n.
Franklin-Silverman n.
Franklin-Silverman biopsy n.
Franklin-Silverman
    prostatic n.
Franklin-Silverman urologic
    biopsy n.
Frazier n.
Frazier ventricular n.
Frederick n.
Frederick pneumothoracic n.
Freenseen liver biopsy n.
Freenseen ultrasound n.
French n.
French-eye n.
French spring-eye n.
Fritz n.
Gallie n.
Gallie fascial n.
ganglion injection n.
Gardner n.
Gardner suture n.
gastrointestinal n.
GC n.
general closure n.

Geuder corneal n.
Geuder keratoplasty n.
Gill n.
Gillmore n.
Girard n.
Girard anterior chamber n.
Girard-Swan n.
Goldbacher n.
Goldbacher rectal n.
Goldmann knife n.
Gordh n.
Gorsch n.
Graefe n.
Graefe iris n.
Graefe knife-n.
Grantham lobotomy n.
Greene n.
Greenfield n.
Green-Gould n.
Grieshaber n.
Grieshaber corneal n.
Grieshaber eye n.
Grieshaber iris n.
Grieshaber ophthalmic n.
Guest n.
n. guide
Haab n.
Haab knife n.
Hagedorn n.
Hagedorn suture n.
Halle n.
Halle septal n.
Halsey n.
harelip n.
Harken n.
Harken heart n.
Harvard n.
Haverhill n.
Hawkins n.
Hearn n.
heart n.
Hegar n.
Hegar-Baumgartner n.
hemorrhoidal n.
Henton n.
Henton suture n.
Henton tonsillar n.
Henton tonsillar suture n.
heparin n.
heparin-flushing n.
Hessburg lacrimal n.
Hey-Groves n.
high-risk n.

needle *(continued)*
Hingson-Edwards n.
Hobbs n.
Hoen n.
Hoen ventricular n.
n. holder (*See* holder)
Holinger n.
Homer n.
Homer localizaton n.
Homerlok n.
Hosford-Hicks n.
Hourin n.
Hourin tonsillar n.
House n.
House-Barbara n.
House-Barbara shattering n.
House-Rosen n.
House stapes n.
Howard Jones n.
Howell biliary aspiration n.
HR n.
Huber n.
Hunt n.
Hurd n.
Hurd suture n.
Hurd tonsillar suturing n.
Hutchins n.
Hutchins biopsy n.
hypodermic n.
Hypospray jet injection n.
Icofly infusion n.
Iliff-Wright n.
Illinois n.
Impex aspiration &
  injection n.
Indian club n.
Infusaid n.
Ingersoll n.
Ingersoll tonsillar n.
injection n.
intestinal n.
intestinal plication n.
intravenous n.
iris knife-n.
irrigating-positioning n.
IV n.
Jalaguier-Reverdin n.
Jameson n.
Jameson strabismus n.
Jamshidi n.
Jamshidi biopsy n.
Jamshidi-Kormed bone
  marrow biopsy n.

Jamshidi liver biopsy n.
Jelco n.
JMS injection n.
Jonesco wire suture n.
Jordan n.
Kader n.
Kader fishhook n.
Kall modification of
  Silverman n.
Kalt n.
Kalt corneal n.
Kalt eye n.
Kalt vein n.
Kaplan n.
Kaplan tracheostomy n.
Kara n.
Kara cataract n.
Karras n.
Karras angiography n.
Keith n.
Keith abdominal n.
Kelly n.
Kelly intestinal n.
Kelman n.
kidney n.
kidney suturing n.
King n.
King suture n.
Klatskin n.
Klatskin biopsy n.
Klatskin liver biopsy n.
Klima-Rosegger sternal n.
Knapp n.
Knapp knife-n.
Knight n.
Knight biopsy n.
Kobak n.
Kocher n.
Kohn n.
Koontz n.
Koontz hernia n.
Kopan n.
Kormed n.
Kormed disposable liver
  biopsy n.
Kronecker n.
Kronecker aneurysm n.
lacrimal n.
Lagleyze n.
Lahey n.
Laminex n.
Lane n.
Lane cleft palate n.

Lane suturing n.
Lapides n.
large-bore n.
Lee n.
Leighton n.
L'Esperance n.
Lewicky n.
Lewy-Holinger n.
Lewy-Holinger Teflon
  injection n.
Lewy-Rubin n.
Lewy-Rubin Teflon
  glycerine-mixture
  injection n.
Lewy Teflon glycerine-
  mixture injection n.
Lichtwicz n.
Lichtwicz antral n.
Lichtwicz-Bier antral n.
ligature n.
Lindeman n.
Lindeman transfusion n.
Linton-Blakemore n.
Lipschwitz n.
List n.
Litvak-Pereyra ligature n.
liver n.
liver biopsy n.
lobotomy n.
lock n.
Long n.
long n.
Longdwel n.
Longdwel catheter n.
Loopuyt n.
Lowell n.
Lowell pleural n.
Lowette n.
Lowette-Verner n.
Lowsley n.
Lowsley ribbon-gut n.
Luer n.
Luer lock n.
lumbar aortography n.
lumbar puncture n.
Lundy n.
Lundy fascial n.
Lundy-Irving n.
Lundy-Irving caudal n.
Luongo n.
Madayag n.
Maddox n.
Maddox caudal n.

Magielski n.
Mahurkar fistular n.
malleable passing n.
Maltz n.
Maltzman n.
Mammalok n.
Mammalok localization n.
Manan n.
Mantoux n.
March laser sclerostomy n.
Marion-Reverdin n.
Markham biopsy n.
Martin n.
Martin uterine n.
Marx n.
Mason-School aspirating n.
Masson n.
Masson fascial n.
Mathieu n.
Maumenee n.
Maumenee vitreous n.
Maumenee vitreous-
  aspirating n.
Mayo n.
Mayo catgut n.
Mayo intestinal n.
Mayo trocar n.
Mayo trocar-point n.
McCurdy n.
McCurdy staphylorrhaphy n.
McDowell n.
McGee prosthesis n.
McGhan plastic surgical n.
McGowan n.
McGregor n.
McIntire n.
McIntyre aspiration n.
McIntyre irrigation n.
mediastinoscopy
  aspirating n.
Medicut n.
Medicut intravenous n.
Medisystems fistular n.
Menghini n.
Menghini biopsy n.
Menghini liver biopsy n.
meniscal repair n.
Mentor prostate biopsy n.
metal n.
Metcoff pediatric biopsy n.
Meyer n.
Meyer cyclodiathermy n.
Microlet electrode n.

needle *(continued)*
micropoint n.
n. microstat set
Microvasive sclerotherapy n.
Millet n.
milliner's n.
Mixter n.
Mixter ventricular n.
Mizzy n.
modified CIF n.
modified spatula n.
MPL dental n.
MPL Hypo intraosseous n.
Mueller n.
Murphy n.
Murphy intestinal n.
myelography n.
Nager palatal n.
Nager tonsillar n.
Nagielski n.
Namic localization n.
nasal n.
nasal suture n.
Nash n.
Nelson n.
Nelson ligature n.
neurosurgical suture n.
Neville ascending aortic air
vent n.
New n.
Newman n.
Newman rectal injection n.
New oral n.
Nichols-Deschamps-Navratil
ligature n.
Noci stimuli n.
noncutting n.
noncutting suture n.
Nordenstrom biopsy n.
O'Brien airway n.
obstetrical anesthesia n.
obstetrical block
anesthesia n.
Ochsner n.
Oldfield n.
Op-Pneu laparoscopy n.
oral n.
Overholt n.
Overholt rib n.
Pace ventricular n.
Page n.
Palmer-Drapier n.
palpating n.

pan disposable n.
Pannett n.
Paparella n.
Paparella straight n.
paracentesis n.
paracervical nerve block n.
Parhad n.
Parhad-Poppen n.
Parker n.
Parker knife-n.
Parker-Pearson n.
Payr vein n.
pediatric biopsy n.
Penfield n.
Penfield biopsy n.
PercuCut biopsy n.
percutaneous n.
Pereyra n.
peribulbar n.
pericardiocentesis n.
Pischel n.
Pitkin n.
plain eye n.
pleural biopsy n.
plication n.
pneumoperitoneum n.
pneumothoracic n.
pneumothoracic injection n.
Politzer paracentesis n.
pop-off n.
Poppen n.
Poppen ventricular n.
positioning n.
postmortem suture n.
Potter n.
Potts n.
Potts-Cournand n.
Potts-Cournand
angiography n.
Presbyterian Hospital n.
Presbyterian Hospital
ventricular n.
n. probe
prostatic biopsy n.
pudendal n.
pudendal block
anesthesia n.
Pulec n.
puncture n.
Quantico n.
quartz n.
Quincke-Babcock n.
radium n.

Radpour n.
Ranfac n.
Rashkind septostomy n.
rectal n.
rectal injection n.
renal n.
retrobulbar n.
retrobulbar prosthesis n.
Retter n.
Retter aneurysm n.
Reverdin n.
Reverdin suturing n.
reverse-cutting n.
Rhoton n.
Rhoton straight point n.
rib n.
ribbon gut n.
Rica aneurysm n.
Rica cerebral angiography
  puncture n.
Rica suturing n.
Rider-Moeller n.
Riedel n.
Riedel corneal n.
Riley n.
Riley arterial n.
Robb n.
Roberts n.
Robinson-Smith n.
Rochester n.
Rochester aortic vent n.
Rochester-Meeker n.
Rolf lance n.
root n.
Rosen n.
Rosenthal n.
Roser n.
Ross n.
Rotex n.
Rotex II biopsy n.
round n.
round body n.
Rubin n.
Rubin-Arnold n.
Rubin knife n.
Ruskin n.
Ruskin antral n.
Ruskin antral trocar n.
Ruskin sphenopalatine
  ganglion n.
Rutner biopsy n.
Sabreloc n.
Sabreloc spatula n.

Sachs n.
Salah n.
Salah sternal n.
Sanders-Brown n.
Sanders-Brown-Shaw n.
Sanders-Brown-Shaw
  aneurysm n.
Sarot n.
Sato cataract n.
Saunders n.
Saunders cataract n.
Saunders-Paparella n.
Saunders-Paparella
  straight n.
Savariaud-Reverdin n.
scalp n.
scalpene n.
Schecter-Bryant aortic
  vent n.
Scheer n.
Scheie n.
Scheie cataract n.
Scheie cataract-aspirating n.
Schmieden n.
Schmieden-Dick n.
Schuknecht n.
scleral spatula n.
sclerotherapy n.
sclerotherapy n.
Scoville n.
Scoville ventricular n.
Seldinger n.
Seldinger arterial n.
septal n.
Septoject n.
Seraflo AV fistular n.
seton n.
Shambaugh n.
Shambaugh palpating n.
shattering n.
Sheldon-Spatz n.
Sheldon-Spatz vertebral
  arteriogram n.
Sheldon-Swann n.
Shirodkar n.
Shirodkar aneurysm n.
Shirodkar cervical n.
short n.
side-cutting spatulated n.
side-flattened n.
sidewall holed n.
Silverman biopsy n.
Silverman-Boeker n.

needle *(continued)*
 Simcoe n.
 Simcoe anterior chamber
  receiving n.
 Simcoe irrigating-
  positioning n.
 Simcoe suture n.
 Simmonds cricothyrotomy n.
 Sims n.
 Sims abdominal n.
 Singer n.
 SITE n.
 ski n.
 skinny n.
 skinny Chiba n.
 Sluder n.
 SMIC suture n.
 Smiley-Williams n.
 Smiley-Williams
  arteriography n.
 spatula split n.
 sphenopalatine n.
 sphenopalatine ganglion n.
 spinal n.
 Spinelli biopsy n.
 spring-eye n.
 spring-hook wire n.
 stab n.
 Stamey n.
 stapes n.
 staphylorrhaphy n.
 sternal n.
 sternal puncture n.
 Stille-Mayo-Hegar n.
 Stille-Seldinger n.
 Stocker n.
 Stocker cyclodiathermy
  puncture n.
 stop n.
 Storz aspiration biopsy n.
 Storz flexible injection n.
 strabismus n.
 straight n.
 straight-point n.
 straight suturing n.
 Strauss n.
 Sturmdorf n.
 Sturmdorf cervical n.
 Sturmdorf pedicle n.
 suction biopsy n.
 Sulze diamond-point n.
 Sure-Cut n.
 Surgicraft suture n.

 Surgineedle
  pneumoperitoneum n.
 Sutton n.
 Sutton biopsy n.
 suture-release n.
 suturing n.
 swaged n.
 swaged-on n.
 Swan knife-n.
 Swedgeon already-
  threaded n.
 Symonds n.
 taper n.
 Tapercut n.
 tapered n.
 taper-point suture n.
 tattooing n.
 Tauber n.
 Teflon n.
 Teflon-covered n.
 Teflon glycerine-mixture
  injection n.
 Teflon injection n.
 Tek-Pro n.
 tendon n.
 Terry-Mayo n.
 Terumo AV fistula n.
 Terumo dental n.
 Terumo hypodermic n.
 TF n.
 TG140 n.
 THI n.
 thin-walled n.
 threaded eye n.
 Ticsay transpubic n.
 n. tip catheter
 tissue desiccation n.
 titanium n.
 Titus n.
 Titus venoclysis n.
 Tocantins bone marrow n.
 Todd n.
 Todd eye cautery n.
 tonsillar n.
 tonsillar suture n.
 Torrington French spring n.
 transpubic n.
 Travenol n.
 Travenol biopsy n.
 Travert n.
 triple-lumen n.
 trocar n.
 Troutman n.

Tru-Cut n.
Tru-Cut biopsy n.
Tru-Cut liver biopsy n.
Trupp ventricular n.
tungsten microdissection n.
Tuohy n.
Tuohy aortography n.
Tuohy lumbar
aortography n.
Tuohy spinal n.
Turkel n.
Turkel liver biopsy n.
Turkel sternal n.
Turner biopsy n.
Turner-Warwick n.
Turner-Warwick
urethroplasty n.
Tworek bone marrow-
aspirating n.
University of Illinois n.
University of Illinois
biopsy n.
University of Illinois
marrow n.
University of Illinois
sternal n.
University of Illinois sternal
puncture n.
Updegraff n.
Updegraff cleft palate n.
Updegraff
staphylorrhaphy n.
urethroplasty n.
uterine n.
Vacutainer n.
vacuuming n.
Veenema-Gusberg n.
Veenema-Gusberg prostatic
biopsy n.
Veirs n.
Venaflo n.
venipuncture n.
venous n.
venting aortic Bengash n.
ventricular n.
Veress n.
Veress-Frangenheim n.
Veress
pneumoperitoneum n.
Veress spring-loaded
laparoscopic n.
Vicat n.
Viking n.

Vim n.
Vim-Silverman n.
Vim-Silverman biopsy n.
Visi-Black n.
Visi-Black surgical n.
Visitec n.
Visitec retrobulbar n.
V. Mueller paracervical
nerve block n.
V. Mueller pudendal nerve
block n.
Vogt-Barraquer corneal n.
Vogt-Barraquer eye n.
Voorhees n.
Walker n.
Walker tonsillar n.
Wang n.
Wangensteen n.
Wangensteen intestinal n.
Wannagat injection n.
Ward n.
Ward French n.
Ward French-eye n.
Watson-Williams n.
wedge-line n.
Weeks n.
Weiss n.
Welsh olive-tipped n.
Wertheim-Navratil n.
Westcott biopsy n.
Westerman-Jansen n.
whirlybird n.
Whitacre n.
Wiener eye n.
Williams n.
Williams cystoscopic n.
Williamson biopsy n.
Wilson-Cook electrode n.
Wolf antral n.
Wolf Veress n.
Wood n.
Wood aortography n.
Wooten eye n.
Wright n.
Wright-Crawford n.
Wright fascial n.
Wright ophthalmic n.
Wright ptosis n.
Yankauer n.
Yankauer septal n.
Yankauer suture n.
Ziegler n.
Zoellner n.

needle holder (*See* holder)
needle-holder forceps
needle-knife
    Girard-Swan n.-k.
    McCaslin n.-k.
    Ziegler n.-k.
needle-nose pliers
needlepoint cautery
Needlescoper endoscope
Neer
    N. II prosthesis
    N. II shoulder system
    N. II total shoulder system
      implant
    N. I prosthesis
    N. shoulder
    N. shoulder prosthesis
Neesone root canal depth indicator
Neff
    N. femorotibial nail system
    N. meniscal knife
Negus
    N. bronchoscope
    N. forceps
    N. laryngoscope
    N. mouth gag
    N. pusher
    N. telescope
    N. tonsillar forceps
Negus-Broyles bronchoscope
Negus-Green forceps
Neibauer-Cutter prosthesis
Neider valvulotome
Neil-Moore
    N.-M. m. e. electrode
    N.-M. m. e. meatotomy
      electrode
    N.-M. m. e. perforator drill
Neiman nasal splint
Neivert
    N. chisel
    N. dissector
    N. double-ended retractor
    N. knife guide
    N. nasal hook
    N. nasal polyp hook
    N. needle holder
    N. osteotome
    N. retractor
    N. rocking gouge
    N. tonsillar knife
Neivert-Anderson osteotome

Neivert-Eves
    N.-E. tonsillar snare
    N.-E. tonsillar wire
Nélaton
    N. bullet probe
    N. catheter
    N. rubber tube drain
Nellcor pulse oximetry telemetry network
Nelson
    N. abdominal puncture
    N. classic plus scissors
    N. empyema trocar
    N. forceps
    N. ligature needle
    N. line keeper
    N. lobectomy scissors
    N. lung-dissecting forceps
    N. lung-dissecting scissors
    N. lung forceps
    N. lung tissue forceps
    N. needle
    N. retractor
    N. rib retractor
    N. rib self-retaining
      retractor
    N. rib spreader
    N. rib stripper
    N. scissors
    N. thoracic trocar
    N. tissue forceps
    N. trocar
    N. Vital dissecting scissors
Nelson-Bethune shears
Nelson-Martin forceps
Nelson-Metzenbaum scissors
Nelson-Patterson empyema trocar
Nelson-Roberts stripper
Nemdi tweezer epilation device
neodymium-doped yttrium-aluminum-garnet laser (Nd:YAG laser)
neodymium laser
Neoguard percussor
neonatal
    n. internal jugular puncture kit
    n. scissors
    n. sternal retractor
    n. vascular clamp
    n. vascular forceps
Neoplex catheter
neoprene dressing

Neos pacemaker
nephrolithotomy forceps
nephroscope
    Cabot n.
Nephross dialyzer
nephrostomy
    n. catheter
    n. clamp
    n. tube
Neplaton catheter
nerve
    n. cuff
    n. dissector
    n. holder
    n. hook
    n. pull hook
    n. retractor
    n. root laminectomy
      dissector
    n. root retractor
    n. root suction retractor
    n. separator spatula
    n. suture
Nesbit
    N. cystoscope
    N. electrode
    N. electrotome
    N. hemostatic bag
    N. resectoscope
    N. tonsillar snare
Nesta stitch suture
nested trocar
Nestor-3
Nestor guiding catheter
Nettleship
    N. canaliculus dilator
    N. dilator
Nettleship-Wilder
    N.-W. dilator
    N.-W. lacrimal dilator
network
    Nellcor pulse oximetry
      telemetry n.
Neubauer
    N. cannula
    N. forceps
    N. foreign body forceps
    N. lancet cannula
    N. vitreous micro-extractor
      forceps
Neubeiser adjustable forearm splint
Neuber bone tube
Neubuser tubal-seizing forceps

Neufeld
    N. driver
    N. nail
    N. pin
    N. plate
    N. tractor
Neumann
    N. calipers block
    N. depth gauge
    N. double-corneal marker
    N. double marker
    N. razor blade fragment
      holder
    N. scissors
Neumann-Shepard
    N.-S. corneal marker
    N.-S. Optical Center corneal
      marker
    N.-S. optical center marker
    N.-S. oval optical center
      marker
Neurain drill
Neurairtome
    N. drill
    Hall N. with Smith
      perforator
neuroendoscope
    Chavantes-Zamorano n.
Neuroguide
    N. camera-processor
    N. interoperative viewing
      system
    N. monitor
    N. optical handpiece
    N. peel-away catheter
      introducer
    N. suction-irrigation adapter
    N. Visicath viewing catheter
Neurolase microsurgical CO_2 laser
neurological
    n. kit
    n. percussion hammer
    n. percussor
    n. sponge
    n. tuning fork
Neurological Institute periosteal
  elevator
Neuromod TENS unit
Neuropath biofeedback device
Neuroprobe pain control system
Neuro-Pulse TENS unit
neurorongeur

neurostimulator
    Jobstens n.
neurosurgical
    n. bur
    n. connector
    n. dissector
    n. dressing forceps
    n. forceps
    n. head holder
    n. headrest
    n. ligature forceps
    n. needle holder
    n. scissors
    n. suction forceps
    n. suture
    n. suture needle
    n. tissue forceps
neurosuture
neurotome
    Bradford enucleation n.
Neurotone biofeedback device
neurovascular
    n. forceps
    n. scissors
neutral
    n. electrode
    n. hook
Neutrocim dental cement
Neuwirth-Palmer forceps
Nevada gonioscope
Neville
    N. ascending aortic air vent needle
    N. tracheal prosthesis
    N. tracheobronchial prosthesis
Nevins
    N. dressing forceps
    N. forceps
    N. tissue forceps
Nevyas
    N. double-sharp cystitome
    N. drape retractor
    N. lens forceps
    N. retractor
New
    N. biopsy forceps
    N. electrode
    N. England Baptist acetabular cup
    N. forceps
    N. Jersey hemiarthroplasty prosthesis

N. Jersey-L.C.S. shoulder prosthesis
N. Jersey-L.C.S. total knee prosthesis
N. Luer-type speaking tube
N. needle
N. oral needle
N. Orleans corneal cutting block
N. Orleans endarterectomy stripper set
N. Orleans Eye and Ear forceps
N. Orleans forceps
N. Orleans lens loop
N. Orleans lens loupe
N. Orleans needle holder
N. Orleans stripper
N. scissors
N. speaking tube
N. suture scissors
N. tenaculum
N. tissue forceps
N. tracheal retractor
N. tracheostomy hook
N. tracheotomy hook
N. Yorker guide wire
N. York erysiphake
N. York Eye and Ear cannula
N. York Eye and Ear fixation forceps
N. York Eye and Ear forceps
N. York Eye and Ear Hospital fixation forceps
N. York glass suction tube
N. York Hospital electrode
N. York Hospital retractor
newborn eyelid retractor
Newell
    N. lid retractor
    N. nucleus hook
Newhart-Casselberry snare
Newhart hook
Newhart-Smith cup
Newkirk mouth gag
New-Lambotte osteotome
Newman
    N. forceps
    N. needle
    N. proctoscope
    N. rectal injection needle

N. tenaculum
N. tenaculum forceps
N. toenail plate
N. uterine forceps
N. uterine knife
N. uterine tenaculum
  forceps
Newport cartilage gouge
Newton
N. guide wire
N. LLT guide wire
Newton-Morgan retractor
**Nezhat-Dorset hydrodissection
  pump**
nibbler
  Schulze anterior capsule n.
Nicati foreign body spud
Niche knife
Nichol clamp
Nichols
N. aortic clamp
N. infundibulectomy rongeur
N. nasal siphon
**Nichols-Deschamps-Navratil
  ligature needle**
**Nichols-Jehle coronary multihead
  catheter**
Nickell cystoscope adapter
Nicola
N. clamp
N. forceps
N. gouge
N. microforceps
N. pituitary rongeur
N. raspatory
N. tendon clamp
Nicoll
N. bone graft
N. plate
N. tendon prosthesis
Niebauer
N. finger-joint replacement
  prosthesis
N. prosthesis
N. trapezium replacement
  prosthesis
Niedner
N. anastomosis clamp
N. clamp
N. commissurotomy knife
N. dissecting forceps
N. forceps
N. pulmonic clamp

NIH
NIH catheter
NIH left ventriculography
  catheter
NIH mitral valve forceps
NIH mitral valve-grasping
  forceps
Niko-Fix
Nikon
N. camera
N. fundus camera
N. slit lamp
Nilsson-Stille abortion suction tube
Nilsson suction tube
**Nimbus Hemopump cardiac assist
  device**
nipper
  anterior crurotomy n.
  cuticle n.
  Dieter n.
  Dieter-House n.
  English nail n.
  Hough anterior
    crurotomy n.
  House-Dieter malleus n.
  House malleus n.
  Lempert malleus n.
  malleus n.
  nail n.
  n. nail drill
  Rica malleus head n.
  SMIC malleus head n.
  Tabb crural n.
  Turnbull nail n.
  Wister n.
Nir Lat male external catheter
Niro
N. arch bars
N. wire-twister forceps
Nisbet
N. eye forceps
N. fixation forceps
Nissen
N. cystic forceps
N. forceps
N. gall duct forceps
N. hassux forceps
N. rib spreader
N. suture
**Nite Train-R enuresis conditioning
  device**
**Ni-Ti Shape Memory alloy
  compression stapler**

NK dental capsule
NL3 guider
Nobetec dental cement
Nobis aortic occluder
Noble
    N. forceps
    N. iris forceps
    N. scissors
Noblock retractor
Noci stimuli needle
nocturnal penile tumescence
    monitor (NPT monitor)
Nogenol dental cement
Noiles prosthesis
Noland-Budd
    N.-B. cervical curette
    N.-B. curette
No-Lok compression screw
Nomos multiprogrammable R-wave
    inhibited demand pacemaker
nonabsorbable
    n. surgical suture
    n. suture
nonadhering dressing
nonadhesive dressing
noncannulated nail
noncompetitive pacemaker
Non-Contact II tonometer
Non-Contact tonometer (NCT)
noncrushing
    n. anterior resection clamp
    n. bowel clamp
    n. clamp
    n. common duct forceps
    n. forceps
    n. gastroenterostomy clamp
    n. gastrointestinal clamp
    n. intestinal clamp
    n. intestinal forceps
    n. liver-holding clamp
    n. pickup forceps
    n. tissue-holding forceps
    n. vascular clamp
noncutting
    n. needle
    n. suture needle
noneverting suture
nonfenestrated
    n. forceps
    n. Moore-type femoral stem
noninvasive continuous cardiac
    output monitor

nonmagnetic
    n. dressing forceps
    n. forceps
    n. tissue forceps
nonperforating
    n. towel clamp
    n. towel forceps
nonpneumatic tourniquet
nonslipping forceps
nontoothed forceps
nontraumatizing
    n. forceps
    n. visceral forceps
nonweightbearing brace
Noon
    N. AV fistular clamp
    N. AV fistular tunneler
    N. modified vascular access
    tunneler
noose suture
Norcross periosteal elevator
Nordan-Colibri forceps
Nordan tying forceps
Nordenstrom biopsy needle
Nordent
    N. amalgam condenser
    N. bone chisel
    N. bone curette
    N. bone file
    N. burnisher
    N. carver
    N. chisel
    N. excavator
    N. explorer
    N. filling instrument
    N. hatchet
    N. hoe
    N. margin trimmer
    N. oral surgery elevator
    N. periodontic knife
    N. scaler
Nordent-Ochsenbein periodontic
    chisel
Nord orthodontic plate
Norelco mucotome
Norfolk aspiration catheter
Norman
    N. tibial bolt
    N. tibial pin
Norplant implant
Norrbacka bone elevator
Norrbacka-Stille lever

Norris
    N. button
    N. sponge forceps
    N. tip magnet
Northbent suture scissors
North-South retractor
Northville brace
Norton
    N. adjustable cup reamer
    N. ball reamer
    N. endotracheal tube
    N. flow-directed Swan-Ganz
      thermodilution catheter
Norwood
    N. forceps
    N. rectal snare
nose
    n. guard splint
    n. splint
Nosik transorbital leukotome
nostril
    n. elevator-retractor
    n. thermistor
notchplasty blade
Noto
    N. dressing forceps
    N. ovum forceps
    N. polypus forceps
    N. sponge forceps
    N. sponge-holding forceps
Nott-Gutmann vaginal speculum
Nott vaginal speculum
Nounton blade
Nourse bladder syringe
Nova
    N. II pacemaker
    N. jaw hook
    N. thermodilution catheter
Novacor left ventricular assist
  device
Novaflex intraocular lens
Novak
    N. biopsy curette
    N. biopsy uterine curette
    N. curette
    N. endometrial biopsy
      suction curette
    N. fixation forceps
    N. gynecology biopsy
      curette
    N. uterine biopsy curette
    N. uterine curette
    N. uterine suction curette

Novak-Schoeckaert endometrial
  curette
Novametrix combination O_2/CO_2
  sensor
Novar oral illuminator
Novito eye implant
Novofil suture
Novoste catheter
Novus 2000 ophthalmoscope
Noyes
    N. chalazion punch
    N. ear forceps
    N. forceps
    N. iridectomy scissors
    N. iris scissors
    N. nasal-dressing forceps
    N. nasal forceps
    N. rongeur
    N. speculum
Noyes-Shambaugh scissors
NPT monitor
    nocturnal penile tumescence
    monitor
N-terface graft dressing
NTS-4 triple-syringe
Nu
nubular blade
nuclear
    n. pacemaker
    n. powered pacemaker
    n. probe
nucleus
    n. cannula
    n. delivery cannula
    n. erysiphake
    n. expressor
    n. loop
    n. removal loop
    n. rotator
    n. spatula
Nu-Comfort colostomy appliance
Nu-Derm dressing
Nu-Form truss
Nu-Gauze dressing
Nu-Gauze sponge
Nu-Gel
    N.-G. dressing
    N.-G. hydrogel wound
      dressing
Nugent
    N. aspirator
    N. erysiphake
    N. fixation forceps

Nugent *(continued)*
    N. forceps
    N. iris hook
    N. soft cataract aspirator
    N. superior rectus forceps
    N. utility forceps
Nugent-Gradle
    N.-G. scissors
    N.-G. stitch scissors
Nugent-Green-Dimitry erysiphake
Nugowski forceps
Nu-Knit absorbable hemostat
NuKO knee orthosis
Nunez
    N. aortic clamp
    N. approximator
    N. auricular clamp
    N. clamp
    N. sternal approximator
    N. ventricular ventilation
      tube
Nunez-Nunez mitral stenosis knife
Nurolon suture
Nussbaum
    N. intestinal clamp
    N. intestinal forceps
nut
    close encounter n.
    healing n.
    locking n.
    nylon n.
    sleeved n.
Nutricath catheter
nutrition
    total parenteral n. (TPN)
Nuttall retractor
Nuva-Lite ultraviolet activator
Nuvistor electronic tonometer
NuVue lens

Nuway in-the-ear hearing aid
Nu-wrap roll dressing
Nyboer esophageal electrode
Nycore
    N. angiography catheter
    N. catheter
Nyhus-Nelson
    N.-N. gastric decompression
      tube
    N.-N. jejunal feeding tube
Nyhus-Potts intestinal forceps
Nylok
    N. bolt
    N. self-locking nail
nylon
    n. face mallet
    n. hand scrub brush
    n. head mallet
    n. loop
    n. monofilament suture
    n. nut
    n. retention suture
    Rica n.
    n. scrub brush
    n. suture
nystagmus
    n. bulb
    n. glasses
Nystroem
    N. abdominal suction tube
    N. hip nail
    N. nail driver
    N. retractor
    N. tumor forceps
Nystroem-Stille
    N.-S. driver
    N.-S. hip nail
    N.-S. retractor

O

O'Beirne sphincter tube
Oberhill
    O. laminectomy retractor
    O. obstetrical forceps
    O. retractor
    O. self-retaining retractor
Ober tendon passer
OB/GYN chair
globular object forceps
oblique
    o. bandage
    o. hook
O'Brien
    O. airway needle
    O. fixation forceps
    O. forceps
    O. foreign body spud
    O. phrenic retractor
    O. rib hook
    O. rib retractor
    O. rongeur
    O. spatula
    O. stitch scissors
    O. suture scissors
O'Brien-Elschnig
    O.-E. fixation forceps
    O.-E. forceps
O'Brien-Mayo scissors
O'Brien-Storz microhemostat
Obstbaum
    O. lens spatula
    O. spatula
    O. synechia spatula
obstetrical
    o. anesthesia needle
    o. block anesthesia needle
    o. decapitating embryotome
    o. decapitating hook
    o. double-armed suture
    o. forceps
    o. hook
    o. retractor
    o. spoon
obturator
    Alcock-Timberlake o.
    Bucy-Frazier coagulating
      suction cannula o.
    cannulated o.
    coagulating suction
      cannula o.

concave o.
convex o.
Cripps o.
distending o.
double-catherizing sheath
  and o.
Ellik-Shaw o.
Fitch o.
Frazier suction tube o.
Leusch atraumatic o.
Rumel tourniquet-eyed o.
sheath and o.
suction tube o.
Thal-Mantel o.
Timberlake o.
tourniquet-eyed o.
ureteral catheter o.
Obwegeser
    O. awl
    O. channel retractor
    O. periosteal retractor
    O. retractor
    O. splitting chisel
occipital suture
occipitomastoid suture
occipitoparietal suture
occipitosphenoidal suture
occluder
    air inflatable vessel o.
      clamp
    aortic o.
    Brockenbrough curved-tip o.
    catheter tip o.
    eye o.
    Goffman o.
    Kean-M-4 o.
    multiple-pin hole o.
    Nobis aortic o.
    Pram combination o.
occluding
    o. clamp
    o. forceps
    o. fracture frame
occlusal rest bar
occlusion
    o. catheter
    o. clamp
    o. multipurpose clamp

occlusive
   o. balloon
   o. dressing
Ochs
  Ochsner
Ochsner (Ochs)
   O. aortic clamp
   O. arterial clamp
   O. arterial forceps
   O. ball-tipped scissors
   O. clamp
   O. diamond-edged scissors
   O. flexible spiral gallstone
    probe
   O. forceps
   O. gallbladder trocar
   O. gallbladder tube
   O. gall duct probe
   O. gallstone probe
   O. hemostatic forceps
   O. malleable retractor
   O. needle
   O. probe
   O. retractor
   O. ribbon retractor
   O. scissors
   O. spiral probe
   O. thoracic clamp
   O. thoracic trocar
   O. trocar
   O. vascular retractor
   O. wire twister
Ochsner-DeBakey spur crusher
Ochsner-Dixon
   O.-D. arterial forceps
   O.-D. forceps
Ochsner-Favaloro self-retaining
  retractor
Ochsner-Fenger gallstone probe
Ockerblad
   O. clamp
   O. forceps
   O. kidney clamp
   O. vessel clamp
O'Connell suture
O'Connor
   O. abdominal retractor
   O. biopsy forceps
   O. clamp
   O.d double-edge curette
   O. drape
   O. eye forceps
   O. finger cup

   O. flat tenotomy hook
   O. forceps
   O. grasping forceps
   O. hook
   O. hook punch
   O. iris forceps
   O. lid clamp
   O. lid forceps
   O. operating arthroscope
   O. rectal finger cot
   O. retractor
   O. scleral depressor
   O. scleral marker
   O. sharp hook
   O. sheath
   O. tenotomy hook
   O. vaginal retractor
O'Connor-Elschnig fixation forceps
O'Connor-O'Sullivan
   O.-O. abdominal retractor
   O.-O. retractor
   O.-O. self-retaining retractor
   O.-O. vaginal retractor
Octopus holder
ocular
   o. cautery
   o. cup
   o. marker
   o. prosthesis
oculocerebrovasculometer (OCVM)
oculogyric stimulator
oculoplethysmograph (OPG)
Oculus lens loupe
ocutome
  disposable o.
   o. probe
   o. vitrector
   o. vitreous blade
OCVM
  oculocerebrovasculometer
O'Dell spicule forceps
Odland ankle prosthesis
Odman-Ledin catheter
O'Donoghue
   O. cartilage feeler
   O. cystourethroscope
   O. dressing
   O. knee splint
   O. stirrup splint
   O. suture passer
odontoid peg-grasping forceps
O'Dwyer tube

OEC
    OEC Dual-Op barrel/plate
      component
    OEC lag screw component
      with keyway
OEC/Kuntscher Interlocking
  Pathfinder nail
Oertli
    O. lid retractor
    O. suture
    O. wire lid retractor
Oettingen
    O. abdominal retractor
    O. abdominal self-retaining
      retractor
offset
    o. hand retractor
    o. hinge
    o. operating laparoscope
O'Gawa
    O. irrigating cannula
    O. needle holder
    O. suture-fixation forceps
    O. suture forceps
    O. two-way aspirating
      cannula
    O. two-way cataract-
      aspirating cannula
    O. two-way irrigating and
      aspirating cannula
    O. tying forceps
O'Gawa-Castroviejo
    O.-C. forceps
    O.-C. tying forceps
Ogden plate system
Ogden-Senturia eustachian inflator
Ogura
    O. forceps
    O. nasal saw
O'Hanlon
    O. forceps
    O. gastrointestinal clamp
    O. intestinal clamp
O'Hanlon-Pool suction tube
O'Hara forceps
O'Harris-Petruso cup
Ohio
    O. critical care ventilator
    O. pressure infuser
    O. safety trap overflow
      bottle
Ohl periosteal elevator
Ohmeda probe

OIC emergency oxygen inhalator
oiled
    o. silk dressing
    o. silk suture
Okmian microneedle holder
Okonek-Yasargil tumor fork
Olbert
    O. balloon
    O. balloon catheter
    O. balloon dilatation
      catheter
Oldberg
    O. brain retractor
    O. dissector
    O. forceps
    O. intervertebral disk
      forceps
    O. intervertebral disk
      rongeur
    O. laminectomy rongeur
    O. pituitary rongeur
    O. pituitary rongeur forceps
    O. straight retractor
Oldfield needle
Oliair
    O. articulator
    O. mouth mirror
oligodonal band
olivary catheter
olive
    Gergoyie o.
    Gergoyie-Guggenheim o.
    interchangeable vein
      stripper o.
    o. wire
Olivecrona
    O. aneurysm clamp
    O. aneurysm forceps
    O. angular scissors
    O. brain spatula
    O. brain spatula-spoon
    O. brain spoon
    O. clip
    O. conchotome
    O. dural scissors
    O. endaural rongeur
    O. forceps
    O. guillotine scissors
    O. rongeur
    O. rongeur forceps
    O. scissors
    O. silver clip
    O. spatula

Olivecrona *(continued)*
   O. trigeminal knife
   O. wire saw
Olivecrona-Gigli
   O.-G. saw
   O.-G. wire saw
Olivecrona-Stille dissector
Olivecrona-Toennis
   O.-T. clip-applying forceps
   O.-T. forceps
Oliver
   O. retractor
   O. scalp retractor
olive-tipped, olive-tip
   o.-t. bougie
   o.-t. catheter
   o.-t. dilator
Olk
   O. membrane peeler
   O. membrane peeler knife
   O. retinal spatula
Ollier
   O. graft
   O. rake retractor
   O. raspatory
   O. retractor
Ollier-Thiersch
   O.-T. graft
   O.-T. implant
Olsen-Hegar needle holder
Olsen self-retaining Laparostat
Olyco
   O. articulator
   O. mouth mirror
Olympia
   O. articulator
   O. mouth mirror
Olympic needle holder
Olympus
   O. alligator-jaw endoscopic forceps
   O. angioscope
   O. basket-type endoscopic forceps
   O. biopsy forceps
   O. camera
   O. colonoscope
   O. diagnostic laparoscope
   O. duodenofiberscope
   O. duodenoscope
   O. endoscope
   O. endoscopic biopsy forceps
   O. ENF-P2 flexible laryngoscope
   O. esophagofiberscope
   O. esophagoscope
   O. fiberoptic bronchoscope
   O. fiberoptic scope
   O. fiberoptic sigmoidoscope
   O. fiberscope
   O. flexible sigmoidoscope
   O. gastrocamera
   O. gastroscope
   O. GIF-D duodenoscope
   O. heat probe
   O. hot biopsy forceps
   O. magnetic extractor forceps
   O. minisnare forceps
   O. OES flexible endoscope
   O. OM-1 endoscopic camera
   O. operating camera
   O. operating laparoscope
   O. pelican-type endoscopic forceps
   O. Pre-OES flexible endoscope
   O. rat-tooth endoscopic forceps
   O. rubber-tip endoscopic forceps
   O. shark-tooth endoscopic forceps
   O. sigmoidoscope
   O. tripod-type endoscopic forceps
   O. W-shaped endoscopic forceps
O'Malley
   O. jaw fracture splint
   O. self-adhering lens implant
   O. vitrector
O'Malley-Heintz cutter
O'Malley-Skia transilluminator
Ombrédanne
   O. forceps
   O. mallet
Omed bulldog vascular clamp
Omega Plus compression hip system
omental
   o. adhevise band
   o. band

Ommaya
    O. CSF reservoir
    O. reservoir implant
      material
    O. ventricular tube
Omni
    O. beam
    O. catheter
    O. knee brace
    O. retractor
Omni-Atricor pacemaker
Omnicor pacemaker
Omni-Ectocor pacemaker
Omnifit
    O. acetabular cup
    O. HA femoral component
    O. HA hip system
    O. HA stem
    O. intraocular lens
Omniflex
    O. balloon catheter
    O. head
    O. impression material
Omni-Orthocor pacemaker
Omnipaque contrast material
OmniPhase penile prosthesis
Omniprep skin prepping paste
Omniscience
    O. cardiac valve prosthesis
    O. heart valve
Omnisil putty
Omni-Stanicor pacemaker
Omni-Theta pacemaker
Omnitone hearing aid
Omni-Ventricor pacemaker
Omron compressor nebulizer
on-edge mattress suture
one-hand speculum
one-horn bridge
O'Neill
    O. cardiac clamp
    O. cardiac operating scissors
    O. clamp
    O. double-curved clamp
one-piece
    o.-p. intraocular lens
    o.-p. shunt
    o.-p. shunt with reservoir
One-Time disposable skin stapler
One-Touch electrolysis

Ono
    O. laryngobronchoscope
      atomizer
    O. loupe for endoscope
Opaca-Garcea ureteral catheter
open
    o. hook
    o. lens
open-end aspirating tube
open-loop intraocular lens
open-side vaginal speculum
operative explorer
OPG
    oculoplethysmograph
Ophthalas laser
ophthalmic
    o. blade
    o. calipers
    o. cautery electrode
    o. cup
    o. hook
    o. pick
    o. sable brush
    o. sponge
ophthalmodynamometer
    Bailliart o.
    dial-type o.
ophthalmoendoscope
    Nebauer o.
    Zylik o.
ophthalmometer
    American Optical o.
    Javal o.
ophthalmoscope
    Alcon indirect o.
    binocular indirect o. with
      SPF
    o. camera
    Ful-Vue o.
    Grafco o.
    Gullstrand o.
    Halberg indirect o.
    halogen o.
    halogen coaxial o.
    indirect o.
    Keeler o.
    May o.
    monocular indirect o.
    Nebauer o.
    Novus 2000 o.
    Propper binocular
      indirect o.
    Reichert o.

ophthalmoscope *(continued)*
    Schepens o.
    Schultz-Crock binocular o.
    Welch Allyn o.
    Zeiss o.
Ophthalon suture
Opiela brace
Opotow
    O. cavity varnish
    O. filling material
Oppenheim brace
Oppenheimer spring wire splint
Op-Pneu laparoscopy needle
Opponens splint
Opraflex
    O. drape
    O. incise drape
Op-Site
    O.-S. drape
    O.-S. dressing
    O.-S. occlusive dressing
Op-Temp cautery
optic
    Boutin o.
    o. cup
Opticaid lens loupe
optical
    o. biopsy forceps
    o. esophagoscope
    o. frames
    o. laryngoscope
    o. radiation intraocular lens
Opticath oximeter catheter
Optic ureterotome
Opti-Fix
    O.-F. acetabular cup
    O.-F. femoral component
    O.-F. total hip system
Optifix acetabular cup
Optiflex intraocular lens
Opti-Gard eye protector
Optilume prostate balloon dilator
Optima
    O. pacemaker
    O. pulse generator
Optipore scrub sponge
Optiray contrast material
Optiscope
    O. angioscope
    O. catheter
Optivisor lens loupe
Opti-Zyme enzymatic cleaner
Optokinetic stimulator

OR-340 imaging system
Orahesive denture adhesive
oral
    o. endoscope
    o. forceps
    o. needle
    o. rongeur forceps
    o. screw
    o. screw mouth gag
    o. screw tongue depressor
    o. speculum mouth gag
Orban curette
orbital
    o. depressor
    o. enucleation compressor
    o. eye implant
    o. floor implant
    o. floor prosthesis
    o. implant
    o. retractor
    o. retractor set
ORC
    ORC intraocular lens
    ORC posterior chamber
        intraocular lens implant
ORC-B Ranfac cholangiographic
   catheter
Oregon prosthesis
Orentreich punch
Oretorp retractable knife
Organdi blade
organizer
    Hunt o.
    Suture VesiBand o.
OR 340 Intraoperative ultrasound
Orion pacemaker
Oris pin
Orley retractor
Orlon vascular prosthesis
Ormco
    O. band pusher-burnisher
    O. band scissors
    O. band setter
    O. ligature director
    O. orthodontic arch-
      expander
    O. orthodontic hemostat
    O. orthodontic pliers
    O. pin
    O. preformed band
    O. wire bracket
oropharyngeal pack

orotome
    Steinhauser o.
Orr
    O. forceps
    O. gall duct forceps
Orr-Buck extension tractor
Orthair oscillating saw
Orthairtome
    AMSCO O.
    Hall O.
    O. II drill
Orth-evac autotransfusion system
Ortho All-Flex diaphragm
Orthoband traction band
OrthoBlend powered bone mill
Orthocor II pacemaker
orthodontic
    o. aligner
    o. appliance
    o. band
    o. band driver
    o. band setter
    o. base plate
    o. bracket
    o. cement
Orthofix
    O. external fixation device
    O. pin
Orthoflex
    O. dressing
    O. elastic plaster bandage
Orthofuse implantable growth
    stimulator
OrthoGen bone growth stimulator
Ortho-Jel impression material
Ortho-last splint
Ortholav irrigation and suction
    device
Ortholen sheet
Ortholoc prosthesis
Orthomedics brace
Ortho-mesh
Orthomite II adhesive
Ortho-Mold spinal brace
orthopaedic
    o. bone file
    o. broach
    o. bur
    o. chisel
    o. curette
    o. cutting instrument
    o. depth gauge

    o. drill
    o. dynamometer
    o. elevator
    o. forceps
    o. goniometer
    o. gouge
    o. hammer
    o. hemostat
    o. impactor
    o. knife
    o. osteotome
    o. pliers
    o. rasp
    o. reamer
    o. retractor
    o. rongeur
    o. scissors
    o. shoulder elevator
    o. stockinette
    o. strap clavicle splint
    o. surgical drill
    o. surgical file
    o. surgical pliers
    o. surgical stripper
    o. Universal drill
OrthoPak II bone growth
    stimulator
Orthoplast
    O. dressing
    O. fracture brace
    O. isoprene splint
    O. jacket
Orthoptic
    O. eye patch
    O. Therapy amblyoscope
orthosis
    A-frame o.
    ankle o. (AO)
    ankle-foot o. (AFO)
    Jousto dropfoot splint,
      skid o.
    NuKo knee o.
    polypropylene glycol-ankle-
      foot o. (PPG-AFO)
    polypropylene glycol-
      thoracolumbosacral orthosis
      (PPG-TLSO)
    standing frame o.
OrthoSorb
    O. absorbable pin
    O. pin
    O. pin fixation

orthotic
- o. attachment implant
- o. device

Ortho-Trac adhesive skin traction bandage
Ortho-Yomy facebow
Ortved stone dislodger
Osada beaver-XL handpiece unit
Osborne
- O. goniometer
- O. osteotomy plate

oscillating saw
oscilloscope
- single-channel electromyograph o.
- single-channel nonfade o.

Oscor pacemaker
Oshar-Newmann 8-line corneal marker
O'Shaughnessy
- O. arterial forceps
- O. clamp
- O. forceps

Osher
- O. air bubble removal cannula
- O. bipolar coaptation forceps
- O. capsular forceps
- O. conjunctival forceps
- O. corneal scissors
- O. diamond knife
- O. foreign body forceps
- O. globe rotator
- O. haptic forceps
- O. internal calipers
- O. iris retractor
- O. iris tuck eliminator
- O. irrigating implant hook
- O. lens vacuuming cannula
- O. lid retractor
- O. malleable microspatula
- O. micro-iris retractor
- O. micrometer cataract knife
- O. needle holder
- O. nucleus lens manipulator
- O. nucleus stab expressor
- O. superior rectus forceps

Osher-Fresnel intraocular lens
Osher-Neumann
- O.-N. corneal marker
- O.-N. marker

Oshukova collapsible bougie guide
Osseodent
- O. dental implant
- O. surgical drill

osseous
- o. implant
- o. pin

ossicle-holding
- o.-h. clamp
- o.-h. forceps

ossicular chain replacement prosthesis
Ossoff-Karlan
- O.-K. laryngoscope
- O.-K. laser forceps
- O.-K. laser laryngeal micro-operating platform
- O.-K. laser laryngoscope
- O.-K. laser suction tube
- O.-K. microlaryngeal laser operating platform
- O.-K. microlaryngeal laser probe
- O.-K. microlaryngeal suction laser operating platform

Ossoff-Karlan-Dedo laryngoscope
Ossoff-Karlan-Jako laryngoscope
Ossoff-Sisson surgical stent
Osteobond vacuum mixing system
osteoclast
- Collin o.
- Phelps-Gocht o.
- Rizzoli o.

Osteogen resorbable osteogenic bone-filling implant
Osteoloc endodontic stabilization kit
Osteon bur
Osteone air drill
Osteonics
- O. prosthesis
- O. reamer

osteoplastic flap clamp
Osteo-Stim apparatus
osteotome
- Albee o.
- Alexander perforating o.
- Anderson-Neivert o.
- Army-pattern o.
- Barsky nasal o.
- Blount scoliosis o.
- Bowen o.
- Box o.

Burton o.
Campbell o.
Carroll o.
Carroll-Legg o.
Carroll-Smith-Petersen o.
Chermel o.
Cherry o.
Cinelli o.
Clayton o.
Cloward o.
Cloward spinal fusion o.
Codman o.
Converse o.
Cottle o.
Cottle chisel o.
Cottle crossbar chisel o.
Crane o.
Cross o.
curved o.
Dautrey o.
Dawson-Yuhl o.
Dingman o.
Epstein o.
flexible blade o.
Fomon o.
Frazier o.
French-pattern o.
hexagonal handle o.
Hibbs o.
Hipps o.
Hoke o.
Houston nasal o.
Howorth o.
Jarit hand surgery o.
Kazanjian action-type o.
Kezerian o.
Lahey Clinic thin o.
Lambotte o.
Lambotte-Henderson o.
lateral o.
Legg o.
Leinbach o.
Lexer o.
Manchester nasal o.
manual o.
Mathews o.
maxillofacial o.
Mayfield bayonet o.
McCollough o.
Meyerding o.
MGH o.
Micro-Aire o.
Miner o.

Moe o.
Moore o.
nasal o.
nasofrontal o.
Neivert o.
Neivert-Anderson o.
New-Lambotte o.
orthopaedic o.
osteotome o.
Parkes o.
Parkes lateral osteotomy o.
Parkes-Quisling o.
Quisling-Parkes o.
Read o.
Rhoton o.
Richards Hibbs o.
Rish o.
Ristow o.
Rowland o.
Rubin o.
Rubin lateral o.
Rubin nasofrontal o.
Sheehan o.
Silver o.
Silver nasal o.
slotting-bur o.
small set o.
Smith-Petersen o.
Stille o.
Stille-pattern o.
Stille-Stiwer o.
straight o.
Tessier o.
Ultra-Cut Hoke o.
Ultra-Cut Smith-Petersen o.
U.S. Army o.
Ward nasal o.
osteotomy pin
Ostic plaster dressing
ostomy
    o. appliance
    o. bag
Ostrum
    O. antral punch
    O. antral punch-tip forceps
    O. forceps
    O. punch
    O. punch forceps
Ostrup vascularized rib graft
O'Sullivan
    O. abdominal retractor
    O. retractor

O'Sullivan *(continued)*
    O. self-retaining abdominal retractor
    O. vaginal retractor
O'Sullivan-O'Connor
    O.-O. abdominal retractor
    O.-O. retractor
    O.-O. self-retaining retractor
    O.-O. vaginal retractor
    O.-O. vaginal speculum
Oswestry-O'Brien spinal stapler
OTE Biomedica Neurograph
Otis
    O. anoscope
    O. bougie
    O. bougie à boule
    O. bougie à boule dilator
    O. ureterotome
    O. urethral sound
    O. urethrotome
Oti Vac lighted suction unit
otoabrader
    Dingman o.
    Elsie-Brown o.
otologic
    o. cup forceps
    o. scissors
otoscope
    acoustic o.
    Bruening o.
    Bruening pneumatic o.
    Brunton o.
    Earscope o.
    fiberoptic o.
    Grafco o.
    halogen o.
    pneumatic o.
    Politzer air bag o.
    Rica pneumatic o.
    Siegel pneumatic o.
    SMIC pneumatic o.
    surgical o.
    Toynbee o.
    video o.
    Welch Allyn dual-purpose o.
    Welch Allyn operating o.
    Wullstein
      ototympanoscope o.
Ototemp 3000
ototome
    o. drill
    o. otological drill

Oto-Wick
    Pope O.-W.
Ottenheimer
    O. common duct dilator
    O. dilator
Ott insufflator filter tubing
Otto
    O. Barkan bident retractor
    O. forceps
    O. tissue forceps
Oughterson forceps
outer
    o. coaxial irrigating cannula
    o. interrupted silk suture
Outerbridge uterine dilator
outflow cannula
outlet
    o. cannula
    o. forceps
output device
oval
    o. cup forceps
    o. cutting bur
    o. esophagoscope
    o. optical zone marker
    o. piston gauge
    o. snare
    o. speculum
oval-open esophagoscope
oval-window
    o.-w. curette
    o.-w. excavator
    o.-w. hook
    o.-w. pick
    o.-w. piston evacuator
ovary forceps
Ovation in-the-ear hearing aid
over-and-over whip suture
over-door traction set
overhead
    o. fracture frame
    o. light
Overholt
    O. dissecting forceps
    O. elevator
    O. forceps
    O. needle
    O. periosteal elevator
    O. raspatory
    O. retractor
    O. rib needle
    O. rib raspatory
    O. rib spreader

Overholt-Finochietto rib spreader
Overholt-Geissendörfer
    O.-G. arterial forceps
    O.-G. forceps
    O.-G. hemostatic forceps
Overholt-Jackson bronchoscope
Overholt-Mixter dissecting forceps
overlapping suture
overlay
    x-ray o.
oversensing pacemaker
Overstreet
    O. endometrial polyp
      forceps
    O. forceps
    O. polyp forceps
over-the-top rasp set
overtube
ovoid
    Hankins lucite o.
    Hockin lucite o.
    Manchester o.
    tandem and o.
ovum
    o. curette
    o. forceps

Owatusi double catheter
Owen
    O. catheter
    O. cloth dressing
    O. gauze dressing
    O. hemostatic bag
    O. Lo-Profile dilation
      catheter
    O. suture
Oxford
    O. nonkinking cuffed tube
    O. prosthesis
oximeter
    ear o.
    pulse o.
oximetric catheter
oximetry catheter
Oxycel
    O. dressing
    O. gauze
    O. oxidized cellulose
Oxyguard mouth block
Oxy-Quik Mark IV oxygen
    inhalator
oxyquinoline dressing
Oyloidin suture

P

PABP
pulmonary artery balloon pump
Pace
P. hysterectomy knife
P. periosteal elevator
P. ventricular needle
pacemaker
AAI p.
AAIR p.
AAI single-chamber p.
AAT p.
Accufix p.
Acculith p.
Activitrax p.
Activitrax single-chamber
responsive p.
Activitrax variable-rate p.
activity-sensing p.
AEC p.
Aequitron p.
AFP p.
AICD p.
AID-B p.
Alcatel p.
American Opitical
Cardiocare p.
American Optic R-
inhibited p.
Amtech-Killeen p.
AOO p.
Arco p.
Arco atomic p.
Arco lithium p.
artificial p.
Arzco p.
Astra p.
ASVIP p.
asynchronous p.
asynchronous mode p.
asynchronous ventricular
VOO p.
atrial p.
atrial synchronous p.
atrial synchronous
ventricular-inhibited p.
atrial tracking p.
atrial triggered ventricular-
inhibited p.
Atricor p.
Atricor Cordis p.

atrioventricular junctional p.
atrioventricular sequential p.
atrioventricular sequential
demand p.
Aurora dual-chamber p.
Autima II p.
Autima II dual-chamber
cardiac p.
Avius sequential p.
AV junctional p.
AV sequential demand p.
AV synchronous p.
Axios p.
Basix p.
Betacel-Biotronik p.
bifocal demand p.
Biotronik demand p.
bipolar p.
bipolar Medtronic p.
bladder p.
burst p.
Byrel p.
cardiac p.
Cardio-Pace Medical
Durapulse p.
p. catheter
Chardack p.
Chardack-Greatbatch p.
Chardack Medtronic p.
Chorus p.
Chronocor IV external p.
Chronos p.
cilium p.
Classix p.
Command PS p.
committed mode p.
Cook p.
cor p.
Coratomic R-wave
inhibited p.
Cordis p.
Cordis Atricor p.
Cordis Chronocor p.
Cordis Ectocor p.
Cordis fixed-rate p.
Cordis Gemini p.
Cordis Multicor p.
Cordis Omnicor Stanicor p.
Cordis Omni Stanicor Theta
transvenous p.

pacemaker *(continued)*

Cordis Sequicor p.
Cordis Ventricor p.
Cortomic p.
Cosmos p.
Cosmos pulse-generator p.
CPI p.
CPI Astra p.
CPI Maxilith p.
CPI Microthin p.
CPI Minilith p.
CPI Ultra II p.
cross-talk p.
Cyberlith p.
Cyberlith demand p.
CyberTach p.
Daig p.
DDD p.
DDI mode p.
Delta p.
demand p.
Devices, Ltd. p.
Diplos p.
dual-chamber p.
dual-chamber AV
  sequential p.
dual-pass p.
Durapulse p.
DVI p.
ECT p.
Ectocor p.
ectopic p.
ectopic atrial p.
Ela p.
Elecath p.
electric cardiac p.
p. electrode
Electrodyne p.
Elema p.
Elema-Schonander p.
Elevath p.
Elgiloy p.
Elgiloy lead-tip p.
Elite p.
Encor p.
endocardial p.
endocardial bipolar p.
Enertrax p.
epicardial p.
escape p.
external p.
external asynchronous p.
external demand p.
external-internal p.
externally-controlled
  noninvasive programmed
  stimulation p.
external transthoracic p.
Fast-Pass lead p.
fixed-rate p.
fixed-rate asynchronous
  atrial p.
fixed-rate asynchronous
  ventricular p.
fully automatic p.
fully automatic
  atrioventricular Universal
  dual-channel p.
Galaxy p.
GE p.
Gemini p.
General Electric p.
Genisis p.
Genisis dual-chamber p.
Guardian p.
heart p.
hermetically-sealed p.
implantable p.
implanted p.
Intermedics p.
Intermedics Cyberlith X
  multiprogrammable p.
Intermedics lithium-
  powered p.
Intermedics Quantum p.
Intermedics Quantum
  unipolar p.
Intermedics Thinlith II p.
Intertach p.
isotopic pulse generator p.
junctional p.
Kalos p.
Kantrowitz p.
Kelvin p.
Lambda p.
Lambda Omni Stanicor p.
latent p.
Laurens-Alcatel nuclear
  powered p.
Legend p.
Leios p.
Leptos p.
Leukos p.
Lillehei p.
lith II p.
lithium p.

lithium-powered p.
Maestro p.
Maestro implantable
  cardiac p.
Malith p.
Mallor p.
malsensing p.
Maxilith p.
Medcor p.
Medtel p.
Medtronic p.
Medtronic Activitrax p.
Medtronic-Alcatel p.
Medtronic Byrel-SX p.
Medtronic corkscrew
  electrode p.
Medtronic Cyberlith p.
Medtronic demand p.
Medtronic
  external/internal p.
Medtronic-Laurens-Alcatel p.
Medtronic Pacette p.
Medtronic Symbios p.
Medtronic-Zyrel p.
Mentor bladder p.
mercury cell-powered p.
Meta MV cardiac p.
Microlith P p.
Microthin P2 p.
Mikros p.
Minilith p.
Minix p.
Mitrothin P2 p.
Multicor cardiac p.
Multicor Gamma p.
Multicor II p.
Multilith p.
multiprogrammable p.
Nathan p.
natural p.
Neos p.
Nomos multiprogrammable
  R-wave inhibited
  demand p.
noncompetitive p.
Nova II p.
nuclear p.
nuclear powered p.
Omni-Atricor p.
Omnicor p.
Omni-Ectocor p.
Omni-Orthocor p.
Omni-Stanicor p.
Omni-Theta p.
Omni-Ventricor p.
Optima p.
Orion p.
Orthocor II p.
Oscor p.
oversensing p.
Pacesetter p.
Pacesetter Synchrony p.
Pacette p.
Paragon p.
Paragon II p.
Pasar p.
Pasar tachycardia
  reversion p.
Pasys p.
permanent p.
permanent myocardial p.
permanent rate-responsive p.
permanent transvenous p.
permanent ventricular p.
Permathane Pacesetter
  lead p.
Phoenix p.
Phoenix single-chamber p.
physiologic p.
Pinnacle p.
PolyFlex implantable pacing
  lead p.
PolyFlex lead p.
Prima p.
Prism-CL p.
Programalith p.
Programalith AV p.
Programalith II p.
Programalith III p.
programmable p.
Programmer III p.
Prolith p.
Pulsar NI p.
Pulsar NI implantable p.
Quantum p.
radiofrequency p.
rate-responsive p.
Reflex p.
Relay p.
rescuing p.
respiratory-dependent p.
reversion p.
RS4 p.
R-synchronous VVT p.
Schaldach electrode p.
Schuletz p.

pacemaker *(continued)*
screw-in lead p.
Seecor p.
Sensolog III p.
sensor-based single-chamber p.
Sensor Kelvin p.
Sequicor p.
Sequicor II p.
Sequicor III p.
Shaldach p.
shifting p.
Siemens-Elema p.
Siemens-Elema multi-programmable p.
Siemens-Pacesetter p.
single-chamber p.
single-pass p.
sinus p.
sinus node p.
Solar p.
Solus p.
Sorin p.
Spectraflex p.
Spectrax p.
Spectrax bipolar p.
Spectrax programmable Medtronic p.
standby p.
Stanicor p.
Stanicor Gamma p.
Stanicor Lambda demand p.
Starr-Edwards p.
Starr-Edwards hermetically sealed p.
Symbios p.
synchronous p.
synchronous burst p.
synchronous mode p.
Synchrony p.
Synchrony II p.
Syticon 5950 bipolar demand p.
tachycardia-terminating p.
Tachylog p.
Telectronics p.
temporary p.
temporary transvenous p.
Thermos p.
Thinlith II p.
tined lead p.
transcutaneous p.

transpericardial p.
transthoracic p.
transvenous p.
transvenous ventricular demand p.
Trios M p.
Ultra p.
Unilith p.
unipolar p.
unipolar atrial p.
unipolar atrioventricular p.
unipolar sequential p.
USCI Vario permanent p.
variable rate p.
VAT p.
VDD p.
Ventak AICD p.
Ventricor p.
ventricular p.
ventricular demand p.
ventricular-suppressed p.
ventricular-triggered p.
Versatrax p.
Versatrax cardiac p.
Versatrax II p.
Vicor p.
Vista p.
Vitatrax II p.
Vitatron p.
Vivalith-10 p.
Vivatron p.
VVI p.
VVI/AAI p.
VVI bipolar Programalith p.
VVIR single-chamber rate-adaptive p.
VVI single-chamber p.
VVT p.
wandering p.
wandering atrial p.
Xyrel p.
Zitron p.
Zoll p.
Zoll NTP p.
pacemeter
Haag-Streit p.
Mishima-Hedbys attachment p.
Paceport catheter
Pace-Potts
P.-P. forceps
P.-P. intestinal clamp set

Pacesetter
P. pacemaker
P. Synchrony pacemaker
Pacette pacemaker
Pach-Pen tonometer
pachymeter
Pacific Coast hearing aid
pacifico
p. cannula
p. catheter
pacing
p. catheter
p. electrode
Hancock bipolar balloon p.
p. wire electrode
pack
Endo Clip ML/Surgiport
System p.
Kirkland periodontal p.
nasal p.
oropharyngeal p.
PCA periodontal p.
Packard intraocular lens
Packer
P. mosquito forceps
P. tunnel silicone sponge
packer
Allport gauze p.
Angell gauze p.
August automatic gauze p.
Bernay gauze p.
gauze p.
Jewett bone chip p.
Kitchen postpartum p.
Kitchen postpartum
gauze p.
Ralks nasal gauze p.
Torpin automatic uterine
gauze p.
Woodson p.
Packiam retractor
packing forceps
Pac-Kit Army-type tourniquet
Packo pars plana cannula
pad
Chaston eye p.
disposable electrode p.
EK-19 p.
p. electrode
Envisan dextranomer p.
Etch-Master felt p.
eye p.
instrument stabilizer p.

Littmann defibrillation p.
Mayfield pediatric
horseshoe p.
Ray-Tec lap p.
Ray-Tec x-ray detectable
lap p.
Sof-Wick lap p.
Spectra p.
Steri-Pad gauze p.
Telfa p.
padded
p. aluminum splint
p. board splint
p. clamp
p. plywood splint
padding
cast p.
splint p.
Padgett
P. blade
P. dermatome
P. dermatome blade
P. electrodermatome
P. graft
P. implant
P. manual dermatome
P. mesh skin graft
P. prosthesis
P. shark-mouth cannula
Padgett-Concorde suction cannula
Padgett-Hood dermatome
Page
P. forceps
P. needle
P. tonsillar forceps
P. tonsillar knife
Pagenstecher
P. lens scoop
P. linen thread suture
P. suture
Pajot decapitating hook
Palacos
P. bone cement
P. cement
P. radiopaque bone cement
Paladon
P. graft
P. implant material
P. prosthesis
palatal bar
palate
p. hook
p. retractor

palate-free activator
palate-type mouth gag
palatine suture
palatoethmoidal suture
palatomaxillary suture
palatorrhaphy elevator
Palex
    P. colostomy irrigation
      starter set
    P. expansion screw
Palfique Estelite tooth shade resin
  material
Palfyn suture
pallesthesiometer
Pallin
    P. lens spatula
    P. spring-assisted syringe
palmar splint
Palmaz
    P. arterial stent
    P. stent
    P. vascular stent
Palmaz-Schatz coronary stent
Palmer
    P. biopsy drill forceps
    P. biopsy forceps
    P. cruciate ligament guide
    P. cutting forceps
    P. dilator
    P. grasping forceps
    P. lens
    P. uterine dilator
Palmer-Buono contact lens
Palmer-Drapier
    P.-D. forceps
    P.-D. needle
palpating needle
palpation probe
palpator
    blunt p.
    Farrior blunt p.
Palumbo
    P. dynamic patellar brace
    P. knee brace
Panasonic hearing aid
Pancoast suture
pancreatic duct stent
pan disposable needle
panendoscope
    p. electrode
    Foroblique p.
    LoPresti p.

panfundoscope
    Rodenstock p.
Pang
    P. biopsy forceps
    P. forceps
    P. nasopharyngeal biopsy
      forceps
    P. nasopharyngeal forceps
Panje
    P. button
    P. implant
    P. prosthesis
    P. tube
    P. voice button
    P. voice prosthesis
Panje-Shagets tracheoesophageal
  fistula forceps
Pannett needle
Pannu
    P. II intraocular lens
    P. intraocular lens
Panoview arthroscopic system
pantoscope
    Keeler p.
pants-over-vest suture
pantyhose
    Glattelast compression p.
Panzer gallbladder scissors
Papanicolaou smear tray
Paparella
    P. angled-ring curette
    P. calipers
    P. canal knife
    P. catheter
    P. curette
    P. drum elevator-knife
    P. duckbill elevator
    P. elevator knife
    P. fenestrometer
    P. footplate pick
    P. incudostapedial joint
      knife
    P. incudostapedial knife
    P. mastoid curette
    P. middle ear instrument
    P. monkey-head holder
    P. myringotomy tube
    P. needle
    P. pick
    P. probe
    P. rasp calipers
    P. retractor
    P. scissors

P. self-retaining retractor
P. sickle knife
P. stapes curette
P. straight needle
P. tissue press
P. ventilation tube
P. wire-cutting scissors
Paparella-Frazier suction tube
Paparella-Hough excavator
Paparella-House
P.-H. curette
P.-H. knife
Paparella-Weitlaner retractor
paper
articulating p.
p. drape
GE Rudischhauser
articulating p.
PD articulating p.
Vimedic articulating p.
papilla drain
papilloma forceps
papillotome
Cremer-Ikeda p.
Frimberger-Karpiel 12
O'Clock p.
Howell Rotatable BII p.
Huibregtse-Katon p.
shark fin p.
Wilson-Cook p.
wire-guided p.
papillotome/sphincterotome
Soehendra BII p./s.
Soehendra Precut p./s.
Swenson wire-guided p./s.
Zimmon p./s.
Papineau bone graft
Pap smear kit
Paquelin cautery
paracentesis
p. knife
p. needle
paracervical nerve block needle
Paracine dressing
Paradentine dental restorative material
paraffin
p. dressing
p. graft
p. implant
p. implant material
Parafil wax
ParaGard intrauterine device

Paragon
P. II pacemaker
P. pacemaker
parallel
p. flow dialyzer
p. pin kit
parallel-loop electrode
Parama pulse wave
ParaMax angled driver
parametrium
p. clamp
p. forceps
Parel-Crock cutter
Paré suture
Parhad needle
Parhad-Poppen needle
Parham band
Parham-Martin
P.-M. band
P.-M. bone clamp
P.-M. bone-holding clamp
P.-M. clamp
P.-M. fracture apparatus
P.-M. fracture-banding
apparatus
parietal suture
parietomastoid suture
parieto-occipital suture
Park
P. blade
P. blade septostomy
catheter
P. eye speculum
P. irrigating cannula
P. lens implantation forceps
P. rectal spreader
Parker
P. clamp
P. double-ended retractor
P. fixation forceps
P. knife-needle
P. micropump insulin
infuser
P. needle
P. retractor
P. serrated discission knife
P. tenotomy knife
P. thumb retractor
P. tube
Parker-Bard
P.-B. blade
P.-B. handle

Parker-Glassman intestinal clamp set
Parker-Kerr
  P.-K. clamp
  P.-K. forceps
  P.-K. intestinal clamp
  P.-K. suture
Parker-Mott double-ended retractor
Parker-Pearson needle
Parkes
  P. hump gouge
  P. lateral osteotomy osteotome
  P. nasal rasp
  P. nasal retractor
  P. osteotome
  P. rasp
Park-Guyton-Callahan eye speculum
Park-Guyton eye speculum
Parkinson head holder
Park-Maumenee speculum
Parks
  P. anal retractor
  P. anal speculum
  P. ileoanal reservoir
  P. ileostomy pouch
  P. nasal rasp
  P. retractor
Parks-Quisling osteotome
Parma band
parotidectomy retractor
Parr closed irrigation system
parrot-beak basket
Par scissors
Parsonnet
  P. aortic clamp
  P. coronary probe
  P. dilator
  P. epicardial retractor
  P. probe
  P. pulse generator pouch
partial
  p. occlusion clamp
  p. occlusion forceps
  p. occlusion inferior vena caval clip
  p. ossicular reconstruction/replacement prosthesis (PORP)
Partipilo
  P. clamp
  P. gastrostomy

Partsch
  P. bone chisel
  P. bone gouge
  P. chisel
  P. gouge
Pasar
  P. pacemaker
  P. tachycardia reversion pacemaker
P.A.S. Port Fluoro-Free peripheral access system
Pasqualini implant
Passavant bar
passer
  Arans pulley p.
  Brand tendon p.
  Bunnell tendon p.
  Carroll tendon p.
  Concept ACL/PCL graft p.
  Concept 2-pin p.
  Crile wire p.
  Dingman wire p.
  Ferszt ligature p.
  Furlow cylinder p.
  Gallie tendon p.
  Garrett vein p.
  Hewson p.
  Holter distal catheter p.
  Joplin tendon p.
  Lahey ligature p.
  ligature p.
  Malis ligature p.
  Ober tendon p.
  O'Donoghue suture p.
  pulley p.
  suture p.
  tendon p.
  Uni-Shunt catheter p.
  wire p.
  Withers tendon p.
  Yankauer ligature p.
passing forceps
Passow chisel
paste
  Coe-Pak periodontal p.
  dextranomer p.
  Envisan dextranomer p.
  p. filler
  Omniprep skin prepping p.
  Stomahesive p.
Pasys pacemaker
patch
  Dacron intracardiac p.

p. dressing
eye p.
Gore-Tex cardiovascular p.
Gore-Tex soft tissue p.
p. graft
p. implant
Ionescu-Shiley pericardial p.
Orthoptic eye p.
polypropylene
intracardiac p.
Pro-Ophta eye p.
Teflon intracardiac p.
Torpedo eye p.
patch-reinforced mattress suture
Patel intraocular magnet
patellar
p. button
p. cement clamp
p. clamp
p. drill guide
p. planer bushing
p. reamer guide
p. resection guide
p. shaft reamer
patella-resurfacing implant
patent
p. ductus clamp
p. ductus forceps
p. ductus retractor
Paterson
P. brain clip forceps
P. cannula
P. laryngeal cannula
P. laryngeal forceps
P. long-shank brain clip
Pathfinder catheter
Patil stereotaxic system
Paton
P. bur
P. corneal dissector
P. corneal forceps
P. corneal knife
P. corneal transplant forceps
P. corneal trephine
P. extra-delicate forceps
P. eye needle holder
P. eye shield
P. forceps
P. needle holder
P. see-through trephine
P. spatula
P. trephine
Paton-Berens mules

Patrick drill
Patten Bottom Perthes brace
pattern
breast reduction p.
p. trephine
p. umbilical scissors
Patterson
P. bronchoscopic biopsy
forceps
P. bronchoscopic forceps
P. double-action biting tip
P. empyema trocar
P. forceps
P. oval biting tip
P. specimen forceps
P. trocar
Patterson-Nelson empyema trocar
Patton
P. bur
P. cannula
P. dilator
P. esophageal dilator
P. septal speculum
patty
Codman surgical p.
Paufique
P. blade
P. corneal knife
P. corneal trephine
P. Duredge knife
P. forceps
P. graft knife
P. suturing forceps
Paul
P. condom bag
P. hemostatic bag
P. intestinal drainage tube
P. lacrimal retractor
P. lacrimal sac retractor
P. retractor
P. tendon hook
Paul-Mixter tube
Paulson
P. infertility microtissue
forceps
P. infertility microtying
forceps
P. knee retractor
Pauwels fracture forceps
Pavlik
P. harness
P. harness splint

Payne-Ochsner
    P.-O. arterial forceps
    P.-O. forceps
Payne-Péan
    P.-P. arterial forceps
    P.-P. forceps
Payne-Rankin
    P.-R. arterial forceps
    P.-R. forceps
Payr
    P. abdominal retractor
    P. clamp
    P. forceps
    P. gastrointestinal clamp
    P. grooved director
    P. intestinal clamp
    P. probe
    P. pylorus clamp
    P. pylorus forceps
    P. resection clamp
    P. retractor
    P. stomach clamp
    P. vein needle
Payr-Schmieden probe
PCA
    porous coated anatomic
    PCA acetabular cup
    PCA hip component
    PCA knee prosthesis
    PCA modular total knee
    PCA periodontal pack
    PCA revision total knee
    PCA total hip
    PCA total hip stem
    PCA total knee system
    PCA unicompartmental knee
PC EEA stapler
PCSD
    prone cranial support device
PD
    PD articulating paper
    PD band
    PD copper band
    PD crown post
    PD dental wax
    PD excavator
    PD orthodontic wire
    PD polishing strip
    PD preformed crown
    PD reamer
    PD root canal post
    PD SS matrix band
PD-10 peritoneal dialysis cycler

PDL intraligamentary syringe
PDS
    peritoneal dialysis system
    polydioxanone
    PDS suture
    PDS Vicryl suture
PDT
    PDT guide wire
    PDT guiding catheter
PE
    PE Plus II balloon
        dilatation catheter
    PE Plus II peripheral
        balloon catheter
PE-60-I-2 implantable pronged unipolar electrode
PE-60-K-10 implantable unipolar endocardial electrode
PE-60-KB implantable unipolar endocardial electrode
PE-85-I-2 implantable pronged unipolar electrode
PE-85-K-10 implantable unipolar endocardial electrode
PE-85-KB implantable unipolar endocardial electrode
PE-85-KS-10 implantable unipolar endocardial electrode
Peabody splint
peacock dressing
Peakometer urinary flow rate meter
Péan
    P. arterial forceps
    P. clamp
    P. forceps
    P. GI forceps
    P. hemostatic clamp
    P. hemostatic forceps
    P. hysterectomy clamp
    P. hysterectomy forceps
    P. intestinal clamp
    P. intestinal forceps
    P. sponge forceps
    P. vessel clamp
peanut
    p. dissector
    p. eye implant
    p. forceps
    p. sponge
    p. sponge-holding forceps
peanut-fenestrated forceps
peanut-grasping forceps

Peanut Secto dissector
peapod
    p. bead-type forceps
    p. chisel
    p. intervertebral disk
      forceps
    p. intervertebral disk
      rongeur
Pearce
    P. coaxial cannula
    P. eye speculum
    P. intraocular glide
    P. posterior chamber
      intraocular lens
    P. Tripod intraocular lens
    P. vaulted-Y lens implant
Pearce-Keates
    P.-K. bifocal intraocular
      lens
    P.-K. bifocal lens
Pearlcast polymer plaster bandage
Pearlon impression material
Pearman
    P. penile implant material
    P. penile prosthesis
    P. transurethral hemostatic
      bag
Pearsall
    P. Chinese twisted suture
    P. silk suture
pear-shaped
    p.-s. bur
    p.-s. fluted bag
    p.-s. fluted hemostatic bag
Pearson
    P. chisel
    P. flexed-knee apparatus
Pease bone drill
Pease-Thomson traction bow
Peaso reamer
Peck
    P. chisel
    P. inlay wax
    P. rake retractor
Peck-Joseph scissors
pectoralis muscle implant
Peczon I & A cannula
Pederson vaginal speculum
pediatric
    p. abdominal retractor
    p. abdominal retractor blade
    p. balloon catheter
    p. biopsy needle

    p. bridge
    p. bulldog clamp
    p. catheter
    p. clamp
    p. dilator
    p. endoscope
    p. esophagoscope
    p. Foley catheter
    p. forceps
    p. Hendren retractor blade
    p. hook retractor blade
    p. mastoid retractor blade
    p. perineal retractor set
    p. pigtail catheter
    p. rectal dilator
    p. retractor
    p. retractor adjustable arm
    p. retractor malleable wire
      hand
    p. retractor oval sprocket
      frame
    p. self-retaining retractor
    p. telescope
pediatric-perineal retractor ring
Pedicat catheter
pedicle
    p. clamp
    p. connector
    p. forceps
    p. hook
    p. implant
    p. screw
peel-away
    p.-a. catheter
    p.-a. introducer
    p.-a. sheath
peeler
    Olk membrane p.
Peeler-Cutter vitrector
peel-off catheter
Peel Pak bag
Peers
    P. clamp
    P. towel clamp
    P. towel forceps
Peeso reamer
Peet
    P. forceps
    P. lighted splanchnic
      retractor
    P. mosquito forceps
    P. splinter forceps

535

PEG
  percutaneous endoscopic
  gastrostomy
  polyethylene glycol
  Gauderer-Ponsky PEG
  PEG self-adhesive elastic
  dressing
  PEG tube
peg
  glenoid alignment p.
  locking p.
Peiper-Beyer bone rongeur
PEJ
  percutaneous endoscopic
  jejunostomy
  PEJ tube
pelican biopsy forceps
Pelkmann
  P. foreign body forceps
  P. gallstone forceps
  P. sponge forceps
  P. uterine-dressing forceps
  P. uterine forceps
pelvic
  p. belt
  p. clamp
  p. reduction forceps
  p. snare
  p. tissue forceps
  p. traction belt
pelvimeter
  Baudelocque p.
  Briesky p.
  Collin p.
  Collyer p.
  DeLee p.
  DeLee-Breisky p.
  Douglas measuring plate p.
  Hanley-McDermott p.
  Martin p.
  Rica p.
  Schneider p.
  Thole p.
  Thomas p.
  Thoms p.
  Williams internal p.
Pemberton
  P. clamp
  P. forceps
  P. retractor
  P. sigmoid anastomosis
  clamp

  P. sigmoid clamp
  P. spur-crushing clamp
pen
  gentian violet marking p.
  marking p.
  p. pump insulin infuser
  skin marking p.
  Skin Skribe p.
  surgical marking p.
  Viomedex surgical
  marking p.
Penberthy double-action aspirator
pencil
  p. cautery
  Cheshire electrosurgical p.
  p. Doppler probe
  electrosurgical p. (ESP)
  Weck electrosurgery p.
pencil-tip cautery
Pendoppler ultrasonic fetal heart
  detector
Pendula cast cutter
pendulum scalpel
penetrating drill
Penfield
  P. biopsy needle
  P. clip
  P. dissector
  P. forceps
  P. needle
  P. retractor
  P. silver clip
  P. suture forceps
  P. watchmaker forceps
penicillin nebulizer
penile
  p. clamp
  p. implant
penis clamp
penlight
Penn
  P. drill
  P. swivel hook
Penn-Anderson fixation forceps
pennate suction catheter
Pennig dynamic wrist fixator
Pennine
  P. leg bag
  P. Nélaton catheter
Pennine-O'Neil urinary catheter
  introducer
Pennington
  P. clamp

P. elevator
P. forceps
P. hemorrhoidal forceps
P. hemostatic forceps
P. rectal speculum
P. septal dissector
P. septal elevator
P. tissue forceps
P. tissue-grasping forceps
Penn tuning fork
Pennybacker rongeur
Penrose drain
Pentax
P. bronchofiberscope
P. bronchoscope
P. choledochocystonephrofiber-
scope
P. colonoscope
P. duodenofiberscope
P. duodenoscope
P. endoscope
P. FC colonofiberscope
P. FD duodenofiberscope
P. FG gastrofiberscope
P. fiberoptic sigmoidoscope
P. fiberscope
P. flexible endoscope
P. flexible sigmoidoscope
P. gastroscope
P. lithotriptor
P. nasopharyngo-
laryngofiberscope
P. side-viewing endoscope
P. sigmoidofiberscope
P. sigmoidoscope
P. Spotmatic camera
Percival gstric balloon
Percor
P. dual-lumen intra-aortic
balloon catheter
P. intra-aortic balloon
catheter
Percor-DL catheter
Percor-Stat-DL catheter
Percor-Stat intra-aortic balloon
PercuCut biopsy needle
Percuflex biliary stent
percussion hammer
percussor
cup palm manual p.
English hospital reflex p.
McGill neurological p.

Neoguard p.
neurological p.
percutaneous
p. aspiration biopsy tray
p. catheter
p. catheter introducer kit
p. dorsal column stimulator
implant
p. endoscopic gastrostomy
(PEG)
p. endoscopic jejunostomy
(PEJ)
p. intra-aortic balloon
counterpulsation (PIBC)
p. needle
p. stent
p. transhepatic biliary
drainge (PTBD)
p. transhepatic pigtail
catheter
p. transhepatic prosthesis
p. transheptatic biliary
drainage catheter
p. transluminal coronary
angioplasty (PTCA)
p. transluminal coronary
angioplasty catheter
Percy
P. amputation retractor
P. bone retractor
P. clamp
P. forceps
P. intestinal forceps
P. retractor
P. tissue forceps
Percy-Wolfson
P.-W. gallbladder forceps
P.-W. gallbladder retractor
P.-W. retractor
Perdue
P. hemostat
P. tonsillar hemostat forceps
Pereyra
P. cannula
P. ligature cannula
P. needle
PerFixation system
perforated
p. Mayo tray
perforating
p. bur
p. drill
p. forceps

perforating *(continued)*
    McGee needle p.
    p. twist drill
perforation rasp
perforator
    Amnihook amniotic
      membrane p.
    antral p.
    Bishop antral p.
    Codman disposable p.
    Cushing cranial p.
    DeLee-Perce membrane p.
    D'Errico p.
    p. drill
    Hillis p.
    Joseph antral p.
    Kalinowski p.
    Lempert p.
    membrane p.
    Royce tympanum p.
    Smellie obstetrical p.
    Smith p.
    spondylophyte annular
      dissector p.
    Stein membrane p.
    Thornwald antral p.
    tympanum p.
    Wellaminski antral p.
    Williams p.
Performance
    P. total knee system
    P. unicompartmental knee
      system
perfusion
    p. cannula
    p. catheter
    p. O ring
periapical curette
peribulbar needle
pericardial snare
pericardiocentesis needle
pericortical clamp
pericostal suture
**Peries medicated hygienic wipe
dressing**
Peri-Guard
    P.-G. guard
    P.-G. vascular graft
    P.-G. vascular graft guard
perimeter
    Goldmann p.
perineal
    p. bandage

    p. prostatectomy retractor
    p. retractor
    p. self-retaining retractor
    p. support suture
Perio
    P. Pik irrigator
    P. Temp dental probe
periodontal probe
periodontimeter
periosteal
    p. comb
    p. elevator
    p. raspatory
    p. spicule sweeper
periosteotome
    Alexander p.
    Alexander costal p.
    Alexander-Farabeuf p.
    Alexander-Farabeuf costal p.
    Ballenger p.
    Brophy p.
    Brown p.
    costal p.
    Dean p.
    Ferris Smith Lyman p.
    Fomon p.
    Freer p.
    Jansen p.
    Joseph p.
    Moorehead p.
    Potts p.
    Speer p.
    Vaughan p.
    West-Beck p.
periotips
    Imax p.
peripheral
    p. atherectomy catheter
    p. atherectomy system
    p. blood vessel forceps
    p. iridectomy forceps
    p. long-line catheter
    p. vascular clamp
    p. vascular forceps
    p. vascular retractor
**peripherally inserted central
catheter (PICC)**
peritoneal
    p. band
    p. button
    p. catheter
    p. clamp
    p. dialysis catheter

p. dialysis system (PDS)
p. forceps
p. reflux control catheter
peritoneoscope
Menghini-Wildhirt p.
Peritronics Medical Inc. fetal monitoring system
Perkins
P. elevator
P. otologic retractor
P. retractor
P. split-weight tractor
P. tonometer
Per-Lee
P.-L. equalizing tube
P.-L. myringotomy tube
P.-L. ventilation tube
Perlon suture
Perma-Cath
P.-C. catheter
P.-C. drain
Perma-Cryl denture base material
Perma-Grip denture adhesive
Perma-Hand
P.-H. braided silk suture
P.-H. silk suture
P.-H. suture
permanent
p. cardiac pacing lead
p. implant
p. myocardial pacemaker
p. pacemaker
p. pacing lead
p. rate-responsive pacemaker
p. silicone catheter
p. transvenous pacemaker
p. ventricular pacemaker
Perman-Stille abdominal retractor
Permathane Pacesetter lead pacemaker
Permatone denture material
peroral gastroscope
Per-Q-Cath percutaneously inserted central venous catheter
Perras mammary prosthesis
Perras-Papillon breast prosthesis
Perritt
P. double-fixation forceps
P. double-fixation suture forceps
P. fixation forceps
P. forceps

P. lens forceps
P. lens implantation forceps
Perry
P. bag
P. catheter
P. forceps
P. ileostomy bag
P. latex Penrose drainage tubing
P. Noz-Stop kit
P. ostomy irrigator
P. pediatric Foley latex catheter
Perry-Foley catheter
personal portable stimulator (PPS)
Personna
P. blade
P. surgical blade
Perspex CQ intraocular lens
Per-Stat-DL catheter
Perthes reamer
perticortical clamp
Pertrach percutaneous tracheostomy tube
pervenous catheter
pessary
Albert Smith p.
Blair modification of Gellhorn p.
blue ring p.
Chambers doughnut p.
Chambers intrauterine p.
cup p.
diaphragm p.
doughnut p.
Dumas p.
Emmet-Gellhorn p.
Findley folding p.
Gariel p.
Gehrung p.
Gellhorn p.
globe prolapsus p.
Gold p.
Gynefold prolapse p.
Gynefold retrodisplacement p.
Hodge p.
hollow lucite p.
intrauterine p.
lever p.
Mayer p.
Menge p.
Menge stem p.

pessary *(continued)*
Milex p.
Plexiglas Gellhorn p.
Prentif p.
Prochownik p.
prolapse ring p.
prolapsus p.
red p.
retrodisplaced p.
retroversion p.
ring p.
safety p.
Smith p.
Smith retroversion p.
stem p.
Thomas p.
Vimule p.
White foam p.
Wylie stem p.
Zwanck radium p.
Pess lid everter
Petanguy-McIndoe gouge
Peter-Bishop forceps
Petersen
P. bag
P. rectal bag
Peterson
P. cervical collar
P. skeletal traction bow
P. trocar
Peters tissue forceps
Petit
P. suture
P. tourniquet
Petralit dental cement
petrobasilar suture
petrolatum
p. dressing
p. gauze dressing
petrosphenobasilar suture
petrosquamous suture
Petz *(See* von Petz)
Peyman
P. special optics for low vision lens
P. vitrector
P. vitreous-grasping forceps
P. vitreous scissors
Peyman-Green
P.-G. vitrectomy lens
P.-G. vitreous forceps
Peyton brain spatula

Pezzer, de Pezzer
P. catheter
P. drain
P. mushroom-tipped catheter
P. self-retaining catheter
P. self-retaining urethral catheter
P. suprapubic cystostomy catheter
PF
PF Lee pediatric goniolens
PF Universal solder
Pfau
P. atticus sphenoidal punch
P. forceps
P. polypus forceps
PFC
Press-Fit component
PFC component
Pfeiffer-Grobety activator
Pfeiffer mechanical dosing pump
Pfister-Schwartz
P.-S. basket forceps
P.-S. sheath
P.-S. stone basket
P.-S. stone dislodger
P.-S. stone retriever
Pfister stone basket
PGA
polyglycolic acid
PGA mesh
PGP flexible nail system
phacodialysis spatula
phacoemulsification
p. cautery
p. handpiece
phacoemulsificator
phacoemulsifier
Alcon p.
Cavitron p.
Kelman p.
MVS p.
Phaco-flex lens
phacofragmatome
phalangeal
p. broach
p. forceps
Phaneuf
P. arterial forceps
P. clamp
P. forceps
P. hysterectomy forceps
P. peritoneal forceps

P. uterine artery forceps
P. uterine artery scissors
P. vaginal forceps
phantom
  p. clamp
  p. guide wire
  Imatron CT bone
    mineral p.
  p. wire
Pharmacia
  P. Intermedics ophthalmics
    intraocular lens
  P. intraocular lens
Pharmaseal
  P. catheter
  P. closed drain
  P. disposable catheter
  P. drain
Pharmex disposable catheter
pharyngeal retractor
pharyngoscope
  Hays p.
  Proud-Beck p.
Phase-A-Caps alloy
Phaseafill dental composite
Phasealloy alloy
Pheifer-Young retractor
Phelan vein stripper
Phelps
  P. brace
  P. splint
Phelps-Gocht osteoclast
Phemister
  P. graft
  P. onlay bone graft
  P. punch
  P. raspatory
  P. raspatory elevator
  P. reamer
Phiefer-Young retractor
Philadelphia collar
Phillips
  P. catheter
  P. clamp
  P. dilator
  P. fixation forceps
  P. forceps
  P. recessed-head screw
  P. rectal clamp
  P. screwdriver
  P. swan neck forceps
  P. urethral catheter

P. urethral whip bougie
P. urologic catheter
phimosis forceps
Phipps forceps
pHisoDerm scrub soap
pHisoHex scrub soap
Phoenix
  P. pacemaker
  P. single-chamber pacemaker
  P. total hip prosthesis
phorometer
phoro-optometer
Phoropter retractor
phoroptors
  A-O minus cylinder p.
  A-O plus cylinder p.
photic-evoked response stimulator
photocoagulator
  American Optics p.
  argon laser p.
  Coherent argon laser p.
  infrared ray p.
  Mira p.
  sapphire crystal infrared p.
  xenon p.
  xenon arc p.
  Zeiss p.
  Zeiss xenon arc p.
photoculdoscope
  Decker p.
photogastroscope *Photon balloon*
  Krentz p.
photolaparoscope
  Lent p.
  Wolf p.
pH probe
phrenicectomy forceps
phrenic retractor
Phynox
  P. clip
  P. cobalt alloy clip
physician's
  p. pickup forceps
  p. splinter forceps
physiologic pacemaker
Phystan implant
piano-wire staff
PIBC
  percutaneous intra-aortic balloon
    counterpulsation
    PIBC catheter

PICC
    peripherally inserted central
    catheter
pick
    anterior footplate p.
    Austin p.
    Bellucci p.
    Burch fixation p.
    Burch ophthalmic p.
    p. chisel
    Cooley p.
    Crabtree dissector p.
    Crane dental p.
    dental p.
    double-ended root tip
      dental p.
    Farrior anterior footplate p.
    Farrior footplate p.
    Farrior oval-window p.
    Farrior posterior
      footplate p.
    footplate p.
    Guilford-Wright footplate p.
    Guilford-Wright stapes p.
    Hayden footplate p.
    Hoffmann scleral fixation p.
    Hough p.
    Hough stapedectomy
      footplate p.
    House p.
    House-Barbara p.
    House-Crabtree dissector p.
    House obtuse p.
    House oval-window p.
    House strut p.
    p. knife
    Kos p.
    McGee footplate p.
    Michels p.
    microsurgical ear p.
    Morgenstein p.
    Morgenstein p.
    ophthalmic p.
    oval-window p.
    Paparella p.
    Paparella footplate p.
    posterior footplate p.
    right-angle p.
    Rosen p.
    Saunders-Paparella p.
    Scheer p.
    Schuknecht p.
    Shea p.

    slightly-curved p.
    slightly-curved ear p.
    small p.
    stapedectomy footplate p.
    stapes p.
    strut p.
    Tabb knife p.
    Trent p.
    Wells scleral suture p.
    Wilder p.
    Wright-Guilford footplate p.
    Wright-Guilford stapes p.
Pickett scissors
Pickrell
    P. hook
    P. retractor
pickup
    Adson p.
    DeBakey p.
    p. forceps
    p. noncrushing forceps
    rat-tooth p.
Picolino monorail catheter
Picot
    P. retractor
    P. vaginal retractor
    P. vaginal speculum
    P. weighted speculum-
      retractor
Pidcock
    P. nail
    P. pin
piece
    Witt fiberoptic hand p.
Piedmont all-cotton elastic dressing
Pie Medical ultrasound system
Pierce
    P. antral trocar
    P. antrum wash tube
    P. attic cannula
    P. cannula
    P. cheek retractor
    P. cryptotome
    P. dissector
    P. elevator
    P. nasal cup
    P. retractor
    P. rongeur
    P. submucous dissector
**Pierce-Donachy ventricular assist
  device**
Pierce-Kyle trocar

Pierse
- P. corneal Colibri-type forceps
- P. corneal forceps
- P. eye speculum
- P. fixation forceps
- P. forceps

Pierse Colibri
- P. C. corneal utility forceps
- P. C. forceps
- P. C.-type corneal forceps
- P. C. utility forceps

Pierse-Hoskins forceps

Pierse-type
- P.-t. Colibri forceps
- P.-t. fine forceps
- P.-t. microforceps
- P.-t. skeleton forceps

Piffard
- P. curette
- P. dermal curette
- P. dermal curette with Luer hub
- P. placental curette

piggyback probe

Pigott forceps

pigskin graft

pigtail
- p. biliary stent
- p. catheter
- p. nephrostomy drain
- p. probe
- p. stent

Pike jawed forceps

Pilcher
- P. bag
- P. bag catheter
- P. catheter
- P. hemostatic bag
- P. hemostatic suprapubic bag
- P. suprapubic hemostatic bag

pile
- p. clamp
- p. forceps

pillar
- p. forceps
- p. retractor

pillar-grasping forceps

Pillet hand prosthesis

Pilling
- P. bronchoscope
- P. clamp
- P. collector
- P. duralite tube
- P. Excalibur gauge
- P. fiberoptic illuminator
- P. forceps
- P. gouge
- P. laryngofissure shears
- P. micro-anastomosis clamp
- P. needle holder
- P. pediatric clamp
- P. retractor
- P. suture

Pilling-Favaloro retractor

Pilling-Hartmann speculum

Pilling-Liston bone utility forceps

Pilling-Negus clamp-on aspirator

Pilling-Ruskin rongeur

Pilling-Wolock approximator

Pilling-Wolvek sternal approximator

pillow
- abduction p.
- cervical p.
- Rubens p.

pilot drill

Pilotip catheter

Pilot point screw

pin
- Ace p.
- Apex p.
- ASIF screw p.
- Asnis p.
- Austin Moore p.
- Barr p.
- beaded hip p.
- Beath p.
- Belos compression p.
- bevel-point Rush p.
- Böhler p.
- Böhler-Knowles hip p.
- Böhler-Steinmann p.
- Bohlman p.
- Breck p.
- calibrated p.
- Canakis beaded hip p.
- cancellous p.
- p. chuck
- cloverleaf p.
- Compere threaded p.
- Conley p.
- cortical p.
- Craig p.

pin *(continued)*
Crowe-tip p.
Crutchfield p.
Davis p.
p. deburring die
Delitala T-p.
deluxe FIN p.
Denham p.
Deyerle p.
duodenal p.
Ender p.
endodontic p.
Fahey p.
Fahey-Compere p.
fixation p.
friction lock p.
Furness-Clute p.
Gardner skull clamp p.
Getz root canal p.
Gouffon hip p.
p. guard
guide p.
p. guide
Hagie p.
Hahnenkratt root canal p.
Hansen-Street p.
Hatcher p.
Haynes p.
p. headrest
Hegge p.
Hewson breakaway p.
hexhead p.
Hoffmann p.
Hoffmann apex fixation p.
Hoffmann transfixion p.
p. holder
p. implant
intramedullary p.
Jones p.
Jurgan p.
Kirschner wire p.
Knowles p.
Knowles hip p.
Kronendonk p.
Kronfeld p.
Küntscher p.
lateral guide p.
Lottes p.
Marble bone p.
Markley retention p.
Mayfield skull p.
Mayfield skull clamp p.
mechanic's p.

medullary p.
metal p.
Modny p.
Moore fixation p.
Moule screw p.
Mt. Sinai skull clamp p.
Neufeld p.
Norman tibial p.
Oris p.
Ormco p.
Orthofix p.
OrthoSorb p.
OrthoSorb absorbable p.
osseous p.
osteotomy p.
Pidcock p.
Pugh hip p.
restorative p.
Rhinelander p.
Rica guide p.
Rica wire guide p.
Riordan p.
Rissler p.
Rissler-Stille p.
Roger Anderson p.
Rush p.
Rush intramedullary
fixation p.
safety p.
Safir p.
Sage p.
Scand p.
Schneider self-broaching p.
Schweitzer p.
self-broaching p.
self-tapering p.
Shantz p.
Shriners p.
skeletal p.
Smillie p.
Smith-Petersen fracture p.
SMo Moore p.
smooth p.
spring p.
Stader p.
Steinmann p.
Steinmann fixation p.
Street p.
strut-type p.
Surgin hemorrhage
occluder p.
p. suture
threaded p.

threaded guide p.
tibial p.
tibial guide p.
trochanteric p.
Turner p.
union broach retention p.
Venable-Stuck fracture p.
p. vise
von Saal medullary p.
Walker hollow quill p.
Watanabe p.
Watson-Jones guide p.
Webb p.
Zimfoam p.
Zimmer p.
Pinard fetal stethoscope
pin-bending forceps
pinchcock clamp
pinch forceps
pinion headrest
Pinkerton catheter
pink twisted cotton suture
Pinnacle
P. introducer set
P. pacemaker
P. sheath
pin-seating forceps
pinwheel
Grafco p.
p. sensation gauge
Wartenberg p.
Pio root canal depth indicator
pipe
fiberoptic light p.
light p.
Storz disposable fiberoptic
light p.
Pipelle
P. endometrial curette
P. endometrial suction
curette
**Pipelle-deCornier endometrial
curette**
Piper
P. forceps
P. lateral wall retractor
P. obstetrical forceps
Pirquet tongue depressor
Pisces
P. device
P. implant
Pischel
P. electrode

P. forceps
P. micropin
P. micropin forceps
P. needle
P. scleral ruler
pistol
suction p.
pistol-grip hand drill
piston
Austin p.
Causse p.
Guilford-Wright Teflon
wire p.
House p.
McGee p.
p. prosthesis
p. wire
Pitanguy forceps
Pitha
P. forceps
P. foreign body forceps
P. urethral forceps
Pitkin
P. dermatome
P. needle
Pittman needle holder
Pittsburgh
P. pelvic triangular external
frame
P. triangular frame
pituitary
p. curette
p. forceps
p. rongeur
p. rongeur forceps
p. spoon
pivot
p. aneurysm clip
p. clip applier
p. lock
p. micro-anastomosis
approximator
pivoting surgical arm board
PKS-25 apparatus stapler
placement forceps
placental
p. clamp
p. curette
placenta previa forceps
placer
Dean bracket p.
plain
p. catgut suture

plain *(continued)*
  p. ear hook
  p. ear spoon
  p. eye needle
  p. forceps
  p. gut suture
  p. interrupted suture
  p. rib shears
  p. rotary scissors
  p. screwdriver
  p. splinter forceps
  p. sterilizer forceps
  p. suture
  p. thumb forceps
  p. tissue forceps
  p. vesical trocar
  p. wire speculum
plain-end grooved director
plain-pattern plate
plane
  corn p.
  p. iris forceps
planer
  calcar p.
plano
  p. lens
  p. T-bandage
planoconcave lens
planoconvex
  p. eye implant
  p. lens
Planustar teeth
plaque retriever
plasma
  p. scalpel
  p. TFE vascular graft
Plastalume
  P. bulb-ended splint
  P. straight splint
plaster
  p. bandage
  p. dressing
  p. knife
  p. pants dressing
  p. saw
  p. shears
  p. spatula
  p. splint
  p. spreader
  p. with lift saw
plaster-of-Paris (POP)
  p.-o.-P. bandage

  p.-o.-P. dressing
  p.-o.-P. jacket
Plastibell
  P. circumcision clamp
  P. circumcision device
  P. clamp
  P. compression instrument
plastic
  p. ball implant
  p. cannula
  p. catheter
  p. cone tip
  p. curette
  p. drape
  p. dressing
  p. forceps
  p. implant
  p. mouth guard
  p. sphere eye implant
  p. surgery scissors
  p. suture
  p. suture-removal forceps
  p. Tiemann catheter
  p. utility scissors
plastic-cuffed tracheostomy tube
Plasticeph cephalometer
Plasticor prosthesis
Plasti-Pore ossicular replacement prosthesis
Plastizote orthotic device
Plastodent
  P. dental impression adhesive
  P. wax
plate
  Alta channel bone p.
  Alta distal fracture bone p.
  Alta proximal-angled bone p.
  Alta supracondylar bone p.
  Anchor p.
  AO compression p.
  ASIF p.
  Babcock p.
  Badgley p.
  Bagby compression p.
  Balser hook p.
  Batchelor p.
  p. bender
  bent blade p.
  Berke-Jaeger lid p.
  blade p.
  Blount p.

bone p.
Bosworth spline p.
buttress p.
Capener nail p.
CAPIS compression p.
CAPIS individual p.
CAPIS reconstruction p.
CHS supracondylar bone p.
coaptation p.
Coffin p.
Crockard midfacial
  osteotomy retractor p.
p. cutter
Deyerle p.
Deyerle bone graft p.
Deyerle II p.
double-angled blade p.
Doughty tongue p.
dynamic compression p.
  (DCP)
Eggers p.
Elliot knee p.
Elliott blade p.
Ellis buttress p.
finger p.
Goidnich bone p.
Hansen-Street anchor p.
Harlow p.
Hicks lugged p.
Hoen skull p.
Hubbard p.
impactor p.
Jaeger lid p.
Jewett double-angled
  osteotomy p.
Jewett slotted p.
Kessel osteotomy p.
keyed supracondylar p.
Kingsley orthodontic p.
Kleer base p.
Laing osteotomy p.
Lane fracture p.
L-buttress p.
lead p.
Letournel acetabular fracture
  bone p.
lid p.
low-contact stress p.
L-plate p.
Luer reconstruction p.
Luhr mandibular p.
Luhr MCS bone p.
Luhr microbone p.

Luhr mini fixation bone p.
Lundholm p.
Lynch mucosa separator p.
Massie II p.
McBride p.
McLaughlin p.
McLaughlin hip p.
Meurig Williams spinal
  fusion p.
Milch resection p.
Moberg bone p.
Moe intertrochanteric p.
Moore blade p.
Moore-Blount p.
mouth gag tooth p.
mucosal separator p.
nail p.
Neufeld p.
Newman toenail p.
Nicoll p.
Nord orthodontic p.
orthodontic base p.
Osborne osteotomy p.
plain-pattern p.
reconstruction p.
Rhinelander p.
Richards sideplate p.
Robin orthodontic p.
Schweitzer spring p.
Senn bone p.
serpentine bone p.
Sherman p.
Sherman bone p.
skull p.
slotted p.
slotted bone p.
Smith-Petersen p.
Smith-Petersen bone p.
SMo p.
snap-on inserter p.
Stahl calipers p.
Temple University p.
Thornton p.
tibial p.
tongue p.
Townsend-Gilfillan p.
trochanteric p.
TSRH p.
tubular p.
Tupman osteotomy p.
V-blade plate p.
VDS p.
Venable bone p.

plate *(continued)*
    Vitallium p.
    Vitallium Elliott knee p.
    Vitallium Hicks radius p.
    Vitallium Wainwright
      blade p.
    Vitallium Walldius
      mechanical knee p.
    VSP p.
    VSP bone p.
    V-type intertrochanteric p.
    Wenger slotted p.
    Wilson spinal fusion p.
    Wright knee p.
    Y-bone p.
    Z-plate p.
    Zuelzer hook p.
plate-holding forceps
platform
    p. forceps
    microlaryngeal laser
      operating p.
    microlaryngeal suction laser
      operating p.
    Ossoff-Karlan laser laryngeal
      micro-operating p.
    Ossoff-Karlan microlaryngeal
      laser operating p.
    Ossoff-Karlan microlaryngeal
      suction laser operating p.
Platina intraocular lens implant
platinum
    p. blade electrode
    p. blade meatotomy
      electrode
    p. spatula
Platorit investment material
Playfair uterine caustic applicator
pledget
    Dacron p.
    p. dressing
    Gelfoam p.
    Meadox Teflon felt p.
    polypropylene p.
    p. sponge
    p. suture
    Teflon p.
pledgeted
    p. Ethibond suture
    p. suture
Plenge foreign body spud
Plenk-Matson raspatory
Plester retractor

plethysmograph
pleural
    p. biopsy needle
    p. biopsy needle shears
    p. biopsy punch
    p. dissector
pleurectomy forceps
Pleur-Evac
    P.-E. autotransfusion system
    P.-E. suction
    P.-E. suction tube
Pleurovac chest catheter
Plexiglas
    P. eye implant
    P. Gellhorn pessary
    P. graft
    P. implant
Pley
    P. capsular forceps
    P. forceps
plicating suture
plication
    p. needle
    p. suture
pliers
    Allen root p.
    Beck p.
    bending p.
    Berbecker p.
    College p.
    crown-crimping p.
    dental p.
    fisherman's p.
    heavy-duty p. with side-
      cutter
    hex nut-holder p.
    Jelenko p.
    K-Y p.
    Mathieu p.
    needle-nose p.
    Ormco orthodontic p.
    orthopaedic p.
    orthopaedic surgical p.
    Power Grip p.
    Reill wire-cutting p.
    Risley p.
    root p.
    Schwarz arrow-forming p.
    slip joint p.
    SMIC p.
    Stille flat p.
    Swan-Jacob goniotomy p.

threader rod holder p.
vise-grip p.
PLIF procedure
posterior lumbar interbody
fusion procedure
Plondke
P. uterine-elevating forceps
P. uterine forceps
plug
Air-Lon decannulation p.
Alcock p.
Biomet p.
Bio-Plug canal p.
bone p.
catheter p.
Concept bone tunnel p.
Corner p.
Counsellor p.
Dittrich p.
Doc's ear p.
Dohlman p.
gastrostomy p.
glass vaginal p.
intramedullary canal p.
Isberg scleral p.
Johnston gastrostomy p.
Kirschner femoral canal p.
Mack ear p.
Reich-Nechtow p.
scleral p.
sealing window p.
Seidel p.
Sims vaginal p.
Teflon p.
Woodson p.
plugger
amalgam p.
endodontic p.
SMIC root canal p.
Plummer
P. bag
P. dilator
P. esophageal dilator
P. hydrostatic bag
P. modified bougie
P. water-filled pneumatic
esophageal dilator
Plummer-Vinson
P.-V. apparatus
P.-V. dilator
P.-V. esophageal dilator
P.-V. radium esophageal
applicator

plus power lens
Plystan
P. graft
P. prosthesis
PMI implant
PMMA
polymethyl methacrylate
all-PMMA intraocular lens
all-PMMA one-piece C-loop
intraocular lens
PMMA centering sleeve
PMMA haptic
PMMA intraocular lens
pneumatic
p. bag
p. balloon catheter
p. balloon dilator
p. cuff
p. dilator
p. drill accessory
p. otoscope
p. tonometer
p. tourniquet
pneumatometer
Semm CO_2 p.
pneumatonograph
Pneumomat laparoscopic insufflator
pneumoperitoneum needle
pneumostatic dilator
pneumotachometer
Rudolph linear p.
pneumothoracic
pneumothoracic apparatus
pneumothoracic injection
needle
pneumothoracic needle
pneumothorax
pneumotome
Wappler p.
pneuPAC
p. resuscitator
p. ventilator
pocket
p. Doppler blood flow
detector
p. probe
**Pocket-Dop II fetal heart rate
monitor**
Poh
P. disclosing gel
P. mouth mirror
point
Crutchfield drill p.

point *(continued)*
>Crutchfield-Raney skull traction tong p.
>drill p.
>p. electrode
>Excell polishing p.
>p. forceps
>G-C "SMOOTH CUT" diamond p.
>gutta-percha p.
>Mathews drill p.
>Raney-Crutchfield drill p.
>Starlite p.
>Universal drill p.
>William Dixon Cratex p.

pointed-tip electrode
Pointer one-piece all-PMMA intraocular lens
Polaris catheter
Polar-Mate bipolar coagulator
Polaroid
>P. camera
>P. CB-100 camera
>P. instant endocamera

Polavision Land camera for endoscopy
Polcyn elevator
Poliak eye retractor
polio laryngoscope
Polisar-Lyons adapted tracheal tube
polisher
>Anis ball capsular p.
>Anis ball reverse-curvature capsular p.
>Anis disk capsular p.
>Bechert capsular p.
>Drews capsular p.
>Freeman capsular p.
>Gill-Welsh capsular p.
>Gill-Welsh curette capsular p.
>Holladay posterior capsular p.
>Jensen capsular p.
>Knolle p.
>Knolle capsular p.
>Kraff capsular p.
>Kratz p.
>Tennessee capsular p.
>Torchia capsular p.

polishing
>p. brush
>p. bur

Politzer
>P. air bag
>P. air bag otoscope
>P. air syringe
>P. angular ear knife
>P. bag
>P. ear knife
>P. ear speculum
>P. paracentesis needle

Politzer-Ralks knife
Polk
>P. placental forceps
>P. sponge forceps

Polley-Bickel trephine
Pollock
>P. double corneal forceps
>P. forceps
>P. sweetheart periosteal elevator
>P. wimp wire impactor
>P. zygoma elevator

Pollock-Dingman septal displacer
Polokoff rasp
polyamide suture
Polybar contrast material
Polycel bone composite prosthesis
polycentric knee prosthesis
Polydek suture
polydioxanone (PDS)
polydioxanone suture
polyester
>p. fiber suture
>p. suture

polyether implant material
polyethylene
>p. cannula
>p. catheter
>p. collar button
>p. drain
>p. eye implant
>p. glycol (PEG)
>p. graft
>p. implant material
>p. liner
>p. retractor tape
>p. seat heart valve
>p. sphere implant
>p. stent
>p. strut
>p. suture

p. talar prosthesis
p. tube
polyfilament suture
PolyFlex
    P. implantable pacing lead
      pacemaker
    P. lead pacemaker
    P. traction dressing
Polyflux hemodialyzer
polyglycolic
    p. acid (PGA)
    p. acid suture
polygoniometer
polymethyl methacrylate (PMMA)
polypectomy snare
polyp forceps
Poly-Plus Dacron vascular graft
polypropylene
    p. button
    p. button suture
    p. glycol (PPG)
    p. glycol-ankle-foot orthosis
      (PPG-AFO)
    p. glycol-thoracolumbosacral
      orthosis (PPG-TLSO)
    p. hand brush
    p. intracardiac patch
    p. intraocular lens
    p. pledget
    p. suture
polypus forceps
Polysil-Foley catheter
polysomnograph
   electroencephalograph 20-channel
   EEG recorder
Polysorb 55 stapler
Polystan
    P. cardiotomy reservoir
    P. catheter
    P. implant
    P. perfusion cannula
    P. venous return catheter
Poly Surgiclip
polytetrafluoroethylene (PTFE)
    p. graft
Polytrac
    P. Gomez retractor
    P. retractor
polyurethane
    p. graft
    p. implant material
polyvinyl
    p. catheter

p. curette
p. drain
p. graft
p. implant material
p. sponge implant
p. tube
p. tubing
Pomeranz
    P. aortic clamp
    P. hiatal hernia retractor
    P. retractor
Pomeroy ear syringe
Ponseti splint
Pool
    P. abdominal suction tube
    P. Pfeiffer self-locking clip
    P. trocar
Poole
    P. abdominal-aspirating tube
    P. abdominal suction tube
    P. suction tube
POP
   plaster-of-Paris
   POP bandage
Pope
    P. halo dressing
    P. Oto-Wick
    P. rectal knife
popliteal retractor
pop-off
    p.-o. needle
    p.-o. suture
Poppen
    P. aortic clamp
    P. clamp
    P. coagulator
    P. electrosurgical coagulator
    P. elevator
    P. forceps
    P. Gigli-saw guide
    P. intervertebral disk
      forceps
    P. intervertebral disk
      rongeur
    P. laminectomy rongeur
    P. monopolar cautery cord
    P. needle
    P. periosteal elevator
    P. pituitary rongeur
    P. suction tube
    P. sympathectomy scissors
    P. ventricular needle

Poppen-Blalock
    P.-B. carotid artery clamp
    P.-B. carotid clamp
    P.-B. clamp
Poppen-Blalock-Salibi
    P.-B.-S. carotid clamp
    P.-B.-S. clamp
Poppen-Gelpi
    P.-G. laminectomy retractor
    P.-G. laminectomy self-
      retaining retractor
Poppers tonsillar guillotine
Poracryl resin
porcine
    p. graft
    p. heart valve
    p. prosthesis
Porex
    P. Medpor implant
    P. nerve locator
    P. PHA implant
Porges stone dislodger
Pori and Rowe EEG receiver
Porocoat material
Porocool prosthesis
Porolon sponge
Poroplastic splint
porous coated anatomic (PCA)
porous coating
Porovin dental resin
PORP
    partial ossicular
      reconstruction/replacement
      prosthesis
port
    side p.
    subcutaneous p.
portable
    p. aspirator
    p. respirator
    p. suction aspirator
Port-A-Cath implantable catheter
Portadial kidney machine
portal
    p. cannula
    p. catheter
    p. vascular bed
Portaray dental x-ray unit
Porter
    P. duodenal forceps
    P. forceps
Porter-Kolpe biliary biopsy set

Porter-O-Surgical cutter
Portex
    P. cannula
    P. chorionic villus sampling
      catheter
    P. nasopharyngeal airway
    P. nylon cannula
    P. tube
Portex-Gibbon catheter
Portmann
    P. drill
    P. retractor
Portnoy
    P. catheter
    P. ventricular cannula
    P. ventricular catheter
Porto-lift
Porto-Vac
    P.-V. catheter
    P.-V. suction tube
Porzett splint
Posada-Vasco orbital retractor
Posey
    P. belt
    P. restraint
    P. sling
    P. snare
Posilok instrument holder
positioner
    beach chair p.
    body p.
    Cook stent p.
    Craniad cup p.
    cup p.
    lateral p.
    McCaffrey p.
    Miller bracket p.
    Schlein shoulder p.
    TMJ head p.
    Vac-Pac p.
positioning needle
Positrol
    P. catheter
    P. II Bernstein catheter
    P. USCI catheter
Posner
    P. diagnostic gonioprism
    P. gonioprism
    P. surgical gonioprism
Post
    P. forceps
    P. washing cannula

post
  Hahnenkratt root canal p.
  PD crown p.
  PD root canal p.
  Stalite root canal p.
  surgical instrument p.
postauricular
  p. ear dressing
  p. hearing aid
  p. retractor
posterior
  p. capsular scrubber
  p. chamber intraocular lens
  p. convex intraocular lens
  p. footplate pick
  p. forceps
  p. fossa retractor
  p. lumbar interbody fusion
    procedure (PLIF procedure)
  p. lumbar retractor set
  p. palatine suture
  p. urethral retractor
Post-Harrington erysiphake
postmortem suture needle
postnasal
  p. balloon
  p. dressing
  p. sponge forceps
postplaced suture
post-TUR
  p.-T. clamp
  p.-T. irrigation clamp
  p.-T. irrigation control
    clamp
post-urethroplasty review speculum
Potain
  P. apparatus
  P. aspirating trocar
  P. aspirator
potassium titanyl phosphate (KTP)
  laser
Potta coarctation forceps
Potter
  P. modified knife
  P. needle
  P. sickle knife
  P. sponge forceps
  P. tonsillar forceps
Potts
  P. aortic clamp
  P. bronchial forceps
  P. bulldog forceps
  P. cardiovascular clamp

  P. clamp
  P. coarctation clamp
  P. coarctation forceps
  P. dental elevator
  P. dilator
  P. dissector
  P. divisional clamp
  P. ductus clamp
  P. expansile dilator
  P. expansile knife
  P. expansile valvulotome
  P. fixation forceps
  P. forceps
  P. infant rib shears
  P. intestinal forceps
  P. needle
  P. patent ductus clamp
  P. patent ductus forceps
  P. periosteotome
  P. pulmonic clamp
  P. scissors
  P. splint
  P. tenaculum
  P. tenotomy scissors
  P. thumb forceps
  P. tie suture
Potts-Cournand
  P.-C. angiography needle
  P.-C. needle
Potts-DeMartel gall duct scissors
Potts-Nevins dressing forceps
Potts-Niedner
  P.-N. aortic clamp
  P.-N. clamp
Potts-Riker
  P.-R. dilator
  P.-R. valvulotome
Potts-Satinsky clamp
Potts-Smith
  P.-S. aortic clamp
  P.-S. aortic occlusion clamp
  P.-S. arterial scissors
  P.-S. dissecting scissors
  P.-S. dressing forceps
  P.-S. forceps
  P.-S. monopolar forceps
  P.-S. needle holder
  P.-S. pulmonic clamp
  P.-S. reverse scissors
  P.-S. scissors
  P.-S. tissue forceps
Potts-Yasargil scissors

pouch
        Bongort urinary diversion p.
        Convatec urostomy p.
        Hollister First Choice p.
        Parks ileostomy p.
        Parsonnet pulse generator p.
        Squibb urostomy p.
        Sur-Fit urostomy p.
        p. type sling
Pousson pigtail catheter
Poutasse
        P. clamp
        P. forceps
        P. renal artery clamp
        P. renal artery forceps
powder
        p. blower
        Chronicure protein
          hydrolysate p.
        Denpac porcelain p.
        Francer porcelain p.
        Stomahesive p.
        Tru-Stain acrylic p.
        Vitadur-N porcelain p.
Power
        P. Grip pliers
        P. Play knee brace
Pozzi
        P. tenaculum
        P. tenaculum forceps
PPG
     polypropylene glycol
         PPG probe
PPG-AFO
     polypropylene glycol-ankle-foot
      orthosis
         PPG-AFO brace
PPG-TLSO
     polypropylene glycol-
      thoracolumbosacral orthosis
         PPG-TLSO brace
PPS
     personal portable stimulator
PPT orthotic device
Praeger iris hook
Pram combination occluder
Pratt
        P. anoscope
        P. antral curette
        P. bivalve retractor
        P. bivalve speculum
        P. crypt hook
        P. curette

        P. cystic hook
        P. dilator
        P. ethmoid curette
        P. forceps
        P. hemostatic forceps
        P. nasal curette
        P. probe
        P. rectal dilator
        P. rectal director
        P. rectal hook
        P. rectal probe
        P. rectal scissors
        P. rectal speculum
        P. T-clamp
        P. tenaculum
        P. tissue forceps
        P. tissue-grasping forceps
        P. T-shaped forceps
        P. T-shaped hemostatic
          forceps
        P. urethral sound
        P. uterine dilator
        P. vulsellum forceps
Pratt-Smith
        P.-S. forceps
        P.-S. hemostatic forceps
        P.-S. tissue-grasping forceps
Precision
        P. eye implant
        P. Osteolock component
        P. Osteolock femoral
          component system
        P. Osteolock hip
Precision-Cosmet intraocular lens
     implant
Preci-Slot dental attachment
Preci-Vertix kit
preclotted graft
precut suture
Predent disclosing solution
Predictor
     CLEARPLAN Easy
      Ovulation P.
Preefer eye speculum
preformed
        p. catheter
        p. clasp
        p. Cordis catheter
Premier irrigation-aspiration unit
Premium
        P. CEEA circular stapling
          device

P. CEEA stapler
P. Poly CS-57 stapler
Prentif pessary
Prentiss forceps
preplaced suture
Preptic dressing
prepuce forceps
presbyopia glasses
Presbyterian
    P. Hospital clamp
    P. Hospital elevator
    P. Hospital forceps
    P. Hospital needle
    P. Hospital occluding clamp
    P. Hospital staphylorrhaphy
      elevator
    P. Hospital T-clamp
    P. Hospital tube clamp
    P. Hospital tube-occluding
      forceps
    P. Hospital tubing clamp
    P. Hospital ventricular
      needle
Prescriptor hearing aid
presection suture
preshaped catheter
Preshaw clamp
press
    Cali-Press graft p.
    House Gelfoam p.
    Paparella tissue p.
    p. plate needle holder
    Sheehy fascial p.
    tissue p.
    tissue graft p.
Press-Fit
    P.-F. component (PFC)
    P.-F. condylar component
    P.-F. total condylar knee
      system
press-fit
    p.-f. implant
    p.-f. prosthesis
Presso-Elastic dressing
Pressoplast compression dressing
Presso-Superior dressing
pressure
    p. bandage
    p. cuff
    p. dressing
    p. forceps
    p. gauge
    p. ring

Preston-Hopkins ligator
Preston ligamentum flavum forceps
Pribram suction tube
Price
    P. muscle biopsy clamp
    P. muscle clamp
Price-Thomas
    P.-T. bronchial clamp
    P.-T. bronchial forceps
    P.-T. bronchus clamp
    P.-T. bronchus forceps
    P.-T. clamp
    P.-T. forceps
    P.-T. rib stripper
Priessnitz
    P. bandage
    P. dressing
Priestley-Smith retinoscope
Priestly catheter
Priest wasp-waist laryngostat
PrimaCast
Primaderm dressing
Primallor alloy
Prima pacemaker
Primapore dressing
primary
    p. suture
    p. trimming bur
Primbs suturing forceps
Prince
    P. advancement forceps
    P. clamp
    P. dissecting scissors
    P. eye cautery
    P. forceps
    P. muscle forceps
    P. rongeur
    P. tonsillar scissors
    P. trachoma forceps
Prince-Potts scissors
Pringle clamp
Printz aspirator
prism
    Allen-Thorpe gonioscopic p.
    Becker gonioscopic p.
    Drews inclined p.
    Jacob-Swan gonioscopic p.
    p. loupe
    Risley p.
    Swan-Jacob gonioscopic p.
Prism-CL pacemaker
Pritchard
    P. cannula

Pritchard *(continued)*
    P. syringe
    P. total elbow prosthesis
Pritikin scleral punch
probe
    Amoils p.
    Amussat p.
    Ando motor-driven p.
    Anel lacrimal p.
    angled p.
    Arbuckle p.
    Arbuckle sinus p.
    Arndorfer esophageal
      motility p.
    back-stop laser p.
    Bakes p.
    Balectrode pacing p.
    Barr p.
    Barr fistular p.
    Barr rectal p.
    Becker p.
    Beckman p.
    Benger p.
    Bermen-Werner p.
    Beyer pigtail p.
    BICAP p.
    biliary balloon p.
    biometry p.
    biplane sector p.
    bipolar p.
    bipolar hemostasis p.
    blood-flow p.
    blunt p.
    blunt-tip p.
    Bodian lacrimal pigtail p.
    Bodian minilacrimal p.
    Bodian pigtail p.
    Bowman p.
    Bowman lacrimal p.
    Brackett p.
    Brackett dental p.
    brain p.
    Brenner rectal p.
    Bresgen p.
    Bresgen frontal sinus p.
    Bresgen sinus p.
    Brock p.
    Brodie p.
    Brodie fistular p.
    bronchoscopic p.
    Bruel-Kjaer transvaginal
      ultrasound p.
    Brunner p.

    Brymill p.
    Brysmill cryosurgical p.
    Buck p.
    Buck ear p.
    Buie p.
    Buie fistula p.
    bullet p.
    Bunnell p.
    Bunnell dissecting p.
    Bunnell forwarding p.
    calibrated p.
    canaliculus p.
    cardiac p.
    cataract p.
    p. catheter
    Chandler V-pacing p.
    Cherry p.
    Cherry brain p.
    chrome p. with eye
    Circon-ACMI
      electrohydraulic
      lithotriptor p.
    coagulation p.
    Coakley p.
    Coakley nasal p.
    Cody magnetic p.
    common duct p.
    conical p.
    Contact Laser bullet p.
    Contact Laser chisel p.
    Contact Laser conical p.
    Contact Laser convex p.
    Contact Laser flat p.
    Contact Laser interstitial p.
    Contact Laser round p.
    continuously perfused p.
    coronary artery p.
    Crawford canaliculus p.
    Criticare sensor p.
    cross-sectional anal
      sphincter p.
    cryogenic p.
    cryotherapy p.
    Desjardins p.
    Desjardins gall duct p.
    Desjardins gallstone p.
    dilating p.
    p. dilator
    dilator p.
    disposable p.
    dissecting p.
    dissection p.
    Dix spud p.

Doppler p.
Doppler flow p.
double-ended p.
double-ended chrome p.
double-ended nickelene p.
double-ended silver p.
drum p.
ear p.
Earle p.
Earle rectal p.
echocardiographic p.
electric p.
electrohydraulic
 lithotriptor p.
electromagnetic flow p.
Ellis p.
Ellis needle p.
Emmet p.
Emmet uterine p.
endocervical p.
endolaser p.
endoscopic BICAP p.
endoscopic heat p.
Esmarch p.
Esmarch tin bullet p.
Esmarch p. with Myrtle
 leaf end
eustachian p.
eye p.
eyed p.
Fenger p.
Fenger gallbladder p.
Fenger gall duct p.
Fenger gallstone p.
Fenger spiral gallstone p.
Ferguson p.
Ferguson esophageal p.
fiberoptic p.
filiform bougie p.
Fish antral p.
Fish sinus p.
fistular p.
flexible p.
flow p.
Fluhrer bullet p.
Fluhrer rectal p.
Fogarty p.
Fogarty biliary p.
Fogarty biliary balloon p.
foreign body p.
forwarding p.
fragmentation p.
Fränkel sinus p.

French-pattern lacrimal p.
Fresgen frontal sinus p.
Frigitronics p.
frontal sinus p.
Gallagher p.
Gallagher bipolar
 mapping p.
gall duct p.
gallstone p.
galvanic p.
Gant p.
Gant rectal p.
Geldmacher tendon-
 passing p.
general p.
Gillquist-Oretorp-Stille p.
Gilmore p.
Girard p.
Girdner p.
Gross p.
Hagar p.
hand-held exploring
 electrode p.
Harms p.
Harms trabeculotomy p.
Hayden p.
heater p.
Heller p.
Henning-Keinkel stomach p.
Hitachi convex-convex
 biplane p.
Hitachi convex
 ultrasound p.
Hitachi fingertip
 ultrasound p.
Hitachi linear ultrasound p.
Hitachi multipurpose
 fingertip ultrasound p.
Hitachi transrectal
 ultrasound p.
Hitachi transvaginal
 ultrasound p.
hot-tipped laser p.
Hotz p.
Hotz ear p.
24-hour esophageal pH p.
illuminated p.
illuminated ureter p.
Injectate p.
irrigating p.
Jackson p.
Jacobson p.
Jacobson blood vessel p.

probe *(continued)*
Jacobson vas deferens p.
Jako p.
Jako laryngeal p.
Jannetta p.
Jansen-Newhart p.
Jansen-Newhart mastoid p.
Jobson-Horne p.
Kalk palpitation p.
Kartch pigtail p.
Kennerdell-Maroon p.
Killian p.
Kirschner guiding p.
Kistner p.
Kleinsasser p.
Knapp p.
Knapp iris p.
Kocher p.
Koenig p.
Kron p.
Kron gall duct p.
Kry-Med 300 p.
lacrimal p.
lacrimal duct p.
Larry p.
Larry rectal p.
laryngeal p.
laser p.
Lente p.
Lente silver nitrate p.
Liebreich p.
Lilienthal p.
Lillie p.
Lillie frontal sinus p.
Linde cryogenic p.
lithotripter p.
lithotripter p.
lithotriptor p.
Lockhart-Mummery p.
Lucae p.
Lucae ear p.
magnetic eye p.
malleable p.
Manhattan Eye and Ear p.
Mannis suture p.
Martin p.
Martin uterine fistula p.
mastoid p.
Max-I-Probe irrigation p.
Mayo p.
Mayo common duct p.
Mayo kidney stone p.
Mayo uterine p.

McKesson mouth p.
Medi-Tech bipolar p.
Meerschaum p.
meniscectomy p.
microballoon p.
microlaryngeal laser p.
Mixter p.
Mixter common duct p.
Mixter Dilaprobe p.
Mixter dilating p.
Mixter gall duct p.
Mixter irrigating p.
Moynihan p.
Moynihan bile duct p.
Moynihan gallstone p.
Muldoon lacrimal p.
multilumen p.
Myrtle leaf p.
nasal p.
nasolacrimal duct p.
needle p.
Nélaton bullet p.
nuclear p.
Ochsner p.
Ochsner-Fenger gallstone p.
Ochsner flexible spiral
  gallstone p.
Ochsner gall duct p.
Ochsner gallstone p.
Ochsner spiral p.
ocutome p.
Ohmeda p.
Olympus heat p.
Ossoff-Karlan microlaryngeal
  laser p.
palpation p.
Paparella p.
Parsonnet p.
Parsonnet coronary p.
Payr p.
Payr-Schmieden p.
pencil Doppler p.
periodontal p.
Perio Temp dental p.
pH p.
piggyback p.
pigtail p.
pocket p.
p. point scissors
PPG p.
Pratt p.
Pratt rectal p.
Quickert p.

Quickert-Dryden p.
Quickert-Dryden lacrimal p.
Quickert lacrimal p.
Quickert lacrimal
 intubation p.
Radiometer p.
rectal p.
reverse-cutting p.
reverse-cutting meniscal p.
Rica ear p.
Richards p.
Rockey p.
Rockey dilating p.
Rohrschneider p.
Rolf lacrimal p.
Rosen p.
Rosen ear p.
Rosen endaural p.
Rubinstein p.
salpingeal p.
Sandhill p.
Sarns temperature p.
Schmieden p.
scissors p.
Sheer p.
Shirodkar p.
Siemens linear p.
Siemens vaginal p.
silver p.
Simpson lacrimal p.
Simpson sterling lacrimal p.
Sims p.
Sims uterine p.
simultaneous thermal
 diffusion blood flow and
 pressure p.
sinus p.
Skillern p.
Skillern sphenoidal p.
SMIC abscess p.
SMIC periodontal p.
spear-ended chrome p.
spear-pointed nickelene p.
Spencer p.
Spencer labyrinth
 exploration p.
sphenoidal p.
Spiesman fistular p.
spiral p.
Stacke p.
Storz-Bowman lacrimal p.
Storz pigtail p.
suction p.

tactile p.
Teflon p.
telephone p.
temperature p.
Theobald p.
Theobald sinus p.
thermistor p.
tin-bullet p.
trabeculotomy p.
transesophageal p.
Tufcote epilation p.
tulip p.
tumor p.
Urrets-Zavalia p.
uterine p.
uterine vertebrated p.
vacuum intrauterine p.
Valliex uterine p.
Versadopp Doppler p.
vertebrated p.
Vibrodilator p.
Wasko p.
Wasko common duct p.
water p.
Weaver sinus p.
Welch Allyn p.
Welch Allyn rectal p.
whalebone eustachian p.
whirlybird p.
Williams p.
Williams lacrimal p.
wire p.
p. with eye
Worst p.
Worst double-ended
 pigtail p.
Worst pigtail p.
Xomed rectal p.
Yankauer p.
Yankauer salpingeal p.
Yellow Springs p.
Yeoman p.
Ziegler p.
Ziegler lacrimal p.
Ziegler needle p.
probe-ended grooved director
probing catheter
Procath electrophysiology catheter
procedure drape
process
 Ti-Nidium surface
 hardening p.
Prochownik pessary

Pro-Comelastic abdominal belt
proctological
- p. ball electrode
- p. cotton carrier
- p. forceps
- p. grasping forceps
- p. polyp forceps

Proctor
- P. cheek retractor
- P. laryngopharyngoscope
- P. laryngostat
- P. mucosal elevator
- P. phrenectomy forceps
- P. phrenicectomy forceps
- P. retractor
- P. suction tube

Proctor-Bruce mastoid searcher
Proctor-Hellens laryngostat
Proctor-Livingston endoprosthesis
proctoscope
- ACMI p.
- Boehm p.
- Fansler p.
- Gabriel p.
- Goldbacher p.
- Hirschman p.
- Hirschman-Martin p.
- Kelly p.
- Lieberman p.
- Montague p.
- Morgan p.
- Morgan-Boehm p.
- National p.
- Newman p.
- Pruitt p.
- Tuttle p.
- Vernon-David p.
- Welch Allyn p.
- Yeoman p.

proctoscopic
- p. electrode
- p. fulguration electrode

proctosigmoid disposable suction tube
proctosigmoidoscope
- ACMI fiberoptic p.
- fiberoptic p.

Proetz
- P. mouth gag
- P. syringe
- P. tongue depressor

Proetz-Jansen mouth gag
Profex finger cot

Profident
Profile
- P. Plus balloon dilatation catheter
- P. Plus catheter
- P. Plus dilatation catheter

profilometer
- Cottle p.
- laryngoscope p.
- Straith p.

Proflex dilatation catheter
Pro-Flo catheter
Progestasert intrauterine device
Programalith
- P. AV pacemaker
- P. II pacemaker
- P. III pacemaker
- P. pacemaker

programmable pacemaker
Programmer III pacemaker
progressive dilators
projector
- fiberoptic light p.

prolapser
- Stone lens nucleus p.

prolapse ring pessary
prolapsus pessary
Prolene
- P. polypropylene suture
- P. suture

Prolith pacemaker
prone cranial support device (PCSD)
3-prong
- 3-p. fork
- 3-p. retractor

pronged retractor
Pro-Ophta
- P.-O. absorbent stick sponge
- P.-O. eye patch
- P.-O. type-K shield
- P.-O. type-S shield

prop
- Hewitt mouth p.

Propel
- Hi-Torque floppy with P.

Proplast
- P. facial implant
- P. graft
- P. II porous implant material
- P. implant

P. I porous implant
material
P. preformed implant
P. prosthesis
P. TORP
Propper
P. binocular indirect
ophthalmoscope
P. retinoscope
Pro Pulse irrigator
propylene dressing
Proscope anoscope
Prospec disposable speculum
prostatectomy
p. bag
p. forceps
prostate retractor
prostatic
p. aluminum electrode
p. biopsy cup
p. biopsy needle
p. catheter
p. dissector
p. driver
p. forceps
p. lobe forceps
p. lobe-holding forceps
p. needle holder
p. retractor
p. tractor
prosthesis
acrylic bar p.
Allen-Brown p.
American Heyer-Schulte p.
American Heyer-Schulte
chin p.
American Heyer-Schulte-
Hinderer malar p.
American Heyer-Schulte
mammary p.
American Heyer-Schulte
Radovan tissue
expander p.
American Heyer-Schulte
rhinoplasty p.
American Heyer-Schulte
testicular p.
AML total hip p.
AMS 700CX Inflatable
penile p.
AMS 700CXM inflatable
penile p.

AMS Malleable 600M
penile p.
AMS Malleable 800
urinary p.
AMS penile p.
AMS Sphincter 800
urinary p.
Anderson columellar p.
Angelchik antireflux p.
ankle p.
Arion rod eye p.
arterial graft p.
Ashley breast p.
Attenborough knee p.
Attenborough total knee p.
Aufranc-Turner hip p.
Austin Moore p.
Austin Moore hip p.
Bateman finger p.
Bechtol system p.
bifurcated seamless p.
Bi-Metric Interlok
femoral p.
Bi-Metric porous primary
femoral p.
Bioclad with pegs reinforced
acetabular p.
Bioglass p.
Bio-Groove femoral p.
Bionic ear p.
Björk p.
Blauth knee p.
Bock knee p.
Bograb Universal offset
ossicular p.
bone p.
Buckholz p.
Byars mandibular p.
Caffinière p.
Calnan-Nicole finger p.
camouflage p.
Canadian hip p.
Carbomedics cardiac
valve p.
Cardona keratoprosthesis p.
Carrion penile p.
Cartwright heart p.
Cathcart orthocentric hip p.
CDH Precoat Plus hip p.
Celestin endoesophageal p.
ceramic ossicular p.
Ceravital incus
replacement p.

prosthesis *(continued)*

Charnley acetabular cup p.
Charnley-Mueller hip p.
Charnley total hip p.
Choyce MK II
  keratoprosthesis p.
Cintor knee p.
combination gel and
  inflatable mammary p.
Conley mandibular p.
constrained hinge knee p.
constrained nonhinged
  knee p.
crimped Dacron p.
Cronin Silastic mammary p.
cruciate-retaining p.
cruciate-sacrificing p.
CUI artificial breast p.
CUI chin p.
CUI eye sphere p.
CUI gel mammary p.
CUI nasal p.
CUI saline mammary p.
CUI tendon p.
CUI testicular p.
Cutter-Smeloff cardiac
  valve p.
cylinder penile p.
cylinder penile
  distendible p.
cylinder penile
  nondistendible p.
Dacron arterial p.
Dacron bifurcation p.
Dacron vessel p.
Dallop-type fascial p.
Deane p.
DeBakey p.
Dee elbow p.
De La Caffiniere Trapezio
  metacarpal p.
DeLaura knee p.
DeLaura-Verner knee p.
Deon hip p.
DePalma hip p.
DePuy hip p. with Scuderi
  head
Deune knee p.
Dilamezinsert penile p.
dual-lock total hip p.
Duocondylar knee p.
Duo-Lock hip p.
Duo-Patellar knee p.

DuraPhase semirigid
  penile p.
Dynaflex penile p.
dynamic penile p.
ear p.
ear pinna p.
ear piston p.
Eaton trapezium finger joint
  replacement p.
Edwards seamless p.
Efteklar-Charnley hip p.
Ehmke ear p.
Eicher hip p.
ELP femoral p.
Endo rotating knee joint p.
endoskeletal p.
Engh porous metal hip p.
Englehardt femoral p.
English-McNab shoulder p.
EPTFE graft p.
Erectaid penile p.
Eric-aid p.
ESKA Jonas silicone-silver
  penile p.
esophageal p.
Esser p.
Estecar p.
Ethicon Polytef paste p.
Ethrone p.
Ewald elbow p.
external breast p.
fascia lata p.
femorofemoral crossover p.
Fett carpal p.
finger p.
Finney p.
Finney-Flexirod p.
Flatt finger p.
Flexi-Flate penile p.
Flexi-rod penile p.
Fountain design p.
Fox p.
Fox-Blazina p.
Fredricks mammary p.
Freeman-Samuelson knee p.
Freeman-Swanson knee p.
Galante hip p.
gel-filled p.
gel-saline Surgitek
  mammary p.
Geomedic knee p.
Geometric total knee p.
Georgiade breast p.

Gilbert p.
Gilfillan humeral p.
Giliberty acetabular p.
Gillies p.
Girard keratoprosthesis p.
Golaski-UMI vascular p.
golf tee-shaped polyvinyl p.
Goodhill p.
Gore-Tex p.
Gott-Daggett heart valve p.
Gott low-profile p.
Gruppe wire p.
GSB elbow p.
GSB knee p.
Guepar knee p.
Guilford-Wright p.
Gunston-Hult knee p.
Gunston polycentric knee p.
Haering esophageal p.
Hall-Kaster tilting-disk
  valve p.
Hamas upper limb p.
Hammersmith mitral
  valve p.
Hancock aortic valve p.
Hanger p.
Hanslik patellar p.
Harken p.
Harris p.
Harris-Galante p.
Harris-Galante porous
  hip p.
Harrison interlocked
  mesh p.
Harris precoat p.
Hartley mammary p.
Helanca seamless tube p.
Henschke-Mauch SNS lower
  limb p.
Herbert knee p.
heterograft p.
Hexcel total condylar p.
Heyer-Schulte breast p.
HG Multilock hip p.
Hinderer malar p.
hinged constrained knee p.
hinged great toe
  replacement p.
hinged-leaflet vascular p.
hinged total knee p.
hinge-knee p.
hingeless heart valve p.
HJB p.

hollow sphere p.
homograft p.
homograft incus p. (HIP)
House piston p.
House tantalum p.
House wire p.
House wire-fat p.
House wire stapes p.
Howmedica p.
Howorth p.
Howse-Coventry p.
HPS II total hip p.
HSS total condylar knee p.
Hufnagel low-profile
  heart p.
Hunter tendon p.
hydraulic knee unit p.
Hydroflex penile p.
hydroxyapatite ossicular p.
I-beam hemiarthroplasty
  hip p.
Image custom external
  breast p.
immediate postoperative p.
  (IPOP)
incus replacement p.
Indong Oh p.
inflatable mammary p.
inflatable Mentor penile p.
inflatable penile p.
Inronail finger or toenail p.
Insall-Burstein knee p.
Integral Interlok femoral p.
internal ear p.
Ionescu-Shiley aortic
  valve p.
Iowa total hip p.
iridium p.
isoelastic pelvic p.
Ivalon p.
Jenny mammary p.
Jewett p.
Jobst p.
Jonas p.
Jonathan Livingston Seagull
  patella p.
Joplin toe p.
Judet p.
Kaufman III anti-
  incontinence p.
Kaufman male urinary
  incontinence p.
Kay-Shiley disk valve p.

prosthesis *(continued)*
Kay-Suzuki p.
Keeler p.
Kessler p.
Kinematic II total knee p.
Kirschner total shoulder p.
knitted p.
knitted Teflon p.
knitted vascular p.
Krause-Wolfe p.
Lacey p.
Lagrange-Letoumel hip p.
Laing hip cup p.
Lanceford p.
Landers-Foulks p.
Lash-Loeffler penile p.
Lattimer Silastic
  testicular p.
Leadbetter-Politano ureteral
  implant p.
Leake Dacron mandible p.
Leinbach p.
Leinbach hip p.
Lillehei-Kaster cardiac
  valve p.
Lillehei valve p.
Lippman hip p.
Lo-Por p.
Lorenzo SMO p.
low-profile p.
MacIntosh tibial plateau p.
Mackler intraluminal
  tube p.
MacNab-English shoulder p.
Macrofit hip p.
Magnuson-Cromie p.
Magnuson valve p.
Magovern-Cromie p.
malleus-incus p.
Mallory-Head hip p.
Mallory-Head porous
  primary femoral p.
mammary p.
Mammatech breast p.
Marlex mesh p.
Marlex methyl
  methacrylate p.
Marmor modular knee p.
Matchett-Brown p.
Mayo elbow p.
Mayo total ankle p.
McBride p.
McBride-Moore p.

McGee ear piston p.
McGhan breast p.
McKee p.
McKee-Farrar hip p.
McKee femoral p.
McKeever patellar cap p.
McNaught p.
Medi-graft vascular p.
Medoc-Celestin
  endoprosthesis p.
Meme breast p.
Mentor breast p.
Mentor inflatable penile p.
Mentor penile p.
Mentor Self-Cath penile p.
Meyerding p.
MGH knee p.
Michael Reese p.
microcrimped p.
Microknit arterial p.
Microvel p.
Miller-Galante hip p.
Milliknit arterial p.
Minneapolis hip p.
Mittlemeir ceramic hip p.
modified Moore hip
  locking p.
modular p.
modular Austin-Moore
  hip p.
modular Iowa Precoat total
  hip p.
Monk p.
Moon-Robinson stapes p.
Moore hip p.
Moretz p.
Moseley glenoid rim p.
Mueller-Charnley hip p.
Mueller total hip p.
Muhlberger orbital p.
Mules p.
Mulligan Silastic p.
Murray knee p.
Naden-Rieth p.
Natural-Lok acetabular
  cup p.
NEB total hip p.
Neer I p.
Neer II p.
Neer shoulder p.
Neibauer-Cutter p.
Neville tracheal p.
Neville tracheobronchial p.

New Jersey
hemiarthroplasty p.
New Jersey-L.C.S.
shoulder p.
New Jersey-L.C.S. total
knee p.
Nicoll tendon p.
Niebauer p.
Niebauer finger-joint
replacement p.
Niebauer trapezium
replacement p.
Noiles p.
ocular p.
Odland ankle p.
OmniPhase penile p.
Omniscience cardiac
valve p.
orbital floor p.
Oregon p.
Orlon vascular p.
Ortholoc p.
ossicular chain
replacement p.
Osteonics p.
Oxford p.
Padgett p.
Paladon p.
Panje p.
Panje voice p.
partial ossicular
reconstruc-
tion/replacement p.
(PORP)
PCA knee p.
Pearman penile p.
percutaneous transhepatic p.
Perras mammary p.
Perras-Papillon breast p.
Phoenix total hip p.
Pillet hand p.
piston p.
Plasticor p.
Plasti-Pore ossicular
replacement p.
Plystan p.
Polycel bone composite p.
polycentric knee p.
polyethylene talar p.
porcine p.
Porocool p.
press-fit p.
Pritchard total elbow p.

Proplast p.
Protasul femoral p.
Protek p.
Proud septal p.
proximal third femoral p.
PTS p.
Radovan tissue expander p.
Rastelli p.
Reverdin p.
Revive system penile p.
Richards p.
Ring hip p.
Ring knee p.
RMC p.
Robert Bent Brigham
knee p.
Robert Brigham p.
Robinson incus
replacement p.
Robinson middle ear p.
Robinson-Moon-Lippy
stapes p.
Robinson-Moon stapes p.
Robinson piston p.
Robinson stapes p.
Rock-Mulligan p.
Rose L-type nose bridge p.
Rosenfeld hip p.
Rosen inflatable urinary
incontinence p.
Rosen urinary
incontinence p.
rotating-hinge knee p.
Ruddy stapes p.
SACH p.
Safian design p.
Safian rhinoplasty p.
Saint George knee p.
Saint Jude p.
Sampson p.
Sauerbruch p.
Sauvage fabric graft p.
Sbarbaro tibial p.
Scarborough p.
SCDT heart valve p.
Scheer Tef-wire p.
Schlein total elbow p.
Schlein trisurface ankle p.
Schuknecht Gelfoam wire p.
Schuknecht Teflon wire
piston p.
Schuknecht Tef-Wire p.
Schurring ossicle cup p.

prosthesis *(continued)*
  Scott penile p.
  Scuderi p.
  Scurasil device p.
  seamless p.
  self-centering Universal
    hip p.
  Shea p.
  Shea polyethylene p.
  Shea Teflon piston p.
  Sheehan knee p.
  Sheehy-House incus p.
  Sheehy-House incus
    replacement p.
  Sheehy incus p.
  Sheehy incus replacement p.
  Shier knee p.
  shoulder p.
  Silastic chin p.
  Silastic fimbrial p.
  Silastic mammary p.
  Silastic otoplasty p.
  Silastic penile p.
  Silastic sheeting keel p.
  Silastic testicular p.
  silicone doughnut p.
  silicone elastomer p.
  Silima breast p.
  Siloxane p.
  Singer-Bloom ossicular p.
  Singh speech system voice
    rehabilitation p.
  Sivash hip p.
  Small-Carrion penile p.
  Smeloff-Cutter ball-valve p.
  Smith p.
  Smith-Petersen hip cup p.
  SMo p.
  p. smooth wire
  Snyder breast p.
  solid ankle cushion heel p.
  solid silicone orbital p.
  Sparks Mandril p.
  Spectron p.
  Speed radius cap p.
  spherocentric knee p.
  S-ROM p.
  stabilocondylar knee p.
  Stanmore shoulder p.
  stapedectomy p.
  Starr p.
  Starr-Edwards p.
  Starr-Edwards heart valve p.

  STD+ Titanium total
    hip p.
  Stenzel rod p.
  Stevens-Street elbow p.
  St. George p.
  St. Jude heart valve p.
  St. Jude Medical p.
  Supramid p.
  Surgitek p.
  Sutter MCP finger joint p.
  Sutter-Smeloff heart
    valve p.
  Swanson finger joint p.
  Swanson flexible hallux
    valgus p.
  Swanson Silastic elbow p.
  Syme p.
  Synatomic total knee p.
  Taperloc femoral p.
  TARA total hip p.
  Teflon tri-leaflet p.
  Tef-wire p.
  tendon p.
  Tevdek p.
  Tharies p.
  Thiersch p.
  T-28 hip p.
  Thompson hemiarthroplasty
    hip p.
  Thompson hip p.
  Thrust femoral p.
  tibial plateau p.
  Ti/CoCr hip p.
  titanium p.
  Tivanium hip p.
  toe p.
  TORP ossicular p.
  torque-type p.
  total ossicular
    replacement p. (TORP)
  Townley total knee p.
  trapeziometacarpal joint
    replacement p.
  Triad p.
  trial p.
  trileaflet p.
  Trilicon external breast p.
  Tri-lock total hip p. with
    Porocoat
  trummion bearing hip p.
  Turner p.
  two-pronged stem finger p.
  Tygon esophageal p.

UCI p.
Ultrex penile p.
Ultrex Plus penile p.
umbrella-type p.
unconstrained p.
unicondylar p.
Universal p.
UPF p.
urinary incontinence p.
UroLume Endourethral
  Wallstent p.
USCI bifurcated Vasculour
  II p.
USCI-DeBakey vascular p.
Usher Marlex mesh p.
Valls p.
Vanghetti limb p.
vascular graft p.
Vascutek vascular p.
Vitallium Moore self-
  locking p.
Vivosil p.
Voltz wrist joint p.
Wada hingeless heart
  valve p.
Wagner resurface p.
Walldius Vitallium
  mechanical knee p.
Waugh p.
Weavenit p.
Weavenit vascular p.
Weck-cel p.
Wehrs incus p.
Weller total hip joint p.
Wesolowski p.
Whiteside p.
Wiles p.
Wilke boot p.
Wilson-Cook esophageal p.
Wilson-Cook esophageal
  balloon p.
wire p.
wire-fat ear p.
wire stapes p.
Wolfe p.
woven-tube vascular graft p.
Wright p.
Wright knee p.
Xenophor femoral p.
Zimaloy femoral head p.
Zimmer shoulder p.

Zimmer tibial p.
Zweymuller hip p.
prosthetic
  p. appliance
  p. device
  p. graft
  p. valve holder
Prosthodont
Protasul femoral prosthesis
protected
  p. bronchoscopic brush
  p. knife handle
protective
  p. bandage
  p. dressing
protector
  Adson dural p.
  alar p.
  Arruga p.
  bite p.
  Cottle alar p.
  Crouch corneal p.
  dural p.
  eye p.
  p. guide
  Joseph saw p.
  Opti-Gard eye p.
  Seraflo transducer p.
  Terumo transducer p.
  tissue p.
Protecto splint
Protek prosthesis
protological biopsy forceps
ProTrac
  P. ACL tibial guide
  P. alignment guide
  P. cruciate reconstruction
    measurement device
  P. endoscopic ACL drill
    guide
protractor
  Harrington p.
  Zimmer p.
protrusio shell
Proud
  P. adenoidectomy forceps
  P. fascia crusher
  P. infant turbinate
    speculum
  P. septal prosthesis
Proud-Beck pharyngoscope
Proud-White uvula retractor

Providence
 P. arterial forceps
 P. Hospital arterial forceps
 P. Hospital clamp
 P. Hospital classic forceps
 P. Hospital forceps
 P. Hospital hemostat
 P. Hospital hemostatic
  forceps
provisional
 Bio-Plug p.
 p. liner
 Morse taper cone p.
Provit filling material
proximal
 p. drill guide assembly
 p. electrode
 p. third femoral prosthesis
Proximate
 P. disposable skin stapler
 P. ILS curved intraluminal
  stapler
 P. stapler
Proximate-ILS circular stapler
Proxi-Strip suture
Pruitt
 P. anoscope
 P. irrigation catheter
 P. occlusion catheter
 P. proctoscope
 P. vascular shunt
Pryor-Péan vaginal retractor
psoas retractor
Psoralite
**PSS Powered disposable skin
 stapler**
PTB brace
PTBD
 percutaneous transhepatic biliary
  drainge
  PTBD catheter
PTCA
 percutaneous transluminal
  coronary angioplasty
  PTCA catheter
pterygium knife
PTFE
 polytetrafluoroethylene
  PTFE Gore-Tex graft
ptosis
 p. clamp
 p. forceps
 p. snare

PTS prosthesis
Puddu
 P. drill guide
 P. tibial aimer
pudendal
 p. block anesthesia needle
 p. block needle and guide
 p. needle
 p. needle guide
Pudenz
 P. barium cardiac catheter
 P. cardiac catheter
 P. connectors
 P. flushing valve
 P. infant cardiac catheter
 P. peritoneal catheter
 P. valve-flushing shunt
 P. ventricular catheter
Pudenz-Heyer
 P.-H. clamp
 P.-H. vascular catheter
Puestow dilator
**Puestow-Olander gastrointestinal
 tube**
Pugh
 P. barrel component
 P. driver
 P. hip pin
 P. self-adjusting nail
 P. tractor
puka chisel
Pulec needle
pull
 p. knife knife
 p. screw
pulley
 p. passer
 p. suture
pull-out
 p.-o. suture
 p.-o. wire suture
pulmonary
 p. arterial catheter
 p. arterial clamp
 p. arterial forceps
 p. arterial snare
 p. artery balloon pump
  (PABP)
 p. balloon
 p. bed
 p. embolism clamp
 p. flotation catheter
 p. retractor

p. triple-lumen catheter
p. vessel clamp
p. vessel forceps
pulmonic
p. clamp
p. stenosis clamp
pulp canal file
Pulpdent cavity liner
pulped muscle dressing
Pulsar
P. NI implantable
pacemaker
P. NI pacemaker
P. obstetrical two-channel
TENS unit
P. TENS unit
pulsatile assist device
pulse
p. lavage
p. oximeter
pulsed angiolaser
Pulvertaft suture
pumice
pump
Asahi blood plasma p.
balloon p.
Basis breast p.
Chicco breast p.
Chid baby breast p.
DeVilbiss suction p.
Dura Neb portable
nebulizer p.
Egnell breast p.
Emerson p.
extracorporeal p.
flexible p.
Grafco breast p.
IABP intra-aortic balloon p.
Infusaid p.
intra-aortic balloon p.
(IABP)
KM-1 breast p.
Kontron intra-aortic
balloon p.
Lactina breast p.
Mary Jane breast p.
Medela breast p.
Mistette nasal spray p.
Nezhat-Dorset
hydrodissection p.
Pfeiffer mechanical
dosing p.

pulmonary artery balloon p.
(PABP)
roller head perfusion p.
surgical suction p.
SynchroMed p.
Talley p.
Unicare breast p.
Pumpette
Master Flow P.
Stat 2 P.
Pump Vac Plus system
punch
Abrams biopsy p.
Abrams pleural biopsy p.
adenoid p.
Adler attic ear p.
Ainsworth p.
Alexander antrostomy p.
antral p.
aortic p.
Bailey p.
Baumgartner p.
Berens corneoscleral p.
Beyer atticus p.
biopsy p.
Brock infundibular p.
Brooks p.
Brooks adenoidal p.
Bruening p.
Bruening cup biting p.
Buerger p.
Casteyer prostatic p.
Castroviejo corneoscleral p.
Cault p.
cervical p.
cigar handle basket p.
Citelli p.
Citelli laminectomy p.
Citelli-Meltzer atticus p.
Cloward bone p.
Cloward-Dowel p.
Cloward-English p.
Cloward-Harper cervical p.
Cloward intervertebral p.
Cloward square p.
Cone bone p.
Cone skull p.
Cordes circular p.
Cordes ethmoidal p.
Cordes semicircular p.
Cordes sphenoidal p.
Cordes square p.
Corgill bone p.

punch *(continued)*
    corneal p.
    corneoscleral p.
    Cottingham p.
    cutaneous p.
    Davol canal wall p.
    Descemet p.
    Deyerle p.
    Dorsey cervical
      foramental p.
    DyoVac suction p.
    Ellison glenoid rim p.
    Eppendorfer p.
    ethmoidal p.
    Ewald-Hensler
      arthroscopic p.
    Faraci p.
    Faraci-Skillern sphenoid p.
    Ferris Smith p.
    Ferris Smith-Kerrison p.
    finned-stem p.
    Flateau oval p.
    fluted stem p.
    p. forceps
    p. forceps tip
    Frangenheim hook p.
    Frenckner-Stille p.
    Gass cervical p.
    Gass corneoscleral p.
    Gass sclerotomy p.
    Gelfoam p.
    Gellhorn uterine biopsy p.
    Gibbs eye p.
    Goldman cartilage p.
    Gosteyer p.
    Graham-Kerrison p.
    Gruenwald p.
    Gruenwald nasal p.
    Grundelach p.
    p. guide
    Gundelach p.
    Gusberg endocervical
      biopsy p.
    Haitz canaliculus p.
    Hajek-Koffler reversible p.
    Hajek-Koffler sphenoidal p.
    Hajek-Skillern p.
    Hajek-Skillern sphenoidal p.
    Hardy sellar p.
    Harper cervical
      laminectomy p.
    Hartmann biopsy p.
    Hartmann-Citelli ear p.

    Hartmann ear p.
    Hartmann nasal p.
    Hartmann tonsillar p.
    Holth p.
    Holth corneoscleral p.
    Holth-Rubin p.
    Housepian sellar p.
    I-beam cement p.
    I-beam press-fit p.
    infundibular p.
    Ingraham skull p.
    Jackson p.
    Jacobson vessel p.
    Jansen-Middleton septal p.
    Johnson-Kerrison p.
    Joseph p.
    Karolinska-Stille p.
    Karp aortic p.
    Kelly p.
    Kelly-Descemet
      membrane p.
    Kerrison p.
    Kerrison-Jacoby p.
    Kerrison laminectomy p.
    Kerrison-Rhoton sellar p.
    Keyes p.
    Keyes biopsy p.
    Keyes cutaneous p.
    Keyes cutaneous biopsy p.
    Keyes dermal p.
    Keyes skin p.
    King adenoidal p.
    Klause antral p.
    Klause-Carmody antral p.
    Knighton-Kerrison p.
    Koffler-Hajek sphenoidal p.
    Krause angular oval p.
    Lange antral p.
    Lebsche sternal p.
    Lempert malleus p.
    Lermoyez nasal p.
    linear scissor p.
    Lineback adenoidal p.
    MacKenty sphenoidal p.
    Mauermayer stone p.
    McGoey Vitallium p.
    Meltzer adenoid p.
    Meltzer tonsillar p.
    Mendez-Schubert aortic p.
    Merz aortic p.
    MGM glenoidal p.
    Mixter brain biopsy p.
    modified sclerectomy p.

Mulligan cervical biopsy p.
Murphy p.
Myerson biting p.
Myles p.
Myles forceps p.
Myles nasal p.
p. myringotomy system
nasal p.
Noyes chalazion p.
O'Connor hook p.
Orentreich p.
Ostrum p.
Ostrum antral p.
Pfau atticus sphenoidal p.
Phemister p.
pleural biopsy p.
Pritikin scleral p.
Raney laminectomy p.
Reaves p.
Rhoton p.
Rhoton sellar p.
Richter laminectomy p.
RME testicular p.
Ronis adenoidal p.
Ronis tonsillar p.
Rowe glenoidal p.
Rubin-Holth modified
  sclerectomy p.
Rubin-Holth sclerectomy p.
Sachs cervical p.
Scheicher laminectomy p.
Scheinmann biting p.
Schlesinger cervical p.
Schmeden tonsillar p.
Schmithhuisen ethmoidal p.
Schmithhuisen sphenoidal p.
Schnaudigel sclerotomy p.
Schubert biopsy p.
Schubert uterine p.
Seiffert grasping p.
Seletz Universal Kerrison p.
sellar p.
skin p.
skull p.
Smeden tonsillar p.
Smillie nail p.
Smithuysen sphenoidal p.
Sokolwski antral p.
Sparks atrioseptal p.
Spencer oval p.
Spencer triangular
  adenoid p.
sphenoidal p.

sphenoidal bone p.
Spies ethmoidal p.
Spurling-Kerrison p.
Spurling-Kerrison
  laminectomy p.
Stammberger antral p.
Stevenson capsular p.
Storz antral p.
Storz intranasal antral p.
Struyken p.
suction p.
Swan corneoscleral p.
Sweet modified sternal p.
Sweet sternal p.
Takahashi p.
Takahashi ethmoidal p.
Takahashi nasal p.
Thompson p.
Thoms-Gaylor biopsy p.
Thoms-Gaylor uterine
  biopsy p.
Thomson adenoidal p.
Tischler cervical biopsy p.
Tomey trabeculectomy p.
tonsillar p.
Townsend biopsy p.
Troutman p.
Turkel prostatic p.
uterine p.
uterine biopsy p.
Van Struyken nasal p.
Veenema-Gusberg
  prostatic p.
vessel p.
Wagner p.
Wagner antral p.
Walton corneoscleral p.
Walton-Schubert p.
Watson-Williams
  ethmoidal p.
Whitcomb-Kerrison
  laminectomy p.
Wilde ethmoidal p.
Wilde nasal p.
Williams-Watson
  ethmoidal p.
Wittner cervical biopsy p.
Yankauer p.
Yankauer antral p.
Yeoman biopsy p.
punctate electrode
punctum dilator

puncture
  p. needle
  Nelson abdominal p.
Puntenney
  P. forceps
  P. tying forceps
Puntowicz arterial forceps
pupillary membrane scissors
pupillometer
Purcell
  P. retractor
  P. self-retaining abdominal
    retractor
Puritan-Bennett ventilator
Purlon suture
pursestring suture
pusher
  Aker lens p.
  p. catheter
  Charnley femoral
    prosthesis p.
  chorda tympani p.
  De La Vega lens p.
  Fresnel lens p.
  hook p.
  Jacobson suture p.
  Jako knot p.
  lens p.
  Mershon band p.
  Negus p.
  Shuletz p.
pusher-burnisher
  Klauber p.-b.
  Ormco band p.-b.
push retractor
Putnam evacuator catheter

Putti
  P. arthroplasty gouge
  P. bone file
  P. bone rasp
  P. frame
  P. rasp
  P. splint
putty
  Omnisil p.
PVB suture
PVC tubing
Pye cannula
pyloric stenosis dilator
pylorodilator
pylorus clamp
Pynchol headband
Pynchon
  P. applicator
  P. cannula
  P. ear snare
  P. mouth gag
  P. nasal speculum
  P. suction tube
  P. tongue depressor
Pynchon-Lillie tongue depressor
pyoktanin
  p. catgut suture
  p. suture
pyramidal
  p. electrode
  p. eye implant
  p. tip
pyrolyte
  p. ball heart valve
  p. cage heart valve
Pyrost bone replacement material

QSA dressing forceps
Quad-Lumen drain
quadpolar W/Damato curve
    catheter
Quadra-Flo infusion catheter
quadraplegic standing frame
quadripolar catheter
Quadro dressing
Qualtex surgical drape
Quantico needle
Quanticor catheter
Quantum
    Q. hearing aid
    Q. pacemaker
quarantine drain
quartz
    q. needle
    q. rod
Queen Anne dressing
Quervain
    Q. abdominal retractor
    Q. cranial forceps
    Q. cranial rongeur forceps
    Q. elevator
    Q. forceps
    Q. rib spreader
Quervain-Sauerbruch retractor
Quevedo
    Q. conjunctival forceps
    Q. forceps
Quickert
    Q. grooved director
    Q. lacrimal intubation
      probe
    Q. lacrimal probe
    Q. probe
    Q. suture

Quickert-Dryden
    Q.-D. lacrimal probe
    Q.-D. probe
Quicket tourniquet
QuickFurl
    Q. double-lumen balloon
    Q. single-lumen balloon
Quick-Lite lamp
Quik splint splint
Quik-Temp thermometer
quilted suture
quilt suture
Quimby
    Q. gum scissors
    Q. scissors
Quincke-Babcock needle
Quinn holder
Quinton
    Q. biopsy catheter
    Q. catheter
    Q. Mahurkar double-lumen
      catheter
    Q. Mahurkar dual-lumen
      peritoneal catheter
    Q. Q-Port catheter
Quire
    Q. automatic finger
    Q. finger forceps
    Q. forceps
    Q. foreign body forceps
    Q. mechanical finger
      forceps
Quires mechanical finger snare
Quisling intranasal hammer
Quisling-Parkes osteotome
Qwik-Clean dressing

Raaf
R. catheter
R. Cath vascular catheter
R. double-lumen catheter
R. dual-lumen catheter
R. flexible lighted spatula
R. forceps
Raaf-Oldberg
R.-O. intervertebral disk
forceps
R.-O. rongeur
Rabiner
R. hammer
R. neurological hammer
Racestyptine
R. cord
R. retraction ring
rack
Bruns sterlizing r.
Cobb sterilizing r.
Fischer sterilizing storage r.
Hibbs-Bruns sterilizing r.
Hoke sterilizing r.
Kidd instrument r.
McKenzie clip r.
McKenzie clip-holding r.
McPherson r.
Saunders instrument r.
Smith-Petersen sterilizing r.
Radcliff
R. perineal retractor
R. retractor
radial
r. arterial catheter
r. bearing
r. keratotomy knife
r. keratotomy marker
r. suture
radial keratotomy (RK)
radiocarpal implant
radiocontrast dye
Radiofocus
R. catheter guide wire
R. Glidewire angiography
catheter
radiofrequency pacemaker
radiographer
Wehmer TMJ r.
radiolucent splint
Radiometer probe

Radionics
R. lesion generator
R. radiofrequency lesion
generator
R. stimulus generator
radiopaque catheter
radium
r. implant
r. needle
radius trial
radix Raney jacket
Radovan
R. breast implant
R. tissue expander
R. tissue expander
prosthesis
R. tissue expander tip
Radpour
R. irrigator
R. needle
Radpour-House
R.-H. irrigator
R.-H. suction irrigator
R.-H. suction tube
RAE endotracheal tube
Ragnell
R. double-ended retractor
R. drain
R. retractor
R. scissors
R. undermining scissors
Ragnell-Davis double-ended
retractor
railway catheter
Raimondi
R. catheter
R. forceps
R. hemostat
R. peritoneal catheter
R. scalp forceps
R. scalp hemostatic forceps
R. shunt
R. ventricular catheter
Rainbow
R. envelope arm snare
R. fracture frame
Raindrop medication nebulizer
Rainen
R. clip-bending spatula
R. iris hook

Rainen *(continued)*
 R. lens hook
 R. spatula
rake retractor
Ralks
 R. bone drill
 R. clamp
 R. drill
 R. ear forceps
 R. ear retractor
 R. eye magnet
 R. fingernail drill
 R. forceps
 R. magnet
 R. mallet
 R. nasal gauze packer
 R. retractor
 R. reversible knife
 R. sinus applicator
 R. splinter forceps
 R. thoracic clamp
 R. tuning fork
 R. wire-cutting forceps
Ralks-Davis mouth gag
Ramdohr suture
Ramel set
Ramirez winged catheter
Ramitec bite material
Rampley
 R. forceps
 R. sponge forceps
Ramsbotham decapitating hook
Ramses
 R. diaphragm
 R. diaphragm introducer
Ramsey County pyoktanin catgut suture
Ramstedt
 R. clamp
 R. dilator
 R. pyloric stenosis dilator
Rand
 R. bayonet ring curette
 R. forceps
 R. microballoon
Randall
 R. biopsy curette
 R. biopsy uterine curette
 R. curette
 R. endometrial biopsy curette
 R. endometrial biopsy suction curette

 R. forceps
 R. kidney stone forceps
 R. stone forceps
 R. uterine biopsy curette
 R. uterine curette
Rand-House suction tube
Rand-Malcolm craniol x-ray frame
Randolph
 R. cannula
 R. cyclodialysis cannula
Rand-Radpour suction tube
Rand-Wells pallidothalmomectomy guide
Raney
 R. bone drill
 R. clip
 R. clip-applying forceps
 R. clip forceps
 R. cranial drill
 R. curette
 R. dissector
 R. drill
 R. flexion jacket brace
 R. forceps
 R. Gigli-saw guide
 R. jacket
 R. laminectomy punch
 R. laminectomy retractor
 R. laminectomy rongeur
 R. perforator drill
 R. periosteal elevator
 R. retractor
 R. rongeur
 R. rongeur forceps
 R. saw guide
 R. scalp clip
 R. scalp clip-applying forceps
 R. scalp clip forceps
 R. scalp hemostasis clip
 R. spinal fusion curette
 R. spring steel clip
 R. stainless steel scalp clip
 R. stirrup-loop curette
 R. straight coagulating forceps
Raney-Crutchfield
 R.-C. drill point
 R.-C. skull tongs
Ranfac
 R. cannula

R. cholangiographic catheter
R. needle
range of motion (ROM)
Ranieri clamp
Rankin
R. anastomosis clamp
R. arterial forceps
R. clamp
R. forceps
R. hemostat
R. hemostatic forceps
R. intestinal anastomosis
clamp
R. intestinal clamp
R. prostatic retractor
R. prostatic tractor
R. retractor
R. stomach clamp
R. suture
Rankin-Crile
R.-C. forceps
R.-C. hemostatic forceps
Rankow forceps
Ranzewski
R. clamp
R. intestinal clamp
Rapazzo intraocular lens
rapid exchange balloon catheter
Rappazzo
R. foreign body scissors
R. haptic scissors
R. intraocular foreign body
forceps
R. intraocular lens forceps
R. iris hook
R. speculum
Rapp forceps
Rashkind
R. balloon
R. balloon catheter
R. catheter
R. septostomy balloon
catheter
R. septostomy needle
rasp (*See also* raspatory)
Aagesen disposable r.
Agris r.
antral r.
Arthrofile orthopaedic r.
Aufricht r.
Aufricht glabellar r.
Aufricht-Lipsett nasal r.
Aufricht nasal r.

Austin Moore r.
Bankart r.
Barsky nasal r.
Bartholdson-Stenstrom r.
Berne nasal r.
Bio-Modular humeral r.
Bio-Moore r.
bone r.
Brawley sinus r.
Brown r.
Cohen sinus r.
compound curved r.
Concept arthroscopy r.
Converse r.
convex r.
Cottle r.
Cottle nasal r.
Dean r.
diamond r.
down-curved r.
ear r.
Eicher r.
Epstein r.
facet r.
Filtzer interbody r.
Fomon r.
Fomon nasal r.
Friedman r.
frontal sinus r.
Gallagher antral r.
Gam-Mer r.
glabellar r.
Gleason r.
Good antral r.
hand surgery r.
interbody r.
interbody fusion r.
Israel r.
Israel nasal r.
Joseph r.
Joseph nasal r.
Kalinowski r.
Kalinowski-Verner r.
Kessler podiatry r.
Lamont nasal r.
Leurs nasal r.
Lewis r.
Lewis nasal r.
Lundsgaard-Burch corneal r.
Maliniac nasal r.
Mallory-Head Interlok r.
Maltz r.
Maltz-Anderson r.

rasp *(continued)*
  Maltz-Anderson nasal r.
  Maltz-Lipsett r.
  Maltz-Lipsett nasal r.
  Maltz nasal r.
  Matchett-Brown stem r.
  McCabe-Farrior r.
  McCabe perforation r.
  McCollough r.
  McGee oval-window r.
  McIndoe r.
  microbayonet r.
  Miller r.
  Moore r.
  Moore stem r.
  nasal r.
  orthopaedic r.
  Parkes r.
  Parkes nasal r.
  Parks nasal r.
  perforation r.
  Polokoff r.
  Putti r.
  Putti bone r.
  Reidy r.
  Ringenberg r.
  Ritter r.
  Robb-Roberts rotary r.
  Rubin oblique r.
  Saunders-Paparella
    window r.
  Schantz sinus r.
  Scheer oval window r.
  side-cutting r.
  Southworth r.
  Spratt r.
  Spratt nasofrontal r.
  straight r.
  Sullivan sinus r.
  surgical general r.
  Thompson r.
  Thompson frontal sinus r.
  Thompson stem r.
  ulnar r.
  V. Mueller diamond r.
  Watson-Williams sinus r.
  Wiener antral r.
  Wiener nasal r.
  Wiener-Pierce antral r.
  Wiener Universal frontal
    sinus r.
  window r.
  Woodward antral r.

raspatory *(See also* rasp)
  Alexander r.
  Alexander rib r.
  Artmann r.
  Babcock r.
  Bacon periosteal r.
  Ballenger r.
  Barsky cleft palate r.
  Bastow r.
  Beck pericardial r.
  Bennett r.
  Berry rib r.
  bronchocele sound r.
  Brunner r.
  cleft palate r.
  Collin r.
  Coryllos r.
  Coryllos rib r.
  Cushing r.
  Davidson-Mathieu rib r.
  Davidson-Sauerbruch rib r.
  Davis r.
  Dolley r.
  Doyen r.
  Doyen rib r.
  Edwards r.
  Edwards-Verner r.
  Farabeuf r.
  Farabeuf-Collin r.
  Farrior mushroom r.
  fishtail spatula r.
  French-pattern r.
  Friedrich r.
  Gam-Mer oblique r.
  Hedbloom rib r.
  Hein r.
  Herczel rib r.
  Hill nasal r.
  Hoen periosteal r.
  Hopkins Hospital
    periosteal r.
  Howarth nasal r.
  Jansen mastoid r.
  Joseph r.
  Joseph periosteal r.
  Joseph-Verner r.
  Kirmisson r.
  Kirmisson r.
  Kirmisson periosteal r.
  Kleesattel r.
  Kocher r.
  Koenig r.
  Kokowicz r.

Ladd r.
Lambert-Berry rib r.
Lambotte r.
Lambotte rib r.
laminectomy r.
Lane periosteal r.
Langenbeck r.
Langenbeck-O'Brien r.
Langenbeck periosteal r.
Lebsche r.
Lewis periosteal r.
Mannerfelt r.
Mathieu r.
Matson r.
Matson-Alexander r.
Matson-Plenk r.
McGee r.
McIndoe r.
Mott r.
Nicola r.
Ollier r.
Overholt r.
Overholt rib r.
periosteal r.
Phemister r.
Plenk-Matson r.
rib r.
Sauerbruch-Frey r.
Sayre periosteal r.
Scheuerlen r.
Schneider r.
Schneider-Sauerbruch r.
Sédillot r.
Semb r.
Semb rib r.
Sewall r.
Shuletz r.
Shuletz-Damian r.
skull r.
Stenstrom r.
Stille-Crafoord r.
Stille-Doyen r.
Stille-Edwards r.
Stillenberg r.
sympathetic r.
Trelat palate r.
Wiberg r.
Willauer r.
Williger r.
Yasargil r.
Zenker r.
Zoellner r.

Rastelli
  R. graft
  R. implant
  R. prosthesis
rat
ratchet
  r. clamp
  r. tourniquet
ratchet-type brace
rate-responsive pacemaker
Ratliff-Blake
  R.-B. forceps
  R.-B. gallstone forceps
Ratliff-Mayo
  R.-M. forceps
  R.-M. gallstone forceps
  R.-M. stone forceps
rat-tail catheter
rat-tooth
  r.-t. forceps
  r.-t. grasping forceps
  r.-t. pickup
  r.-t. rongeur
Rauchfuss snare
Ravich
  R. bougie
  R. clamp
  R. dilator
  R. lithotriptoscope with
    Luer lock
  R. lithotrite
  R. needle holder
  R. ureteral dilator
Ray
  R. brain spatula
  R. brain spoon
  R. curette
  R. forceps
  R. kidney stone forceps
  R. nasal speculum
  R. pituitary curette
  R. rhizotomy electrode
  R. screw
  R. screw
Raybar 75 contrast material
Raylor
  R. bone impactor
  R. malleable retractor
Rayner-Choyce
  R.-C. eye implant
  R.-C. intraocular lens
Raypaque resin

Ray-Parsons-Sunday
  staphylorrhaphy elevator
Rayport
  R. dural knife
  R. muscle biopsy clamp
  R. muscle clamp
Ray-Tec
  R.-T. band
  R.-T. dressing
  R.-T. lap pad
  R.-T. sponge
  R.-T. x-ray detectable lap
    pad
  R.-T. x-ray detectable
    sponge
Rayvist contrast material
Raz double-prong ligature carrier
Razi cannula introducer
razor
  r. blade
  r. bladebreaker
  r. blade holder
  Castroviejo r.
  Castroviejo oscillating r.
  Detroit Receiving
    Hospital r.
  Emir r.
  r. scalpel
  Weck-Prep orderly r.
R&B portable pneumothorax
  apparatus
RC1 catheter
RC2 catheter
reach-and-pin forceps
Read
  R. chisel
  R. facial curette
  R. forceps
  R. oral curette
  R. osteotome
  R. periosteal elevator
Real scissors
reamer
  Anatomic/Intracone r.
  Aufranc finishing ball r.
  Aufranc finishing cup r.
  Aufranc offset r.
  Austin Moore r.
  r. awl
  bone r.
  r. bushing
  calcar r.
  canal r.

cannulated r.
cannulated four-flute r.
Charnley r.
r. clamp
debris-retaining acetabular r.
Dentatus r.
DePuy cannulated r.
Duthie r.
end-cutting r.
endodontic r.
expanding r.
femoral shaft r.
final-cut acetabular r.
flexible r.
flexible-wire bundle r.
fluted r.
Green-Armytage r.
Gruca hip r.
Harris brace-type r.
Hewson-Richards r.
humeral r.
Indiana r.
intramedullary r.
Jergensen r.
Jergensen-Trinkle r.
Jewett socket r.
K r.
Küntscher r.
Lorenzo r.
Lottes r.
MacAusland r.
MacAusland finishing-ball r.
MacAusland finishing-cup r.
Mallory-Head Interlok r.
Marin r.
medullary canal r.
Mira-Charnley r.
Mira female trochanteric r.
Mira femoral head r.
Moore bone r.
Murphy ball r.
Norton adjustable cup r.
Norton ball r.
orthopaedic r.
Osteonics r.
patellar shaft r.
PD r.
Peaso r.
Peeso r.
Perthes r.
Phemister r.
revision conical r.
Rowe glenoidal r.

Rush awl r.
shaft r.
shelf r.
Smith-Petersen hip r.
Sovak r.
spiral trochanteric r.
spot face r.
straight r.
Sturmdorf cervical r.
Swanson r.
tapered r.
T-handle r.
Tinel tapered r.
rear-entry ACL drill guide
rear-tip extender
Reaves punch
REB
rubber-reinforced bandage
rebreathing bag
Récamier
R. curette
R. uterine curette
receiver
Pori and Rowe EEG r.
telemetry r.
recessed balloon septostomy
catheter
recession forceps
rechargeable nerve stimulator
battery pack
reciprocating saw
Recklinghausen tonometer
Recon
R. nail
R. proximal drill guide bolt
reconstruction plate
reconstructive suture
recorder
Angus-Esterline r.
Honeywell r.
Leeds-Northrup
Speedomax r.
polysomnograph
electroencephalograph 20-
channel EEG r.
recording electrode
rectal
r. balloon
r. biopsy forceps
r. catheter
r. cautery snare
r. cautery wire
r. clamp

r. curette
r. dilator
r. finger cot
r. forceps
r. hook
r. hook retractor
r. injection cannula
r. injection needle
r. muscle cuff
r. needle
r. probe
r. retractor
r. snare
r. snare hinged-loop wire
r. snare insulated stem
r. snare replacement wire
r. snare stem brush
r. speculum
r. trocar
r. tube
rectangle
Harshill r.
rectangular tapper
rectoromanoscope
rectoscope
Storz continuous flow r.
rectosigmoidoscope
rectosphincteromanometric study
rectus
r. retractor
r. traction suture
recurrent bandage
Red
R. Cross adhesive dressing
R. Witch bur
red
r. laser
r. pessary
r. Robinson catheter
r. rubber catheter
Reddick cystic duct cholangiogram
catheter
Redi-Around finger splint
RediFurl
R. catheter
R. double-lumen balloon
R. single-lumen balloon
Reditron refractometer
Redivac
R. drain
R. suction tube
R. tube
Redo intestinal clamp

Redon drain
red-tip aspirator
reduced small fragment set
reducing fracture frame
reduction
    r. instrument
    r. ring
Redy
    R. 2000 dialysis system
    R. hemodialysis
    R. Sorbent dialysis system
Reece PO shoe
Reed cast belt
reefed vaginal cuff
reef knot suture
Reeh stitch scissors
Rees
    R. disposable battery-driven
      lighted retractor
    R. lighted retractor
Reese
    R. advancement forceps
    R. dermatome
    R. dermatome blade
    R. forceps
    R. muscle forceps
    R. ptosis knife
Reese-Drum dermatome
reference electrode
Reflex
    R. pacemaker
    R. skin stapler
    R. SuperSoft steerable guide
      wire
reform
    r. eye implant
    r. implant
refractometer
    AMO r.
    Reditron r.
refractor
    ARK-Juno r.
    Marco ARK-2000 r.
    Ultramatic Rx master
      phoroptor r.
Regaud radium colpostat
regular
    r. forceps
    r. forceps with teeth
Rehbein
    R. infant abdominal
      retractor
    R. internal steel strut

Rehfuss duodenal tube
Rehne
    R. abdominal retractor
    R. retractor
Reich curette
Reichert
    R. antroscope
    R. camera
    R. fiberoptic sigmoidoscope
    R. flexible sigmoidoscope
    R. Ful-Vue spot retinoscope
    R. ophthalmoscope
    R. sigmoidoscope
    R. slit lamp
    R. steriotaxic brain
      apparatus
    R. tonometer
Reichling scissors
Reich-Nechtow
    R.-N. arterial clamp
    R.-N. cervical biopsy
      curette
    R.-N. clamp
    R.-N. curette
    R.-N. dilator
    R.-N. forceps
    R.-N. hypogastric artery
      forceps
    R.-N. hysterectomy forceps
    R.-N. plug
Reid retinoscope
Reidy rasp
Reif
    R. catheter
    R. design catheter
Reill
    R. forceps
    R. needle holder
    R. wire-cutting pliers
reimplanted electrode
Reinecke-Carroll lacrimal tube
Reiner
    R. curette
    R. ear syringe
    R. knife
    R. plaster knife
    R. rongeur
Reiner-Alexander
    R.-A. ear syringe
    R.-A. syringe
Reiner-Beck tonsillar snare

Reiner-Knight
  R.-K. ethmoid-cutting
    forceps
  R.-K. forceps
reinforcing suture
Reinhoff
  R. forceps
  R. rib spreader
  R. swan neck clamp
  R. thoracic scissors
Reinhoff-Finochietto rib spreader
Reipe-Bard gastric balloon
Reipen
  R. cannula
  R. speculum
Reisinger
  R. forceps
  R. lens-extracting forceps
  R. lens forceps
Relat vaginal speculum
relaxation suture
Relay pacemaker
Release
  R. dressing
  R. nonadhering dressing
Reliavac
  R. closed wound suction
    set
  R. drain
reliner
  Brimms denture r.
  Coe-Rect denture r.
  Coe-Soft denture r.
  Simpa denture r.
  Super-Soft denture r.
Reliquet lithotrite
Relton-Hall frame
Rema-Exakt investment material
Remak band
Remaloy wire
Remanium
  R. alloy
  R. wire
Remedy
  R. colostomy appliance
  R. ileostomy appliance
Remine mastectomy skin flap
  retractor
removable
  r. appliance
  r. implant
removal of drain
Removatron epilator

remover
  Alger brush rust ring r.
  Atwood crown and
    bridge r.
  Bailey foreign body r.
  Braithwaite clip r.
  clip r.
  Concept Ophtho-bur corneal
    rust ring r.
  Damon-Julian ring r.
  DMV II contact lens r.
  Ferrolite crown r.
  Mead bridge r.
  Mead crown r.
  modular head r.
  Richwil crown and
    bridge r.
  ring r.
  Tott ring r.
  Universal clip r.
  Wölfe-Böhler cast r.
Remy separator
renal
  r. artery clamp
  r. artery forceps
  r. clamp
  r. needle
  r. pedicle clamp
  r. retractor
  r. sinus retractor
Renatron II dialyzer reprocessing
  system
Renografin contrast material
Rentrop
  R. catheter
  R. infusion catheter
Reo Macrodex suture
replacement
  r. collection bag
  Manchester knee r.
  Müller-type femoral head r.
  total ossicular r.
replacer
  Smith-Fisher iris r.
Replogle catheter
repositioner
  Wilson-Cook prosthesis r.
repositor
  iris r.
  Knapp iris r.
Reprodent
Repro head halter

Resano
    R. sigmoid forceps
    R. thoracic scissors
rescuing pacemaker
resection
    r. clamp
    r. intestinal forceps
    submucous r. (SMR)
    transurethral r. (TUR)
    transurethral r. of prostate
      (TURP)
resector
    Dyonics full-radius r.
    Friedrich-Petz machine r.
    full-radius r.
    Stryker r.
resectoscope
    ACMI r.
    r. adapter
    Bard r.
    Baumrucker r.
    r. curette
    Ellik r.
    Foroblique r.
    Foroblique microlens r.
    Iglesias r.
    Iglesias continuous flow r.
    Iglesias fiberoptic r.
    Iglesias microlens r.
    Kaplan r.
    Mauermayer r.
    McCarthy continuous-flow r.
    McCarthy microlens r.
    McCarthy miniature r.
    McCarthy multiple r.
    Nesbit r.
    Scott rotating r.
    r. sheath
    Stern-McCarthy r.
    Stern-McCarthy
      electrotome r.
    Storz r.
    Storz direct-view r.
    Storz laser r.
    Streak r.
    Thompson direct full-
      vision r.
    Timberlake obturator r.
    Wappler r. with microlens
      optics
reservoir
    Accu-Flo r.
    Accu-Flo CSF r.

    Braden flushing r.
    Cardiometrics cardiotomy r.
    cardiotomy r.
    Cobe cardiotomy r.
    CSF r.
    Denver r.
    double-dome r.
    flat bottom r.
    flushing r.
    Foltz flushing r.
    Heyer-Schulte r.
    Heyer-Schulte Jackson-Pratt
      wound-drainage r.
    Heyer-Schulte-Ommaya
      CSF r.
    Heyer-Schulte wedge-
      suction r.
    H-H Rickham cerebrospinal
      fluid r.
    Holter r.
    Holter-Rickham
      ventriculostomy r.
    Holter-Salmon-Rickham
      ventriculostomy r.
    Holter-Selker
      ventriculostomy r.
    Holter ventriculostomy r.
    Intersept cardiotomy r.
    Jackson-Pratt large-volume
      suction r.
    Jostra cardiotomy r.
    J-Vac bulb suction r.
    large-volume suction r.
    Ommaya CSF r.
    Parks ileoanal r.
    Polystan cardiotomy r.
    Resipump pump r.
    Rickham r.
    Salmon-Rickham
      ventriculostomy r.
    Sci-Med extracorporeal
      silicone rubber r.
    Selker ventriculostomy r.
    Shiley cardiotomy r.
    UNI r.
    Uni-Shunt with r.
    Uni-Shunt with elliptical r.
    William Harvey
      cardiotomy r.
    wound drainage r.
resin
    Aclec r.
    Astron r.

Astron dental r.
Brilliant Dentin r.
Brilliant light-cured r.
Coe orthodontic r.
Dentalon R r.
Dentsply r.
Ivocryl r.
Lee orthodontic r.
Myerson r.
Poracryl r.
Porovin dental r.
Raypaque r.
RM orthodontic acrylic r.
Royale III denture r.
Shur r.
Vynacron r.
Vynagel dental r.
Resipump pump reservoir
Resnick
R. button bipolar coagulator
R. speech teacher
R. Tone Emitter I intraoral electrolarynx device
respirator
Ambu r.
BABYbird r.
Bath r.
Bear r.
Bennett r.
Bird Mark 8 r.
Bourns infant r.
Bragg-Paul r.
Clevedan positive pressure r.
cuirass r.
Dann r.
Drinker r.
Emerson r.
Engstrom r.
Gill r.
Huxley r.
Kirmisson r.
mechanical r.
Med-Neb r.
Merck r.
Monaghan r.
Morch r.
Morsch-Retec r.
Moynihan r.
portable r.
Sanders jet ventilation device r.
respiratory-dependent pacemaker

respiratory function monitor
Respitrace
rest
Cedar anesthesia face r.
face r.
Muirhead pelvic r.
neck r.
Reston
R. dressing
R. foam dressing
restorative pin
restraint
Posey r.
vacuum-operated viscous r.
restrictor
Buck femoral cement r.
cement r.
Charnley cement r.
Resuscitaire neonatal resuscitation unit
resuscitator
pneuPAC r.
retained suture
retainer
r. arch bar
r. closure
Hahnenkratt r.
Hawley r.
r. insert
McNealey-Glassman visceral r.
r. ring
Tofflemire r.
viscera r.
retaining
r. device
r. retractor
retention
Ackerman overdenture r.
r. catheter
r. drill
r. ring
r. suture
r. suture bolster
r. suture bridge
retinal
r. diathermy electrode
r. Gelfilm implant
retinoscope
Boilo r.
Copeland r.
Copeland streak r.
electric r.

retinoscope *(continued)*
Ful-Vue spot r.
Ful-Vue streak r.
Macula r.
Priestley-Smith r.
Propper r.
Reichert Ful-Vue spot r.
Reid r.
spot r.
streak r.
Welch Allyn standard r.
Welch Allyn streak r.
Retract-A-Cord
retracting rod
retraction ring
Grieshaber-Balfour retractor
retractor
Abadie self-retaining r.
abdominal r.
r. abdominal blade
abdominal ring r.
abdominal vascular r.
Ablaza r.
Ablaza aortic wall r.
Ablaza-Blanco r.
Ablaza-Blanco cardiac
  valve r.
Abramson r.
Adams r.
Adamson r.
r. adjustable arm
Adson r.
Adson-Beckman r.
Adson brain r.
Adson cerebellar r.
Adson splanchnic r.
Agrikola r.
Agrikola lacrimal sac r.
Aim r.
airgun r.
alar r.
Alden r.
Alexander r.
Alexander-Ballen orbital r.
Alexander-Matson r.
Alexian Hospital model r.
Alfreck r.
Allen r.
Allis r.
Allis lung r.
Allison r.
Allison lung r.
Allport r.

Allport-Babcock r.
Allport-Gifford r.
Allport mastoid r.
Allport mastoid bayonet r.
Alm r.
Alm microsurgery r.
Alm minor surgery r.
Alm self-retaining r.
Alter lip r.
aluminum cortex r.
Amenabar r.
American Heyer-Schulte
  brain r.
Amoils r.
Amoils iris r.
amputation r.
anal r.
Anderson-Adson r.
Anderson-Adson scalp r.
Anderson-Adson self-
  retaining r.
Andrews r.
Andrews tracheal r.
angled decompression r.
angled vein r.
Ankeney r.
Ankeney sternal r.
Ann Arbor r.
Ann Arbor phrenic r.
anterior r.
anterior prostatic r.
Anthony r.
Anthony pillar r.
antral r.
AOR collateral ligament r.
aortic r.
aortic r.
aortic valve r.
Apfelbaum cerebellar r.
apicolysis r.
appendectomy r.
appendiceal r.
arch rake r.
Arem-Madden r.
Aren r.
arm r.
Army-Navy r.
Aronson r.
Aronson esophageal r.
Aronson lateral
  sternomastoid r.
Aronson medical
  esophageal r.

Arruga r.
Arruga eye r.
Arruga globe r.
Ashley r.
atrial r.
atrial septal r.
Aufranc r.
Aufranc cobra r.
Aufranc femoral neck r.
Aufranc hip r.
Aufranc psoas r.
Aufranc push r.
Aufricht r.
Aufricht nasal r.
Austin r.
Austin dental r.
automatic skin r.
Auvard weighted vaginal r.
Azar iris r.
Babcock r.
baby r.
baby Adson brain r.
baby Balfour r.
baby Collin abdominal r.
baby Roux r.
baby Senn-Miller r.
baby Weitlaner r.
baby Weitlaner self-
  retaining r.
Backmann thyroid r.
Bacon r.
Bacon cranial r.
Badgley r.
Badgley laminectomy r.
Bahnson r.
Bahnson sternal r.
Bakelite r.
Balfour r.
Balfour abdominal r.
Balfour baby r.
Balfour center-blade r.
Balfour center-blade
  abdominal r.
Balfour detachable-blade
  abdominal r.
Balfour malleable center-
  blade abdominal r.
Balfour pediatric r.
Balfour pediatric
  abdominal r.
Balfour self-retaining r.
Balfour r. with fenestrated
  blade

Ballantine
  hemilaminectomy r.
Ballen-Alexander r.
Ballen-Alexander orbital r.
ball-type r.
Bankart r.
Bankart rectal r.
Bankart shoulder r.
Baron r.
Barr r.
Barraquer lid r.
Barrett-Adson r.
Barrett-Adson cerebellum r.
Barron r.
Barr rectal r.
Barr rectal crypt hook r.
Barr self-retaining r.
Barsky r.
Barsky nasal r.
Beardsley esophageal r.
Beatty pillar r.
Beaver r.
Bechert-Kratz cannulated
  nucleus r.
Becker r.
Beckman r.
Beckman-Adson r.
Beckman-Adson
  laminectomy r.
Beckman-Eaton r.
Beckman-Eaton
  laminectomy r.
Beckman goiter r.
Beckman self-retaining r.
Beckman thyroid r.
Beckman-Weitlaner r.
Beckman-Weitlaner
  laminectomy r.
B.E. glass abdominal r.
Bellfield wire r.
Bellman r.
Belluci-Wullstein r.
Beneventi r.
Beneventi self-retaining r.
Bennett r.
Bennett bone r.
Bennett tibial r.
Berens r.
Berens esophageal r.
Berens eye r.
Berens lid r.
Berens mastectomy r.

retractor *(continued)*

Berens mastectomy skin flap r.
Berens skin flap r.
Berens thyroid r.
Bergen r.
Bergman tracheal r.
Bergman wound r.
Berkeley r.
Berkeley-Bonney r.
Berkeley-Bonney self-retaining abdominal r.
Berlind-Auvard r.
Berna r.
Berna infant abdominal r.
Bernay r.
Bernay tracheal r.
Bernstein r.
Bernstein nasal r.
Bethune r.
Bethune phrenic r.
Bicek r.
Bicek vaginal r.
bident r.
Biestek thyroid r.
bifid r.
bifid gallbladder r.
bifurcated r.
Biggs r.
Biggs mammaplasty r.
biliary r.
Billroth r.
Billroth-Stille r.
bivalved r.
Black r.
bladder r.
blade r.
r. blade
Blair r.
Blair-Brown r.
Blair-Brown vacuum r.
Blair four-prong r.
Blakesley r.
Blakesley uvular r.
Blanco r.
Bland perineal r.
Blount r.
Blount bone r.
Blount double-prong r.
Blount hip r.
Blount knee r.
Blount single-prong r.
blunt r.

blunt rake r.
boardlike r.
Bodnar knee r.
Boley r.
bone r.
Bookwalter r.
Bookwalter-Balfour r.
Bookwalter-Harrington r.
Bookwalter-Kelly r.
Bookwalter-Magrina vaginal r.
Bose r.
Bosworth r.
Bosworth nerve root r.
bowel r.
Boyd r.
Boyes-Goodfellow hook r.
Braastad r.
Braastad costal arch r.
brain r.
brain silicone-coated r.
Brantley-Turner r.
Brantley-Turner vaginal r.
Brawley r.
Brawley scleral wound r.
Breen r.
Breisky vaginal r.
Brewster r.
Brewster phrenic r.
Briggs r.
Brinker hygienic tissue r.
Bristow-Bankart humeral r.
Bristow-Bankart soft tissue r.
Brompton Hospital r.
Bronson-Turtz iris r.
Brophy r.
Brophy tenaculum r.
Brown r.
Brown-Burr modified Gillies r.
Brown uvula r.
Bruch mastoid r.
Bruening r.
Brunner r.
Brunschwig r.
Brunschwig visceral r.
Bucy r.
Bucy spinal cord r.
Budde halo neurosurgical r.
Buie r.
Buie-Smith r.
Buie-Smith anal r.

bulb r.
Bulnes-Sanchez r.
Burford r.
Burford-Finochietto r.
Burford-Finochietto rib r.
Burford rib r.
Butler r.
Butler dental r.
Butler pillar r.
buttonhook r.
buttonhook nerve r.
Bycroft-Brunswick thyroid r.
Byford r.
Cairns r.
Cairns scalp r.
Callahan r.
Campbell r.
Campbell lacrimal sac r.
Campbell nerve root r.
Campbell self-retaining r.
Campbell suprapubic r.
Canadian chest r.
Cardens r.
Cardillo r.
cardiovascular r.
Carlens-Stille tracheal r.
Carlens tracheotomy r.
Caroline finger r.
Carroll r.
Carroll-Bennett finger r.
Carroll offset hand r.
Carroll self-retaining
  spring r.
Carter r.
Carter mitral valve r.
Caspar r.
Castallo r.
Castallo eyelid r.
Castallo lid r.
Castaneda r.
Castaneda infant sternal r.
Castroviejo r.
Castroviejo adjustable r.
cat's paw r.
Cave r.
Cave knee r.
cecostomy r.
r. center blade
cerebellar r.
cerebral r.
cervical r.
cervical disk r.
chalazion r.

Chamberlain-Fries
  atraumatic r.
Chandler r.
Chandler laminectomy r.
channel r.
Charnley r.
Charnley knee r.
Cheanvechai-Favaloro r.
cheek r.
Cherry r.
Cherry laminectomy self-
  retaining r.
Cherry S-shaped brain r.
Cheyne r.
Children's Hospital r.
Children's Hospital
  pediatric r.
Chitten-Hill r.
Christie gallbladder r.
Cibis-Vaiser muscle r.
claw r.
Clayman lid r.
Clevedent r.
r. clip
Cloward r.
Cloward blade r.
Cloward brain r.
Cloward cervical r.
Cloward-Cushing vein r.
Cloward dural r.
Cloward-Hoen r.
Cloward-Hoen
  laminectomy r.
Cloward nerve root r.
Cloward self-retaining r.
Cloward tissue r.
Cobb r.
cobra r.
Cocke large flap r.
Cohen r.
Cole r.
Cole duodenal r.
Coleman r.
collar button iris r.
Collin abdominal r.
Collin-Hartmann r.
Collins-Mayo mastoid r.
Collin sternal self-
  retaining r.
Collis anterior cervical r.
Collis posterior lumbar r.
Collis-Taylor r.
Colonial r.

Chevalier–Delacroix

retractor *(continued)*
    Colver r.
    Colver tonsillar r.
    Comyns-Berkeley r.
    Cone r.
    Cone laminectomy r.
    Cone scalp r.
    Cone self-retaining r.
    contour r.
    contour scalp r.
    Converse r.
    Converse alar r.
    Converse blade r.
    Converse double-ended r.
    Converse nasal r.
    Conway eye r.
    Conway lid r.
    Cook r.
    Cook rectal r.
    Cooley r.
    Cooley atrial r.
    Cooley atrial valve r.
    Cooley carotid r.
    Cooley femoral r.
    Cooley-Marz sternal r.
    Cooley mitral valve r.
    Cooley MPC
     cardiovascular r.
    Cooley neonatal r.
    Cooley neonatal sternal r.
    Cooley rib r.
    Cooley sternotomy r.
    Cope double-ended r.
    corner r.
    cortex r.
    Coryllos r.
    costal arch r.
    Costenbader r.
    Coston-Trent cryo r.
    Cottle r.
    Cottle alar r.
    Cottle four-prong r.
    Cottle hook r.
    Cottle-Joseph r.
    Cottle-Neivert r.
    Cottle pillar r.
    Cottle pronged r.
    Cottle sharp-prong r.
    Cottle single-blade r.
    Cottle soft palate r.
    Cottle upper lateral
     exposing r.
    Cottle weighted r.

    Crafoord r.
    Craig-Sheehan r.
    cranial r.
    Crawford r.
    Crawford aortic r.
    Crego r.
    Crego periosteal r.
    Crile r.
    Crile angle r.
    Crile thyroid double-
     ended r.
    Crockard hard-palate r.
    Crockard pharyngeal r.
    Crotti r.
    Crotti goiter r.
    Crotti thyroid r.
    Cushing r.
    Cushing aluminum r.
    Cushing aluminum cortex r.
    Cushing angled r.
    Cushing angled
     decompression r.
    Cushing brain r.
    Cushing decompression r.
    Cushing-Kocher r.
    Cushing nerve r.
    Cushing S-r.
    Cushing self-retaining r.
    Cushing straight r.
    Cushing vein r.
    dacryocystorhinostomy r.
    Dallas r.
    Danis r.
    Darling popliteal r.
    Darrach r.
    Dautrey r.
    Davidoff r.
    Davidoff trigeminal r.
    Davidson r.
    Davidson erector spinae r.
    Davidson scapular r.
    Davis r.
    Davis brain r.
    Davis double-ended r.
    Davis pillar r.
    Davis scalp r.
    Davis self-retaininig scalp r.
    Deaver r.
    Deaver pediatric r.
    Deaver-type r.
    DeBakey r.
    DeBakey-Balfour r.
    DeBakey chest r.

DeBakey-Cooley r.
DeBakey-Cooley-Deaver r.
DeBakey-Cooley Deaver-
  type r.
Decker r.
decompressive r.
Dedo laser r.
deep r.
deep abdominal r.
deep Deaver r.
deep rake r.
DeLaginiere abdominal r.
Delaney r.
Delaney phrenic r.
DeLee r.
DeLee corner r.
DeLee Universal r.
DeLee vaginal r.
DeLee vesical r.
DeMartel r.
DeMartel self-retaining
  brain r.
Denis Browne r.
Denis Browne adjustable-
  arm r.
Denis Browne pediatric r.
Denis Browne ring r.
dental r.
DePuy r.
D'Errico-Adson r.
D'Errico nerve r.
D'Errico nerve root r.
Desmarres r.
Desmarres cardiovascular r.
Desmarres lid r.
Desmarres vein r.
Deucher abdominal r.
Devine-Millard-Aufricht r.
Di-Main r.
Dingman r.
Dingman flexible r.
Dingman Flexsteel r.
Dingman-Senn r.
Dingman zygoma hook r.
disposable r.
disposable iris r.
Dixon center-blade r.
Doane knee r.
Dockhorn r.
dog chain r.
Dohn-Carton brain r.
Dorsey r.
Dorsey nerve root r.

Dorton self-retaining r.
Dott r.
double-angled r.
double-cobra r.
double-crank r.
double-ended r.
Downing r.
Downing II laminectomy r.
Doyen r.
Doyen abdominal r.
Doyen child abdominal r.
Doyen vaginal r.
Drews iris r.
Drews-Rosenbaum r.
dull r.
dull-pronged r.
Dumont r.
duodenal r.
dural r.
90° dural root suction r.
dural suction r.
Duryea r.
Eastman r.
Eastman vaginal r.
East-West r.
East-West soft tissue r.
easy-out r.
Echols r.
Eddey parotid r.
Edinburgh r.
Edinburgh brain r.
Effenberger r.
Elias lid r.
Elschnig r.
Elschnig lid r.
Emmet r.
Emmet obstetrical r.
endaural r.
Enker brain r.
Enker self-retaining brain r.
epicardial r.
epiglottis r.
erector spinae r.
esophageal r.
examination r.
externofrontal r.
eye r.
eyelid r.
face-lift r.
Falk r.
Falk vaginal r.
Farabeuf r.
Farabeuf double-ended r.

retractor *(continued)*
Farmingdale r.
Farr r.
Farr self-retaining r.
Farr spring r.
Farr wire r.
Fasanella r.
Fasanella double-ended r.
Fasanella iris r.
fat-pad r.
Favaloro atrial r.
Favaloro self-retaining
    sternal r.
Federspiel cheek r.
Feldman r.
Feldman lip r.
femoral neck r.
Ferguson r.
Ferguson-Moon r.
Ferguson-Moon rectal r.
Fernstroem bladder r.
Fernstroem-Stille r.
Ferris Smith r.
Ferris Smith orbital r.
Ferris Smith-Sewall r.
Ferris Smith-Sewall
    orbital r.
fiberoptic r.
finger r.
finger rake r.
Fink r.
Fink lacrimal r.
Finochietto r.
Finochietto-Geissendorfer
    rib r.
Finochietto hand r.
Finochietto infant rib r.
Finochietto laminectomy r.
Finochietto rib r.
Finsen r.
Fisch dural r.
Fisher r.
Fisher double-ended r.
Fisher fenestrated lid r.
Fisher lid r.
Fisher-Nugent r.
Fisher solid-blade r.
Fisher tonsillar r.
flexible r.
flexible shaft r.
Flexsteel r.
Flexsteel ribbon r.
Foerster abdominal r.

Foerster abdominal ring r.
Fomon r.
Fomon hook r.
Fomon nasal r.
Fomon nostril r.
force fulcrum r.
Ford-Deaver r.
Foss r.
Foss bifid r.
Foss bifid gallbladder r.
Foss biliary r.
Foss gallbladder r.
four-prong r.
Fowler self-retaining r.
r. frame
Franklin r.
Franklin malleable r.
Franz r.
Franz abdominal r.
Frater r.
Frater intracardiac r.
Frazier r.
Frazier cerebral r.
Frazier-Fay r.
Frazier laminectomy r.
Frazier lighted r.
Freeman r.
Freeman face-lift r.
Freer r.
Freer dural r.
Freer skin r.
Freer submucous r.
Freiberg r.
Freiberg hip r.
Freiberg nerve root r.
Freidrich-Ferguson r.
French r.
French brain r.
French S-shaped r.
French S-shaped brain r.
French-Stern-McCarthy r.
Friederich-Ferguson r.
Friedman r.
Friedman perineal r.
Friedman vaginal r.
Fritsch r.
Fritsch abdominal r.
Fulton r.
Gabarro r.
Gabarro plate skin r.
gallbladder r.
gallows-type r.

Gam-Mer medial
esophageal r.
Gam-Mer occipital r.
Gant gallbladder r.
Garrett r.
Garrett peripheral
vascular r.
Garrigue vaginal r.
gastric resection r.
Gaubatz rib r.
Gauthier r.
Geissendorfer rib r.
Gelpi r.
Gelpi abdominal r.
Gelpi perineal r.
Gelpi self-retaining r.
Gelpi vaginal r.
general r.
Gerbode sternal r.
Ghazi rib r.
Gibson-Balfour r.
Gibson-Balfour abdominal r.
Gifford r.
Gifford-Jansen mastoid r.
Gifford mastoid r.
Gifford scalp r.
Gillies single-hook skin r.
Gil-Vernet r.
Gil-Vernet lumbotomy r.
Gil-Vernet renal r.
Gil-Vernet renal sinus r.
Givner eye r.
Glaser r.
Glaser laminectomy r.
Glass r.
Glass abdominal r.
Glenner r.
Glenner vaginal r.
Goelet r.
Goelet double-ended r.
goiter r.
Goldstein r.
Goldstein lacrimal sac r.
Goligher r.
Goligher modification of
the Berkeley-Bonney r.
Goligher sternal-lifting r.
Gomez r.
Gomez gastric r.
Gooch r.
Gooch mastoid r.
Good r.
Goodhill r.

Goodyear r.
Goodyear tonsillar r.
Gossert self-retaining r.
Gosset r.
Gosset abdominal r.
Gosset appendectomy r.
Gosset self-retaininig r.
Goulet r.
Gradle r.
Gradle eyelid r.
Graether r.
Graether collar-button r.
Graether collar-button iris r.
Grant r.
Grant gallbladder r.
Green r.
Greenberg r.
Greenberg Universal r.
Greene r.
Greene goiter r.
Greene thyroid r.
Green goiter r.
Grieshaber r.
Grieshaber-Balfour r.
Grieshaber spring wire r.
Grieshaber wire r.
Groenholm r.
Groenholm lid r.
Gross r.
Gross iris r.
Gross patent ductus r.
Gross-Pomeranz-Watkins r.
Gross-Pomeranz-Watkins
atrial r.
Gruenwald r.
Guilford-Wright meatal r.
Guthrie r.
Guttmann r.
Guttmann obstetrical r.
Guttmann vaginal r.
Guzman-Blanco epiglottic r.
Haight r.
Haight baby r.
Haight-Finochietto r.
Haight-Finochietto rib r.
Haight pulmonary r.
Haight rib r.
Hajek r.
Hajek antral r.
Hajek lip r.
half-moon r.
halo r.

593

retractor *(continued)*
    Hamburger-Brennan-
      Mahorner thyroid r.
    Hamby r.
    Hamby brain r.
    Hamby-Hibbs r.
    hand r.
    hand-held r.
    hard palate r.
    Hardy r.
    Hardy-Duddy r.
    Hardy-Duddy vaginal r.
    Hardy lip r.
    Harken r.
    Harken rib r.
    Harrington r.
    Harrington bladder r.
    Harrington Britetrac r.
    Harrington-Pemberton r.
    Harrington-Pemberton
      sympathectomy r.
    Harrington splanchnic r.
    Harrington
      sympathectomy r.
    Harrison r.
    Harrison chalazion r.
    Hartstein r.
    Hartstein iris r.
    Hartstein irrigating iris r.
    Hartzler rib r.
    Haslinger r.
    Haslinger palate r.
    Haslinger uvula r.
    Hasson r.
    Haverfield r.
    Haverfield
      hemilaminectomy r.
    Haverfield-Scoville r.
    Haverfield-Scoville
      hemilaminectomy r.
    Hayes r.
    Haynes r.
    Hays finger r.
    Hays hand r.
    Heaney r.
    Heaney hysterectomy r.
    Heaney-Simon r.
    Heaney-Simon
      hysterectomy r.
    Heaney-Simon vaginal r.
    Heaney vaginal r.
    Hedblom r.
    Hedblom rib r.

Heifitz r.
Heiss r.
Heiss mastoid r.
Heiuss soft tissue r.
Helfrick r.
Helfrick anal r.
Helfrick anal ring r.
hemilaminectomy r.
Henderson r.
Henderson self-retaining r.
Henley r.
Henley carotid r.
Henner r.
Henner endaural r.
Henner T-model endaural r.
Henrotin r.
hernia r.
Hertzler baby r.
Hertzler rib r.
Hess nerve root r.
Heyer-Schulte r.
Heyer-Schulte brain r.
Hibbs r.
Hibbs laminectomy r.
Hibbs self-retaining r.
Hill r.
Hill-Ferguson r.
Hill-Ferguson rectal r.
Hillis eyelid r.
Hillis lid r.
Hill rectal r.
Himmelstein r.
Himmelstein sternal r.
hip r.
Hipps self-retaining r.
Hirschman r.
Hoen r.
Hoen hemilaminectomy r.
Hoen scalp r.
Hohmann r.
Holman r.
Holman lung r.
Holscher nerve r.
Holscher nerve root r.
Holzbach r.
Holzbach abdominal r.
Holzheimer r.
Holzheimer mastoid r.
Holzheimer skin r.
r. hook
hook r.
r. hook blade
Horgan r.

horizontal r.
horizontal flexible bar r.
Hosel r.
House r.
House hand r.
House hand-held r.
House-Urban r.
House-Urban middle
  fossa r.
Howorth r.
Howorth toothed r.
Huang Universal arm r.
Hubbard r.
Hudson r.
Hudson bone r.
humeral r.
Hunt r.
Hunt bladder r.
Hupp r.
Hupp tracheal r.
Hurd r.
Hurd pillar r.
Hurd tonsillar pillar r.
Hurson flexible r.
Hutchinson iris r.
hysterectomy r.
incision r.
infant r.
infant abdominal r.
infant eyelid r.
infant rib r.
Inge r.
Inge laminar r.
Inge laminectomy r.
initial incision r.
intestinal occlusion r.
intracardiac r.
iris r.
iris disposable r.
Iron interne r.
irrigating mushroom r.
Israel r.
Israel blunt rake r.
Israel rake r.
Jackson r.
Jackson double-ended r.
Jackson goiter r.
Jackson right-angle r.
Jackson self-retaining
  goiter r.
Jackson tracheal r.
Jackson vaginal r.
Jacobson r.

Jacobson bladder r.
Jacobson goiter r.
Jaeger r.
Jaeger lid r.
Jaeger lid plate r.
Jaffe-Givner lid r.
Jaffe lid r.
Jaffe wire lid r.
Jako laser r.
Jannetta r.
Jannetta posterior fossa r.
Jansen r.
Jansen-Gifford r.
Jansen-Gifford mastoid r.
Jansen mastoid r.
Jansen scalp r.
Jansen-Wagner r.
Jansen-Wagner mastoid r.
Jarit cross-action r.
Jarit-Deaver r.
Jarit renal sinus r.
Jarit spring wire r.
Jefferson r.
Jefferson self-retaining r.
Joe's hoe r.
Johns Hopkins r.
Johns Hopkins
  gallbladder r.
Johnson r.
Johnson cheek r.
Johnson hook r.
Johnson ventriculogram r.
Jones r.
Jones IMA epicardial r.
Jorgenson r.
Joseph hook r.
Joseph skin r.
Joseph skin hook r.
Joseph wound r.
Judd-Allis intestinal r.
Judd-Mason r.
Judd-Mason bladder r.
Judd-Mason prostatic r.
Kalamarides dural r.
Kanavel-Senn r.
Karmody vascular spring r.
Kaufer type II r.
Keizer r.
Keizer eye r.
Keizer lid r.
Kel r.
Kelly r.
Kelly abdominal r.

retractor *(continued)*
   Kelly-Sims r.
   Kelly-Sims vaginal r.
   Kelman r.
   Kelman iris r.
   Kennerdell-Maroon orbital r.
   Kennerdell medial orbital r.
   Kerrison r.
   kidney r.
   Killey molar r.
   Killian-King r.
   Killian-King goiter r.
   Kilner r.
   Kilner nasal r.
   Kilner skin hook r.
   Kilner skin wound r.
   Kilpatrick r.
   King r.
   King goiter r.
   King goiter self-retaining r.
   King-Hurd r.
   Kirby r.
   Kirby lid r.
   Kirchner r.
   Kirkland r.
   Kirklin atrial r.
   Kirschner abdominal r.
   Kirschner-Balfour
     abdominal r.
   Kitner r.
   Kleinert-Kutz hook r.
   Kleinert-Ragnell r.
   Kleinsasser r.
   Klemme r.
   Klemme appendectomy r.
   Klemme gasserian
     ganglion r.
   Klemme laminectomy r.
   Kliners alar r.
   Knapp r.
   Knapp lacrimal r.
   Knapp lacrimal sac r.
   knee r.
   Knighton r.
   Knighton hemilaminectomy
     self-retaining r.
   Kocher r.
   Kocher bladder r.
   Kocher blade r.
   Kocher bone r.
   Kocher-Crotti r.
   Kocher-Crotti goiter r.

   Kocher-Crotti goiter self-
     retaining r.
   Kocher gallbladder r.
   Kocher goiter self-
     retaining r.
   Kocher-Langenbeck r.
   Kocher-Wagner r.
   Koenig r.
   Koenig vein r.
   Koerte r.
   Koneg r.
   Korte r.
   Korte-Wagner r.
   Kozlinski r.
   Krasky r.
   Kretschmer r.
   Kristeller r.
   Kristeller vaginal r.
   Kronfeld r.
   Kronfeld eyelid r.
   Krönlein-Berke r.
   Kuglen r.
   Kwapis subcondylar r.
   Lack tongue r.
   lacrimal r.
   lacrimal sac r.
   Lahey r.
   Lahey Clinic r.
   Lahey Clinic nerve root r.
   Lahey goiter r.
   Lahey thyroid r.
   laminectomy r.
   laminectomy self-retaining r.
   Landau vaginal r.
   Landon narrow-bladed r.
   Lane r.
   Lange r.
   Langenbeck r.
   Langenbeck-Cushing vein r.
   Langenbeck-Green r.
   Langenbeck-Mannerfelt r.
   Langenbeck periosteal r.
   Laplace r.
   Laplace liver r.
   laryngeal r.
   laryngofissure r.
   lateral r.
   Latrobe r.
   Latrobe soft palate r.
   Laufe r.
   Lawton-Balfour self-
     retaining r.
   leaflet r.

Leasure tracheal r.
Leatherman trochanteric r.
Lee double-ended r.
Legen self-retaining r.
Legueu r.
Legueu bladder r.
Legueu kidney r.
Lemmon self-retaining
  sternal r.
Lemmon sternal r.
Lemole atrial valve self-
  retaining r.
Lemole mitral valve r.
Lempert r.
Lempert-Colver r.
Levinthal surgery r.
Levy perineal r.
Lewis r.
Leyla r.
Leyla brain r.
Leyla self-retaining brain r.
Leyla-Yasargil r.
Leyla-Yasargil self-
  retaining r.
lid r.
Liddicoat aortic valve r.
lighted r.
Lilienthal-Sauerbruch r.
Lillehei r.
Lillie r.
Lillie pillar r.
Linton r.
Linton splanchnic r.
lip r.
Little r.
liver r.
Lockhart-Mummery r.
Lofberg thyroid r.
Logan r.
Logan lacrimal sac self-
  retaining r.
London r.
London narrow-bladed r.
loop r.
Lorie r.
Lorie cheek r.
Lothrop r.
Lothrop tonsillar r.
Lothrop uvula r.
Love r.
Lovejoy r.
Love nasopharyngeal r.
Love nerve r.

Love nerve root r.
Love uvula r.
Lowman r.
Lowman hand r.
Lowsley r.
Lowsley prostate r.
Luer r.
Luer "S" r.
Luer tracheal r.
Luer tracheal double-
  ended r.
Lukens r.
Lukens epiglottic r.
Lukens thymus r.
Lukens tracheal r.
Lukens tracheal double-
  ended r.
lumbar r.
lumbotomy r.
lung r.
Luongo r.
Luongo hand r.
Luther-Peter r.
MacAusland r.
MacAusland-Kelly r.
MacAusland muscle r.
MacKay r.
MacKay contour r.
MacKay contour self-
  retaining r.
MacKool capsule r.
Magrina-Bookwalter
  vaginal r.
Mahorner r.
Mahorner thyroid r.
Maison r.
Maliniac r.
Maliniac nasal r.
Malis r.
Malis cerebellar r.
Malis cerebral r.
malleable r.
malleable blade r.
malleable copper r.
r. malleable copper blade
malleable ribbon r.
malleable stainless steel r.
r. malleable wire hand
Maltz r.
Mannerfelt r.
Manning r.
manual r.
Markham-Meyerding r.

retractor *(continued)*

Markham-Meyerding
hemilaminectomy r.
Mark II Chandler r.
Markley r.
Martin r.
Martin abdominal r.
Martin cheek r.
Martin lip r.
Martin nerve root r.
Martin palate r.
Martin rectal hook r.
Martin vaginal r.
Mason-Judd r.
Mason-Judd bladder r.
Mason-Judd self-retaining r.
mastectomy skin flap r.
mastoid r.
r. mastoid blade
mastoid-retaining r.
mastoid self-retaining r.
Mathieu r.
Mathieu double-ended r.
Matson-Mead apicolysis r.
Mattison-Upshaw r.
Mayfield r.
Mayo r.
Mayo abdominal r.
Mayo-Adams r.
Mayo-Adams
appendectomy r.
Mayo-Adams self-retaining r.
Mayo-Collins r.
Mayo-Collins
appendectomy r.
Mayo-Collins double-
ended r.
Mayo-Collins mastoid r.
Mayo-Lovelace r.
Mayo-Lovelace abdominal r.
Mayo-Simpson r.
McBurney r.
McBurney fenestrated r.
McBurney thyroid r.
McCabe antral r.
McCabe parotidectomy r.
McCabe posterior fossa r.
McCullough r.
McCullough externofrontal r.
McGannon r.
McGannon eye r.
McGannon iris r.
McGill r.

McIndoe r.
McNealey visceral r.
meat hook r.
Medicon rib r.
Meigs r.
Meller r.
Meller lacrimal sac r.
meniscal r.
Merrill-Levassier r.
metacarpal double-ended r.
Meyer biliary r.
Meyerding r.
Meyerding-Deaver r.
Meyerding finger r.
Meyerding laminectomy r.
Meyerding laminectomy self-
retaining r.
Meyerding self-retaining r.
microlumbar r.
microlumbar diskectomy r.
microsurgical r.
microvascular modified
Alm r.
Middledorpf r.
Middlesex-Pointe r.
Mikulicz r.
Mikulicz abdominal r.
Mikulicz liver r.
Miles r.
Milex r.
Miller r.
Miller-Senn r.
Miller-Senn double-ended r.
Milligan self-retaining r.
Millin r.
Millin-Bacon r.
Millin-Bacon bladder r.
Millin-Bacon bladder self-
retaining r.
Millin-Bacon retropubic
prostatectomy r.
Millin bladder r.
Millin retropublic bladder r.
Millin self-retaining r.
Miltex r.
mini-Hohmann r.
Minnesota r.
Miskimon cerebellar r.
Miskimon cerebellar self-
retaining r.
mitral valve r.
Moberg r.
Moberg-Stille r.

Mollison r.
Mollison self-retaining r.
Moon rectal r.
Moore r.
Moore bone r.
Moore elevator r.
Moorehead r.
Moorehead cheek r.
Moorehead dental r.
Morris r.
Morrison-Hurd r.
Morrison-Hurd pillar r.
Morse r.
Morse modified
  Finochietto r.
Morse sternal r.
Morse valve r.
Morson r.
Mosher r.
Mosher lifesaver r.
Mott r.
Mott double-ended r.
Mueller r.
Mueller-Balfour r.
Mueller-Balfour self-
  retaining r.
Mueller lacrimal sac r.
Mufson-Cushing r.
Muldoon lid r.
multipurpose r.
Munro r.
Munro self-retaining r.
Murless head r.
Murphy r.
Murphy-Balfour r.
Murphy gallbladder r.
Murphy rake r.
Murtagh self-retaining infant
  scalp r.
Myers r.
Myers knee r.
Naclerio diaphragm r.
narrow r.
nasal r.
nasopharyngeal r.
Neivert r.
Neivert double-ended r.
Nelson r.
Nelson rib r.
Nelson rib self-retaining r.
neonatal sternal r.
nerve r.
nerve root r.

nerve root suction r.
Nevyas r.
Nevyas drape r.
newborn eyelid r.
Newell lid r.
Newton-Morgan r.
New tracheal r.
New York Hospital r.
Noblock r.
North-South r.
Nuttall r.
Nystroem r.
Nystroem-Stille r.
Oberhill r.
Oberhill laminectomy r.
Oberhill self-retaining r.
O'Brien phrenic r.
O'Brien rib r.
obstetrical r.
Obwegeser r.
Obwegeser channel r.
Obwegeser periosteal r.
Ochsner r.
Ochsner-Favaloro self-
  retaining r.
Ochsner malleable r.
Ochsner ribbon r.
Ochsner vascular r.
O'Connor r.
O'Connor abdominal r.
O'Connor-O'Sullivan r.
O'Connor-O'Sullivan
  abdominal r.
O'Connor-O'Sullivan self-
  retaining r.
O'Connor-O'Sullivan
  vaginal r.
O'Connor vaginal r.
Oertli lid r.
Oertli wire lid r.
Oettingen abdominal r.
Oettingen abdominal self-
  retaining r.
offset hand r.
Oldberg brain r.
Oldberg straight r.
Oliver r.
Oliver scalp r.
Ollier r.
Ollier rake r.
Omni r.
orbital r.
Orley r.

retractor *(continued)*
orthopaedic r.
Osher iris r.
Osher lid r.
Osher micro-iris r.
O'Sullivan r.
O'Sullivan abdominal r.
O'Sullivan-O'Connor r.
O'Sullivan-O'Connor
 abdominal r.
O'Sullivan-O'Connor self-
 retaining r.
O'Sullivan-O'Connor
 vaginal r.
O'Sullivan self-retaining
 abdominal r.
O'Sullivan vaginal r.
Otto Barkan bident r.
r. oval sprocket frame
Overholt r.
Packiam r.
palate r.
Paparella r.
Paparella self-retaining r.
Paparella-Weitlaner r.
Parker r.
Parker double-ended r.
Parker-Mott double-ended r.
Parker thumb r.
Parkes nasal r.
Parks r.
Parks anal r.
parotidectomy r.
Parsonnet epicardial r.
patent ductus r.
Paul r.
Paul lacrimal r.
Paul lacrimal sac r.
Paulson knee r.
Payr r.
Payr abdominal r.
Peck rake r.
pediatric r.
pediatric abdominal r.
pediatric self-retaining r.
Peet lighted splanchnic r.
Pemberton r.
Penfield r.
Percy r.
Percy amputation r.
Percy bone r.
Percy-Wolfson r.
Percy-Wolfson gallbladder r.

perineal r.
perineal prostatectomy r.
perineal self-retaining r.
peripheral vascular r.
Perkins r.
Perkins otologic r.
Perman-Stille abdominal r.
pharyngeal r.
Pheifer-Young r.
Phiefer-Young r.
Phoropter r.
phrenic r.
Pickrell r.
Picot r.
Picot vaginal r.
Pierce r.
Pierce cheek r.
pillar r.
Pilling r.
Pilling-Favaloro r.
Piper lateral wall r.
Plester r.
Poliak eye r.
Polytrac r.
Polytrac Gomez r.
Pomeranz r.
Pomeranz hiatal hernia r.
popliteal r.
Poppen-Gelpi
 laminectomy r.
Poppen-Gelpi laminectomy
 self-retaining r.
Portmann r.
Posada-Vasco orbital r.
postauricular r.
posterior fossa r.
posterior urethral r.
Pratt bivalve r.
Proctor r.
Proctor cheek r.
3-prong r.
4-prong r.
6-prong r.
pronged r.
2-prong rake r.
prostate r.
prostatic r.
Proud-White uvula r.
Pryor-Péan vaginal r.
psoas r.
pulmonary r.
Purcell r.

Purcell self-retaining abdominal r.
push r.
Quervain abdominal r.
Quervain-Sauerbruch r.
Radcliff r.
Radcliff perineal r.
Ragnell r.
Ragnell-Davis double-ended r.
Ragnell double-ended r.
rake r.
Ralks r.
Ralks ear r.
Raney r.
Raney laminectomy r.
Rankin r.
Rankin prostatic r.
Raylor malleable r.
rectal r.
rectal hook r.
rectus r.
Rees disposable battery-driven lighted r.
Rees lighted r.
Rehbein infant abdominal r.
Rehne r.
Rehne abdominal r.
Remine mastectomy skin flap r.
renal r.
renal sinus r.
retaining r.
retropubic r.
retropubic prostatectomy r.
rib r.
ribbon r.
ribbon malleable r.
Rica brain r.
Rica mastoid r.
Rica multipurpose r.
Rica posterior cranial fossa r.
Ricard abdominal r.
Rica scalp r.
Richards abdominal r.
Richardson r.
Richardson abdominal r.
Richardson appendectomy r.
Richardson-Eastman r.
Richardson-Eastman double-ended r.
Richter r.

Richter vaginal r.
Rigby r.
Rigby abdominal r.
Rigby appendectomy r.
Rigby bivalve r.
Rigby rectal r.
Rigby vaginal r.
right-angle r.
ring abdominal r.
Rissler kidney r.
Rizzo r.
Rizzuti r.
Rizzuti iris r.
Roberts thumb r.
Robin-Masse abdominal r.
Robinson r.
Robinson lung r.
Rochester r.
Rochester atrial r.
Rochester atrial septal r.
Rochester atrial septal defect r.
Rochester colonial r.
Rochester-Ferguson r.
Rochester-Ferguson double-ended r.
Rochester rake r.
Rogers vaginal r.
Rollet r.
Rollet eye r.
Rollet lacrimal sac r.
Rollet lake r.
Rollet skin r.
Roos r.
Roos brachial plexus root r.
Rose double-ended r.
Rosenbaum-Drews r.
Rosenbaum-Drews iris r.
Rosenbaum-Drews plastic r.
Rosenbaum iris r.
Rosenberg r.
Rosenberg full-radius blade synovial r.
Rosenberg-Sampson r.
Rose tracheal r.
Ross r.
Ross aortic r.
Ross aortic valve r.
Rotalok skin r.
Roux r.
Roux double-ended r.
Rowe r.
Rowe boathook r.

retractor *(continued)*
Rowe scapular neck r.
Rowe scapular neck
spike r.
Row humeral head r.
Rudolph trowel r.
Rumel r.
Ryecroft r.
Ryerson r.
Ryerson bone r.
S r.
Sachs r.
Sachs angled vein r.
Sachs-Cushing r.
Sachs vein r.
Sanchez-Bulnes r.
Sanchez-Bulnes lacrimal sac
self-retaining r.
Sato lid r.
Sauerbruch r.
Sauerbruch-Zukschwerdt r.
Sauerbruch-Zukschwerdt
rib r.
Sawyer r.
Sawyer rectal r.
Sayre r.
scalp r.
scalp self-retaining r.
Scanlan r.
Scanlan pediatric r.
scapular r.
Schepens r.
Schepens eye r.
Schepens orbital r.
Schindler r.
Schnitker scalp r.
Schoenborn r.
Schuknecht r.
Schuknecht postauricular r.
Schuknecht postauricular
self-retaining r.
Schuknecht-Wullstein r.
Schultz r.
Schultz iris r.
Schultz irrgating iris r.
Schwartz r.
Schwartz laminectomy r.
Schwartz laminectomy self-
retaining r.
scleral wound r.
Scott peds r.
Scoville r.
Scoville Britetrac r.

Scoville cervical disk r.
Scoville cervical disk self-
retaining r.
Scoville-Haverfield
hemilaminectomy r.
Scoville-Haverfield
laminectomy r.
Scoville hemilaminectomy r.
Scoville hemilaminectomy
self-retaining r.
Scoville laminectomy r.
Scoville nerve r.
Scoville nerve root r.
Scoville psoas muscle r.
Scoville-Richter r.
Scoville-Richter self-
retaining r.
Scoville self-retaining r.
Seen r.
Segond r.
Segond abdominal r.
Seldin dental r.
Seletz-Gelpi r.
Seletz-Gelpi laminectomy r.
Seletz-Gelpi self-retaining r.
self-retaining r.
self-retaining abdominal r.
self-retaining skin r.
self-retaining spring r.
Semb r.
Semb lung r.
Semb self-retaining r.
Semm abdominal r.
Senn r.
Senn-Dingman r.
Senn-Dingman double-
ended r.
Senn double-ended r.
Senn-Green r.
Senn-Kanavel r.
Senn-Kanavel double-
ended r.
Senn mastoid r.
Senn-Miller r.
Senn self-retaining r.
Senturia r.
serrated r.
serrefine r.
r. set
Sewall r.
Sewall orbital r.
Shambaugh r.
Shambaugh endaural r.

Shambaugh endaural self-
retaining r.
sharp-pronged r.
Shearer r.
Shearer lip r.
Sheehan r.
Sheldon r.
Sheldon-Gosset r.
Sheldon-Gosset self-
retaining r.
Sheldon hemilaminectomy r.
Sheldon hemilaminectomy
self-retaining r.
Sheldon laminectomy r.
Sherwin self-retaining r.
Sherwood r.
short Heaney r.
Shriners Hospital r.
Shriners Hospital
interlocking r.
Shriners interlocking r.
Shuletz-Paul rib r.
Shurly r.
Shurly tracheal r.
r. side blade
Silverstein lateral venous
sinus r.
Simon r.
Simon vaginal r.
Sims r.
Sims double-ended r.
Sims-Kelly r.
Sims-Kelly vaginal r.
Sims rectal r.
Sims vaginal r.
single blade r.
Sisson-Love r.
Sisson spring r.
Sistrunk r.
Sistrunk band r.
Sistrunk double-ended r.
six-prong rake r.
skin r.
skin flap r.
skin hook r.
skin self-retaining r.
Sloan r.
Sloan goiter r.
Sloan goiter self-retaining r.
Sluder r.
Sluder palate r.
Small rake r.
Small tissue r.

SMIC cheek r.
Smillie r.
Smillie knee joint r.
Smith r.
Smith anal r.
Smith-Buie r.
Smith-Buie anal r.
Smith-Buie rectal r.
Smith-Buie rectal self-
retaining r.
Smith nerve root suction r.
Smith-Petersen r.
Smith-Petersen capsular r.
Smith rectal r.
Smith rectal self-retaining r.
Smith vaginal r.
Smith vaginal self-
retaining r.
Smithwick r.
Snitman r.
Snitman endaural r.
Snitman endaural self-
retaining r.
Sofield r.
soft palate r.
spike r.
spinal r.
spinal cord r.
Spivey iris r.
splanchnic r.
spoon r.
spring r.
spring-wire r.
Spurling r.
S-shaped r.
S-shaped brain r.
Stack r.
stay suture r.
Steiner-Auvard vaginal r.
sternal r.
sternotomy r.
Stevens lacrimal r.
Stevenson r.
Stevenson lacrimal r.
Stevenson lacrimal sac r.
Stille-Broback knee r.
Stille cheek r.
Stille heart r.
Stiwer r.
St. Luke's r.
St. Mark's Hospital r.
St. Mark's lipped r.
St. Mark's pelvis r.

retractor *(continued)*

Stookey r.
Storer r.
Storer thoracoabdominal r.
Storz r.
straight r.
Strandell r.
Strandell-Stille r.
Struck laminectomy r.
Strully r.
Strully nerve root r.
Stuck laminectomy self-
  retaining r.
submucous r.
suprapubic r.
suprapubic self-retaining r.
surgical r.
Sweeney r.
Sweeney posterior vaginal r.
Sweet r.
Sweet amputation r.
sweetheart r.
Symmonds hysterectomy r.
sympathectomy r.
table-fixed r.
Tara retropubic r.
Taylor r.
Taylor Britetrac r.
Taylor fiberoptic r.
Taylor spinal r.
Temple-Fay r.
Temple-Fay laminectomy r.
Tepas r.
Theis r.
Theis self-retaining r.
Theis vein r.
Thoma tissue r.
Thompson r.
Thorlakson r.
Thorlakson deep
  abdominal r.
Thorlakson multipurpose r.
Thornton iris r.
three-prong r.
thumb r.
Thurmond r.
Thurmond iris r.
thymus r.
thyroid r.
tibial r.
Tiko rake r.
Tillary r.
Tillary double-ended r.

tissue r.
T-malleable r.
T-model endaural r.
Toennis r.
tonsillar r.
tonsillar pillar r.
toothed r.
Tower r.
Tower interchangeable r.
Tower rib r.
Tower spinal r.
tracheal r.
transoral r.
Trent eye r.
trigeminal r.
trigeminal self-retaining r.
Tubinger self-retaining r.
Tucker-Levine vocal cord r.
Tuffier r.
Tuffier abdominal r.
Tuffier-Raney r.
Tuffier-Raney
  laminectomy r.
Tuffier rib r.
Turner-Doyen r.
Turner-Warwick r.
Turner-Warwick posterior
  urethral r.
Turner-Warwick prostate r.
two-prong rake r.
Tyrer nerve root r.
Tyrell hook r.
Ullrich r.
Ullrich laminectomy r.
Ullrich self-retaining r.
Ullrich-St. Gallen self-
  retaining r.
Universal r.
upper-hand r.
upper-lateral exposing r.
Urban r.
USA r.
U.S. Army r.
U.S. Army double-ended r.
U.S. Army-pattern r.
U-shaped r.
uvular r.
Vacher r.
Vacher self-retaining r.
vacuum r.
vaginal r.
vagotomy r.
Vail lid r.

Vaiser-Dibis muscle r.
Valin hemilaminectomy r.
Valin hemilaminectomy self-
retaining r.
Vasco-Posada orbital r.
vascular r.
vascular spring r.
Veenema r.
Veenema retropubic r.
Veenema retropubic self-
retaining r.
vein r.
ventriculogram r.
Verbrugge r.
vertical r.
vertical bone self-
retaining r.
vesical r.
vessel r.
Viboch graft r.
Viboch iliac graft r.
Vinke r.
V. Mueller-Balfour
abdominal r.
V. Mueller fiberoptic r.
Volkmann r.
Volkmann finger r.
Volkmann hand r.
Volkmann pocket r.
Volkmann rake r.
Wachtenfeldt-Stille r.
Walker r.
Walker gallbladder r.
Walker lid r.
Walter-Deaver r.
Wangensteen r.
Weary nerve root r.
Webb r.
Webb-Balfour r.
Webb-Balfour abdominal r.
Webb-Balfour self-
retaining r.
Weber r.
Webster r.
Webster abdominal r.
Weder r.
Weder-Solenberger r.
Weder-Solenberger pillar r.
Weder-Solenberger
tonsillar r.
Weder-Solenberger tonsillar
pillar r.
weighted r.

weighted posterior r.
Weinberg r.
Weinberg "Joe's hoe"
double-ended r.
Weinberg vagotomy r.
Weinstein horizontal r.
Weinstein intestinal r.
Weitlaner r.
Weitlaner brain r.
Weitlaner hinged r.
Weitlaner microsurgery r.
Weitlaner self-retaining r.
Wellington Hospital
vaginal r.
Wesson r.
Wesson perineal r.
Wesson perineal self-
retaining r.
Wesson vaginal r.
Wexler r.
Wexler abdominal r.
Wexler-Balfour r.
Wexler-Bantam r.
Wexler-Deaver blade
abdominal r.
Wexler deep-spreader blade
abdominal r.
Wexler expandable-blade
abdominal r.
Wexler large-frame
abdominal r.
Wexler lateral side-blade
abdominal r.
Wexler malleable-blade
abdominal r.
Wexler self-retaining r.
Wexler standard
abdominal r.
Wexler standard-frame
abdominal r.
Wexler Universal-joint
abdominal r.
Wexler vaginal r.
Wexler X-P large
abdominal r.
White-Proud r.
White-Proud uvular r.
Wieder dental r.
Wieder pillar r.
Wieder-Solenberger pillar r.
Wiet r.
Wigderson ribbon r.
Wilauer-Deaver r.

retractor *(continued)*
    Wilder r.
    Wilder scleral r.
    Wilder scleral self-
      retaining r.
    Wilder scleral wound r.
    Wilkes self-retaining r.
    Wilkinson r.
    Wilkinson abdominal r.
    Wilkinson abdominal self-
      retaining r.
    Wilkinson-Deaver blade
      abdominal r.
    Wilkinson ring-frame
      abdominal r.
    Willauer-Deaver r.
    Williams microlumbar r.
    Williams microlumbar
      diskectomy r.
    Williams microlumbar
      diskectomy suction r.
    Wills eye lacrimal r.
    Wilmer r.
    Wilmer-Bagley r.
    Wilmer cryosurgical iris r.
    Wilmer iris r.
    Wilson r.
    Wilson hand r.
    Wiltse-Bankart r.
    Wiltse-Gelpi r.
    Wiltse-Gelpi self-retaining r.
    Wiltse iliac r.
    Winsburg-White r.
    wiring r.
    Wise r.
    Wise orbital r.
    Wolf meniscal r.
    Wolfson r.
    Wolfson gallbladder r.
    Woodward r.
    Worrall r.
    Worrall deep r.
    Wort antral r.
    Wullstein r.
    Wullstein ear self-
      retaining r.
    Wullstein-Weitlaner r.
    Wullstein-Weitlaner self-
      retaining r.
    Wylie r.
    Wylie renal vein r.
    Wylie splanchnic r.
    X-ray translucent r.
    Yasargil r.
    Young r.
    Young anterior r.
    Young anterior prostatic r.
    Young bifid r.
    Young bladder r.
    Young bulb r.
    Young lateral r.
    Young lateral prostatic r.
    Young prostatic r.
    Z r.
    Zalkind-Balfour center-
      blade r.
    Zalkind-Balfour self-
      retaining r.
    Zalkind lung r.
    Zenker r.
    Zimberg esophageal hiatal r.
    Zylik-Michaels r.

retractor-contractor
retractor-speculum
    Aufricht r.-s.
retrieval
    r. forceps
    r. loop
Retriever
    Golden R.
retriever
    basket r.
    Brimfield magnetic r.
    Carroll tendon r.
    Kleinert-Kutz tendon r.
    magnetic r.
    Pfister-Schwartz stone r.
    plaque r.
    Soehendra stent r.
    stone r.
    ureteral stone r.
    Vantec loop r.
    Warren-Wilder r.
    Wilson-Cook ministent r.
retrobulbar
    r. needle
    r. prosthesis needle
retrodisplaced pessary
retrograde
    r. Beaver blade
    r. blade
    r. bougie
    r. curette
    r. electrode
    r. knife

r. meniscal blade
r. valvulotome
retroperfusion catheter
retropubic
r. prostatectomy retractor
r. retractor
retrospective telescope
retroversion pessary
Retter
R. aneurysm needle
R. needle
return-flow
r.-f. cannula
r.-f. catheter
r.-f. hemostatic catheter
r.-f. retention catheter
Reul
R. aortic clamp
R. coronary artery scissors
R. coronary forceps
reusable vein stripper
Reuse Expanda-graft dermatome
Reuter
R. bobbin collar button
R. bobbin implant
R. bobbin ventilation tube
R. button
Revelation handpiece
Reverdin
R. graft
R. holder
R. implant
R. needle
R. prosthesis
R. spatula
R. suturing needle
reverse
r. adenotome
r. bandage
r. cystotome
r. intraocular lens
r. knuckle-bender splint
r. scissors
reverse-action hypophysectomy forceps
reverse-angle skid curette
reverse-bevel laryngoscope
reverse-curve
r.-c. adenoid curette
r.-c. clamp
reverse-cutting
r.-c. meniscal probe
r.-c. needle

r.-c. probe
r.-c. scissors
r.-c. suture
reversed bandage
reverse-shaped eye implant
reverse-threaded screw
reversion pacemaker
revision conical reamer
Revivac catheter
Revive system penile prosthesis
Revots vulsellum tenaculum
Rew-Wyly
R.-W. blade
R.-W. mouth gag
Rexton hearing aid
Reynolds
R. clamp
R. dissecting clamp
R. dissecting scissors
R. infusion catheter
R. resection clamp
R. scissors
R. skull traction tongs
R. vascular clamp
Reynolds-Jameson vessel scissors
Rezek forceps
Rezifilm dressing
Reziplast spray-on dressing
RF balloon catheter
rhabdoid suture
Rheinstaedter
R. curette
R. flushing curette
R. uterine curette
Rhinelander
R. clamp
R. guide
R. pin
R. plate
rhinolaryngoscope
rhinolarynx stroboscope
rhinoplasty
r. diamond bur
r. implant
rhinoscope
Wolf-Post r.
Wylie-Post r.
rhinoscopic mirror
Rhode Island
R. I. dissector
R. I. Secto dissector
Rhoton
R. ball dissector

Rhoton *(continued)*
R. bayonet bipolar forceps
R. bayonet needle holder
R. bayonet scissors
R. bipolar forceps
R. cup forceps
R. curette
R. dissector
R. dressing forceps
R. dural forceps
R. elevator
R. enucleator
R. forceps
R. general purpose elevator
R. grasping forceps
R. hook
R. horizontal ring curette
R. loop curette
R. microcup forceps
R. microcurette
R. microdissecting forceps
R. microforceps
R. microneedle holder
R. microscissors
R. microsurgical scissors
R. microtying forceps
R. microvascular forceps
R. needle
R. needle holder
R. nerve hook
R. osteotome
R. pituitary curette
R. 3-prong fork
R. punch
R. ring tumor forceps
R. round dissector
R. scissors
R. sellar punch
R. spatula dissector
R. spoon curette
R. straight point needle
R. tissue forceps
R. transsphenoidal bipolar
forceps
R. tumor forceps
R. tying forceps
R. vertical ring curette
Rhoton-Adson
R.-A. dressing forceps
R.-A. tissue forceps
Rhoton-Cushing
R.-C. dressing forceps

R.-C. forceps
R.-C. tissue forceps
Rhoton-Merz
R.-M. rotatable coupling
head
R.-M. suction tube
Rhoton-Tew bipolar forceps
rhytidectomy scissors
Riahl coronary compressor
rib
r. brad awl
r. contractor
r. drill
r. edge stripper
r. needle
r. raspatory
r. retractor
r. rongeur forceps
r. shears
r. spreader (*See* spreader)
r. stripper
Riba
R. electrical ureteral
meatotome
R. electrourethrotome
electrode
R. urethrotome
Riba-Valeira forceps
Ribble
R. bandage
R. dressing
ribbon
r. gut needle
r. gut suture
r. malleable retractor
r. retractor
Rica
R. anesthetic laryngoscope
R. aneurysm needle
R. anterior commissure
laryngoscope
R. arterial clamp
R. bone drill
R. bone hammer
R. bone mallet
R. bone rongeur
R. brain retractor
R. brain spatula
R. cerebral angiography
puncture needle
R. cerumen hook
R. clamp
R. clip-applying forceps

R. cotton carrier
R. cranial rongeur
R. cranioclast
R. cross-action towel clip
R. dermatome
R. ear curette
R. ear polypus scissors
R. ear probe
R. ear speculum
R. esophagoscopy set
R. eustachian catheter
R. forceps holder
R. gouge
R. guide pin
R. hemostatic forceps
R. hook
R. infant laryngoscope
R. laminectomy rongeur
R. laryngoscope
R. lipoma curette
R. malleus head nipper
R. mastoid chisel
R. mastoid curette
R. mastoid gouge
R. mastoid retractor
R. mastoid rongeur
R. mastoid suction tube
R. micro-arterial clamp
R. multipurpose retractor
R. myringotome
R. nasal periosteal elevator
R. nasal septal speculum
R. nasal speculum
R. nylon
R. pelvimeter
R. pneumatic otoscope
R. posterior cranial fossa retractor
R. powder blower
R. scalp retractor
R. silver clip
R. skull perforator set
R. spinal rongeur
R. stem clamp
R. surgical catgut
R. suture clip
R. suturing needle
R. tracheostomy cannula
R. trigeminal knife
R. tuning fork
R. Universal trocar
R. uterine curette
R. uterine sound

R. vaginal speculum
R. vessel clamp
R. wire guide pin
R. wire saw
Rica-Adson forceps
Ricard abdominal retractor
Richard
R. Gruber speculum
R. Wolf arthroscope
R. Wolf laparoscope
R. Wolf Medical Instruments diagnostic laparoscope
R. Wolf Medical Instruments operating laparoscope
Richard-Allan surgical ruler
Richards
R. abdominal retractor
R. Andrews forceps
R. bone clamp
R. bone curette
R. bone hook
R. bone tap
R. chisel
R. clamp
R. classic compression hip screw
R. Cobb spinal elevator
R. Cobb spinal gouge
R. Colles fracture frame
R. combination mallet
R. compression device
R. compression screw
R. curette
R. drill guide
R. ethmoid curette
R. fixation staple
R. fixator system
R. forceps
R. headrest
R. Hibbs gouge
R. Hibbs osteotome
R. hip endoprosthesis system
R. Lovejoy bone drill
R. mastoid curette
R. ministaple
R. Phillips screwdriver
R. pistol-grip drill
R. probe
R. prosthesis
R. sideplate plate

Richards *(continued)*
   R. Solcotrans orthopaedic drainage-reinfusion system
   R. Solcotrans Plus drainage system
   R. tonsil-grasping forceps
   R. tonsillar forceps
   R. tonsil-seizing forceps
   R. wire twister
Richards-Hibbs chisel
Richards-Moeller pneumatic air-filled dilator
Richardson
   R. abdominal retractor
   R. angle suture
   R. appendectomy retractor
   R. periosteal elevator
   R. polyethylene tube introducer
   R. retractor
   R. suture
Richardson-Eastman
   R.-E. double-ended retractor
   R.-E. retractor
Riches diathermy forceps
Richet
   R. bandage
   R. dressing
Rich forceps
Richmond
   R. bolt
   R. forceps
   R. subarachnoid screw
   R. subarachnoid screw sensor
   R. subarachnoid twist drill
   R. subarachnoid wrench
Richnau-Holmgren ear speculum
Richter
   R. bone drill
   R. bone screwdriver
   R. forceps
   R. laminectomy punch
   R. retractor
   R. scissors
   R. screwdriver
   R. suture
   R. suture clip-removing forceps
   R. vaginal retractor
Richter-Heath
   R.-H. clip forceps
   R.-H. clip-removing forceps
   R.-H. forceps
   R.-H. suture-removing forceps
Richwil crown and bridge remover
Rickett facebow
Rickham
   R. cup
   R. reservoir
   R. reservoir shunt
Riddle coagulator
Rider-Moeller
   R.-M. cardia dilator
   R.-M. needle
   R.-M. pneumatic dilator
ridged
   r. lenses intraocular lens
   r. lenses lens
   r. posterior chamber intraocular lens
ridge forceps
Ridley
   R. anterior chamber implant
   R. forceps
   R. Mark II lens implant
Ridlon
   R. plaster knife
   R. spreader
Ridpath
   R. curette
   R. ethmoid curette
Riecker-Kleinsasser laryngoscope
Riecker respiration bronchoscope
Riedel
   R. corneal needle
   R. needle
Rienhoff
   R. arterial clamp
   R. arterial forceps
   R. clamp
   R. dissector
   R. rib spreader
Rienhoff-Finochietto rib contractor
Rienhoff-Finochietto rib spreader
Rigal suture
Rigby
   R. abdominal retractor
   R. appendectomy retractor
   R. bivalve retractor
   R. rectal retractor
   R. retractor
   R. vaginal retractor
Rigenberg forceps

Rigg cannula
right
   r. atrial cuff
   r. coronary catheter
   r. ventricular assist device
right-angle
   r.-a. chest catheter
   r.-a. clamp
   r.-a. colon clamp
   r.-a. curette
   r.-a. elevator
   r.-a. erysiphake
   r.-a. examining telescope
   r.-a. forceps
   r.-a. hook
   r.-a. knife
   r.-a. mattress suture
   r.-a. pick
   r.-a. retractor
   r.-a. scissors
   r.-a. telescope
rigid
   r. biopsy forceps
   r. curette
   r. endoscope
   r. holding rod
   r. intraocular lens
   r. kidney stone forceps
   r. sigmoidoscope
   r. sound
Rigident denture adhesive
Rigiflex
   R. balloon
   R. balloon dilator
   R. dilator
Riley
   R. arterial needle
   R. needle
Ring
   R. biliary drainage catheter
   R. catheter
   R. hip prosthesis
   R. knee prosthesis
ring
   r. abdominal retractor
   adult retractor set r.
   r. bayonet Rand curette
   r. biliary stent
   r. blade
   blepharostat r.
   Bonaccolto-Flieringa
    scleral r.
   Bookwalter retractor r.

Bookwalter round r.
Bookwalter segmented r.
Bookwalter vaginal
  retractor r.
Budde halo hinged r.
carbon fiber half r.
Carpentier r.
r. cataract mask eye shield
r. clamp
Crawford suture r.
r. curette
r. cutters
Duran annuloplasty r.
Falope r.
Falope tubal sterilization r.
fixation r.
Flieringa r.
Flieringa fixation r.
Flieringa-Legrand fixation r.
Flieringa scleral r.
r. forceps
Girard scleral expander r.
gold r.
half r.
Katena r.
laparotomy r.
laparotomy sponge r.
laparotomy sponge r.
Magrina-Bookwalter vaginal
  retractor r.
Martinez scleral centering r.
Mayo perfusing "O" r.
McKinney fixation r.
McNeil-Goldman
  blepharostat r.
McNeil-Goldman scleral r.
Mertz keratoscopy r.
Moran-Karaya r.
Nakayama r.
pediatric-perineal retractor r.
perfusion O r.
r. pessary
pressure r.
Racestyptine retraction r.
reduction r.
r. remover
retainer r.
retention r.
retraction r.
r. retractor blade
sponge r.
St. Jude annuloplasty r.
r. stripper

ring *(continued)*
    suture r.
    symblepharon r.
    tantalum r.
    tantalum "O" r.
    Thornton fixating r.
    r. tongue blade
    Tru-Arc blood vessel r.
    Turner-Waru r.
    Turner-Warwick adult
      retractor r.
    Turner-Warwick pediatric
      perineal retractor r.
    vacuum fixation r.
    Valtrac anastomosis r.
    Walsh pressure r.
    Wolf-Yoon r.
    Yoon r.
    Yoon tubal sterilization r.
ring-cutting saw
Ring-Derlan TM biliary
  endoprosthesis
Ringenberg
    R. ear forceps
    R. electrode
    R. rasp
    R. stapedectomy forceps
ring-handled bulldog clamp
ring-jawed holding clamp
Ring-McLean catheter
ring-rotation forceps
Rionet hearing aid
Riordan
    R. flexible silver cannula
    R. pin
Ripstein
    R. arterial forceps
    R. forceps
    R. tissue forceps
Rish
    R. cartilage knife
    R. chisel
    R. osteotome
Risley
    R. pliers
    R. prism
Risser wedging jacket
Rissler
    R. kidney retractor
    R. mallet
    R. periosteal elevator
    R. pin
    R. vein sound

Rissler-Stille pin
Ristow osteotome
Ritch
    R. contact lens
    R. trabeculoplasty laser lens
Ritchey nail starter
Ritchie cleft palate tenaculum
Ritch-Krupin Denver eye valve
  insertion forceps
Ritisch suture
Ritter
    R. Bovie
    R. coagulator
    R. coagulator electrosurgical
      unit
    R. dilator
    R. drain
    R. forceps
    R. meatal dilator
    R. rasp
    R. sound
    R. suprapubic suction drain
    R. suprapubic suction tube
Ritter-Bantam
    R.-B. Bovie coagulator
    R.-B. Bovie electrosurgical
      unit
Riverbank Laboratories tuning fork
Riwomat respirator jet
Rizzoli osteoclast
Rizzo retractor
Rizzuti
    R. double-prong forceps
    R. eye expressor
    R. graft carrier spatula
    R. iris expressor
    R. iris retractor
    R. keratoplasty scissors
    R. lens expressor
    R. retractor
    R. scleral fixation forceps
    R. scleral forceps
    R. stitch-removal knife
    R. superior rectus forceps
Rizzuti-McGuire scissors
Rizzuti-Spizziri
    R.-S. cannula knife
    R.-S. knife
Rizzuti-Verhoeff forceps
Rizzutti forceps
Rizzutti-Furness cornea-holding
  forceps

RK
  radial keratotomy
  RK marker
RM
  RM crown
  RM orthodontic acrylic
    resin
RMC prosthesis
RME testicular punch
R-N clamp
Robb
  R. antral cannula
  R. cannula
  R. forceps
  R. needle
  R. sponge-holding forceps
  R. tonsillar forceps
  R. tonsillar knife
  R. tonsillar sponge forceps
Robbins automatic tourniquet
Robb-Roberts rotary rasp
Robert
  R. Bent Brigham knee
    prosthesis
  R. Brigham prosthesis
  R. Jones bandage
  R. Jones compressive
    dressing
  R. Jones dressing
  R. Jones splint
  R. nasal snare
Roberts
  R. abdominal trocar
  R. applicator
  R. arterial forceps
  R. bronchial biopsy forceps
  R. bronchial forceps
  R. chisel
  R. dental implant
  R. episiotomy scissors
  R. esophageal speculum
  R. esophagoscope
  R. folding esophagoscope
  R. forceps
  R. hemostatic forceps
  R. hip dissecting chisel
  R. laryngoscope
  R. needle
  R. oval esophagoscope
  R. oval speculum
  R. self-retaining
    laryngoscope
  R. thumb retractor

Roberts-Jesberg esophagoscope
Roberts-Nelson
  R.-N. lobectomy tourniquet
  R.-N. rib stripper
Robertson
  R. corneal trephine
  R. forceps
  R. suprapubic drain
  R. tonsillar forceps
  R. tonsillar knife
  R. tonsil-seizing forceps
Roberts-Singley
  R.-S. dressing forceps
  R.-S. thumb forceps
Robinject needle injector
Robin-Masse abdominal retractor
Robin orthodontic plate
Robinson
  R. artifical apparatus
  R. artificial pneumothorax
    apparatus
  R. bag
  R. catheter
  R. dislodger
  R. equalizing tube
  R. flap knife
  R. incus replacement
    prosthesis
  R. lung retractor
  R. middle ear prosthesis
  R. piston prosthesis
  R. retractor
  R. stapes prosthesis
  R. stone basket
  R. stone dislodger
  R. strut
  R. urethral catheter
Robinson-Moon
  R.-M. prosthesis inserter
  R.-M. stapes prosthesis
**Robinson-Moon-Lippy stapes
  prosthesis**
Robinson-Smith
  R.-S. needle
  R.-S. tamp
Robot Starr II camera
Robson intestinal forceps
Roch
  Rochester
Rochester (Roch)
  R. aortic vent needle
  R. atrial retractor

Rochester *(continued)*
R. atrial septal defect
   retractor
R. atrial septal retractor
R. awl
R. clamp
R. colonial retractor
R. dissector
R. dressing
R. elevator
R. forceps
R. gallstone forceps
R. hook clamp
R. laminar dissector
R. mitral stenosis knife
R. needle
R. needle holder
R. oral forceps
R. rake retractor
R. retractor
R. scissors
R. sigmoid clamp
R. sternum-perforating awl
   set
R. suction tube
R. syringe
R. tissue forceps
R. tracheal tube
Rochester-Carmalt
R.-C. forceps
R.-C. hemostatic forceps
R.-C. hysterectomy forceps
Rochester-Davis forceps
Rochester-Ewald
R.-E. forceps
R.-E. tissue forceps
Rochester-Ferguson
R.-F. double-ended retractor
R.-F. retractor
R.-F. scissors
Rochester-Harrington forceps
Rochester-Kocher clamp
Rochester-Meeker needle
Rochester-Mixter
R.-M. arterial forceps
R.-M. forceps
R.-M. gall duct forceps
Rochester-Müller forceps
Rochester-Ochsner (Roch-Ochs)
R.-O. forceps
R.-O. hemostat
R.-O. hemostat forceps
R.-O. scissors

Rochester-Péan
R.-P. clamp
R.-P. forceps
R.-P. hemostat
R.-P. hemostatic forceps
R.-P. hysterectomy forceps
Rochester-Rankin
R.-R. arterial forceps
R.-R. forceps
R.-R. hemostatic forceps
Rochester-Russian forceps
Roch-Ochs
Rochester-Ochsner
Rock endometrial suction curette
rocker-bottom cast boot shoe
rocket
Rockey
R. cannula
R. clamp
R. dilating probe
R. endoscope
R. forceps
R. mediastinal cannula
R. probe
R. tracheal cannula
R. vascular clamp
Rockey-Thompson catheter
Rock-Mulligan prosthesis
Rockwood shoulder screw
rod
Alta femoral
   intramedullary r.
r. bender
Biofix fixation r.
cloverleaf r.
cold rolled r.
colostomy r.
r. cutter
Edwards Universal r.
r. electrode
Ender r.
flared spinal r.
glass retracting r.
Green-Armytage polythene r.
Hamby r.
Harrington r.
r. holder
Hough measuring r.
House measuring r.
Hunter r.
Instra-Rack security r.
intramedullary alignment r.
intramedullary Rush r.

Knodt distraction r.
Küntscher r.
laser r.
Lincoff sponge r.
Maddox r.
McLaughlin laser r.
McLaughlin laser vaginal
  measuring r.
McLaughlin quartz r.
measuring r.
Meckel r.
Moe subcutaneous r.
Mouradian humeral r.
quartz r.
retracting r.
rigid holding r.
Rogozinski r.
round extension r.
Rush r.
Schneider r.
slotted intramedullary r.
Stader connecting r.
Stenzel fracture r.
telescoping r.
r. template
threaded r.
vaginal laser measuring r.
Veirs canaliculus r.
Wissinger r.
Zickel II subtrochanteric r.
Zickel supracondylar r.
Rodenstock
  R. lens
  R. panfundoscope
Rodin
  R. implant
  R. orbital implant
Rodriguez-Alvarez catheter
Rodriguez catheter
rod-sleeve
Roe
  R. aortic clamp
  R. aortic tourniquet clamp
Roeder
  R. clamp
  R. forceps
  R. towel clamp
  R. towel forceps
Roeltsch forceps
Roger
  R. Anderson apparatus
  R. Anderson appliance

R. Anderson external
  skeletal fixation device
R. Anderson fixation bar
R. Anderson pin
R. Anderson well-leg splint
R. dissector
R. elevator
R. forceps
R. hysterectomy forceps
R. septal elevator
R. septal knife
R. submucous dissector
R. vascular-toothed
  hysterectomy forceps
R. wire-cutting scissors
Rogers
  R. mammotone
  R. needle holder
  R. vaginal retractor
  R. wire cutter
Rogge sterilizing forceps
Rogozinski
  R. hook
  R. rod
  R. screw system
  R. spinal rod system
**Rohm and Haas PMMA
  intraocular lens**
Rohrschneider
  R. cannula
  R. probe
Roland dilator
Rolf
  R. dilator
  R. forceps
  R. jeweler's forceps
  R. lacrimal probe
  R. lance needle
  R. muscle hook
  R. punctum dilator
  R. utility forceps
Rolf-Jackson cannula
roll
  ACCO cotton r.
  Celluron dental r.
  intrascapular r.
  Lakeside cotton r.
  Veratex cotton r.
roller
  r. ball
  r. bandage
  Devonshire r.
  r. dressing

roller *(continued)*
   r. electrode
   r. forceps
   r. head perfusion pump
   r. knife
   Spence cranioplastic r.
   tubing hand r.
Roller pump suction tube
Rollet
   R. chisel
   R. eye retractor
   R. lacrimal sac retractor
   R. lake retractor
   R. retractor
   R. rugine
   R. skin retractor
   R. strabismus hook
Rollett anterior chamber irrigator
Rolnel catheter
Rolodermatome
Rolyan
   R. brace
   R. tibial fracture brace
ROM
   range of motion
Roman laryngostat
romanoscope
Rommel-Hildreth cautery
Rondic sponge dressing
rongeur
   Adson r.
   Adson bone r.
   Adson cranial r.
   Andrews-Hartmann r.
   Bacon r.
   Bacon cranial r.
   Bacon cranial bone r.
   Bailey aortic r.
   Bailey aortic valve r.
   Bane r.
   Bane-Hartmann r.
   Bane mastoid r.
   Belz lacrimal r.
   Belz lacrimal sac r.
   Beyer r.
   Beyer bone r.
   Beyer endaural r.
   Beyer-Lempert r.
   biting r.
   Blakesley laminectomy r.
   Blumenthal r.
   Blumenthal bone r.
   Bogle r.

Böhler r.
Boies-Lombard mastoid r.
bone r.
bone-cutting r.
Bruening-Citelli r.
Cairns r.
Callahan lacrimal r.
Campbell laminectomy r.
Campbell nerve r.
Carroll r.
Caspar r.
Cherry-Kerrison
   laminectomy r.
Cicherelli r.
Cicherelli bone r.
Citelli r.
Citelli sphenoid r.
Cloward r.
Cloward-English r.
Cloward-Harper r.
Cloward-Harper
   laminectomy r.
Cloward intervertebral
   disk r.
Cloward laminectomy r.
Cloward pituitary r.
Cloward-type r.
Codman cervical r.
Codman-Kerrison r.
Codman-Kerrison
   laminectomy r.
Codman laminectomy r.
Codman-Leksell r.
Codman-Leksell
   laminectomy r.
Codman-Schlesinger r.
Codman-Schlesinger cervical
   laminectomy r.
Colclough r.
Colclough laminectomy r.
Colclough Love-Kerrison
   laminectomy r.
Converse-Lange r.
Converse nasal root r.
Costen-Kerrison r.
Cottle-Jansen r.
cranial r.
cranial bone r.
Cushing r.
Cushing bone r.
Cushing intervertebral
   disk r.
Cushing laminectomy r.

Cushing pituitary r.
Dahlgren r.
Dale first rib r.
Dale rib r.
Dale thoracic r.
Dawson-Yuhl-Kerrison r.
Dawson-Yuhl-Leksell r.
Dean r.
Dean bone r.
Decker r.
Decker microsurgical r.
Defourmental nasal r.
delicate intervertebral
 disk r.
Dench r.
dental r.
DePuy pituitary r.
DeVilbiss r.
DeVilbiss cranial r.
double-action r.
down-cutting r.
duckbill r.
Duggan r.
Echlin duckbill r.
Echlin laminectomy r.
Falconer r.
Ferris Smith r.
Ferris Smith disk r.
Ferris Smith-Gruenwald r.
Ferris Smith intervertebral
 disk r.
Ferris Smith-Kerrison r.
Ferris Smith-Kerrison
 disk r.
Ferris Smith-Kerrison
 laminectomy r.
Ferris Smith pituitary r.
Ferris Smith-Spurling r.
Ferris Smith-Takahashi r.
r. forceps
Friedman r.
Friedman bone r.
Frykholm bone r.
Fulton laminectomy r.
Gam-Mer r.
Glasgow-pattern r.
Glover r.
Goldman-Kazanjian r.
Gruenwald-Love
 intervertebral disk r.
Gruenwald pituitary r.
Guleke bone r.
Hajek antral r.

Hajek-Claus r.
Hajek downbiting r.
Hajek-Koffler r.
Hajek-Koffler
 laminectomy r.
Hajek-Koffler sphenoidal r.
Hajek upbiting r.
Hakansson r.
Hakansson bone r.
Hakansson-Olivecrona r.
Hartmann r.
Hartmann bone r.
Hartmann ear r.
Hartmann-Herzfeld ear r.
Hein r.
Henny laminectomy r.
Hoen r.
Hoen intervertebral disk r.
Hoen laminectomy r.
Hoffmann ear r.
Horsley bone r.
Houghton r.
Husk r.
Husk mastoid r.
intervertebral disk r.
IVD r.
Ivy mastoid r.
Jackson r.
Jansen bayonet r.
Jansen bone r.
Jansen-Cottle r.
Jansen-Middleton r.
Jansen-Zaufel r.
Jarit-Kerrison r.
Jarit-Ruskin r.
jaw r.
Juers-Lempert r.
Juers-Lempert endaural r.
Kazanjian-Goldman r.
Kerrison r.
Kerrison cervical r.
Kerrison-Costen r.
Kerrison-Ferris Smith r.
Kerrison lumbar r.
Kerrison mastoid r.
Kerrison-Morgenstein r.
Kerrison-Schwartz r.
Kerrison-Spurling r.
Killearn r.
Kleinert-Kutz r.
Kleinert-Kutz bone r.
Koffler-Hajek
 laminectomy r.

rongeur *(continued)*
    laminectomy r.
    Lange-Converse nasal
      root r.
    Lebsche r.
    Leksell r.
    Leksell bone r.
    Leksell laminectomy r.
    Leksell-Stille r.
    Lempert r.
    Lempert bone r.
    Lempert endaural r.
    Lempert-Juers r.
    Lillie r.
    Liston-Luer-Whiting r.
    Littauer r.
    Lombard r.
    Lombard-Beyer r.
    Lombard-Boies mastoid r.
    Love-Gruenwald r.
    Love-Gruenwald
      intervertebral disk r.
    Love-Gruenwald
      laminectomy r.
    Love-Gruenwald pituitary r.
    Love-Kerrison r.
    Luer r.
    Luer bone r.
    Luer-Friedmann r.
    Luer-Hartmann r.
    Luer-Liston-Wheeling r.
    Luer-Stille r.
    Luer thoracic r.
    Markwalder rib r.
    Marquardt bone r.
    mastoid r.
    Mead bone r.
    Mead dental r.
    Mollison mastoid r.
    Montenovesi cranial r.
    Morgenstein-Kerrison r.
    Nichols infundibulectomy r.
    Nicola r.
    Noyes r.
    O'Brien r.
    Oldberg intervertebral
      disk r.
    Oldberg laminectomy r.
    Oldberg pituitary r.
    Olivecrona r.
    Olivecrona endaural r.
    orthopaedic r.
    peapod intervertebral disk r.

    Peiper-Beyer bone r.
    Pennybacker r.
    Pierce r.
    Pilling-Ruskin r.
    pituitary r.
    Poppen intervertebral
      disk r.
    Poppen laminectomy r.
    Poppen pituitary r.
    Prince r.
    Raaf-Oldberg r.
    Raney r.
    Raney laminectomy r.
    rat-tooth r.
    Reiner r.
    Rica bone r.
    Rica cranial r.
    Rica laminectomy r.
    Rica mastoid r.
    Rica spinal r.
    Ronjair air-powered r.
    Röttgen-Ruskin bone r.
    Rowland r.
    Rowland nasal r.
    Ruskin r.
    Ruskin bone r.
    Ruskin duckbill r.
    Ruskin-Jay r.
    Ruskin mastoid r.
    Ruskin multiple-action r.
    Ruskin-Storz r.
    Sauerbruch r.
    Sauerbruch-Coryllos rib r.
    Sauerbruch-Lebsche r.
    Scaglietti r.
    Schlesinger r.
    Schlesinger cervical r.
    Schlesinger intervertebral
      disk r.
    Schlesinger laminectomy r.
    Schwartz-Kerrison r.
    Selverstone intervertebral
      disk r.
    Selverstone laminectomy r.
    Semb r.
    Semb-Sauerbruch r.
    Shearer r.
    Shearer bone r.
    SMIC bone r.
    SMIC cranial r.
    SMIC laminectomy r.
    SMIC mastoid r.
    Smith-Petersen r.

Smith-Petersen
laminectomy r.
Smolik curved r.
Smolinski endaural r.
Spence intervertebral disk r.
Spence intervertebral disk r.
Spurling r.
Spurling intervertebral
disk r.
Spurling-Kerrison r.
Spurling laminectomy r.
Spurling-Love-Gruenwald-
Cushing r.
Spurling pituitary r.
Stellbrink synovectomy r.
Stille-Beyer r.
Stille bone r.
Stille-Horsley r.
Stille-Leksell r.
Stille-Liston r.
Stille-Luer r.
Stille-Luer angled r.
Stille-Luer angular
duckbill r.
Stille-Luer bone r.
Stille-Luer-Echlin r.
Stille-Ruskin r.
Stille-Zaufal-Jansen r.
St. Luke's double-action r.
Stookey r.
Stookey cranial r.
Storz duckbill r.
Struempel r.
Strully-Kerrison r.
synovectomy r.
Takahashi r.
taper-jaw r.
Tobey ear r.
Universal Kerrison r.
Urschel r.
Urschel-Leksell r.
von Seemen r.
Voris intervertebral disk r.
Wagner r.
Walton r.
Walton-Ruskin r.
Watson-Williams
intervertebral disk r.
Weil-Blakesley r.
Weil pituitary r.
Weingartner r.
Whitcomb-Kerrison r.
Whiting mastoid r.

Wilde r.
Wilde intervertebral disk r.
Young r.
Young cystoscopic r.
Zaufel-Jansen r.
Zaufel-Jansen bone r.
Ronis
R. adenoidal punch
R. cutting forceps
R. tonsillar punch
Ronjair air-powered rongeur
Roos
R. brachial plexus root
retractor
R. first rib shears
R. retractor
Roosevelt
R. clamp
R. gastroenterostomy clamp
R. gastrointestinal clamp
R. intestinal clamp
root
r. canal broach
r. canal drill
r. canal file
r. canal spreader
r. needle
r. pliers
Roper
R. alpha-chymotrypsin
cannula
R. cannula
Roper-Rumel tourniquet
Rosa-Berens eye implant
rosary bougie
Rosato fascial splitter
Rosch catheter
Roschke dropper sponge
Rose
R. bed dressing
R. disimpaction forceps
R. double-ended retractor
R. L-type nose bridge
prosthesis
R. tracheal retractor
Rosebud dissector
Rosen
R. angular elevator
R. bayonet separator
R. bur
R. cartilage knife
R. curette
R. dissector

Rotablator (handwritten)

Rosen *(continued)*
R. ear incision knife
R. ear probe
R. endaural probe
R. fenestrator
R. fenestrometer
R. guide wire
R. hone
R. incision knife
R. incontinence device
R. inflatable urinary incontinence prosthesis
R. J-guide wire
R. knife curette
R. middle ear instrument
R. needle
R. pick
R. probe
R. separator
R. suction
R. suction tube
R. urinary incontinence prosthesis
Rosenbaum-Drews
R.-D. iris retractor
R.-D. plastic retractor
R.-D. retractor
Rosenbaum iris retractor
Rosenberg
R. full-radius blade synovial retractor
R. meniscal repair kit
R. retractor
Rosenberg-Sampson retractor
Rosenblatt scissors
Rosenfeld hip prosthesis
Rosenmüller, Rosenmueller
R. curette
R. fossa curette
Rosenthal
R. needle
R. urethral speculum
Rosenthal-French nebulization dosimeter
Roser
R. mouth gag
R. needle
Roser-Koenig mouth gag
rosette blade
Ross
R. aortic retractor
R. aortic valve retractor
R. catheter

R. needle
R. retractor
Rosser crypt hook
Rotalok
R. cup
R. skin retractor
R. wrist strap
rotary
r. basket
r. dissector
r. hub saw
r. scissors with cigar handle
r. scissors with loop handle
rotatable
r. coupling head
r. polypectomy snare
r. transsphenoidal enucleator
r. transsphenoidal horizontal ring curette
r. transsphenoidal knife handle
r. transsphenoidal right-angle hook
r. transsphenoidal round dissector
r. transsphenoidal spatula dissector
r. transsphenoidal vertical ring curette
rotating
r. adapter
r. anoscope
r. forceps
r. laryngoscope
r. speculum anoscope
r. transilluminator
rotating-hinge knee prosthesis
rotation
r. device
r. forceps
rotational
r. ablation laser
r. atherectomy device
rotation-stop washer
rotator
Bechert r.
Bechert-Hoffer nucleus r.
Bechert-Kratz nucleus r.
Bechert nucleus r.
r. cuff
Jaffe-Bechert nucleus r.
nucleus r.
Osher globe r.

Rotex
  R. II biopsy needle
  R. needle
Roth dental cement
Rothene catheter
Rothman Institute porous femoral component
Roticulator
  R. 55 Poly stapler
  R. stapler
  R. 30 stapler
  R. 55 stapler
Roto-extractor extractor
Roto Kinetic bed
Roto-Rest bed
rotosteotome rotary handpiece
Röttgen-Ruskin bone rongeur
Roubaix forceps
round
  r. body needle
  r. bur
  r. chuck-end Kirschner wire
  r. cutting bur
  r. diamond bur
  r. dissector
  r. extension rod
  r. Gigli saw
  r. knife
  r. needle
  r. optical zone marker
  r. punch forceps
  r. PVC drain
  r. ruby knife
  r. speculum
  r. tapper
round-end cutter
round-loop electrode
round-tip
  r.-t. catheter
  r.-t. microscissors
round-wire electrode
Roush tonometer
Roussel-Fankhauser contact lens
router
  trochanteric r.
Roux
  R. double-ended retractor
  R. retractor
  R. spatula
Roveda eversor

Rovenstine
  R. catheter-introducing forceps
  R. forceps
Rowe
  R. boathook retractor
  R. bone-drilling forceps
  R. bone elevator
  R. disimpaction forceps
  R. forceps
  R. glenoidal punch
  R. glenoidal reamer
  R. maxillary forceps
  R. retractor
  R. scapular neck retractor
  R. scapular neck spike retractor
Rowe-Killey forceps
Rowen spinal fusion gouge
Row humeral head retractor
Rowland
  R. double-action forceps
  R. double-action hump forceps
  R. forceps
  R. hump forceps
  R. keratome
  R. nasal hump forceps
  R. nasal rongeur
  R. osteotome
  R. rongeur
Rowland-Hughes osteotomy spline
Rowsey
  R. cannula
  R. fixation cannula
Royal
  R. crown
  R. disposable skin stapler
  R. Flush angiographic flush catheter
  R. Hospital dilator
  R. spoon
Royale III denture resin
Royalite body jacket
Royalt-Street bougie
Royce
  R. bayonet ear knife
  R. ear knife
  R. forceps
  R. tympanum perforator
RS4 pacemaker
R-synchronous VVT pacemaker

rubber
- r. acorn tip
- r. airway
- r. bite liner
- r. catheter
- r. dam clamp
- r. dam drain
- r. drain
- r. finger cot
- r. Scan spray dressing
- r. shod clamp
- r. sponge
- r. suture

rubber-dam
- r.-d. clamp forceps
- r.-d. drain

rubber-reinforced bandage (REB)
rubber-shod
- r.-s. catheter
- r.-s. forceps

Rubbs aortic dilator
Rubens pillow
Rubgy deep-surgery forceps
Rubin
- R. bronchial clamp
- R. cannula
- R. clamp
- R. fallopian tube cannula
- R. gouge
- R. knife needle
- R. lateral osteotome
- R. morcellizer
- R. nasal chisel
- R. nasofrontal osteotome
- R. needle
- R. oblique rasp
- R. osteotome
- R. septal morcellizer

Rubin-Arnold needle
Rubin-Holth
- R.-H. modified sclerectomy punch
- R.-H. sclerectomy punch

Rubin-Lewis periosteal elevator
Rubinstein probe
Rubin-Wright forceps guard
Rubio
- R. needle holder
- R. scissors
- R. wire-holding clamp

Rubovits clamp
ruby
- r. knife

- r. knife scalpel
- r. laser

Rudd
- R. Clinic forceps
- R. Clinic hemorrhoidal forceps
- R. ligator

Rudderman "Frelevator" fragment elevator
Ruddock laparoscope
Ruddy
- R. dissector
- R. stapes calipers
- R. stapes prosthesis

Rudolf-Buck suturing device
Rudolph
- R. breathing system
- R. calibrated super syringe
- R. linear pneumotachometer
- R. mask
- R. one-way respiratory valve
- R. trowel retractor

Ruedemann
- R. eye implant
- R. lacrimal dilator

Ruedemann-Todd tendon tucker
Ruel
- R. aortic clamp
- R. forceps

Ruese bone graft
Rugby
- R. deep-surgery forceps
- R. forceps

Rugelski arterial forceps
Ruggles microcurette
rugine
- Farabeuf r.
- Rollet r.

Ruiz
- R. adjustable marker
- R. fundus contact lens
- R. fundus laser lens
- R. plano fundus lens
- R. plano fundus lens implant

Ruiz-Shepard marker
rule
- bronchoscopic r.
- steel r.

ruler
- Berndt hip r.
- r. calipers

centimeter subtraction r.
Charnow notched r.
Hyde astigmatism r.
Joseph measuring r.
Krinsky-Prince
  accommodation r.
metal r.
millimeter r.
Pischel scleral r.
Richard-Allan surgical r.
stainless steel flexible r.
Tabb r.
Tabb 3-millimeter r.
Thornton r.
Thornton corneal press-
  on r.
ulnar r.
V. Mueller r.
Walker scleral r.
Webster r.
Weck astigmatism r.

Rumel
R. aluminum bridge splint
R. cardiovascular tourniquet
R. catheter
R. clamp
R. dissecting forceps
R. forceps
R. hemostatic forceps
R. lobectomy forceps
R. myocardial clamp
R. ratchet tourniquet
R. ratchet tourniquet eyed
  stylet
R. retractor
R. rubber clamp
R. thoracic artery forceps
R. thoracic clamp
R. thoracic-dissecting forceps
R. thoracic forceps
R. tourniquet
R. tourniquet-eyed obturator

Rumel-Belmont tourniquet

running
r. chromic suture
r. continuous suture
r. imbricating suture
r. nylon suture
r. subcuticular suture
r. suture

running-locked suture

ruptured disk curette

Rusch
R. bougie
R. bronchial catheter
R. catheter
R. cleaning brush
R. coudé catheter
R. esophageal stethoscope
R. external catheter
R. filiform
R. follower
R. head strap
R. laryngectomy tube
R. laryngoscope
R. laryngoscope blade
R. laryngoscope handle
R. laryngoscope lamp
R. leg bag
R. mucous trap
R. nephrostomy catheter
R. perineal drape
R. tube

Ruschelit
R. catheter
R. urethral bougie

Rusch-Foley catheter

Rush
R. awl reamer
R. bone clamp
R. clamp
R. driver
R. extractor
R. intramedullary fixation
  pin
R. mallet
R. nail
R. pin
R. pin reamer awl
R. rod

Rushkin balloon

Ruskin
R. antral needle
R. antral trocar
R. antral trocar needle
R. bone-cutting forceps
R. bone rongeur
R. bone-splitting forceps
R. duckbill rongeur
R. forceps
R. mastoid rongeur
R. multiple-action rongeur
R. needle
R. rongeur
R. rongeur forceps

Ruskin *(continued)*
R. sphenopalatine ganglion needle
Ruskin-Jay rongeur
Ruskin-Liston
R.-L. bone-cutting forceps
R.-L. forceps
Ruskin-Rowland forceps
Ruskin-Storz rongeur
Russell
R. dilator
R. forceps
R. frame
R. gastrostomy tray
R. hydrostatic dilator
R. hysterectomy forceps
R. percutaneous endoscopic gastrostomy
R. suction tube
R. traction device
Russell-Beck extension tractor
Russell-Davis forceps
Russell-Taylor
R.-T. femoral interlocking nail system
R.-T. interlocking nail instrumentation
R.-T. nail
R.-T. screw
Russian
R. fixation hook
R. forceps
R. four-pronged fixation hook
R. thumb forceps
R. tissue forceps
Russian-Péan forceps

Russ-model
R.-m. tumor forceps
R.-m. vascular forceps
Rust amputation saw
Ruth-Hedwig
R.-H. pneumothorax apparatus
R.-H. splitter
Rutner
R. biopsy needle
R. catheter
R. nephrostomy balloon catheter
R. stone basket
R. stone extractor
R. wedge catheter
Rutzen bag
Ruuska meniscotome
RVAD centrifugal right ventricular assist device
Rychener-Weve electrode
Rycroft
R. cannula
R. lamp
R. tying forceps
Rydel-Seiffert tuning fork
Ryder
R. needle holder
R. scissors
Ryecroft retractor
Ryerson
R. bone retractor
R. bone skid
R. retractor
R. tenotome
R. tenotome knife
Ryle duodenal tube

S
S. retractor
S. root canal file
Saalfeld comedo extractor
Sabbatsberg septum elevator
saber-back scissors
sable brush
Sableflex anterior chamber
    intraocular lens
Sabreloc
S. needle
S. spatula needle
S. suture
SAC
stable access cannula
SACH
solid ankle cushion heel
SACH implant
SACH prosthesis
Sachs
S. angled vein retractor
S. brain-exploring cannula
S. bur
S. cannula
S. cervical punch
S. dural hook
S. dural separator
S. forceps
S. needle
S. nerve separator
S. nerve separator-spatula
S. retractor
S. skull bur
S. spatula
S. suction tube
S. tissue forceps
S. tube
S. urethrotome
S. vein retractor
Sachs-Cushing retractor
Sachs-Freer dissector
Sacks biliary drain
Sacks-Vine PEG tube
sacral screw
saddle locator
Sadler
S. bone hook
S. cartilage scissors
S. scissors

Saenger
S. ovum forceps
S. placental forceps
S. suture
Safar-S airway
Safar ventilation bronchoscope
Safco
S. alloy
S. diamond instrument
S. polycarbonate crown
Safestretch incontinence system
Safe-T-Coat heparin-coated
    thermodilution catheter
Safe-T-Tube
Montgomery-Lofgren
    tapered S.-T.-T.
safety
s. handle
s. handles tray
s. pessary
s. pin
s. pin closer
s. pin splint
safety-bolt suture
Safian
S. design prosthesis
S. nasal splint
S. rhinoplasty prosthesis
Safir pin
Saf-T-Coil intrauterine device
Saf-T-Fit amalgamator capsule
Saf-T J guide wire
Saf-T-Sound uterine sound
Sage
S. pin
S. tonsillar snare
S. wire
sagittal
s. oscillating saw
s. saw
s. suture
Saint George knee prosthesis
Saint Jude prosthesis
Saint Mark dilator
Sajou laryngeal forceps
Sakler erysiphake
Salah
S. needle
S. sternal needle

Salem
  S. sump action nasogastric
    tube
  S. sump drain
Salenius meniscal knife
Salibi carotid artery clamp
saline dressing
Saling amnioscope
Salinger reduction instrument
saliva
  Glandosane synthetic s.
salivary bypass tube
**Salmon-Rickham ventriculostomy
  reservoir**
salpingeal
  s. curette
  s. probe
salpingograph
  Schultze s.
Salvatore-Maloney tracheotome
Salvatore umbilical cord ligator
Samiento brace
sampler
  Cervex-Brush cervical cell s.
  Endopap endometrial s.
  Isaacs endometrial cell s.
  Johnson's swab s.
Sampson prosthesis
Sam Roberts
  S. R. bronchial biopsy
    forceps
  S. R. bronchial forceps
  S. R. esophagoscope
  S. R. forceps
  S. R. headrest
  S. R. laryngoscope
  S. R. self-retaining
    laryngoscope
Samson-Davis
  S.-D. infant suction tube
  S.-D. infant tube
SAM splint
Samuels
  S. forceps
  S. hemoclip-applying forceps
  S. vein stripper
Samway tourniquet
Sana-Lok syringe
Sanchez-Bulnes
  S.-B. lacrimal sac self-
    retaining retractor
  S.-B. retractor
sandbag

Sanders
  S. bed
  S. forceps
  S. intubation laryngoscope
  S. jet ventilation device
    respirator
  S. laryngoscope
  S. valve
  S. vasectomy forceps
  S. ventilation adapter
Sanders-Brown needle
Sanders-Brown-Shaw
  S.-B.-S. aneurysm needle
  S.-B.-S. needle
Sanders-Castroviejo forceps
Sandhill
  S. esophageal motility
    system
  S. probe
sandpaper dermabrader
Sandt
  S. suture forceps
  S. utility forceps
Sanford ligator
Santa Casa wrench
Santulli clamp
Santy
  S. dissecting forceps
  S. forceps
  S. ring-end forceps
saphenous-aorta tissue forceps
saphenous vein cannula
sapphire
  s. crystal infrared
    photocoagulator
  s. knife
  s. lens
Saqalain dressing forceps
Saratoga sump catheter
Sargis uterine tenaculum
Sarnoff
  S. aortic clamp
  S. clamp
Sarns
  S. aortic arch cannula
  S. cannula
  S. temperature probe
  S. two-stage cannula
  S. venous drainage cannula
Sarot
  S. arterial clamp
  S. arterial forceps
  S. bronchial clamp

S. clamp
S. forceps
S. intrathoracic forceps
S. knife
S. needle
S. needle holder
S. pleurectomy forceps
S. thoracoscope
S. Vital needle holder
Satelite ear endoscope
Satinsky
S. anastomosis clamp
S. aortic clamp
S. clamp
S. forceps
S. pediatric clamp
S. scissors
S. tangential occlusion
  forceps
S. vascular clamp
S. vena caval clamp
S. vena caval scissors
Sato
S. cataract needle
S. corneal knife
S. lid retractor
S. speculum
Satterlee
S. advancement forceps
S. amputating saw
S. aseptic saw
S. bone saw
S. bone saw blade
S. muscle forceps
S. saw
Sauer
S. corneal debrider
S. eye speculum
S. forceps
S. hemostatic tonsillectome
S. infant eye speculum
S. infant speculum
S. outer ring forceps
S. suture forceps
S. suturing forceps
S. tonometer
S. tonsillectome
Sauerbruch
S. forceps
S. implant
S. pickup forceps
S. prosthesis
S. retractor

S. rib rongeur forceps
S. rib shears
S. rongeur
Sauerbruch-Britsch rib shears
Sauerbruch-Coryllos
S.-C. rib rongeur
S.-C. rib shears
Sauerbruch-Frey
S.-F. raspatory
S.-F. rib elevator
S.-F. rib shears
Sauerbruch-Lebsche
S.-L. rib shears
S.-L. rongeur
Sauerbruch-Lillienthal rib spreader
Sauerbruch-Zukschwerdt
S.-Z. retractor
S.-Z. rib retractor
Sauer-Sluder tonsillectome
Sauer-Storz
S.-S. tonometer
S.-S. tonsillectome
Saunders
S. cataract needle
S. eye speculum
S. instrument rack
S. needle
Saunders-Paparella
S.-P. marker
S.-P. needle
S.-P. pick
S.-P. stapes hook
S.-P. straight needle
S.-P. window rasp
Saurex spreader
Sauvage
S. Bionit graft
S. Dacron graft
S. fabric graft prosthesis
Savage intestinal decompressor
Savariaud-Reverdin needle
Savary
S. dilator
S. esophageal dilator
S. tapered thermoplastic
  dilator
Savary-Gilliard
S.-G. dilator
S.-G. dilator set
S.-G. esophageal dilator
S.-G. wire guide
Savlon splint

saw

Adams s.
air s.
Albee s.
amputating s.
aseptic s.
Bailey conductor s.
Becker-Joseph s.
Bergman plaster s.
Bishop oscillatory bone s.
Bodenham s.
Bodenham surgical s.
bone s.
Bosworth s.
Bosworth Joseph nasal s.
Brown s.
Brown-Joseph s.
Butcher s.
chain s.
Charnley s.
Charriere s.
Charriere amputation s.
Charriere aseptic
  metacarpal s.
Charriere bone s.
Clerf laryngeal s.
Codman sternal s.
Converse s.
Converse nasal s.
Cottle-Joseph s.
Cottle Universal nasal s.
Crego-Gigli s.
Crown s.
crurotomy s.
DeMartel conductor s.
DeMartel T-wire s.
electric laryngofissure s.
Engel plaster s.
Farabeuf s.
Farrior-Joseph s.
Farrior-Joseph bayonet s.
finger ring s.
Gigli s.
Gigli solid-handle s.
Gigli wire s.
Goldman s.
Gottschalk transverse s.
Guilford-Wright bur s.
Guilford-Wullstein bur s.
s. handle
helical tube s.
Hetherington circular s.
Hey skull s.

Hill-Bosworth s.
Hough bur-crurotomy s.
Hough-Wullstein bur s.
Hub s.
humeral s.
Joseph s.
Joseph bayonet s.
Joseph-Farrior s.
Joseph-Maltz angular s.
Joseph-Maltz nasal s.
Joseph nasal s.
Joseph-Stille s.
Joseph-Verner s.
Lamont nasal s.
Langenbeck amputation s.
Langenbeck metacarpal s.
laryngeal s.
Lebsche s.
Lell laryngofissure s.
Luck-Bishop s.
Luck bone s.
Macewen s.
Magnuson circular twin s.
Magnuson double counter-
  rotating s.
Magnuson single circular s.
Maltz bayonet s.
McCabe crurotomy s.
metacarpal s.
Micro-Aire bone s.
micro-oscillating s.
microreciprocating s.
microsagittal s.
Mueller s.
Myerson laryngectomy s.
nasal s.
Ogura nasal s.
Olivecrona-Gigli s.
Olivecrona-Gigli wire s.
Olivecrona wire s.
Orthair oscillating s.
oscillating s.
plaster s.
plaster with lift s.
reciprocating s.
Rica wire s.
ring-cutting s.
rotary hub s.
round Gigli s.
Rust amputation s.
sagittal s.
sagittal oscillating s.
Satterlee s.

Satterlee amputating s.
Satterlee aseptic s.
Satterlee bone s.
Schwartz antral trocar s.
Seltzer s.
Shrady s.
Slaughter nasal s.
sternal s.
Stille-Gigli wire s.
Stiwer finger ring s.
Stryker s.
Stryker autopsy s.
surgical s.
Tuke bone s.
Tyler Gigli s.
Tyler spiral Gigli s.
Universal nasal s.
V. Mueller amputating s.
V. Mueller Gigli s.
Wigmore plaster s.
wire s.
Woakes nasal s.
Xomed micro-oscillating s.
sawdust bed
Sawtell
  S. applicator
  S. arterial forceps
  S. forceps
  S. gallbladder forceps
  S. hemostat
  S. hemostatic forceps
  S. laryngeal applicator
  S. tonsillar artery forceps
  S. tonsillar forceps
Sawtell-Davis
  S.-D. forceps
  S.-D. hemostat
  S.-D. tonsillar hemostat
    forceps
saw-toothed curette
Sawyer
  S. rectal retractor
  S. rectal speculum
  S. retractor
Sayre
  S. apparatus
  S. bandage
  S. double-end periosteal
    elevator
  S. dressing
  S. elevator
  S. head snare
  S. jacket

  S. periosteal elevator
  S. periosteal raspatory
  S. retractor
  S. splint
Sbarbaro tibial prosthesis
Scaglietti rongeur
scale
  Digitron dialysis chair s.
scaler
  Amdent ultrasonic s.
  Brahler ultrasonic dental s.
  Buffalo ultrasonic s.
  Densco ultrasonic s.
  dental s.
  Ellman rotary s.
  loop s.
  Nordent s.
  Sonatron ultrasonic s.
  Steele s.
  Tamsco periodontic s.
  Titan s.
  ultrasonic s.
  Vivant ultrasonic s.
  XGT ultrasonic s.
Scaler curette
scalp
  s. clip
  s. clip-applying forceps
  s. clip forceps
  s. electrode
  s. forceps
  s. hemostasis clip
  s. needle
  s. retractor
  s. self-retaining retractor
  s. suture
scalpel
  ASR s.
  Bard-Parker s.
  Bergman s.
  blade s.
  bone s.
  carbon dioxide (CO_2)
    laser s.
  Cavitron s.
  Contact Laser s.
  Dieffenbach s.
  disposable s.
  Downing cartilage s.
  feather s.
  Green pendulum s.
  Hamer s.
  s. handle

scalpel *(continued)*
    Jackson s.
    Jackson tracheal s.
    John Green pendulum s.
    laser s.
    LaserSonics Nd:YAG
      LaserBlade s.
    lid s.
    long s.
    pendulum s.
    plasma s.
    razor s.
    ruby knife s.
    sculpturing s.
    Shaw s.
    tracheal s.
    ultrasonic harmonic s.
    water s.
scalpene needle
scan
    Meckel s.
Scand pin
Scanlan
    S. aneurysm clip
    S. bipolar coagulator
    S. laproscopic forceps
    S. ligator
    S. ligature guide
    S. microforceps
    S. microneedle holder
    S. micronerve hook
    S. microrasp
    S. microscissors
    S. microvessel hook
    S. pediatric retractor
    S. plaster shears
    S. retractor
    S. rib shears
    S. scissors
    S. vascular tunneler
    S. vessel dilator
Scanlan-Crafoord contractor
scanner
    diagnostic ultrasound
      linear s.
    Interad whole body CT s.
    Sinvision ultrasound s.
    Sonoline Siemens
      ultrasound s.
    Tomomatic brain s.
    Toshiba brain s.
Scanpor surgical tape
Scan spray dressing

Scanzoni forceps
scaphoid screw guide
scapular retractor
Scarborough prosthesis
scarf bandage
scarifier
    Desmarres s.
    Graefe s.
    s. knife
scarifying curette
scarlet red gauze dressing
scattergram
SCDK heart valve
SCDT
    SCDT heart valve
    SCDT heart valve
      prosthesis
Schaaf foreign body forceps
Schachar blepharostat
Schacht colostomy appliance
Schaedel
    S. clip
    S. towel clamp
    S. towel forceps
Schaeffer
    S. curette
    S. ethmoid curette
    S. mastoid curette
Schafer cortical hearing instrument
Schaldach electrode pacemaker
Schall laryngectomy tube
Schamberg
    S. comedo extractor
    S. extractor
Schantz sinus rasp
Schanz
    S. brace
    S. collar brace
    S. screw
Schanzioni craniotomy forceps
Scharff bipolar forceps
Schatz utility forceps
Schecter-Bryant aortic vent needle
Schede
    S. bone curette
    S. curette
Scheer
    S. crimper forceps
    S. elevator knife
    S. hook
    S. knife elevator
    S. middle ear instrument
    S. needle

S. oval window rasp
S. pick
S. Tef-wire prosthesis
Scheer-Wullstein cutting bur
Scheicher laminectomy punch
Scheie
S. anterior chamber cannula
S. cannula
S. cataract-aspirating cannula
S. cataract-aspirating needle
S. cataract needle
S. goniopuncture knife
S. goniotomy knife
S. needle
S. ophthalmic cautery
Scheie-Graefe
S.-G. fixation forceps
S.-G. forceps
Scheie-Westcott
S.-W. corneal section scissors
S.-W. scissors
Scheimpflug camera
Scheinmann
S. biting punch
S. biting tip
S. esophagoscopy forceps
S. forceps
S. laryngeal forceps
Schein syringe
Schepens
S. binocular indirect camera
S. boat silicone
S. clip
S. depressor
S. electrode
S. eye cautery
S. eye retractor
S. forceps
S. grooved rubber silicone
S. hollow hemisphere implant
S. hollow silicone hemisphere implant material
S. ophthalmoscope
S. orbital retractor
S. pad silicone
S. retractor
S. scleral depressor
S. surface electrode
S. tantalum clip

Scherback-Porges vaginal speculum set
Scheuerlen raspatory
Schick forceps
Schillinger suture support
Schimelbusch inhaler
Schindler
S. esophagoscope
S. forceps
S. gastroscope
S. optical esophagoscope
S. peritoneal forceps
S. retractor
Schink dermatome
Schiøtz tonometer
Schirmer tear test
Schivitz tenometer
Schlein
S. clamp
S. shoulder positioner
S. total elbow prosthesis
S. trisurface ankle prosthesis
Schlesinger
S. cervical punch
S. cervical punch forceps
S. cervical rongeur
S. clamp
S. forceps
S. Gigli-saw guide
S. intervertebral disk forceps
S. intervertebral disk rongeur
S. laminectomy rongeur
S. meniscus-grasping forceps
S. rongeur
Schmeden
S. dural scissors
S. tonsillar punch
Schmidt
S. clamp
S. hemostatic forceps
Schmidt-Rumpler forceps
Schmid vascular spatula
Schmieden
S. needle
S. probe
Schmieden-Dick needle
Schmieden-Taylor
S.-T. dissector
S.-T. dural scissors
Schmiedt tube

Schmithhuisen
    S. ethmoidal punch
    S. sphenoidal punch
Schmuth modification activator
Schnaudigel sclerotomy punch
Schneider
    S. catheter
    S. intramedullary nail
    S. nail driver
    S. pelvimeter
    S. raspatory
    S. rod
    S. self-broaching pin
Schneider-Sauerbruch raspatory
Schneider-Shiley
    S.-S. catheter
    S.-S. dilatation catheter
Schneider-Wallstent endoprosthesis
Schnidt
    S. clamp
    S. forceps
    S. gall duct forceps
    S. hemostat
    S. thoracic forceps
    S. tonsillar forceps
    S. tonsillar hemostatic
      forceps
Schnidt-Rumpler forceps
Schnieder wall stent
Schnitker scalp retractor
Schnitman skin hook
Schocket scleral depressor
Schoemaker
    S. intestinal clamp
    S. scissors
Schoemaker-Loth scissors
Schoenberg
    S. forceps
    S. intestinal forceps
    S. uterine-elevating forceps
    S. uterine forceps
Schoenborn retractor
Scholl meniscal knife
Schoonmaker
    S. catheter
    S. femoral catheter
    S. multipurpose catheter
Schroeder
    S. curette
    S. episiotomy scissors
    S. forceps
    S. interlocking sound
    S. operating scissors

    S. tenaculum
    S. tenaculum forceps
    S. tissue forceps
    S. uterine curette
    S. uterine scoop
    S. uterine tenaculum
    S. uterine tenaculum forceps
    S. uterine vulsellum forceps
    S. vulsellar forceps
    S. vulsellum
    S. vulsellum uterine
      tenaculum
Schroeder-Braun
    S.-B. forceps
    S.-B. uterine forceps
Schroeder-Van Doren tenaculum
forceps
Schrotter catheter
Schubert
    S. biopsy forceps
    S. biopsy punch
    S. biopsy punch forceps
    S. cervical biopsy forceps
    S. forceps
    S. uterine biopsy forceps
    S. uterine biopsy punch
      forceps
    S. uterine punch
    S. uterine tenaculum forceps
Schuknecht
    S. chisel
    S. crimper
    S. cutter
    S. elevator
    S. excavator
    S. footplate hook
    S. Gelfoam wire prosthesis
    S. gouge
    S. middle ear instrument
    S. needle
    S. pick
    S. postauricular retractor
    S. postauricular self-retaining
      retractor
    S. retractor
    S. roller knife
    S. scissors
    S. sickle knife
    S. spatula
    S. stapes hook
    S. suction tip
    S. suction tube

S. Teflon wire piston
prosthesis
S. Tef-Wire prosthesis
S. temporal trephine
S. whirlybird excavator
S. wire-bending die
S. wire crimper
S. wire-cutting scissors
Schuknecht-Paparella wire-bending
die
Schuknecht-Wullstein retractor
Schulec silver clip
Schuler aspiration/irrigation tube
Schuletz
S. antral curette
S. pacemaker
Schuletz-Simmons ethmoidal
curette
Schultz
S. iris retractor
S. irrgating iris retractor
S. retractor
Schultz-Crock binocular
ophthalmoscope
Schultze
S. ambryotomy knife
S. salpingograph
Schulze anterior capsule nibbler
Schumacher, Schumaker
S. aortic clamp
S. biopsy forceps
S. forceps
S. sternal shears
S. umbilical cord scissors
Schumann giant eye magnet
Schumann-Schreus dermabrader
Schurring ossicle cup prosthesis
Schutte basket
Schutz
S. clamp
S. clip
S. forceps
Schwarten balloon-dilatation
catheter
Schwartz
S. antral trocar saw
S. arterial aneurysm clamp
S. bulldog clamp
S. cervical tenaculum hook
S. clamp
S. clip
S. clip applier
S. clip-applying forceps

S. cordotomy knife
S. curette
S. endocervical curette
S. forceps
S. intracranial clamp
S. laminectomy retractor
S. laminectomy self-retaining
retractor
S. obstetrical forceps
S. retractor
S. temporary clip
S. temporary intracranial
artery clamp
S. temporary vessel clamp-
applying forceps
S. trocar
S. vascular clamp
Schwartz-Kerrison rongeur
Schwarz
S. arrow-forming pliers
S. bow-type activator
S. modification activator
S. traction bow
Schwasser
S. brain clip
S. microclip clip
Schweigger
S. capsular forceps
S. extracapsular forceps
S. forceps
Schweitzer
S. pin
S. spring plate
Schweizer
S. cervix-holding forceps
S. forceps
S. speculum
S. uterine forceps
Scialom dental implant material
Science-Med balloon catheter
Scientronics magnet
Sci-Med
S.-M. angioplasty catheter
S.-M. extracorporeal silicone
rubber reservoir
S.-M. guiding catheter
S.-M. Life Systems, Inc.
membrane artificial lung
S.-M. skinny catheter
scimitar blade
scintigraphic balloon
scintillation camera

scissors (*See also* shears)
 abdominal s.
 Abeli corneal s.
 Ada s.
 Adson s.
 Adson ganglion s.
 Aebli corneal s.
 Aebli corneal section s.
 Aebli-Manson s.
 Aebli tenotomy s.
 alligator s.
 American umbilical s.
 angled s.
 angular s.
 Anis corneal s.
 arteriotomy s.
 Arthro Force hook s.
 Aston face-lift s.
 Atkinson-Walker s.
 Aufricht s.
 Azar corneal s.
 baby Metzenbaum s.
 Bahama suture s.
 Bakst cardiac s.
 ball tipped s.
 Baltimore nasal s.
 bandage s.
 Bantam wire cutting s.
 Barkan s.
 Barnes vessel s.
 Barraquer corneal section s.
 Barraquer-DeWecker iris s.
 Barraquer iris s.
 Barraquer-Karakashian s.
 Barraquer vitreous strand s.
 Barsky nasal s.
 Baruch circumcision s.
 bayonet s.
 bayonet-shaped s.
 beaded-tip s.
 Beall s.
 Beall circumflex artery s.
 Becker s.
 Becker septal s.
 Becker spatulated corneal
  section s.
 Beckman nasal s.
 Beebe wire s.
 Bellucci s.
 Bellucci alligator s.
 Berens corneal transplant s.
 Berens iridocapsulotomy s.
 Bergman plaster s.

 Blanco s.
 Blum arterial s.
 Boettcher s.
 Boettcher tonsillar s.
 Bonn iris s.
 Bowman strabismus s.
 Boyd s.
 Boyd dissecting s.
 Boyd-Stille tonsillar s.
 Boyd tonsillar s.
 Bozeman s.
 brain s.
 Braun episiotomy s.
 Braun-Stadler s.
 Braun-Stadler episiotomy s.
 Brooks gallbladder s.
 Brophy s.
 Brown s.
 Brown dissecting s.
 Bruns plaster s.
 Buerger-McCarthy s.
 Buie ractal s.
 bulldog s.
 Bunge s.
 Burnham s.
 Burnham bandage s.
 Busch umbilical cord s.
 calcified tissue s.
 canalicural s.
 cannular s.
 Caplan s.
 Caplan angular s.
 Caplan dorsal s.
 Caplan nasal s.
 capsulotomy s.
 Carb-Edge s.
 cardiovascular s.
 cartilage s.
 Castanares face-lift s.
 Castroviejo s.
 Castroviejo anterior
  synechia s.
 Castroviejo corneal s.
 Castroviejo corneal
  section s.
 Castroviejo iris s.
 Castroviejo keratoplasty s.
 Castroviejo-McPherson
  keratectomy s.
 Castroviejo microcorneal s.
 Castroviejo minicorneal s.
 Castroviejo tenotomy s.
 Castroviejo-Troutman s.

Castroviejo-Vannas s.
Castroviejo-Vannas
  capsulotomy s.
cataract s.
Caylor s.
Chadwick s.
Charnley cup-trimming s.
Cherry S-shape s.
Chevalier Jackson s.
Church s.
Church pediatric s.
Cinelli-Fomon s.
circumflex s.
circumflex artery s.
Classon pediatric s.
Clayman-Troutman
  corneal s.
Clayman-Vannas s.
Clayman-Westcott s.
clip-removing s.
Cohan-Vannas iris s.
Cohan-Westcott s.
Cohney s.
collar s.
conjunctival s.
Converse s.
Converse-Wilmer
  conjunctival s.
Cooley s.
Cooley arteriotomy s.
Cooley cardiovascular s.
Cooley neonatal s.
Cooley reverse-cut s.
corneal s.
corneal section s.
corneal section-enlarging s.
corneal transplant s.
corneoscleral s.
coronary s.
coronary artery s.
Costa wire suture s.
Cottle s.
Cottle angular s.
Cottle bulldog s.
Cottle dorsal s.
Cottle dressing s.
Cottle heavy septal s.
Cottle nasal s.
Cottle spring s.
Crafoord s.
Crafoord lobectomy s.
Crafoord lung s.
Crafoord thoracic s.

Craig s.
craniotomy s.
crown s.
curved-on-flat s.
curved operating s.
cuticle s.
Dahlgren iris s.
Dandy neurosurgical s.
Dandy trigeminal s.
Davis rhytidectomy s.
Dean s.
Dean dissecting s.
Dean tonsillar s.
Dean-Trussler s.
Deaver s.
Deaver operating s.
DeBakey s.
DeBakey endarterectomy s.
DeBakey-Metzenbaum s.
DeBakey-Potts s.
DeBakey stitch s.
DeBakey valve s.
DeBakey vascular s.
Decker microsurgical s.
delicate s.
delicate operating s.
DeMartel neurosurgical s.
DeMartel vascular s.
Derf s.
DeWecker s.
DeWecker iris s.
DeWecker-Pritikin iris s.
diamond-edge s.
diathermy s.
Diethrich s.
Diethrich circumflex
  artery s.
Diethrich coronary artery s.
Diethrich-Hegemann s.
Diethrich valve s.
dissecting s.
dorsal angled s.
Douglas nasal s.
Doyen abdominal s.
Doyen dissecting s.
Doyen-Ferguson s.
dressing s.
Dubois decapitation s.
Duffield s.
Dumont thoracic s.
dural s.
Durotip s.
ear s.

635

scissors *(continued)*
    East Grinstead s.
    Edelstein s.
    Eiselsberg ligature s.
    Emmet uterine s.
    endarterectomy s.
    enterotomy s.
    enucleation s.
    episiotomy s.
    E-Series s.
    Esmarch s.
    Esmarch bandage s.
    esophageal s.
    Essrig dissecting s.
    eye s.
    eye stitch s.
    eye suture s.
    face-lift s.
    Favaloro s.
    Favaloro coronary s.
    Federspiel s.
    Ferguson s.
    Ferguson abdominal s.
    Ferguson-Metzenbaum s.
    Ferguson uterine s.
    Fine s.
    Finochietto s.
    Fisch microcrurotomy s.
    fistular s.
    Fomon s.
    Fomon angular s.
    Fomon lower lateral s.
    Fomon saber-back s.
    Fomon upper lateral s.
    s. forceps
    Foster s.
    Frahur s.
    Frazier dural s.
    Freeman rhytidectomy s.
    Freeman-Schepens s.
    Fulton pediatric s.
    gallbladder s.
    ganglion s.
    gauze s.
    gauze pattern s.
    Gellquist s.
    general utility s.
    Giardet corneal s.
    Gillies suture s.
    Gill-Welsh s.
    Gill-Welsh-Vannas s.
    Gill-Welsh-Vannas
      capsulotomy s.

    Glasscock s.
    Glassman thin-point s.
    goiter s.
    Goldman-Fox gum s.
    Goldman septal s.
    Good-Reiner s.
    Good tonsillar s.
    Gorney rhytidectomy s.
    Gradle stitch s.
    Graham s.
    Graham pediatric s.
    Guggenheim s.
    Guggenheim-Schuknecht s.
    Guilford s.
    Guilford-Schuknecht wire-
      cutting s.
    Guilford-Wright s.
    guillotine s.
    Guist enucleation s.
    Guyton s.
    Haglund plaster s.
    Haimovici arteriotomy s.
    Halsted strabismus s.
    Harrington s.
    Harrington deep surgical s.
    Harrington-Mayo s.
    Harrison suture-removing s.
    Harvey wire s.
    Haynes s.
    Heath clip-removing s.
    Heath suture s.
    Heath suture-cutting s.
    Heath wire-cutting s.
    heavy septal s.
    Hegemann s.
    Heyman nasal s.
    Heyman-Paparella s.
    Heyman-Paparella angular s.
    Hipp & Sohn dental s.
    Hoen laminectomy s.
    Holinger curved s.
    Holmes s.
    hook s.
    hook rotary s.
    Hooper pediatric s.
    Hough s.
    House s.
    House alligator s.
    House-Bellucci s.
    House-Bellucci-Shambaugh s.
    House-Bellucci-Shambaugh
      alligator s.
    Huey s.

Huger diamond-back
    nasal s.
IMA s.
insitu valve s.
iridocapsulotomy s.
iris s.
iris with Barraquer
    handle s.
Irvine s.
Jabaley s.
Jackson esophageal s.
Jackson laryngeal s.
Jackson turbinate s.
Jacobson s.
Jacobson bayonet-shaped s.
Jacobson spring-handled s.
Jako microlaryngeal s.
Jameson s.
Jameson-Metzenbaum s.
Jameson-Werber s.
Jannetta s.
Jannetta bayonet-shaped s.
Jannetta-Kurze s.
Jannetta-Kurze dissecting s.
Jarit dissecting s.
Jarit endarterectomy s.
Jarit flat-tip s.
Jarit lower lateral s.
Jarit microstitch s.
Jarit microsurgery s.
Jarit peripheral vascular s.
Jarit stitch s.
Jesco s.
Jones dissecting s.
Jones IMA s.
Jorgenson s.
Jorgenson dissecting s.
Jorgenson gallbladder s.
Joseph s.
Joseph-Maltz s.
Kahn s.
Katzeff cartilage s.
Katzin corneal transplant s.
Katzin-Troutman s.
Kaye s.
Kaye fine-dissecting s.
Kelly s.
Kelly fistular s.
Kelly uterine s.
keratoplasty s.
Kitner dissecting s.
Kleinsasser microlaryngeal s.
Klinkenbergh-Loth s.

Knapp iris s.
Knapp strabismus s.
Knight nasal s.
Knowles bandage s.
Koenig-Stille s.
Kreuscher s.
Kreuscher semilunar
    cartilage s.
Kurze dissecting s.
Lagrange s.
Lagrange sclerectomy s.
Lahey s.
Lahey Carb-Edge s.
Lahey delicate s.
Lahey operating s.
Lakeside nasal s.
laparoscopic s.
laryngeal s.
laser tubal s.
Lawrie s.
Lawrie modified
    circumflex s.
Lawton corneal s.
Leather-Karmody in-situ
    valve s.
Lexer s.
Lexer dissecting s.
Lexer-Durotip dissecting s.
ligature s.
Lillie s.
Lillie tonsillar s.
Lincoln s.
Lincoln-Metzenbaum s.
Lincoln pediatric s.
Lindley s.
Lister s.
Lister bandage s.
Liston plaster-of-Paris s.
Littauer s.
Littauer stitch s.
Littauer suture s.
Littler s.
Littler suture-carrying s.
Little suture s.
Litwak general utility s.
Litwak mitral valve s.
Litwin s.
Litwin angled s.
Lloyd-Davis rectal s.
lobectomy s.
lung dissecting s.
Lynch s.
MacKenty s.

scissors *(continued)*
Maclay tonsillar s.
Maki s.
Malis s.
Malis neurosurgical s.
Mancusi-Ungaro s.
Manson-Aebli corneal s.
Marbach episiotomy s.
marking s.
Martin ballpoint s.
Martin cartilage s.
Martin throat s.
Mattis s.
Mattis corneal s.
Mattox-Potts s.
Maunoir s.
Mayo s.
Mayo curved s.
Mayo dissecting s.
Mayo-Harrington s.
Mayo-Harrington
dissecting s.
Mayo-Lexer s.
Mayo long dissecting s.
Mayo-New s.
Mayo-Noble s.
Mayo-Noble dissecting s.
Mayo operating s.
Mayo-Potts dissecting s.
Mayo round blade s.
Mayo-Sims s.
Mayo-Sims dissecting s.
Mayo-Stille s.
Mayo-Stille operating s.
Mayo straight s.
Mayo uterine s.
McAllister s.
McClure iris s.
McGuire corneal s.
McIndoe s.
McLean capsulotomy s.
McPherson-Castroviejo
corneal s.
McPherson-Castroviejo
microcorneal s.
McPherson corneal
section s.
McPherson
microconjunctival s.
McPherson
microtenotomy s.
McPherson micro-utility
suture s.

McPherson-Vannas s.
McPherson-Vannas micro-
iris s.
McPherson-Westcott s.
McPherson-Westcott
conjunctival s.
McPherson-Westcott stitch s.
McReynolds pterygium s.
meniscal hook s.
meniscectomy s.
Metzenbaum s.
Metzenbaum delicate s.
Metzenbaum dissecting s.
Metzenbaum-Lipsett s.
Metzenbaum long s.
Metzenbaum operating s.
microconjunctival s.
microcorneal s.
micro-infertility s.
micro-infertility dissecting s.
micro-iris s.
microlaryngeal s.
micropituitary s.
microscopic s.
microsurgical s.
Microtek s.
microtenotomy s.
micro-utility s.
microvascular s.
Microvit s.
Microwec s.
Miller dissecting s.
Miller operating s.
Miller rectal s.
Millesi s.
Mills s.
Mills circumflex s.
Milteck s.
mitral valve s.
Mixter operating s.
Moore-Troutman corneal s.
Morse s.
Morse backward-cutting
aortic s.
Munro brain s.
Nadler s.
nail s.
s. nail drill
nail-nipper s.
nasal s.
Nelson s.
Nelson classic plus s.
Nelson lobectomy s.

Nelson lung-dissecting s.
Nelson-Metzenbaum s.
Nelson Vital dissecting s.
neonatal s.
Neumann s.
neurosurgical s.
neurovascular s.
New s.
New suture s.
Noble s.
Northbent suture s.
Noyes iridectomy s.
Noyes iris s.
Noyes-Shambaugh s.
Nugent-Gradle s.
Nugent-Gradle stitch s.
O'Brien-Mayo s.
O'Brien stitch s.
O'Brien suture s.
Ochsner s.
Ochsner ball-tipped s.
Ochsner diamond-edged s.
Olivecrona s.
Olivecrona angular s.
Olivecrona dural s.
Olivecrona guillotine s.
O'Neill cardiac operating s.
Ormco band s.
orthopaedic s.
Osher corneal s.
otologic s.
Panzer gallbladder s.
Paparella s.
Paparella wire-cutting s.
Par s.
pattern umbilical s.
Peck-Joseph s.
Peyman vitreous s.
Phaneuf uterine artery s.
Pickett s.
plain rotary s.
s. plaster shears
plastic surgery s.
plastic utility s.
Poppen sympathectomy s.
Potts s.
Potts-DeMartel gall duct s.
Potts-Smith s.
Potts-Smith arterial s.
Potts-Smith dissecting s.
Potts-Smith reverse s.
Potts tenotomy s.
Potts-Yasargil s.

Pratt rectal s.
Prince dissecting s.
Prince-Potts s.
Prince tonsillar s.
s. probe
probe point s.
pupillary membrane s.
Quimby s.
Quimby gum s.
Ragnell s.
Ragnell undermining s.
Rappazzo foreign body s.
Rappazzo haptic s.
Real s.
Reeh stitch s.
Reichling s.
Reinhoff thoracic s.
Resano thoracic s.
Reul coronary artery s.
reverse s.
reverse-cutting s.
Reynolds s.
Reynolds dissecting s.
Reynolds-Jameson vessel s.
Rhoton s.
Rhoton bayonet s.
Rhoton microsurgical s.
rhytidectomy s.
Rica ear polypus s.
Richter s.
right-angle s.
Rizzuti keratoplasty s.
Rizzuti-McGuire s.
Roberts episiotomy s.
Rochester s.
Rochester-Ferguson s.
Rochester-Ochsner s.
Roger wire-cutting s.
Rosenblatt s.
rotary s. with cigar handle
rotary s. with loop handle
Rubio s.
Ryder s.
saber-back s.
Sadler s.
Sadler cartilage s.
Satinsky s.
Satinsky vena caval s.
Scanlan s.
Scheie-Westcott s.
Scheie-Westcott corneal
  section s.
Schmeden dural s.

scissors *(continued)*

Schmieden-Taylor dural s.
Schoemaker s.
Schoemaker-Loth s.
Schroeder episiotomy s.
Schroeder operating s.
Schuknecht s.
Schuknecht wire-cutting s.
Schumacher umbilical
  cord s.
Scott dissecting s.
Scott right-angle s.
Scoville s.
Sealy dissecting s.
Seiler turbinate s.
Semm dissecting s.
serrated s.
Serratex s.
Seutin s.
Sharpshay-Healy laryngeal s.
Shea-Bellucci s.
shears s.
Shea vein graft s.
Shepard-Westcott s.
Shortbent s.
Shortbent suture s.
Siebold uterine s.
Sims s.
Sims-Siebold uterine s.
Sims uterine s.
Sistrunk s.
Sistrunk dissecting s.
Slip-N-Snip s.
small spring s.
Smart enucleation s.
Smellie obstetrical s.
SMIC s.
SMIC collar s.
SMIC ear polypus s.
Smith s.
Smith bandage s.
Smith suture s.
Smith suture wire s.
Snowden-Pencer Supercut s.
Southbent s.
Spencer s.
Spencer eye suture s.
Spencer suture s.
Spetzler s.
spring s.
spring-handled s.
Stalzner rectal s.
Stevens s.

Stevens eye s.
Stevenson alligator s.
Stevens stitch s.
Stevens tenotomy s.
Stille s.
Stille dissecting s.
Stille-Mayo s.
Stille-Mayo dissecting s.
Stille Super Cut s.
stitch s.
Stiwer s.
Storz intraocular s.
Storz iris s.
Storz stitch s.
Storz-Westcott s.
Storz wire-cutting s.
strabismus s.
straight s.
Strully s.
Strully cardiovascular s.
Strully dissecting s.
Strully dural s.
Strully hook s.
Strully neurosurgical s.
Sullival gum s.
surgical s.
Sutherland s.
Sutherland eye s.
suture s.
suture-carrying s.
suture-removing s.
suture wire s.
suture wire-cutting s.
Sweet s.
Sweet delicate pituitary s.
Sweet esophageal s.
Tamsco wire-cutting s.
Taylor brain s.
Taylor dural s.
tenotomy s.
Thomson-Walker s.
thoracic s.
Thorek s.
Thorek-Feldman
  gallbladder s.
Thorek gallbladder s.
Thorek thoracic s.
Thorpe-Castroviejo
  cataract s.
Thorpe pupillary
  membrane s.
Thorpe-Westcott cataract s.
Tindall s.

Toennis-Adson s.
Toennis-Adson dural s.
Toennis dissecting s.
tonsillar s.
Torchia conjunctival s.
Torchia microcorneal s.
Torchia-Vannas micro-iris s.
trigeminal s.
Troutman-Castroviejo s.
Troutman-Castroviejo
  corneal section s.
Troutman conjunctival s.
Troutman corneal s.
Troutman-Katzin s.
Troutman-Katzin corneal
  transplant s.
Trusler-Dean s.
tubal s.
turbinate s.
Turner-Warwick
  diathermy s.
umbilical s.
Universal wire s.
upper lateral s.
U.S. Army gauze s.
U.S. Army-pattern
  umbilical s.
uterine s.
utility s.
utility bandage s.
valve leaflet excision s.
Vannas s.
Vannas capsulotomy s.
Vannas corneal s.
Vannas iridocapsulotomy s.
vascular s.
Verhoeff dissecting s.
Verner-Joseph s.
Vernon s.
Vernon wire-cutting s.
Vezien abdominal s.
Vital Cooley operating s.
Vital Cooley wire-cutting s.
Vital Cottle dorsal angled s.
Vital Fomon angular s.
Vital Knapp iris s.
Vital Knapp strabismus s.
Vital Mayo dissecting s.
Vital Metzenbaum s.
Vital Metzenbaum
  dissecting s.
Vital Nelson dissecting s.
Vital operating s.

Vital wire-cutting s.
vitreous s.
V. Mueller curved
  operating s.
V. Mueller laser tubal s.
V. Mueller operating s.
V. Mueller-Vital laser Mayo
  dissecting s.
Wadsworth s.
Walker-Apple s.
Walker-Atkinson s.
Walker corneal s.
Walton s.
Weber tissue s.
Weck iris s.
Weck-Spencer suture s.
Weck suture s.
Weck suture-removal s.
Weck wire-cutting s.
Weller cartilage s.
Werb s.
Westcott s.
Westcott conjunctival s.
Westcott double-end s.
Westcott-Scheie s.
Westcott spring-action s.
Westcott stitch s.
Westcott tenotomy s.
Westcott-type stitch s.
Westcott utility s.
Wester meniscectomy s.
White s.
Wiechel s.
Wiechel-Stille bile duct s.
Wiet otologic s.
Willauer s.
William Dixon collar s.
Wilmer s.
Wilmer-Converse
  conjunctival s.
Wilmer iris s.
Wilson intraocular s.
Wincor enucleation s.
wire s.
wire-cutting s.
wire suture s.
Wullstein s.
Wullstein ear s.
Wutzler s.
Yankauer s.
Yasargil s.
Yasargil bayonet s.

scissors *(continued)*
    Yasargil microvascular
      bayonet s.
    Zoellner s.
    Zylik-Michaels s.
scleral
    s. band
    s. bed
    s. buckle eye implant
    s. buckler implant
    s. buckling catheter
    s. depressor
    s. eye implant
    s. implant
    s. marker
    s. plug
    s. shell
    s. spatula needle
    s. twist fixation hook
    s. wound retractor
sclerectomy punch forceps
sclerotherapy needle
sclerotherapy needle
sclerotome
    Alvis-Lancaster s.
    Atkinson s.
    s. blade
    Castroviejo s.
    Curdy s.
    Guyton-Lundsgaard s.
    Lancaster s.
    Lundsgaard s.
    Lundsgaard-Burch s.
    Walker-Lee s.
Scobee
    S. muscle hook
    S. oblique muscle hook
Scobee-Allis forceps
scoliosis brace
scoop
    Abbott s.
    abdominal s.
    abortion s.
    Arlt fenestrated lens s.
    Arlt lens s.
    Asch uterine secretion s.
    Beck abdominal s.
    Berens common duct s.
    Berens lens s.
    Bruus s.
    common duct s.
    common duct stone s.
    Councill stone s.

cystic duct s.
Daviel lens s.
Desjardins gall duct s.
Desjardins gallstone s.
duct s.
Elschnig s.
Elschnig lens s.
enucleation s.
Ferguson gall duct s.
Ferguson gallstone s.
Ferris common duct s.
French s.
gallbladder s.
gall duct s.
gallstone s.
Goudet uterine s.
Green lens s.
Hess lens s.
Hibb s.
Klebanoff gallstone s.
Knapp lens s.
Lang eye s.
lens s.
lens enucleation s.
Lewis lens s.
Luer fenestrated lens s.
Luer-Koerte gallstone s.
Mayo s.
Mayo common duct s.
Mayo cystic duct s.
Mayo gallbladder s.
Mayo gall duct s.
Mayo gallstone s.
Mayo-Robson gallstone s.
microbayonet s.
Moore gall duct s.
Moore gallstone s.
Moynihan gallstone s.
Mules s.
Pagenstecher lens s.
Schroeder uterine s.
Simon uterine s.
Snellen lens s.
Syrrat s.
uterine s.
Volkmann s.
Wallich abortion s.
Wallich placental s.
Weber lens s.
Wells enucleation s.
Wilder lens s.
Yasargil s.
Zarski gallstone s.

Scoop transtracheal catheter
scope
    endocervicometer s.
    fixed-focus s.
    Keymed fiberoptic s.
    Olympus fiberoptic s.
    variable-focus s.
    Welch Allyn s.
Scopemaster hysteroscope
Scott
    S. attic cannula
    S. cannula
    S. dissecting scissors
    S. ear speculum
    S. humeral splint
    S. nasal suction tube
    S. peds retractor
    S. penile prosthesis
    S. right-angle scissors
    S. rotating resectoscope
    S. rubber ventricular
      cannula
    S. ventricular cannula
Scott-Harden tube
Scottish
    S. Rite brace
    S. Rite splint
Scott-McCracken elevator
Scoville
    S. blade
    S. blunt hook
    S. brain forceps
    S. brain spatula
    S. brain spatula forceps
    S. Britetrac retractor
    S. cervical disk retractor
    S. cervical disk self-
      retaining retractor
    S. clip
    S. clip applier
    S. clip-applying forceps
    S. curette
    S. curved nerve hook
    S. dural hook
    S. flat brain spatula
    S. forceps
    S. hemilaminectomy
      retractor
    S. hemilaminectomy self-
      retaining retractor
    S. laminectomy retractor
    S. needle
    S. nerve retractor

    S. nerve root retractor
    S. psoas muscle retractor
    S. retractor
    S. retractor blade
    S. retractor hook
    S. retractor hook with cross
      blade
    S. ruptured disk curette
    S. scissors
    S. self-retaining retractor
    S. skull trephine
    S. ventricular needle
Scoville-Drew clip applier
Scoville-Greenwood
    S.-G. Bayonet neurosurgical
      bipolar forceps
    S.-G. forceps
Scoville-Haverfield
    S.-H. hemilaminectomy
      retractor
    S.-H. laminectomy retractor
Scoville-Hurteau forceps
Scoville-Lewis
    S.-L. aneurysm clip
    S.-L. clamp
    S.-L. clip
Scoville-Richter
    S.-R. retractor
    S.-R. self-retaining retractor
scraper
    amalgam s.
    capsular s.
    Charnley acetabular s.
    drum s.
    Hough drum s.
    Knolle s.
    Knolle capsular s.
    Kratz s.
    Kratz capsular s.
    Lewicky capsular s.
    Simcoe capsular s.
scratcher
    Knolle capsular s.
    Kratz s.
    Kratz capsular s.
screen
    Bernell tangent s.
    Bjerrum s.
    Grey-Hess s.
    Hess s.
    tangent s.
screw
    Alta cancellous s.

screw *(continued)*
  Alta cortical s.
  Alta cross-locking s.
  Alta lag s.
  Alta transverse s.
  Aten olecranon s.
  Basile hip s.
  bone s.
  Bosworth coracoclavicular s.
  Buttress thread s.
  cancellous s.
  cancellous bone s.
  cannulated s.
  CAPIS s.
  carpal scaphoid s.
  Carrel-Girard s.
  Collison s.
  s. compressor
  cortex s.
  Crites laryngeal cotton s.
  crown drill s.
  cruciate head s.
  cruciate head bone s.
  cruciform head bone s.
  Cubbins s.
  Demuth hip s.
  s. depth calibrator
  s. depth gauge
  Deyerle s.
  Doyen myoma s.
  Doyen tumor s.
  Duo-Drive cortical s.
  Dwyer spinal s.
  Eggers s.
  encased s.
  expansion s.
  Fabian s.
  foreign body s.
  Gardner-Wells traction
    tongs s.
  Geckeler s.
  glenoid fixation s.
  Hall spinal s.
  Heck s.
  Integrity acetabular cup s.
  interference s.
  intracranial pressure
    monitor s.
  Jewett pick-up s.
  Johannsen lag s.
  Johannsen-Stille lag s.
  Kristiansen eyelet lag s.
  Kurosaka s.

  lag s.
  Leinbach olecranon s.
  Leone expansion s.
  Lewis tonsillar s.
  locking s.
  Lorenzo s.
  Luhr s.
  Luhr implant s.
  Lundholm s.
  Marion s.
  maxillofacial bone s.
  McLaughlin carpal
    scaphoid s.
  Morris biphase s.
  myoma s.
  No-Lok compression s.
  s. occlusive clamp
  oral s.
  Palex expansion s.
  pedicle s.
  Phillips recessed-head s.
  Pilot point s.
  pull s.
  Ray s.
  Ray s.
  reverse-threaded s.
  Richards classic compression
    hip s.
  Richards compression s.
  Richmond subarachnoid s.
  Rockwood shoulder s.
  Russell-Taylor s.
  sacral s.
  Schanz s.
  Scuderi s.
  self-tapping bone s.
  Sherman bone s.
  Simmons double-hole
    spinal s.
  Simmons-Martin s.
  Stryker s.
  Stryker lag s.
  Synthes s.
  s. tap
  Thatcher s.
  s. tip
  titanium s.
  tonsillar s.
  Townley bone graft s.
  Townsend-Gilfillan s.
  traction tongs s.
  transfixion s.
  tumor s.

Venable s.
Virgin hip s.
Vitallium s.
VLC compression s.
Weise jack s.
Wood s.
Woodruff s.
Yuan s.
Zimmer s.
screwdriver
Allen-headed s.
automatic s.
Becker s.
CAPIS s.
Children's Hospital s.
Collison s.
cross-slot s.
cruciform s.
Cubbins s.
Cubbins bone s.
DePuy s.
Dorsey s.
Dorsey screw-holding s.
Hall s.
heavy cross-slot s.
hexhead s.
Johnson s.
Ken s.
Lane s.
light cross-slot s.
Lok-it s.
Lok-screw s.
Lok-screw double-slot s.
Massie s.
Master s.
Moore-Blount s.
Phillips s.
plain s.
Richards Phillips s.
Richter s.
Richter bone s.
Shallcross s.
Sherman s.
Sherman-Pierce s.
single cross-slot s.
skull plate s.
straight hex s.
Stryker s.
Trinkle s.
Universal s.
Universal hex s.
V. Mueller s.
White s.

Williams s.
Woodruff s.
Zimmer s.
screw-holding forceps
screw-in lead pacemaker
scrotal
s. dressing
s. truss
scrub
s. brush
s. file
scrubber
capsular s.
posterior capsular s.
Simcoe anterior chamber
capsular s.
Simcoe capsular s.
Simcoe posterior capsular s.
scrub soap
benzoin s. s.
Betadine s. s.
Derma surgical s. s.
Envisan cleaning pad s. s.
Envisan wound cleaning
paste s. s.
G-11 s. s.
Gamophen s. s.
Germa-medica s. s.
Germicide C.R.I. s. s.
G.S.I. s. s.
Hexa-germ s. s.
Hibiclens s. s.
Hibiscrub s. s.
Instasan s. s.
Ioprep s. s.
pHisoDerm s. s.
pHisoHex s. s.
Septisol s. s.
Scudder
S. clamp
S. forceps
S. intestinal clamp
S. intestinal forceps
S. skid
S. stomach clamp
Scuderi
S. bipolar coagulating
forceps
S. forceps
S. prosthesis
S. screw
Scuderi-Callahan flange
sculpturing scalpel

scultetus
    s. bandage
    s. binder band
    s. binder dressing
    s. dressing
Scurasil device prosthesis
Scutan temporary splint material
SD-1 stone disintegrator
seal
    Ilex stomal s.
sealer
    endodontic s.
    Hydroset root canal s.
    Terumo tube s.
sealing window plug
Sealy dissecting scissors
seamless
    s. graft
    s. prosthesis
seam-sealer gun
searcher
    Allport-Babcock mastoid s.
    Allport mastoid s.
    mastoid s.
    Proctor-Bruce mastoid s.
    Shea s.
    Shuletz s.
Searcy
    S. capsular forceps
    S. chalazion trephine
    S. erysiphake
    S. fixation anchor
    S. fixation hook
    S. forceps
    S. oval cup erysiphake
    S. tonsillectome
seat
    Heffington lumbar s.
Sebileau elevator
Sebra arm tourniquet
Sechrist
    S. infant ventilator
    S. neonatal ventilator
secondary suture
Secto
    S. dissector
    S. tonsillar sponge
Secu clip
seculum
Securat suction tube
Secure denture adhesive
Seddon nerve graft

Sédillot
    S. elevator
    S. periosteal elevator
    S. raspatory
Seecor pacemaker
seed implant
Seeman-Seiffert mouth gag
Seen retractor
Seep-Pruf ileostomy appliance
Segond
    S. abdominal retractor
    S. forceps
    S. hysterectomy forceps
    S. myomatome
    S. retractor
    S. tumor forceps
    S. vaginal spatula
Segond-Landau hysterectomy
    forceps
Segura-Dretler stone basket
Segura stone basket
Sehrt
    S. clamp
    S. compressor
Seidel
    S. bone-holding clamp
    S. catheter
    S. plug
Seiffert
    S. double-articulated
      grasping forceps tip
    S. esophagoscopy forceps
    S. forceps
    S. grasping punch
    S. grasping tip
    S. laryngeal forceps
    S. suturing instrument
    S. tonsillectome
Seiler
    S. tonsillar knife
    S. turbinate scissors
seizing forceps
Seldin dental retractor
Seldinger
    S. apparatus
    S. arterial needle
    S. cardiac catheter
    S. catheter
    S. needle
Selective-HI catheter
selector
    sleeve s.

Seletz
- S. cannula
- S. catheter
- S. foramen-plugging forceps
- S. forceps
- S. Universal Kerrison punch
- S. ventricular cannula

Seletz-Gelpi
- S.-G. laminectomy retractor
- S.-G. retractor
- S.-G. self-retaining retractor

Selfast dental cement

self-broaching pin

self-centering Universal hip prosthesis

self-inflating tissue expander

self-injurious-behavior inhibiting system (SIBIS)

self-opening
- s.-o. forceps
- s.-o. rigid snare
- s.-o. snare

self-retaining
- s.-r. abdominal retractor
- s.-r. bone forceps
- s.-r. brain retractor set
- s.-r. catheter
- s.-r. chamber maintainer
- s.-r. infusion cannula
- s.-r. laryngoscope
- s.-r. retractor
- s.-r. retractor blade
- s.-r. skin retractor
- s.-r. spring retractor
- s.-r. sternal retractor set

self-tapering pin

self-tapping bone screw

Selker ventriculostomy reservoir

sellar punch

Sellheim
- S. elevating spoon
- S. obstetrical lever
- S. uterine catheter

Sellor
- S. clamp
- S. contractor
- S. mitral valve knife
- S. rib contractor
- S. valvulotome

Selman
- S. clamp
- S. clip
- S. forceps

- S. nonslip tissue forceps
- S. peripheral blood vessel forceps
- S. tissue forceps
- S. vessel forceps

Selofix dressing

Selopor dressing

Selrodo
- S. bulb
- S. nebulizer

Selsi sport telescope

Seltzer saw

Selverstone
- S. carotid artery clamp
- S. carotid clamp
- S. clamp
- S. cordotomy hook
- S. embolus forceps
- S. forceps
- S. intervertebral disk forceps
- S. intervertebral disk rongeur
- S. intervertebral disk rongeur forceps
- S. laminectomy rongeur

Semb
- S. bone-cutting forceps
- S. bone-holding clamp
- S. bone-holding forceps
- S. bronchus clamp
- S. dissecting forceps
- S. forceps
- S. ligature-carrying forceps
- S. ligature forceps
- S. lung retractor
- S. raspatory
- S. retractor
- S. rib raspatory
- S. rongeur
- S. rongeur forceps
- S. self-retaining retractor
- S. shears
- S. vaginal speculum

Semb-Ghazi
- S.-G. dissecting forceps
- S.-G. forceps

Semb-Sauerbruch rongeur

SEMI
- S. bulb irrigation syringe
- S. leg bag

semicircular gouge

semicompressive dressing

semifinished glass
semiflat tip electrode
semiflexible endoscope
semiflexible intraocular lens
semilunar cartilage knife
semilunar-tip blade
seminal suture
semipermeable membrane dressing
semipressure dressing
semirigid
   s. catheter
   s. endoscope
semirigid intraocular lens
semishell eye implant
Semken
   S. bipolar forceps
   S. dressing forceps
   S. forceps
   S. infant forceps
   S. microbipolar
     neurosurgical forceps
   S. thumb forceps
   S. tissue forceps
Semm
   S. abdominal retractor
   S. cannula
   S. CO_2 pneumatometer
   S. dissecting scissors
   S. pneumoperitoneum
     apparatus
   S. uterine cannula
   S. uterine catheter
   S. vacuum
   S. vacuum cannula
   S. vacuum catheter
Semmes
   S. dural forceps
   S. spinal curette
   S. spinal fusion curette
Sengstaken
   S. balloon
   S. nasogastric tube
Sengstaken-Blakemore
   S.-B. balloon
   S.-B. device
   S.-B. esophageal varices
     balloon
   S.-B. tube
Senn
   S. bone plate
   S. double-ended retractor
   S. forceps
   S. mastoid retractor

S. retractor
S. self-retaining retractor
Senn-Dingman
   S.-D. double-ended retractor
   S.-D. retractor
Senn-Green retractor
Senning
   S. bulldog clamp
   S. cardiovascular forceps
   S. clamp
   S. featherweight bulldog
     clamp
   S. forceps
Senning-Stille clamp
Senn-Kanavel
   S.-K. double-ended retractor
   S.-K. retractor
Senn-Miller retractor
Senoran aspirator
Sens dissector
Sensimatic electrosurgical unit
sensing catheter
Sensolog III pacemaker
sensor
   Albin-Bunegin pressure s.
   Novametrix combination
     $0_2/C0_2$ s.
   Richmond subarachnoid
     screw s.
sensor-based single-chamber
  pacemaker
Sensor Kelvin pacemaker
Senstaken esophageal tube
Senturia
   S. forceps
   S. pharyngeal speculum
   S. retractor
Senturia-Alden specimen collector
separator
   Asahi Plasmaflo plasma s.
   bayonet s.
   Benson baby pyloric s.
   Davis nerve s.
   Dorsey dural s.
   dural s.
   Elast-O-Chain s.
   Frazier dural s.
   Grant dural s.
   Harris s.
   head/stem spoon s.
   Hoen dural s.
   Horsley dural s.
   House s.

House ear s.
Hunter s.
iliac graft s.
Kirby s.
Kirby curved zonular s.
Kirby cylindrical zonular s.
Kirby double-ball s.
Kirby flat zonular s.
Lig-A-Ring s.
Luys s.
Remy s.
Rosen s.
Rosen bayonet s.
Sachs dural s.
Sachs nerve s.
Sep-A-Ring s.
Silverstein nerve s.
Woodson dural s.
zonule s.
separator-spatula
Sachs nerve s.-s.
Sep-A-Ring separator
septal
s. bone forceps
s. chisel
s. clamp
s. compression forceps
s. dissector
s. elevator
s. forceps
s. knife
s. needle
s. ridge forceps
s. straightener
Septisol
S. scrub soap
S. soap dressing
Septoject needle
Septopack periodontal dressing
Septosil impression material
septostomy balloon catheter
septum-cutting forceps
septum-straightening forceps
sequential compression stockings
sequestrum forceps
Sequicor
S. II pacemaker
S. III pacemaker
S. pacemaker
Seraflo
S. AV fistular needle
S. transducer protector
Seraphim clip

Seraton dialysis control system
Serature
S. clip
S. spur clip
Seroma-cath feeding tube
seromuscular suture
seromuscular-to-edge suture
seroserosal
s. silk suture
s. suture
seroserous suture
serpentine bone plate
serrated
s. blade
s. curette
s. fine-cutting knife
s. forceps
s. grasping tip
s. retractor
s. scissors
s. suture
s. T-spatula
Serratex scissors
Serrator
serrefine
Blair s.
Brunswick s.
s. clamp
Dieffenbach s.
s. forceps
Hess s.
s. implant
Lemoine s.
Mack s.
s. retractor
servo-controlled
Servo ventilator
Servox hearing aid
sesamoidectomy dissector
set
Acland-Banis arteriotomy s.
adult retractor s.
Amicon arteriovenous blood tubing s.
anterior cervical retractor s.
Arnold-Bruening intracordal injection s.
arthroscopic meniscus repair instrument s.
arthroscopy bur s.
auditory canal dissector s.
Bantam irrigation s.

set *(continued)*
  Bio-Medicus percutaneous
    cannula s.
  Biostil blood transfusion s.
  bone biopsy trephine s.
  bone drill s.
  bone forceps standard s.
  bone plating s.
  Borst side-arm introducer s.
  Brodmerkel colon
    decompression s.
  bronchial brush biopsy s.
  bronchography s.
  Bruening-Arnold intracordal
    injection s.
  Bruening intracordal
    injection s.
  Bruening otoscope s.
  bucket handle tear s.
  butterfly winged infusion s.
  Catalano intubation s.
  cervical accessory s.
  Cheshire suture removal s.
  clamp s.
  Cliniset infusion s.
  Cloward cervical retractor s.
  Codman external drainage
    ventricular s.
  Colapinto transjugular
    biopsy s.
  Collis anterior cervical
    retractor s.
  Collis anterior lumbar
    accessory s.
  Collis cervical TDR
    accessory s.
  Collis lumbar TDR
    accessory s.
  Collis posterior lumbar
    retractor s.
  Collis Universal
    laminectomy s.
  Cone-Bucy suction
    cannula s.
  Cook peelaway introducer s.
  Cooley neonatal
    instrument s.
  Cope gastrointestinal suture
    anchor s.
  corneal trephine s.
  coronary endarterectomy s.
  Corpak enteral Y
    extension s.

  Cotton-Huibregtse biliary
    stent s.
  Cotton-Leung biliary stent s.
  Craig vertebral biopsy s.
  Craig vertebral body biopsy
    instrument s.
  Crampton-Tsang
    percutaneous endoscopic
    biliary stent s.
  dacryocystorhinostomy s.
  Dansac colostomy
    irrigation s.
  Dujovny microsuction
    dissection s.
  Dynacor vaginal irrigator s.
  Eiken-Kizai hemodialysis
    blood tubing s.
  endarterectomy stripper s.
  endometrial biopsy s.
  Endo-Suction sinus
    microstat s.
  Entera Flo spike s.
  Erlangen s.
  esophageal dilating s.
  eustachian filiform s.
  Freiburg biopsy s.
  Garcia endometrial
    biopsy s.
  Grandon cortex extractor s.
  Grieshaber global control
    tubing s.
  Guibor canaliculus
    intubation s.
  Halogen Lite s.
  Harris leg length calipers s.
  Hartmann tuning fork s.
  Harvard microbore
    intravenous extension s.
  Hawkins transhepatic
    cholangiography needle s.
  Hobbs stent s.
  Huibregtse biliary stent s.
  Inpersol peritoneal
    dialysis s.
  insitu bypass instrument s.
  Jackson lacrimal
    intubation s.
  Jackson magnification
    ruler s.
  laser microsurgery s.
  laser surgery s.
  Leather in-situ bypass
    instrument s.

Lehman wire-guided biliary manometry catheter s.

Leung endoscopic nasal biliary drainage s.

Liguory endoscopic nasal biliary drainage s.

liver biopsy s.

Loversan infusion s.

lumbar accessory s.

Malis irrigation tubing s.

Marcon Colon Decompression s.

Mardis-Dangler ureteral stent s.

Marino rotatable transsphenoidal instrument s.

McIntyre guarded irrigating cystitome s.

McIntyre infusion s.

Menghini s.

Mentanium vitreoretinal instrument s.

Mills coronary endarterectomy s.

Moore nail s.

mouth gag s.

Nagaraja endoscopic nasal biliary drainage s.

nail s.

nasal tenaculum s.

needle microstat s.

New Orleans endarterectomy stripper s.

orbital retractor s.

over-door traction s.

over-the-top rasp s.

Pace-Potts intestinal clamp s.

Palex colostomy irrigation starter s.

Parker-Glassman intestinal clamp s.

pediatric perineal retractor s.

Pinnacle introducer s.

Porter-Kolpe biliary biopsy s.

posterior lumbar retractor s.

Ramel s.

reduced small fragment s.

Reliavac closed wound suction s.

retractor s.

Rica esophagoscopy s.

Rica skull perforator s.

Rochester sternum-perforating awl s.

Savary-Gilliard dilator s.

Scherback-Porges vaginal speculum s.

self-retaining brain retractor s.

self-retaining sternal retractor s.

Simcoe lens-positioning s.

Sippy esophageal dilating s.

small fragment and implant s.

small osteotome s.

Smillie cartilage s.

Soehendra lithotripsy s.

Stille bone drill s.

Stille-pattern trephine and bone drill s.

Storz ear knife s.

transcricothyroid selective bronchography s.

trocar s.

Turkel bone biopsy trephine s.

Universal laminectomy s.

ureteral pigtail stent s.

vaginal dilating s.

vascular access s.

Veirs dacryocystorhinostomy s.

Vennes pancreatic dilation s.

VPI-Jacobellis microhematuria catheter s.

Wiegerinck culdocentesis puncture s.

Wilson-Cook Carey capsule s.

Wilson-Cook low-profile esophageal prosthesis s.

wire-guided biliary manometry catheter s.

Wissinger s.

Wylie endarterectomy s.

Young vaginal dilator s.

Zimmon endoscopic biliary stent s.

Zimmon endoscopic pancreatic stent s.

Setacure denture repair acrylic
seton
  s. drain
  s. hip brace
  s. needle
  s. suture
setter
  Eby band s.
  Klauber band s.
  Ormco band s.
  orthodontic band s.
Seutin
  S. bandage
  S. plaster shears
  S. scissors
severance
  s. transurethral bag
  s. transurethral hemostatic
    bag
Severin multiple closed-loop
  intraocular lens
Sewall
  S. antral cannula
  S. antral trocar
  S. brain clip-applying
    forceps
  S. cannula
  S. chisel
  S. ethmoidal chisel
  S. ethmoidal elevator
  S. forceps
  S. mucoperiosteal periosteal
    elevator
  S. orbital retractor
  S. raspatory
  S. retractor
sewing-machine stitch suture
sewn-in waterproof drape
Sexton ear knife
Seyand vulsellum
Seyfert forceps
Seyffert vaginal speculum
SFB-I right-angled bronchoscope
SGIA
  SGIA 50 disposable stapler
  SGIA stapling device
Shaaf
  S. eye forceps
  S. forceps
  S. foreign body forceps
shadow-free laryngoscope
Shadow-Stripe catheter

Shaffer modification of Barkan
  knife
shaft
  biopsy forceps s.
  bladder specimen forceps s.
  Braasch bladder specimen
    forceps s.
  Cloward drill s.
  cup pusher s.
  s. eamer
  s. reamer
  slide hammer s.
Shah
  S. aural dressing
  S. grommet
  S. nasal splint
  S. ventilation tube
Shahan thermopore
Shahinian lacrimal cannula
Shah-Shah intraocular lens
shaking sound
Shaldach pacemaker
Shallcross
  S. cystic duct forceps
  S. forceps
  S. gallbladder forceps
  S. hemostat
  S. hemostatic forceps
  S. nasal forceps
  S. nasal-packing forceps
  S. screwdriver
Shallcross-Dean gall duct forceps
Shambaugh
  S. adenoidal curette
  S. adenotome
  S. elevator
  S. endaural hook
  S. endaural retractor
  S. endaural self-retaining
    retractor
  S. fistula hook
  S. hook
  S. irrigator
  S. knife
  S. microscopic hook
  S. narrow elevator
  S. needle
  S. palpating needle
  S. retractor
  S. reverse adenotome
Shambaugh-Derlacki
  S.-D. chisel
  S.-D. duckbill elevator

S.-D. elevator
S.-D. microhook
Shambaugh-Lempert knife
Shampaine head holder
shank
Bi-Metric tapered reamer
with Zimmer-Hudson s.
calcar trimmer with
Zimmer-Hudson s.
Crowley s.
grater-type reamer with
Zimmer-Hudson s.
Hudson s.
taper with Zimmer s.
Zimmer-Hudson s.
Shank electrode
Shantz
S. dressing
S. pin
shaper
interspace s.
Shapleigh
S. curette
S. ear curette
Shapshay-Healy laryngoscope
Sharbaro driver
shark
s. fin papillotome
s. fin sphincterotome
shark-tooth forceps
Sharman curette
Sharp
S. dermal curette
S. point-tip cystitome
sharp
s. curette
s. hook
s. knife
s. trocar
Sharplan
S. CO_2 laser
S. laser
S. Medilas Nd:YAG surgical
laser
S. surgical laser
SharpLase Nd:YAG laser
Sharplav laparoscope
Sharpley hook
Sharpoint V-lance blade
sharp-pointed forceps
sharp-pronged retractor

Sharpshay-Healy
S.-H. laryngeal alligator
forceps
S.-H. laryngeal-cutting
forceps
S.-H. laryngeal-grasping
forceps
S.-H. laryngeal scissors
Sharpshay laser bronchoscope
Shasta alloy
shattering needle
shaver
s. catheter
Concept s.
Stryker s.
Shaw
S. carotid artery clot
stripper
S. scalpel
Shea
S. bur
S. curette
S. drill
S. ear drill
S. elevator
S. fenestration hook
S. fistular hook
S. headrest
S. hook
S. incision knife
S. irrigator
S. knife
S. long back-handed
elevator
S. microdrill
S. middle ear instrument
S. oblique hook
S. pick
S. polyethylene prosthesis
S. prosthesis
S. prosthesis placement
instrument
S. searcher
S. speculum
S. speculum holder
S. stapes hook
S. Teflon piston prosthesis
S. vein graft scissors
Shea-Anthony
S.-A. bag
S.-A. balloon
Shea-Bellucci scissors
Shealy facet rhizotomy electrode

Shearer
S. bone rongeur
S. chicken-bill forceps
S. forceps
S. lip retractor
S. retractor
S. rongeur
S. rongeur forceps
Shearing
S. intraocular lens
S. J-Loop intraocular lens
S. posterior chamber
implant material
S. posterior chamber
intraocular lens
S. S-style anterior chamber
intraocular lens
shears (*See also* scissors)
Bacon s.
bandage s.
bandage plaster s.
Bethune-Coryllos rib s.
Bethune rib s.
Bortone s.
Braun-Stadler sternal s.
Brunner rib s.
Brun plaster s.
Bruns plaster s.
Clayton laminectomy s.
Collin s.
Cooley first rib s.
Cooley-Pontius sternal s.
Coryllos s.
Coryllos-Bethune s.
Coryllos-Moure rib s.
Coryllos rib s.
Coryllos-Shoemaker rib s.
Duval-Coryllos rib s.
Eccentric lock rib s.
Endo s.
Esmarch plaster s.
first rib s.
Frey-Sauerbruch rib s.
Giertz rib s.
Giertz-Stille rib s.
Gluck rib s.
Hercules plaster s.
Horgan-Coryllos-Moure
rib s.
Horgan-Wells rib s.
infant rib s.
Jackson esophageal s.
Jackson-Moore s.

Jarit plaster s.
Jarit utility s.
Lebsche sternal s.
Lefferts rib s.
Liston s.
Liston-Ruskin s.
Moure-Coryllos rib s.
Nelson-Bethune s.
Pilling laryngofissure s.
plain rib s.
plaster s.
pleural biopsy needle s.
Potts infant rib s.
rib s.
Roos first rib s.
Sauerbruch-Britsch rib s.
Sauerbruch-Coryllos rib s.
Sauerbruch-Frey rib s.
Sauerbruch-Lebsche rib s.
Sauerbruch rib s.
Scanlan plaster s.
Scanlan rib s.
Schumacher sternal s.
s. scissors
scissors plaster s.
Semb s.
Seutin plaster s.
Shoemaker rib s.
Shuletz rib s.
sternal s.
Stille-Aesculap plaster s.
Stille-Ericksson rib s.
Stille-Giertz s.
Stille-Horsley s.
Stille plaster s.
Stille-Stiwer plaster s.
Thompson rib s.
Thomsen rib s.
Tudor-Edwards rib s.
utility s.
Walton rib s.
Weck s.

sheath
Amplatz renal dilator
and s.
arterial s.
beaked s.
concave s.
convex s.
double-channel operating s.
fiberoptic s.
French s.
hysteroscope s.

incandescent s.
irrigating s.
IVT percutaneous catheter
  introducer s.
Medi-Tech s.
s. and obturator
O'Connor s.
peel-away s.
Pfister-Schwartz s.
Pinnacle s.
resectoscope s.
single-channel operating s.
Storz s.
tear away introducer s.
UMI Cath-Seal s.
venous s.
Warne penile s.
s. with side-arm adapter
sheathed flexible gastric forceps
Sheehan
S. chisel
S. knee prosthesis
S. nasal chisel
S. osteotome
S. retractor
Sheehan-Gillies needle holder
Sheehy
S. button
S. canal knife
S. collar button
S. collar button tube
S. fascial press
S. forceps
S. incus prosthesis
S. incus replacement
  prosthesis
S. myringotomy knife
S. ossicle-holding clamp
S. ossicle-holding forceps
S. round knife
S. Tytan ventilation tube
S. weapon
Sheehy-House
S.-H. chisel
S.-H. curette
S.-H. incus prosthesis
S.-H. incus replacement
  prosthesis
S.-H. knife
S.-H. knife curette
Sheen tip graft
sheepskin dressing

Sheer
S. probe
S. wire crimper
sheer spot Band-Aid dressing
sheet
Abanda drape s.
casting wax s.
s. holder
Moran-Karaya s.
Ortholen s.
s. rubber drain
Subortholen s.
Teknamed drape s.
Sheets
S. cannula
S. closed-loop posterior
  chamber intraocular lens
S. eye glide
S. glide
S. intraocular glide
S. iris hook
S. irrigating vectis
S. irrigating vectis cannula
S. lens cutter
S. lens forceps
S. lens-inserting forceps
S. lens spatula
S. micro-iris hook
S. spatula
S. two flexible closed loops
  intraocular lens
Sheets-Hirsch spatula
Sheets-McPherson angled forceps
Sheets-McPherson tying forceps
sheet-wadding dressing
Sheffield splint
Sheinmann laryngeal forceps
Sheldon
S. catheter
S. clamp
S. hemilaminectomy
  retractor
S. hemilaminectomy self-
  retaining retractor
S. laminectomy retractor
S. retractor
S. spreader
Sheldon-Gosset
S.-G. retractor
S.-G. self-retaining retractor
Sheldon-Pudenz dissector
Sheldon-Spatz
S.-S. needle

Sheldon-Spatz *(continued)*
    S.-S. vertebral arteriogram
      needle
Sheldon-Swann needle
shelf reamer
shell
    aluminum s.
    s. eye implant
    Harris protrusio s.
    s. implant
    s. implant material
    Integrity s.
    KM-4 s.
    KM-3A s.
    protrusio s.
    scleral s.
shellac-covered catheter
shell-type eye implant
Shepard
    S. bipolar forceps
    S. calipers block
    S. cannula
    S. curved intraocular lens
      forceps
    S. depth gauge
    S. drain tube
    S. flexible anterior chamber
      intraocular lens
    S. forceps
    S. grommet
    S. grommet ventilation tube
    S. hook
    S. incision depth gauge
    S. incision irrigating
      cannula
    S. intraocular lens forceps
    S. intraocular lens implant
    S. intraocular lens-inserting
      forceps
    S. intraocular utility forceps
    S. iris hook
    S. lens forceps
    S. lens-inserting forceps
    S. micro-iris hook
    S. optical center marker
    S. radial keratotomy
      irrigating cannula
    S. tying forceps
    S. Universal intraocular lens
Shepard-Kramer calipers block
Shepard-Reinstein intraocular lens
    forceps
Shepard-Westcott scissors

shepherd's hook catheter
Sherman
    S. bone plate
    S. bone screw
    S. plate
    S. screwdriver
    S. suction tube
Sherman-Pierce screwdriver
Sherman-Stille drill
Sherwin self-retaining retractor
Sherwood retractor
shield
    aluminum eye s.
    American Medical
      Electronics, Inc. PinSite s.
    Atkins-Tucker surgical s.
    Barraquer eye s.
    binocular s.
    bronchoscopic face s.
    Buller eye s.
    Carapace face s.
    Cartella eye s.
    circumcisional s.
    collagen s.
    corneal light s.
    Dacron s.
    eye s.
    face s.
    Faraday s.
    Fox eye s.
    Fuller s.
    Fuller perianal s.
    Garter s.
    Goffman blue eye garter s.
    gonad s.
    Gottesman splash s.
    Grafco eye s.
    Green eye s.
    Guibor Expo eye bubble s.
    Jardon eye s.
    Jet s.
    metal Fox s.
    Mueller s.
    Paton eye s.
    Pro-Ophta type-K s.
    Pro-Ophta type-S s.
    ring cataract mask eye s.
    Simmons eye s.
    Storz s.
    Storz Easy s.
    Universal eye s.
shielded open-end cone
Shier knee prosthesis

Shiffrin bone wire tightener
shifting pacemaker
Shiley
    S. cardiotomy reservoir
    S. catheter
    S. convexoconcave heart
      valve
    S. French sump tube
    S. guiding catheter
    S. irrigation catheter
    S. JL-4 guiding catheter
    S. monostrut heart valve
    S. MultiPro catheter
    S. saphenous vein irrigation
      and pressurization device
    S. soft-tip guiding catheter
    S. sump tube
    S. Tetraflex vascular graft
Shiley-Ionescu catheter
Shimadzu ultrasound system
Shimstock occlusion foil
Ship arthroplasty implant
Shirlee spline
Shirley
    S. sump type drain
    S. wound drain
Shirodkar
    S. aneurysm needle
    S. cervical needle
    S. needle
    S. probe
    S. suture
SHJR4s catheter
shocker
    Take-Me-Along Personal
      Shocker pocket s.
shoe
    beach bum rocker-bottom
      cast sandle s.
    Darby surgical s.
    decubitus boot s.
    Gard-all boot s.
    Mala-paedic s.
    Reece PO s.
    rocker-bottom cast boot s.
shoehorn speculum
Shoemaker
    S. intestinal clamp
    S. rib shears
Shofu
    S. dental cement
    S. porcelain stain kit

short
    s. bold
    s. C-loop intraocular lens
    s. Heaney retractor
    s. needle
Shortbent
    S. scissors
    S. suture scissors
Short bridge
shorthand vertical mattress stitch
   suture
short-leg brace
short-tip
    s.-t. bag
    s.-t. hemostatic bag
short-tooth forceps
shot compressor
shotted suture
shoulder
    s. blade
    s. brace
    Neer s.
    s. prosthesis
    s. subluxation inhibitor
      (SSI)
    s. subluxation inhibitor
      brace
Shrady saw
Shriners
    S. Hospital interlocking
      retractor
    S. Hospital retractor
    S. interlocking retractor
    S. pin
Shulec adenotome
Shuletz
    S. pusher
    S. raspatory
    S. rib shears
    S. searcher
    S. spring
Shuletz-Damian raspatory
Shuletz-Paul rib retractor
Shulitz catheter
shunt
    Accura hydrocephalus s.
    Ames ventriculoperitoneal s.
    Austin endolymph
      dispersement s.
    Brenner carotid bypass s.
    Cobe AV s.
    CSF T-tube s.
    CUI s.

shunt *(continued)*
   Denver s.
   Denver pleuroperitoneal s.
   Denver valve s.
   Gore-Tex s.
   Gott s.
   Hakim s.
   Heyer-Schulte
    hydrocephalus s.
   Heyer-Schulte-Spetzler
    lumbar peritoneal s.
   Holter s.
   House endolymphatic s.
   Javid s.
   Javid carotid s.   *Inahara-*
   s. kit   *Pruitt*
   LeVeen s. *Shunt*
   LeVeen ascites s.
   LeVeen peritoneal s.
   loop s.
   mesocaval H-graft s.
   Mischer-Pudenz s.
   Mischler s.
   one-piece s.
   one-piece s. with reservoir
   Pruitt vascular s.
   Pudenz valve-flushing s.
   Raimondi s.
   Rickham reservoir s.
   Silastic Ames s.
   Silastic
    ventriculoperitoneal s.
   Spetzler s.
   Sundt s.
   Sundt carotid
    endarterectomy s.
   TDMAC heparin s.
   Thomas femoral s.
   Torkildsen s.
   UNI s.
   Uresil carotid s.
   Uresil Vascu-Flo carotid s.
   Vascushunt carotid
    balloon s.
Shuppe biting forceps
Shurly
   S. retractor
   S. tracheal retractor
Shur resin
Shuster
   S. forceps
   S. suture forceps
   S. tonsillar forceps

Shute forceps
shutoff clamp
Shutt
   S. Aggressor forceps
   S. alligator forceps
   S. blunt tip forceps
   S. B-scoop forceps
   S. forceps
   S. grasping forceps
   S. microscissors
   S. Mini-Aggressor forceps
   S. minibasket
   S. minitip forceps
   S. retrograde forceps
   S. shovel nose forceps
   S. suction forceps
shuttle forceps
SIBIS
   self-injurious-behavior inhibiting
    system
Sichel
   S. implant
   S. iris knife
   S. movable implant
   S. orbital implant
sickle knife
sickle-shaped
   s.-s. Bever blade
   s.-s. blade
side
   s. blade
   s. mouth gag
   s. port
side-arm adapter
side-biting clamp
side-curved forceps
side-cutting
   s.-c. basket forceps
   s.-c. blade
   s.-c. bur
   s.-c. irrigating cystitome
   s.-c. rasp
   s.-c. spatula
   s.-c. spatulated needle
side-flattened needle
side-grasping
   s.-g. forceps
   s.-g. tissue forceps
side-hole
   s.-h. catheter
   s.-h. Judkins right, curved
    4, short catheter
   s.-h. pigtail catheter

side-port cannula
side-viewing
    s.-v. endoscope
    s.-v. fiberscope
sidewall
    s. holed needle
    s. infusion cannula
sidewinder
    s. aortic clamp
    s. catheter
    s. percutaneous intra-aortic
      balloon catheter
Sidney Stephenson corneal
  trephine
Siebold uterine scissors
Siegel pneumatic otoscope
Sieger insufflator
Siegle
    S. ear speculum
    S. speculum
Siegler
    S. biopsy forceps
    S. forceps
Siegler-Hellman clamp
Sielaff gastroscope
Siemens
    S. linear probe
    S. PTCA open-heart suture
    S. Servo ventilator
    S. vaginal probe
Siemens-Elema
    S.-E. multi-programmable
      pacemaker
    S.-E. pacemaker
Siemens-Pacesetter pacemaker
Siepser intraocular lens
Sierra alloy
Sierra-Sheldon tracheotome
sieve graft
sigmoid
    s. anastomosis clamp
    s. clamp
sigmoidofiberscope
    Pentax s.
sigmoidoscope
    ACMI flexible s.
    adult s.
    s. biopsy forceps
    Boehm s.
    Buie s.
    disposable s.
    Eder s.
    ESI s.

    fiberoptic s.
    flexible s.
    Frankfeldt s.
    Fujinon flexible s.
    Gorsch s.
    Heinkel s.
    Hopkins s.
    Kelly s.
    KleenSpec s.
    KleenSpec fiberoptic
      disposable s.
    Lieberman s.
    Lieberman s. with swinging
      window
    s. light carrier
    Lloyd-Davis s.
    Montague s.
    Olympus s.
    Olympus fiberoptic s.
    Olympus flexible s.
    Pentax s.
    Pentax fiberoptic s.
    Pentax flexible s.
    Reichert s.
    Reichert fiberoptic s.
    Reichert flexible s.
    s. replacement lamp
    rigid s.
    Solow s.
    Strauss s.
    Turrell s.
    Tuttle s.
    Vernon David s.
    Visiline disposable s.
    Welch Allyn s.
    Welch Allyn fiberoptic s.
    Welch Allyn flexible s.
    Welch Allyn KleenSpec
      fiberoptic disposable s.
    Yeoman s.
Signet disposable skin stapler
Signorini tourniquet
Sigvaris medical stockings
Siker mirror laryngoscope
Silastic
    S. Ames shunt
    S. band
    S. bur hole cover
    S. cannula
    S. catheter
    S. chin implant
    S. chin prosthesis
    S. corneal eye implant

Silastic *(continued)*
S. coronary artery cannula
S. Cronin implant
S. cup extractor
S. drain
S. dressing
S. elastomer infusion catheter
S. eustachian tube
S. eye implant
S. fimbrial prosthesis
S. finger implant
S. graft
S. grommet
S. ileal reservoir catheter
S. implant
S. intestinal tube
S. mammary prosthesis
S. medical adhesive
S. mold
S. mushroom catheter
S. obstetrical vacuum cup
S. otoplasty prosthesis
S. penile implant
S. penile prosthesis
S. rhinoplasty implant
S. scleral buckler eye implant
S. sheeting keel prosthesis
S. silicone rubber implant
S. sponge
S. stent
S. subdermal implant
S. sucker suction tube
S. suture button
S. testicular implant
S. testicular prosthesis
S. thoracic drain
S. thyroid drain
S. toe implant
S. tracheostomy tube
S. ventriculoperitoneal shunt

Silber
S. clamp
S. microneedle holder
S. microvascular clamp
S. needle holder
S. vasovasostomy clamp
Silcath subclavian catheter
Silcock dissection forceps
Silesian bandage
silica contact lens

silicone
s. adhesive
s. ball heart valve
s. buckling implant
s. button eye implant
s. cannula
s. disk heart valve
s. doughnut prosthesis
s. drain
s. dressing
s. elastomer
s. elastomer band
s. elastomer catheter
s. elastomer infusion catheter
s. elastomer prosthesis
s. explant
s. eye implant
s. flat drain
s. hubless flat drain
s. implant
s. meshed motility implant
s. mold
s. nasal strut implant
s. oil cannula
s. pad eye implant
s. rod implant
s. round drain
s. rubber Dacron-cuffed catheter
Schepens boat s.
Schepens grooved rubber s.
Schepens pad s.
s. sleeve eye implant
s. sponge implant
s. strip eye implant
s. sump drain
s. support cradle
s. thoracic drain
s. tip cannula
s. tire eye implant
tire-grooved s.
s. T-tube
s. tube
silicone-filled breast implant
silicone-spiked mat
silicone-treated
s.-t. surgical silk suture
s.-t. suture
Silicore catheter
Sili-Gel impression material
Silima breast prosthesis

Silitek
  S. catheter
  S. ureteral stent
silk
  s. braided suture
  s. guide wire
  s. interrupted mattress suture
  s. nonabsorbable suture
  s. pop-off suture
  s. stay suture
  s. suture
  s. traction suture
silk-and-wax catheter
silkworm gut suture
Silky Polydek suture
Silovi saphenous vein graft
Siloxane
  S. graft
  S. implant
  S. prosthesis
Siltex mammary implant
Silva-Packer
Silver
  S. cannula
  S. chisel
  S. curved cannula
  S. endaural forceps
  S. forceps
  S. knife
  S. nasal osteotome
  S. osteotome
silver
  s. clip
  s. probe
  s. suture
silvered contact lens
silverized catgut suture
Silverman biopsy needle
Silverman-Boeker
  S.-B. cannula
  S.-B. needle
Silverstein
  S. arachnoid dissector
  S. auditory canal dissector
  S. dressing
  S. dural elevator
  S. lateral venous sinus retractor
  S. micromirror
  S. micro-utility knife
  S. nerve separator

  S. permanent aeration tube (SPAT)
  S. round knife
  S. sickle knife
Simcoe
  S. -ens positioning set
  S. anterior chamber capsular scrubber
  S. anterior chamber receiving needle
  S. anterior chamber-retaining wire
  S. capsular scraper
  S. capsular scrubber
  S. C-loop intraocular lens
  S. connecting tubing
  S. corneal marker
  S. cortex cannula
  S. cortex extractor
  S. double-barreled cannula
  S. double cannula
  S. double-end lens loop
  S. eye implant
  S. eye speculum
  S. I&A cannula
  S. I&A system
  S. implant
  S. implantation forceps
  S. intraocular lens implant
  S. irrigating-positioning needle
  S. irrigation-aspiration system
  S. lens forceps
  S. lens implant forceps
  S. lens-inserting forceps
  S. lens-positioning set
  S. loop
  S. microhook
  S. needle
  S. notched irrigating spatula
  S. notched spatula
  S. nucleus delivery cannula
  S. nucleus delivery loop
  S. nucleus erysiphake
  S. nucleus forceps
  S. nucleus intraocular removal forceps
  S. nucleus lens loop
  S. nucleus lens loupe
  S. nucleus loop
  S. nucleus spatula

Simcoe *(continued)*
- S. posterior capsular scrubber
- S. posterior chamber forceps
- S. posterior chamber lens forceps
- S. reverse aperture cannula
- S. reverse irrigating-aspirating cannula
- S. spatula
- S. speculum
- S. superior rectus forceps
- S. suture needle
- S. wire speculum

Simcoe-Amo eye implant

Simcoe-Barraquer eye speculum

Simmonds
- S. cricothyrotomy needle
- S. vaginal speculum

Simmons
- S. catheter
- S. chisel
- S. double-hole spinal screw
- S. eye shield
- S. plating system

Simmons-Kimbrough glaucoma spatula

Simmons-Martin screw

Simon
- S. bone curette
- S. cup uterine curette
- S. dermatome
- S. expansion arch
- S. fistula hook
- S. fistula knife
- S. retractor
- S. spinal curette
- S. suture
- S. uterine scoop
- S. vaginal retractor

Simonart
- S. band
- S. bar

Simones spinal curette

Simon-Nitinol
- S.-N. filter
- S.-N. inferior vena caval filter

Simons
- S. cleft palate knife
- S. stone-removing forceps

Simpa denture reliner

simple suture

Simplus
- S. catheter
- S. dilatation catheter

Simpson
- S. antral curette
- S. atherectomy catheter
- S. AtheroCath catheter
- S. coronary AtheroCath catheter
- S. curette
- S. directional coronary atherectomy device
- S. epistaxis balloon
- S. forceps
- S. lacrimal dilator
- S. lacrimal probe
- S. obstetrical forceps
- S. PET balloon atherectomy device
- S. sterling lacrimal probe
- S. suction catheter
- S. sugar-tong splint
- S. Ultra Lo-Profile balloon catheter
- S. uterine dilator
- S. uterine sound

Simpson-Braun obstetrical forceps

Simpson-Luikart
- S.-L. forceps
- S.-L. obstetrical forceps

Simpson-Robert
- S.-R. ACS dilatation catheter
- S.-R. catheter
- S.-R. vascular dilation system

Simpulse lavage system

Simrock speculum

Sims
- S. abdominal needle
- S. anoscope
- S. cannula
- S. curette
- S. dilator
- S. double-ended retractor
- S. double-ended vaginal speculum
- S. irrigating uterine curette
- S. needle
- S. plain uterine sound
- S. probe

S. rectal retractor
S. rectal speculum
S. retractor
S. scissors
S. sponge holder
S. suture
S. uterine curette
S. uterine depressor
S. uterine dilator
S. uterine probe
S. uterine scissors
S. uterine sound
S. vaginal plug
S. vaginal retractor
S. vaginal speculum
Sims-Kelly
S.-K. retractor
S.-K. vaginal retractor
Sims-Maier
S.-M. clamp
S.-M. sponge and dressing
forceps
Sims-Siebold uterine scissors
simultaneous thermal diffusion
blood flow and pressure probe
Sinexon dilator
Singer
S. needle
S. portable apparatus
S. portable pneumothorax
apparatus
Singer-Bloom
S.-B. ossicular prosthesis
S.-B. tube
Singh speech system voice
rehabilitation prosthesis
single
s. blade retractor
s. bridge
s. clamp
s. cross-slot screwdriver
s. hook
s. patient system (SPS)
s. Softjaw clamp
s. Softjaw handleless clamp
s. tenaculum
single-armed suture
single-chamber pacemaker
single-channel
s.-c. electromyograph
oscilloscope
s.-c. nonfade oscilloscope
s.-c. operating sheath

single-fiber EMG electrode
single-handed knot suture
single-hinged speculum
single-J urinary diversion stent
single-lumen
s.-l. balloon stone extractor
catheter
s.-l. catheter
s.-l. infusion catheter
single-pass pacemaker
single-stage catheter
Singleton empyema trocar
single-tooth
s.-t. forceps
s.-t. tenaculum
single-use
s.-u. dermatome
s.-u. electrode (SUE)
single-wire electrode
Singley
S. clamp
S. forceps
S. intestinal clamp
S. intestinal forceps
S. intestinal tissue forceps
S. tissue forceps
Singley-Tuttle
S.-T. dressing forceps
S.-T. forceps
S.-T. intestinal forceps
S.-T. tissue forceps
Siniscal eyelid clamp
Siniscal-Smith lid everter
sinoscopy
s. cannula
s. trocar
Sinskey
S. forceps
S. hook
S. intraocular lens
S. intraocular lens forceps
S. iris hook
S. lens
S. lens hook
S. lens implant
S. lens-manipulating hook
S. lens manipulator
S. micro-iris hook
S. microlens hook
S. microtying forceps
S. needle holder
S. nucleus spatula
Sinskey-McPherson forceps

**Sinskey-style J-loop intraocular
  lens**
Sinskey-Wilson
  S.-W. forceps
  S.-W. foreign body forceps
sinus
  s. antral cannula
  s. balloon
  s. biopsy forceps
  s. bur
  s. cannula
  s. chisel
  s. curette
  s. dilator
  s. irrigator
  s. node pacemaker
  s. pacemaker
  s. probe
  s. trephine
  s. tympani excavator
sinus-irrigating cannula
Sinvision ultrasound scanner
siphon
  Nichols nasal s.
  s. suction tube
Sippy
  S. dilator
  S. esophageal dilating set
  S. esophageal dilator
  S. esophageal dilator coiled
    spiral pusher wire
  S. esophageal dilator piano-
    wire staff
Sisler lacrimal trephine
Sisson
  S. forceps
  S. hemostatic forceps
  S. spring hook
  S. spring retractor
Sisson-Cottle speculum
Sisson-Love retractor
Sisson-Vienna speculum
sister
  s. hook forceps
  twisted s.
Sistrunk
  S. band retractor
  S. dissecting scissors
  S. double-ended retractor
  S. retractor
  S. scissors
SITE
  S. argon laser

  S. I&A instrument
  S. irrigating-aspirating unit
  S. laser
  S. needle
  S. TXR phacoemulsification
    system
sitz bath
Sivash hip prosthesis
six-eye catheter
six-prong rake retractor
sixty-degree valve heart valve
sizer
  Björk-Shiley heart valve s.
  Meadox graft s.
Skeele
  S. chalazion curette
  S. corneal curette
  S. curette
  S. eye curette
skeletal pin
Skene
  S. catheter
  S. forceps
  S. tenaculum
  S. tenaculum forceps
  S. uterine curette
  S. uterine forceps
  S. uterine spoon
  S. uterine spoon curette
  S. uterine tenaculum
  S. uterine tenaculum forceps
  S. uterine vulsellum forceps
  S. vulsellum
  S. vulsellum forceps
skid
  acetabular s.
  Austin Moore-Murphy
    bone s.
  bone s.
  s. curette
  Davis s.
  Davis bone s.
  hip s.
  MacAusland s.
  MacAusland hip s.
  Meyerding s.
  Meyerding bone s.
  Meyerding hip s.
  Meyerding shoulder s.
  Murphy bone s.
  Murphy-Lane s.
  Murphy-Lane bone s.
  Ryerson bone s.

Scudder s.
Yund s.
Yund acetabular s.
Skillern
S. cannula
S. curette
S. forceps
S. phimosis forceps
S. probe
S. sinus curette
S. sphenoidal cannula
S. sphenoidal probe
Skillman
S. arterial forceps
S. forceps
S. hemostatic forceps
S. mosquito forceps
S. mosquito hemostatic
forceps
S. prepuce forceps
skin
s. clip
s. elevator
s. flap retractor
s. forceps
s. graft expander mesh
s. graft mesher
s. grinder
s. hook
s. hook retractor
s. marker
s. marking pen
s. punch
s. retractor
s. self-retaining retractor
s. splint
s. staple
s. suture
ski needle
skinfold calipers
Skinny
S. balloon catheter
skinny
s. Chiba needle
s. needle
Skin Skribe pen
Sklar
S. anoscope
S. brush
S. cutter
S. evacuator
S. medical breast stamp
S. scribe skin marker

S. sinus cleanser
S. tonometer
Sklar-Junion Tompkins aspirator
Sklar-Schitz jewel tonometer
Skoog nasal chisel
skull
s. bur
s. clamp
s. elevator
s. plate
s. plate screwdriver
s. punch
s. raspatory
s. traction drill
s. traction tongs
s. trephine
Skylark
S. surface electrode
S. TENS unit
Skytron air-fluidized bed
slaphammer
BIAS s.
Slatis frame
Slaughter nasal saw
Sled implant
sleeper suture
sleeve
s. adapter
s. bag
Bi-Metric PMMA
centering s.
Cunningham-Cotton s.
Ken Drive s.
laparoscopic s.
Mentor Foley catheter with
comfort s.
PMMA centering s.
s. selector
Supramid eye muscle s.
Sur-Fit colostomy
irrigation s.
Surgigrip s.
tri-point K-Wire s.
Watzke s.
sleeved nut
sleeve-spreading
s.-s. dilating forceps
s.-s. forceps
slide
s. hammer
s. hammer shaft
Slidewire extension guide

sliding
- s. capsular forceps
- s. hammer
- s. laryngoscope
- s. lock
- s. stapler

slightly-curved ear pick
slightly-curved pick
Slimfit lens
slimline blade
sling
- Ampoxen s.
- arm elevator s.
- Böhler-Braun leg s.
- cradle arm s.
- s. dressing
- hanging cast s.
- Harris splint s.
- Kodel s.
- leg s.
- Mersilene s.
- Posey s.
- pouch type s.
- slinger-style envelope s.
- sling and swathe s.
- s. suture
- Thomas Kodel s.
- triangular arm s.
- Uni-Versatil s.
- Weil pelvic s.
- Westfield-style envelope s.

sling-and-swathe bandage
slinger-style envelope sling
Slinky
- S. balloon
- S. balloon catheter
- S. PTCA catheter

slip joint pliers
Slip-N-Snip scissors
slit
- s. blade
- s. illuminator
- s. illuminator slit lamp
- s. lamp

Sloan
- S. dissector
- S. goiter flap dissector
- S. goiter retractor
- S. goiter self-retaining retractor
- S. retractor

Slocum meniscal clamp
Slocum-Smith-Petersen nail

slotted
- s. bone plate
- s. intramedullary rod
- s. laryngoscope
- s. mallet
- s. nail
- s. plate
- s. suture
- s. whisker
- s. wrench

slotting bur
slotting-bur osteotome
SLT
- SLT CL100 Contact laser
- SLT CL MD/110 Contact laser
- SLT CL MD/Dual contact laser
- SLT Contact ArthroProbe
- SLT Contact laser
- SLT FiberTact/Contact laser fiber

Sluder
- S. adenotome
- S. cautery electrode
- S. headband
- S. knife
- S. needle
- S. palate retractor
- S. retractor
- S. sphenoidal hook
- S. sphenoidal speculum
- S. tonometer
- S. tonsillar guillotine
- S. tonsillar tonsillectome

Sluder-Ballenger
- S.-B. tonsillar punch forceps
- S.-B. tonsillectome
- S.-B. tonsillotome

Sluder-Demarest
- S.-D. tonometer
- S.-D. tonsillectome

Sluder-Ferguson mouth gag
Sluder-Jansen mouth gag
Sluder-Mehta electrode
Sluder-Sauer
- S.-S. tonsillar guillotine
- S.-S. tonsillectome

Small
- S. rake retractor
- S. tissue retractor

small
- s. bone chisel

s. bone-cutting forceps
s. bone-holding forceps
s. fragment and implant set
s. joint forceps
s. osteotome set
s. pick
s. set osteotome
s. spring scissors
s. tray

Small-Carrion
S.-C. penile implant
material
S.-C. penile prosthesis
S.-C. Silastic rod for penile
implant

small-loop electrode
Smart
S. chalazion forceps
S. enucleation scissors
S. forceps
S. nonslipping chalazion
forceps

smart
s. laser
s. position-sensing catheter

SM disposable loading unit
Smead-Jones suture
Smedberg
S. brace
S. dilator
S. drill

Smeden tonsillar punch
Smellie
S. obstetrical forceps
S. obstetrical hook
S. obstetrical perforator
S. obstetrical scissors
S. perforater

Smeloff-Cutter
S.-C. ball-valve prosthesis
S.-C. heart valve

Smeloff heart valve
SMI
SMI cannula
SMI Surgi-Med CPM device

SMIC
SMIC abdominal spatula
SMIC abscess probe
SMIC anterior commisure
laryngoscope
SMIC auricular tourniquet
SMIC bone chisel
SMIC bone file

SMIC bone hammer
SMIC bone rongeur
SMIC brain spatula
SMIC burnisher
SMIC carver
SMIC cerumen hook
SMIC cheek retractor
SMIC collar scissors
SMIC cranial rongeur
SMIC curette
SMIC dermatome
SMIC ear curette
SMIC ear polypus scissors
SMIC ear speculum
SMIC eustachian catheter
SMIC excavator
SMIC explorer
SMIC gouge
SMIC hook
SMIC intestinal clamp
SMIC laminectomy rongeur
SMIC laryngoscope
SMIC malleus head nipper
SMIC mastoid chisel
SMIC mastoid curette
SMIC mastoid gouge
SMIC mastoid rongeur
SMIC mastoid suction tube
SMIC mouth mirror
SMIC myringotome
SMIC nasal septal speculum
SMIC nasal speculum
SMIC nylon thread
SMIC periodontal file
SMIC periodontal probe
SMIC periosteal elevator
SMIC pituitary curette
SMIC pliers
SMIC pneumatic otoscope
SMIC powder blower
SMIC root canal plugger
SMIC scissors
SMIC sternal chisel
SMIC sternal drill
SMIC sternal knife
SMIC surgical catgut
SMIC surgical mallet
SMIC suture needle
SMIC tonsillar guillotine
SMIC tuning fork

Smiley-Williams
S.-W. arteriography needle
S.-W. needle

Smillie
- S. cartilage chisel
- S. cartilage instrument
- S. cartilage knife
- S. cartilage set
- S. chisel
- S. knee joint retractor
- S. knife
- S. meniscal knife
- S. meniscotome
- S. nail
- S. nail punch
- S. pin
- S. retractor

Smirmaul eyelid speculum

Smith
- S. anal retractor
- S. anal speculum
- S. aneurysm clip
- S. anoscope
- S. bandage scissors
- S. bone clamp
- S. cataract knife
- S. clamp
- S. clip
- S. cordotomy clamp
- S. cordotomy knife
- S. dissector
- S. drill
- S. electrode
- S. endoscopic electrode
- S. endoscopic electrode handle
- S. expressor
- S. expressor hook
- S. eye speculum
- S. forceps
- S. grasping forceps
- S. lens expressor
- S. lid expressor
- S. lid hook
- S. lid lens expressor
- S. lid-retracting hook
- S. lion-jaw forceps
- S. marginal clamp
- S. nerve root suction retractor
- S. obstetrical forceps
- S. orbital floor implant
- S. perforator
- S. pessary
- S. posterior cartilage stripper
- S. prosthesis
- S. rectal retractor
- S. rectal self-retaining retractor
- S. retractor
- S. retroversion pessary
- S. scissors
- S. suture scissors
- S. suture wire scissors
- S. tonsillar dissector
- S. total ankle
- S. tube
- S. vaginal retractor
- S. vaginal self-retaining retractor

Smith-Buie
- S.-B. anal retractor
- S.-B. rectal retractor
- S.-B. rectal self-retaining retractor
- S.-B. rectal speculum
- S.-B. retractor

Smith-Fisher
- S.-F. cataract knife
- S.-F. cataract spatula
- S.-F. iris replacer
- S.-F. iris spatula

Smith-Green
- S.-G. cataract knife
- S.-G. double-ended spatula
- S.-G. eye knife

Smith-Leiske lens manipulator

Smith-Miller-Patch cryosurgical instrument

Smith-Petersen
- S.-P. arthrosplasty gouge
- S.-P. bone gouge
- S.-P. bone plate
- S.-P. cannulated nail
- S.-P. capsular retractor
- S.-P. chisel
- S.-P. cup
- S.-P. curette
- S.-P. elevator
- S.-P. extractor
- S.-P. forceps
- S.-P. fracture pin
- S.-P. gouge
- S.-P. hip cup prosthesis
- S.-P. hip reamer
- S.-P. laminectomy rongeur
- S.-P. mallet
- S.-P. osteotome

S.-P. plate
S.-P. retractor
S.-P. rongeur
S.-P. spatula
S.-P. sterilizing rack
Smithuysen sphenoidal punch
Smithwick
S. anastomotic clamp
S. button hook
S. buttonhook button
S. clamp
S. clip
S. clip-applying forceps
S. dissector
S. forceps
S. nerve dissector
S. nerve hook
S. retractor
S. silk buttonhook button
S. silver clip
S. sympathectomy hook
Smithwick-Hartmann forceps
SMo
stainless steel with molybdenum
SMo Moore pin
SMo plate
SMo prosthesis
Smoke
S. Controller device
S. Control Porta-Pack
aversive stimulator
Smolik curved rongeur
Smolinski endaural rongeur
smooth
s. dressing forceps
s. pin
s. tissue forceps
s. transfixion wire
smooth-tooth forceps
SMR
submucous resection
SMR speculum
SMS investment material
Smuckler tucker
snap band
snap-lock brace
snap-on inserter plate
snare
Alfred s.
Amplatz retinal s.
automatic ratchet s.
Banner enucleation s.
Beck-Schenck tonsillar s.

Beck-Storz tonsillar s.
Bobath s.
Boettcher-Farlow s.
Bosworth nasal s.
Brown tonsillar s.
Bruening ear s.
Bruening nasal s.
Bruening tonsillar s.
Buerger s.
Castroviejo enucleation s.
cautery s.
Colles s.
Cox polypectomy s.
Crapeau nasal s.
crescent s.
Douglas nasal s.
Douglas tonsillar s.
ear s.
ear polyp s.
EUE tonsillar s.
Eves-Neivert tonsillar s.
Eves tonsillar s.
Farlow-Boettcher s.
Farlow tonsillar s.
fascial s.
Foerster enucleation s.
Foster s.
Foster enucleation s.
Frankfeldt s.
Frankfeldt diathermy s.
Frankfeldt rectal s.
Freidenwald-Guyton s.
frontalis s.
Glegg nasal polyp s.
Glisson s.
Goebel-Stoeckel s.
hand cock-up s.
Harris s.
hexagon s.
Hobbs polypectomy s.
Hoyer s.
Jarvis s.
Krause ear s.
Krause ear polyp s.
Krause laryngeal s.
Krause nasal s.
Krause nasal polyp s.
laryngeal s.
levator s.
Lewis tonsillar s.
Marlex mesh s.
Martin s.
Mason-Allen s.

snare *(continued)*
Meek s.
Microvena Amplatz s.
Milwaukee s.
Myles tonsillectome s.
nasal s.
Neivert-Eves tonsillar s.
Nesbit tonsillar s.
Newhart-Casselberry s.
Norwood rectal s.
oval s.
pelvic s.
pericardial s.
polypectomy s.
Posey s.
ptosis s.
pulmonary arterial s.
Pynchon ear s.
Quires mechanical finger s.
Rainbow envelope arm s.
Rauchfuss s.
rectal s.
rectal cautery s.
Reiner-Beck tonsillar s.
Robert nasal s.
rotatable polypectomy s.
Sage tonsillar s.
Sayre head s.
self-opening s.
self-opening rigid s.
Stewart lenticular nuclear s.
Stiegler unipolar nasal s.
Storz-Beck tonsillar s.
Stutsman nasal s.
Supramid s.
surgical s.
Teare s.
tonsillar s.
Tydings automatic ratchet s.
Tydings tonsillar s.
Veeder tip s.
Velpeau s.
Wappler polypectomy s.
Weil pelvic s.
Weston rectal s.
Wilde-Bruening ear s.
Wilde-Bruening nasal s.
Wilde ear polyp s.
Wilde nasal s.
Wilson-Cook polypectomy s.
s. wire
wire s.
Wright nasal s.

Wright tonsillar s.
Zimmer s.
Snellen
S. conventional reform eye implant
S. entropion forceps
S. eye implant
S. forceps
S. lens loop
S. lens scoop
S. suture
S. test
Snitman
S. endaural retractor
S. endaural self-retaining retractor
S. retractor
Snowden-Pencer
S.-P. laparoscopic cholecystectomy instrument
S.-P. Supercut scissors
Snowflake laparotomy sponge
Snug denture cushion
Snyder
S. breast prosthesis
S. deep-surgery forceps
S. forceps
S. Hemovac drain
S. Hemovac evacuator
S. Hemovac silicone sump drain
S. Hemovac suction tube
S. Hemovac tube
S. mini-Hemovac drain
S. Surgivac suction tube
S. Urevac suction tube
S. Urevac trocar
S. Urevac tube
soap
infant s.
Weck-Prep infant s.
socket
floating shoulder s.
s. wrench
sodium
s. alginate wool mold
s. hyaluronate viscoelastic
Soehendra
S. BII papillotome/sphincterotome
S. endoscopic biliary stent system
S. lithotripsy set

S. Precut papillotome/sphincterotome
S. stent retriever
S. Universal catheter
Sof-Band bulky bandage
Sofield
   S. retractor
   S. retractor blade
   S. retractor clip
Sof-Kling
   S.-K. bandage
   S.-K. conforming bandage
Soflens enzymatic contact lens cleaner
Sofnet cleaner
Sof-Rol dressing
Soft
   S. Mate disinfection and storage solution
soft
   s. cataract aspirator
   s. catheter
   s. intraocular lens
   s. palate retractor
   s. rubber curette
   s. rubber drain
   s. scrub brush
   s. silicone sphere implant
   s. wire loop
Softepil tweezer epilation device
SOF-T guiding catheter
Softgut
   S. chromic suture
   S. surgical chromic catgut suture
   S. suture
Softip
   S. arteriography catheter
   S. catheter
   S. diagnostic catheter
Softjaw
   S. clamp
   S. handleless clamp
   S. insert
Softouch
   S. Cobra 1 catheter
   S. Cobra 2 catheter
   S. guiding catheter
   S. Headhunter 1 catheter
   S. Multipurpose B2 catheter
   S. Simmons 1 catheter
   S. Simmons 2 catheter

S. spinal angiography catheter
Sof-Wick
   S.-W. drain
   S.-W. dressing
   S.-W. lap pad
   S.-W. sponge
Soileau Tytan ventilation tube
Sokolec elevator
Sokolwski antral punch
Solar pacemaker
SOLA VIP lens
Solcotrans Plus drainage reinfusion system
solder
   PF Universal s.
soldering tweezers
solid
   s. ankle cushion heel (SACH)
   s. ankle cushion heel prosthesis
   s. buckling implant material
   s. copper head mallet
   s. hex bolt
   s. silicone exoplant implant material
   s. silicone implant material
   s. silicone orbital prosthesis
   s. silicone with Supramid mesh implant
solid-center malleable blade
solid-state
   s.-s. esophageal manometry catheter
   s.-s. silk suture
solid-tip catheter
Solos Endoscopy diagnostic laparoscope
Solow sigmoidoscope
Soluset device
Solus pacemaker
solution
   balanced salt s. (BSS)
   Barnes-Hind contact lens cleaning and soaking s.
   Barnes-Hind wetting s.
   Cidex s.
   cold soak s.
   DCI hemolyte s.
   electrolyte s.
   Etch-Master electrolyte s.

solution *(continued)*
    McCarey-Kaufman s.
    Predent disclosing s.
    Soft Mate disinfection and
      storage s.
    Soquette contact lens
      soaking s.
    Sporicidin cold soak s.
    Visalens contact lens
      cleaning and soaking s.
Solvang graft
Somatics mouth guard
Somers
    S. clamp
    S. forceps
    S. uterine clamp
    S. uterine-elevating forceps
    S. uterine elevator
    S. uterine forceps
Somerset bur
SOMI
    sternal occipital mandibular
      immobilization
    SOMI brace
Sommers compression dressing
Sonatron ultrasonic scaler
Sones
    S. Cardio-Marker catheter
    S. catheter
    S. coronary catheter
    S. hemostatic bag
    S. Hi-Flow catheter
    S. Positrol catheter
    S. vent catheter
Songer tonsillar forceps
**Sonicaid SYSTEM 8000 fetal
  monitor**
sonic curette
Sonnenschein nasal speculum
**Sonoline Siemens ultrasound
  scanner**
Sonop
    S. handpiece
    S. ultrasonic aspirator
Soonawalla vasectomy forceps
**Soquette contact lens soaking
  solution**
Sorbiclear dialyzer
Sorbothane orthotic device
Sorbsan
    S. dressing
    S. wound dressing
Sorbtrate dialysate concentrate

Soresi cannula
Sorin pacemaker
sound
    Allport mastoid s.
    Bellocq s.
    Béniqué s.
    bladder s.
    bronchocele s.
    Campbell-French s.
    Campbell miniature s.
    Campbell miniature
      urethral s.
    Davis interlocking s.
    Dittel urethral s.
    Dittel uterine s.
    Ellik s.
    female s.
    flexible s.
    Fowler urethral s.
    French s.
    Gouley tunneled urethral s.
    Guyon-Benique urethral s.
    Guyon dilating s.
    Guyon urethral s.
    Hishida pine-needle s.
    Hunt metal s.
    interlocking s.
    Jewett urethral s.
    Jewett uterine s.
    Klebanoff common duct s.
    Kocher bronchocele s.
    Korotkoff s.
    lacrimal s.
    LeFort s.
    LeFort urethral s.
    LeFort uterine s.
    Mark-7 intrauterine s.
    Martin uterine s.
    McCrea s.
    McCrea infant s.
    meatal s.
    miniature s.
    Otis urethral s.
    Pratt urethral s.
    Rica uterine s.
    rigid s.
    Rissler vein s.
    Ritter s.
    Saf-T-Sound uterine s.
    Schroeder interlocking s.
    shaking s.
    Simpson uterine s.
    Sims plain uterine s.

Sims uterine s.
urethral s.
uterine s.
Van Buren canvas roll s.
Van Buren dilating s.
Van Buren urethral s.
Walther urethral s.
Winternitz s.
Woodward s.
sounder
mini-echo s.
soundgraph
Korotkoff s.
source
fiberoptic light s.
xenon light s.
**Souter Strathclyde total elbow
system**
Southbent scissors
**Southern Eye Bank corneal cutting
block**
Southey
S. anasarca trocar
S. cannula
S. capillary drainage tube
Southey-Leech trocar
Southwick
S. clamp
S. screw extractor
Southworth rasp
Souttar
S. cautery
S. esophageal conductor
S. tube
Sovak reamer
**Sovally suprapubic suction cup
drain**
Soviet
S. mechanical bronchial
stapler
S. stapler
spacer
Bio-Moore II provisional
neck s.
spaghetti drain
Spaide depressor
Spanish blue virgin silk suture
spanner
Codman s.
s. wrench
Sparks
S. atrioseptal punch
S. Mandril prosthesis

Sparta
S. microforceps
S. micro-iris forceps
SPAT
Silverstein permanent aeration
tube
spatula
Allison lung s.
Ayre cervical s.
Bakelite s.
Bangerter angled iris s.
Barraquer cyclodialysis s.
Barraquer iris s.
Bechert s.
brain s.
Castroviejo s.
Castroviejo cyclodialysis s.
Castroviejo double-end s.
Castroviejo synechia s.
Cave scaphoid s.
cement s.
Children's Hospital brain s.
Clayman s.
Cleasby iris s.
corneal graft s.
coronary endarterectomy s.
Crile s.
Culler iris s.
Cushing brain s.
Cushing S-shaped brain s.
cyclodialysis s.
Davis s.
Davis brain s.
D'Errico brain s.
s. dissector
Dixey s.
Dorsey s.
Doyen s.
Drews-Sato capsular
fragment s.
Elschnig cyclodialysis s.
endarterectomy s.
Fisher-Smith s.
fishtail s.
flat s.
Freer s.
Freer nasal s.
French-pattern s.
Galin lens s.
Garron s.
Girard synechia s.
Green s.
Green lens s.

673

spatula *(continued)*
    Gross brain s.
    Haberer s.
    Halle vascular s.
    Heifitz s.
    Hirschman s.
    Hirschman iris s.
    Hirschman lens s.
    Hough s.
    Interstate s.
    iris s.
    irrigating s.
    irrigating notched s.
    Jacobson endarterectomy s.
    Jaffe s.
    Jaffe lens s.
    Johnson s.
    Kader intestinal s.
    Kallmorgen vaginal s.
    Katena s.
    Kellman-Elschnig s.
    Kennerdell s.
    Killian laryngeal s.
    Kimura platinum s.
    Kirby iris s.
    Knapp cyclodialysis s.
    Knapp iris s.
    Knolle lens s.
    Knolle lens cortex s.
    Knolle lens nucleus s.
    Kocher s.
    Kocher bladder s.
    Korte abdominal s.
    Krause-Davis s.
    Kummel intestinal s.
    Kwitko lens s.
    Laird s.
    Legueu s.
    lens s.
    Leriche s.
    Lewicky IOL s.
    Lieppman s.
    Lindner cyclodialysis s.
    lingual s.
    Lynch s.
    malleable s.
    Manhattan Eye and Ear s.
    Maumenee-Barraquer
      vitreous sweep s.
    Mayfield malleable brain s.
    McIntyre s.
    McIntyre irrigating s.
    McPherson iris s.

    McReynolds eye s.
    Meller cyclodialysis s.
    microvitreoretinal s.
    Mikulicz s.
    Milex s.
    Millin bladder s.
    Mills coronary
      endarterectomy s.
    Morgenstein s.
    s. needle suture
    nerve separator s.
    nucleus s.
    O'Brien s.
    Obstbaum s.
    Obstbaum lens s.
    Obstbaum synechia s.
    Olivecrona s.
    Olivecrona brain s.
    Olk retinal s.
    Pallin lens s.
    Paton s.
    Peyton brain s.
    phacodialysis s.
    plaster s.
    platinum s.
    Raaf flexible lighted s.
    Rainen s.
    Rainen clip-bending s.
    Rainin lens s.
    Ray brain s.
    Reverdin s.
    Rica brain s.
    Rizzuti graft carrier s.
    Roux s.
    Sachs s.
    Schmid vascular s.
    Schuknecht s.
    Scoville brain s.
    Scoville flat brain s.
    Segond vaginal s.
    serrated T-s.
    Sheets s.
    Sheets-Hirsch s.
    Sheets lens s.
    side-cutting s.
    Simcoe s.
    Simcoe notched s.
    Simcoe notched irrigating s.
    Simcoe nucleus s.
    Simmons-Kimbrough
      glaucoma s.
    Sinskey nucleus s.
    SMIC abdominal s.

SMIC brain s.
Smith-Fisher cataract s.
Smith-Fisher iris s.
Smith-Green double-ended s.
Smith-Petersen s.
s. split needle
S-shaped brain s.
stainless s.
Sterling iris s.
Suker cyclodialysis s.
surgical s.
"T" s.
Tan s.
Tauber vaginal s.
Tennant s.
Thomas s.
Troutman-Barraquer iris s.
Troutman lens s.
Tuffier abdominal s.
University of Kansas s.
vaginal s.
wax-removing s.
Weary brain s.
Wecker iris s.
Wheeler cyclodialysis s.
Wheeler iris s.
Wills s.
Woodson s.
Woodson elevator s.
Wullstein transplant s.
Wurmuth s.
Wylie s.

spatula-spoon
Cushing brain s.-s.
Olivecrona brain s.-s.

speaking tube
spear blade
Speare dural hook
spear-ended chrome probe
spear-pointed nickelene probe
spears
eye s.

special
s. blade
s. Colles splint
s. distance measure

specimen
s. forceps

Speck-Ange cutter
Speck introducer
spectacles
bronchoscopic s.
Fresnel nystagmus s.

Spectra-Bond
Spectra-Cath
Spectraflex pacemaker
Spectra pad
Spectra-Physics
S.-P. argon laser
S.-P. microsurgical laser
Spectraprobe-PLS laser angioplasty catheter
Spectrax
S. bipolar pacemaker
S. pacemaker
S. programmable Medtronic pacemaker
S. SXT pulse generator
Spectron
S. EF total hip system
S. prosthesis
spectroscopy-directed laser
speculum, pl. specula
adolescent vaginal s.
Adson s.
Agrikola s.
Agrikola eye s.
Alfonso eye s.
Allen-Heffernan nasal s.
Allingham rectal s.
anal s.
s. anoscope
Arruga eye s.
Arruga globe s.
Aufricht septal s.
aural s.
Auvard s.
Auvard-Britetrac s.
Auvard-Remine vaginal s.
Auvard vaginal s.
Auvard weighted s.
Auvard weighted vaginal s.
Bárány s.
Barr anal s.
Barraquer s.
Barraquer-Colibri eye s.
Barraquer-Douvas eye s.
Barraquer eye s.
Barraquer-Floyd s.
Barraquer solid s.
Barraquer wire s.
Barr rectal s.
Barr-Shuford s.
Beard eye s.
Becker-Park s.
Beckman s.

speculum *(continued)*

Beckman-Colver nasal s.
Beckman nasal s.
Bedrossian eye s.
Berens eye s.
Berlind-Auvard s.
Berlind-Auvard vaginal s.
bivalved s.
bivalved anal s.
Bodenheimer s.
Bodenheimer rectal s.
Bosworth nasal wire s.
Boucheron s.
Boucheron ear s.
Bovin-Stille vaginal s.
Bovin vaginal s.
Bowman eye s.
Bozeman s.
Braun s.
Breisky-Navratil s.
Breisky-Navratil vaginal s.
Breisky-Stille s.
Breisky vaginal s.
Brewer vaginal s.
Brinkerhoff rectal s.
Britetrac s.
Bronson s.
Bronson-Turtz s.
Brown ear s.
Bruening s.
Bruner vaginal s.
Buie-Smith rectal s.
Burnett Sani-Spec
  disposable s.
Callahan modification s.
Carter septal s.
Caspar s.
Castallo eye s.
Castroviejo eye s.
Chelsea-Eaton anal s.
Chelsea-Eaton rectal s.
Chevalier Jackson
  laryngeal s.
Clark eye s.
Coakley nasal s.
Coldlite s.
Coldlite-Graves s.
Collin vaginal s.
Converse nasal s.
Conway lid s.
Cook eye s.
Cook eye infection s.
Cook rectal s.

Cottle s.
Cottle nasal s.
Cottle septal s.
Critchett eye s.
Culler s.
Culler iris s.
Cusco vaginal s.
Cushing-Landolt s.
Cushing-Landolt
  transsphenoidal s.
David rectal s.
DeLee s.
DeRoaldes s.
Desmarres eye s.
Desmarres lid s.
DeVilbiss-Stacy s.
DeVilbiss vaginal s.
Disposo-Spec disposable s.
Docherty cheek s.
Douglas mucosal s.
Doyen vaginal s.
duckbill s.
Dudley-Smith rectal s.
Duplay-Lynch nasal s.
Duplay nasal s.
Dynacor vaginal s.
ear s.
Eaton nasal s.
Eisenhammer s.
endaural s.
ENT s.
Erhardt ear s.
Erosa-Spec vaginal s.
eye s.
Fansler rectal s.
Fanta s.
Farkas urethral s.
Farrior s.
Farrior ear s.
Farrior oval s.
Ferguson tubular vaginal s.
Ferguson vaginal s.
Fergusson s.
Fergusson tubular vaginal s.
fiberoptic vaginal s.
Flannery ear s.
Flint glass s.
Floyd-Barraquer s.
Floyd-Barraquer wire s.
Forbes eosphageal s.
s. forceps
Foster-Ballenger nasal s.
four-prong finger s.

Fox eye s.
Fränkel s.
Garrigue vaginal s.
Garrigue weighted vaginal s.
Gerzog nasal s.
Gilbert-Graves s.
Gleason s.
Goldbacher anoscope s.
Goldstein septal s.
Goligher s.
Graefe s.
Graefe eye s.
Graves s.
Graves bivalve s.
Graves Britetrac vaginal s.
Graves open-side vaginal s.
Graves vaginal s.
Gruber s.
Gruber ear s.
Guild-Pratt rectal s.
Guilford-Wright bivalve s.
Guist-Black eye s.
Guist eye s.
Gutter s.
Guttmann vaginal s.
Guyton-Park s.
Guyton-Park eye s.
Gyn-A-Lite vaginal s.
Haglund-Stille vaginal s.
Haglund vaginal s.
Halle nasal s.
Halle-Tieck nasal s.
Hardy bivalve s.
Hardy-Duddy s.
Hardy nasal bivalve s.
Hartmann s.
Hartmann dewaxer s.
Hartmann ear s.
Hartmann nasal s.
Hayes vaginal s.
Heffernan nasal s.
Helmholtz s.
Helmont s.
Henrotin vaginal s.
Henrotin weighted
  vaginal s.
Hertel nephrostomy s.
Higbee vaginal s.
Hinkle-James rectal s.
Hirschman anoscope
  rectal s.
s. holder

Holinger infant
  esophageal s.
Hood-Graves vaginal s.
Hough-Boucheron ear s.
House stapes s.
Huffman-Graves adolescent
  vaginal s.
Huffman-Graves vaginal s.
Huffman infant vaginal s.
Iliff-Park s.
illuminated s.
s. illuminator
  transilluminator
Ingals nasal s.
Ives rectal s.
Jackson vaginal s.
Jaffe eyelid s.
Jaffe lid s.
Jarit-Graves vaginal s.
Jarit-Pederson vaginal s.
Jonas-Graves vaginal s.
Kahn-Graves vaginal s.
Kalinowski ear s.
Kalinowski-Verner ear s.
Keizer-Lancaster eye s.
Kelly rectal s.
Killian-Halle nasal s.
Killian nasal s.
Killian rectal s.
Killian septal s.
Klaff septal s.
KleenSpec disposable s.
KleenSpec disposable
  vaginal s.
Knapp s.
Knapp-Culler s.
Knapp eye s.
Kogan s.
Kogan endocervical s.
Kogan endospeculum s.
Kogan urethra s.
Kramer ear s.
Kratz-Barraquer s.
Kratz-Barraquer wire eye s.
Kristeller vaginal s.
Kyle nasal s.
Lancaster s.
Lancaster eye s.
Lancaster-O'Connor s.
Landau s.
Lange eye s.
Lawford s.

speculum *(continued)*
   Lempert-Beckman-Colver
     endaural s.
   Lempert-Colver endaural s.
   Lester-Burch eye s.
   lid s.
   lighted s.
   Lillie nasal s.
   Lister-Burch eye s.
   Lofberg vaginal s.
   Lucae ear s.
   Luer eye s.
   Macon Hospital s.
   Mahoney intranasal antral s.
   Martin rectal s.
   Martin vaginal s.
   Mason-Auvard weighted
     vaginal s.
   Mathews rectal s.
   Matzenauer s.
   Matzenauer vaginal s.
   Maumenee-Park eye s.
   McBratney aspirating s.
   McHugh oval s.
   McKee s.
   McKinney s.
   McKinney eye s.
   McLaughlin s.
   McPherson s.
   McPherson eye s.
   Mellinger-Axenfeld eye s.
   Mellinger eye s.
   Mellinger fenestrated
     blades s.
   Merz-Vienna s.
   Merz-Vienna nasal s.
   Metcher eye s.
   Miller vaginal s.
   Milligan s.
   Montgomery-Bernstine s.
   Montgomery vaginal s.
   Mosher nasal s.
   Mosher urethral s.
   Mueller s.
   Mueller eye s.
   Muir rectal s.
   Murdock eye s.
   Murdock-Wiener eye s.
   Murdoon eye s.
   Myles nasal s.
   Myles-Ray s.
   nasal s.
   nasal bivalve s.

   Nasa-Spec nasal s.
   nasopharyngeal s.
   National ear s.
   National Graves vaginal s.
   Nott-Gutmann vaginal s.
   Nott vaginal s.
   Noyes s.
   one-hand s.
   open-side vaginal s.
   O'Sullivan-O'Connor
     vaginal s.
   oval s.
   Park eye s.
   Park-Guyton-Callahan eye s.
   Park-Guyton eye s.
   Park-Maumenee s.
   Parks anal s.
   Patton septal s.
   Pearce eye s.
   Pederson vaginal s.
   Pennington rectal s.
   Picot vaginal s.
   Pierse eye s.
   Pilling-Hartmann s.
   plain wire s.
   Politzer ear s.
   post-urethroplasty review s.
   Pratt bivalve s.
   Pratt rectal s.
   Preefer eye s.
   Prospec disposable s.
   Proud infant turbinate s.
   Pynchon nasal s.
   Rappazzo s.
   Ray nasal s.
   rectal s.
   Reipen s.
   Relat vaginal s.
   Rica ear s.
   Rica nasal s.
   Rica nasal septal s.
   Rica vaginal s.
   Richard Gruber s.
   Richnau-Holmgren ear s.
   Roberts esophageal s.
   Roberts oval s.
   Rosenthal urethral s.
   round s.
   Sato s.
   Sauer eye s.
   Sauer infant s.
   Sauer infant eye s.
   Saunders eye s.

Sawyer rectal s.
Schweizer s.
Scott ear s.
Semb vaginal s.
Senturia pharyngeal s.
Seyffert vaginal s.
Shea s.
shoehorn s.
Siegle s.
Siegle ear s.
Simcoe s.
Simcoe-Barraquer eye s.
Simcoe eye s.
Simcoe wire s.
Simmonds vaginal s.
Simrock s.
Sims double-ended
    vaginal s.
Sims rectal s.
Sims vaginal s.
single-hinged s.
Sisson-Cottle s.
Sisson-Vienna s.
Sluder sphenoidal s.
SMIC ear s.
SMIC nasal s.
SMIC nasal septal s.
Smirmaul eyelid s.
Smith anal s.
Smith-Buie rectal s.
Smith eye s.
SMR s.
Sonnenschein nasal s.
stapes s.
Stearnes s.
Steiner-Auvard s.
Stop eye s.
Storz nasal s.
Storz septal s.
Storz Vienna nasal s.
Storz-Vienna nasal s.
Sweeney posterior vaginal s.
Swiss-pattern s.
Swolin self-retaining
    vaginal s.
Tauber s.
Taylor vaginal s.
Terson s.
Thornton s.
Thornton open-wire lid s.
Thudichum nasal s.
Tieck-Halle infant nasal s.
Tieck-Halle nasal s.

Tieck nasal s.
Torchia eye s.
Toynbee s.
Toynbee ear s.
transsphenoidal s.
Trelat vaginal s.
Troeltsch ear s.
Turner-Warwick s.
Turner-Warwick post-
    urethroplasty review s.
Ullrich vaginal s.
Universal s.
vaginal s.
Vaginard metal s.
Vauban s.
Verner s.
Verner-Kalinowski s.
Vernon-David rectal s.
Vienna s.
Vienna nasal s.
Vienna original nasal s.
Vienns Britetrac nasal s.
Voltolini s.
Voltolini nasal s.
Watson s.
Weck eye s.
Weeks eye s.
weighted s.
weighted vaginal s.
Weiner s.
Weisman-Graves vaginal s.
Weiss s.
Weissbarth vaginal s.
Welch Allyn illuminated s.
Welch Allyn KleenSpec
    vaginal s.
Wellington Hospital
    vaginal s.
Wiener s.
Williams eye s.
Williams pediatric eye s.
Wilson-Kirbe s.
wire s.
wire bivalve vaginal s.
wire lid s.
Worcester City Hospital s.
Yankauer nasopharyngeal s.
Ziegler eye s.
Zower s.
Zylik-Michaels s.
speculum-retractor
    Picot weighted s.-r.
    weighted s.-r.

Speed
S. hand splint
S. osteotomy graft
S. radius cap prosthesis
S. splint
Speed-E-Rim denture bite block
Speed-Sprague knife
Speer
S. periosteotome
S. suture hook
Spence
S. cranioplastic roller
S. forceps
S. intervertebral disk rongeur
S. intervertebral disk rongeur
S. rongeur forceps
Spence-Adson
S.-A. clip-introducing forceps
S.-A. forceps
Spencer
S. cannula
S. chalazion forceps
S. eye suture scissors
S. forceps
S. incontinence device
S. labyrinth exploration probe
S. oval punch
S. oval tip
S. plication forceps
S. probe
S. scissors
S. silicone subimplant
S. suture scissors
S. trachelotome
S. triangular adenoid punch
S. triangular tip
S. Universal adenoid punch tip
Spencer-Wells
S.-W. arterial forceps
S.-W. chalazion forceps
S.-W. forceps
S.-W. hemostatic forceps
Spenco
S. external breast form
S. orthotic device
spermatocele implant
Sperm Select system
Spero
S. forceps

S. meibomian expressor forceps
S. meibomian forceps
Spetzler
S. catheter
S. clip applier
S. dissector
S. forceps
S. MacroVac surgical suction device
S. needle holder
S. scissors
S. shunt
S. subarachnoid catheter
sphenoethmoidal suture
sphenofrontal suture
sphenoidal
s. bone punch
s. bur
s. cannula
s. probe
s. punch
s. punch forceps
sphenomalar suture
sphenomaxillary suture
spheno-occipital suture
spheno-orbital suture
sphenopalatine
s. ganglion needle
s. needle
sphenoparietal suture
sphenopetrosal suture
sphenosquamous suture
sphenotemporal suture
sphenozygomatic suture
sphere
American Heyer-Schulte s.
s. eye implant
s. implant
s. introducer
spherical
s. bur
s. eye implant
s. head hex drive
s. implant
spherocentric knee prosthesis
sphincter
AMD urinary s.
s. dilator
sphincteroscope
Kelly s.
sphincterotome
Cremer-Ikeda s.

Doubilet s.
Frimberger-Karpiel 12
  O'Clock s.
Howell Rotatable BII s.
Huibregtse-Kato s.
Koch-Julian s.
shark fin s.
Ultratome s.
Wilson-Cook wire-guided s.
wire-guided s.
sphygmomanometer
  s. cuff
sphyncteroscope
spica
  s. bandage
  s. cast boss
  s. dressing
  s. splint
spicule forceps
Spiegel-Wycis stereoencephalotome
Spielberg
  S. dilator
  S. sinus cannula
Spies ethmoidal punch
Spiesman
Spiesman fistular probe
Spigelman baseball finger splint
spigot
  catheter s.
spiked washer
spike retractor
spinal
  s. arthroscope
  s. cord retractor
  s. curette
  s. fusion chisel
  s. fusion curette
  s. fusion gouge
  s. needle
  s. retractor
  s. retractor blade
  s. rongeur forceps
  s. slip wrench
spinal-perforating forceps
spincterotomy basket
Spinelli biopsy needle
Spinhaler Turbo-Inhaler
spinous process spreader
spiral
  s. bandage
  s. drill
  s. electrode
  s. filler

s. forceps
s. probe
s. reverse bandage
s. stone dislodger
s. suture
s. trochanteric reamer
s. or twist drill
s. vein stripper
spiral-tipped
  s.-t. bougie
  s.-t. catheter
Spirec drill
spirometer
  Barnes s.
Spitz-Holter
  S.-H. flushing device
  S.-H. valve
  S.-H. valve implant material
Spivey iris retractor
Spizziri
  S. cannula knife
  S. knife
Spizziri-Simcoe cannula
splanchnic retractor
splice
  breakaway s.
spline
  Bosworth osteotomy s.
  Keys-Briston type s.
  Rowland-Hughes
    osteotomy s.
  Shirlee s.
splint
  abduction s.
  abduction finger s.
  abduction pillow cover s.
  abduction thumb s.
  acrylic cap s.
  Adam and Eve rib belt s.
  aeroplane s.
  Agnew s.
  Ainslie acrylic s.
  air s.
  airfoam s.
  air foam s.
  airplane s.
  Alumafoam nasal s.
  aluminum s.
  aluminum fence s.
  aluminum finger cot s.
  aluminum wire s.
  anchor s.
  Anderson s.

splint *(continued)*
    angle s.
    ankle-foot orthotic s.
    anterior acute flexion
      elbow s.
    Asch nasal s.
    Ashhurst leg s.
    Atkins nasal s.
    Balkan femoral s.
    ball-peen s.
    banjo s.
    baseball finger s.
    Basswood s.
    Bavarian s.
    Baylor adjustable cross s.
    Baylor metatarsal s.
    board s.
    Böhler-Braun s.
    Böhler wire s.
    Bond arm s.
    boutonniere s.
    Bowlby arm s.
    bracketed s.
    Brady balanced
      suspension s.
    Brant aluminum s.
    Browne s.
    Brown nasal s.
    Buck extension s.
    Buck traction s.
    Bunnell knuckle bender s.
    Bunnell outrigger s.
    Cabot leg s.
    calibrated clubfoot s.
    Campbell airplane s.
    Campbell traction s.
    Cannon Bio-Flek nasal s.
    cap s.
    Carl P. Jones traction s.
    Carter intranasal s.
    cartilage elastic pullover
      kneecap s.
    cast lingual s.
    Cawood nasal s.
    Chandler felt collar s.
    Chatfield-Girdleston s.
    coaptation s.
    cock-up s.
    cock-up arm s.
    COH hip abduction s.
    Colles s.
    composite spring elastic s.
    Converse s.

Cordon Colles fracture s.
Cramer wire s.
Culley ulna s.
Curry walking s.
Davis metacarpal s.
Denis Browne clubfoot s.
Denis Browne hip s.
Denver nasal s.
DePuy s.
DePuy aeroplane s.
DePuy any-angle s.
DePuy coaptation s.
DePuy open-thimble s.
DePuy-Pott s.
DePuy rocking leg s.
DePuy rolled Colles s.
dorsal wrist s. with
  outrigger
double-occlusal s.
drop-foot s.
dynamic s.
Easton cock-up s.
Eggers contact s.
Engelmann thigh s.
Erich maxillary s.
Erich nasal s.
fence s.
Ferciot tip-toe s.
Fillauer night s.
finger s.
finger cot s.
finger extension
  clockspring s.
fold-over finger s.
Formatray mandibular s.
Forrester head s.
four-prong finger s.
Fox clavicular s.
Frac-Sur s.
Fractomed s.
fracture s.
Frejka s.
frog-leg s.
Froimson s.
Fruehevald s.
full-hand s.
full-occlusal s.
Funsten supination s.
Gallows s.
Galveston s.
Gibson s.
Gilmer dental s.
Gooch s.

Granberry s.
Gunning jaw s.
Hammond orthodontic s.
hand s.
hand cock-up s.
Hare compact traction s.
Hart extension finger s.
Haynes-Griffin
  mandibular s.
Hexcelite s.
Hexcelite sheet s.
hinged Thomas s.
Hirschtick utility shoulder s.
Hodgen hip s.
Hodgen leg s.
infant abduction s.
inflatable s.
interdental s.
intranasal bivalve s.
Jelenko s.
Jonell countertraction
  finger s.
Jonell thumb s.
Jones arm s.
Jones forearm s.
Jones metacarpal s.
Jones nasal s.
Joseph nasal s.
Joseph septal s.
Kanavel cock-up s.
Kazanjian nasal s.
Keller-Blake leg s.
Kerr abduction s.
Keystone s.
Klenzak double-upright s.
knee s.
knee brace s.
knee immobilizer s.
knuckle-bender s.
Lambrinudi s.
Levis arm s.
Lewin baseball finger s.
Lewin finger s.
Lewin-Stern finger s.
Lewin-Stern thumb s.
s. liner
Liston s.
live s.
Love nasal s.
Lynch septal s.
Lytle metacarpal s.
MacKay nasal s.

Magnuson abduction
  humeral s.
Mason s.
Mason-Allen hand s.
Mason-Allen Universal
  hand s.
Mayer nasal s.
McGee s.
McIntire s.
McLeod padded
  clavicular s.
metal s.
Mohr finger s.
Murphy s.
Murray-Jones arm s.
Murray-Thomas arm s.
nasal s.
Neiman nasal s.
Neubeiser adjustable
  forearm s.
nose s.
nose guard s.
O'Donoghue knee s.
O'Donoghue stirrup s.
O'Malley jaw fracture s.
Oppenheimer spring wire s.
Opponens s.
Ortho-last s.
orthopaedic strap clavicle s.
Orthoplast isoprene s.
padded aluminum s.
padded board s.
padded plywood s.
s. padding
palmar s.
Pavlik harness s.
Peabody s.
Phelps s.
Plastalume bulb-ended s.
Plastalume straight s.
plaster s.
Ponseti s.
Poroplastic s.
Porzett s.
Potts s.
Protecto s.
Putti s.
Quik splint s.
radiolucent s.
Redi-Around finger s.
reverse knuckle-bender s.
Robert Jones s.
Roger Anderson well-leg s.

splint *(continued)*
Rumel aluminum bridge s.
safety pin s.
Safian nasal s.
SAM s.
Savlon s.
Sayre s.
Scott humeral s.
Scottish Rite s.
Shah nasal s.
Sheffield s.
Simpson sugar-tong s.
skin s.
special Colles s.
Speed s.
Speed hand s.
spica s.
Spigelman baseball finger s.
spreading hand s.
spring cock-up s.
spring wire safety pin s.
Stack s.
Stader s.
Stax s.
Stax fingertip s.
Stock finger splint s.
Strampelli eye s.
strap clavicle s.
Stromeyer s.
Stuart Gordon hand s.
sugar-tong s.
Supramead nose s.
Swanson dynamic toe
splint s.
Swanson hand s.
Taylor s.
Teare arm s.
tennis elbow s.
T-finger s.
therapeutic s.
Thomas full-ring s.
Thomas hinged s.
Thomas knee s.
Thomas leg s.
Thomas posterior s.
Thomas suspension s.
Thomas s. with Pearson
attachment
Thompson modification of
Denis Browne s.
Ticonium s.
Titus forearm s.
Titus wrist s.

Toad finger s.
Tobruk s.
Toronto s.
torsion bar s.
Universal support s.
Urias pressure s.
Valentine s.
Van Rosen s.
Velcro extenders s.
Volkmann s.
Wertheim s.
Winter s.
wire s.
Xomed Doyle nasal
airway s.
Xomed Silastic s.
Yucca wood s.
Zimfoam s.
Zimmer s.
Zimmer airplane s.
Zimmer clavicular cross s.
Zim-Trac traction s.
Zim-Zip rib belt s.
Zollinger s.
Zucker s.
splinter forceps
Splintline acrylic
split drape
split-sheath catheter
splitter
Rosato fascial s.
Ruth-Hedwig s.
Tooke angled s.
Troutman corneal s.
Zeiss small beam s.
split-thickness implant
splitting
s. chisel
s. forceps
S-P needle holder
spondylophyte
s. annular dissector
perforator
s. impactor
sponge
Accu-Sorb gauze s.
Accu-Sorb laparotomy s.
Alcon s.
Bicol collagen s.
Bohm dropper s.
Boston gauze s.
bronchoscopic s.
s. carrier

cherry s.
s. clamp
Codman Bicol s.
Collostat s.
cotton ball s.
Curity disposable
  laparotomy s.
cylindrical s.
s. dissector
s. ear curette
s. forceps
Fuller silicone s.
Gardlok neurosurgical s.
gauze s.
gauze dissector s.
gauze rosebud s.
s. graft
Graham Clark silicone s.
grooved silicone s.
Helistat collagen
  hemostatic s.
Heros chiropody s.
Hibbs s.
s. implant
Ivalon s.
Johnson gauze s.
K dissector s.
Kenwood laparotomy s.
Kerlix laparotomy s.
laminectomy wedge s.
laparotomy s.
Lincoff s.
Masciuli silicone s.
Mediskin hemostatic s.
Merocel s.
nasal tampon s.
Naso-Tamp nasal packing s.
neurological s.
Nu-Gauze s.
ophthalmic s.
Optipore scrub s.
Packer tunnel silicone s.
peanut s.
pledget s.
Porolon s.
Pro-Ophta absorbent stick s.
Ray-Tec s.
Ray-Tec x-ray detectable s.
s. ring
Roschke dropper s.
rubber s.
Secto tonsillar s.
Silastic s.

s. silicone implant material
Snowflake laparotomy s.
Sof-Wick s.
s. stick
strip and point s.
tonsillar s.
Topper s.
Topper dressing s.
tracheotomy s.
two-by-two strung s.
Vistec x-ray detectable s.
Weck s.
Weck-cel s.
Weck-cel surgical spear s.
Wextran s.
x-ray detectable
  laparotomy s.
sponge-and-dressing forceps
sponge-holding forceps
sponger
  Wannagat s.
sponging forceps
spongiosa bone graft
spoon
  s. anastomosis clamp
  Ballance mastoid s.
  Bunge evisceration s.
  Bunge exenteration s.
  Castroviejo s.
  cataract s.
  s. clamp
  Coyne s.
  Culler lens s.
  s. curette
  Cushing pituitary s.
  Cushing spatula s.
  Daviel cataract s.
  Daviel lens s.
  ear s.
  Elschnig cataract s.
  Elschnig lens s.
  enucleation s.
  exenteration s.
  Falk appendectomy s.
  Fisher s.
  Fisher eye s.
  Fisher spoon needle s.
  gallbladder s.
  Graefe cataract s.
  Gross ear s.
  Hardy pituitary s.
  Hatt s.
  Hess lens s.

spoon *(continued)*
    Hiebert esophageal suture s.
    Hoke s.
    Hoke-Roberts s.
    Kalt eye s.
    Kirby lens s.
    Knapp cataract s.
    Knapp lens s.
    Kocher brain s.
    lens s.
    MacNamara cataract s.
    meniscal s.
    Moore gallbladder s.
    obstetrical s.
    Olivecrona brain s.
    pituitary s.
    plain ear s.
    Ray brain s.
    s. retractor
    Royal s.
    Sellheim elevating s.
    Skene uterine s.
    spoon and spatula s.
    Turner-Warwick malleable s.
    Volkmann s.
    Wells enucleation s.
    Wills s. with spatula
    Woodson obstetrical s.
spoon-shaped forceps
Sporicidin cold soak solution
spot
    s. face reamer
    s. retinoscope
spotlight
    examining s.
Sprague ear curette
Spratt
    S. bone curette
    S. curette
    S. ear curette
    S. mastoid curette
    S. nasofrontal rasp
    S. rasp
spray
    s. bandage
    Forrester s.
Spray Band dressing
spreader
    baby Inge bone s.
    baby Inge laminar s.
    Bailey rib s.
    s. bar
    Beeson cast s.

    Beeson plaster cast s.
    Benson pylorus s.
    Blanco valve s.
    Bores incision s.
    Burford s.
    Burford-Finochietto infant
        rib s.
    Burford-Finochietto rib s.
    Burford rib s.
    cast s.
    Cloward s.
    Cloward vertebral s.
    Costenbader incision s.
    Davis modified Finochietto
        rib s.
    DeBakey infant and child
        rib s.
    Finochietto s.
    Finochietto-Burford rib s.
    Finochietto rib s.
    Finochietto-Stille rib s.
    Gerbode s.
    Gerbode modified Burford
        rib s.
    Gill incision s.
    Gross ductus s.
    Haglund s.
    Haglund-Stille plaster s.
    Haight-Finochietto rib s.
    Haight pediatric rib s.
    Haight rib s.
    Harken rib s.
    Henning cast s.
    Henning plaster cast s.
    Hertzler rib s.
    incision s.
    Inge s.
    Inge laminar s.
    intervertebral s.
    Jarit three-prong cast s.
    jaw s.
    Kimpton vein s.
    Kwitko conjunctival s.
    laminar s.
    Landolt s.
    Lefferts rib s.
    Lemmon sternal s.
    Lilienthal rib s.
    Lilienthal-Sauerbruch rib s.
    McGuire rib s.
    Millin-Bacon bladder
        neck s.
    Millin bladder neck s.

Miltex rib s.
Morris mitral valve s.
Morse sternal s.
Nelson rib s.
Nissen rib s.
Overholt-Finochietto rib s.
Overholt rib s.
Park rectal s.
plaster s.
Quervain rib s.
Reinhoff-Finochietto rib s.
Reinhoff rib s.
rib s.
Ridlon s.
Rienhoff-Finochietto rib s.
Rienhoff rib s.
root canal s.
Sauerbruch-Lillienthal rib s.
Saurex s.
Sheldon s.
spinous process s.
sternal s.
Stille plaster s.
Stille-Quervain s.
Struck s.
Suarez s.
Sweet-Burford rib s.
Sweet rib s.
Theis infant rib s.
Tudor-Edwards s.
Tudor-Edwards rib s.
Tuffier rib s.
Turek spinous process s.
Turner-Warwick bladder
neck s.
USA plaster s.
Ventura s.
Weinberg rib s.
Wilson rib s.
Wiltberger spinous
process s.
Wölfe-Böhler plaster cast s.
spreading hand splint
spring
s. clip
s. cock-up splint
Gruca s.
s. holder
s. hook
Kesling tooth-spacing s.
Mershon s.
s. needle holder
s. pin

s. retractor
s. scissors
Shuletz s.
Strach s.
Weiss s.
s. wire loop
s. wire safety pin splint
spring-assisted syringe
spring-eye needle
spring-handled
s.-h. forceps
s.-h. needle holder
s.-h. scissors
spring-hook wire needle
spring-loaded vascular stent
spring-wire retractor
Sprong suture
SPS
single patient system
SPTU Soviet stapler
spud
Alvis s.
Alvis foreign body s.
Bennett foreign body s.
Bishop-Harman s.
Corbett foreign body s.
corneal s.
curved needle s.
Davis foreign body s.
s. dissector
Dix s.
Dix eye s.
Dix foreign body s.
Ellis s.
Ellis foreign body s.
Fisher s.
flat s.
flat needle s.
foreign body s.
Francis knife s.
golf-club s.
golf-club knife s.
Gross ear s.
Hosford foreign body s.
knife s.
LaForce s.
LaForce golf-club knife s.
LaForce knife "golf-club" s.
Levine curetting s.
Levine foreign body s.
Nicati foreign body s.
O'Brien foreign body s.
Plenge foreign body s.

spud *(continued)*
    Walter corneal s.
    Walton round gauge s.
    Whittle s.
spur-crushing clamp
Spurling
    S. forceps
    S. intervertebral disk forceps
    S. intervertebral disk rongeur
    S. laminectomy rongeur
    S. periosteal elevator
    S. pituitary rongeur
    S. retractor
    S. rongeur
    S. rongeur forceps
    S. tissue forceps
Spurling-Kerrison
    S.-K. forceps
    S.-K. laminectomy punch
    S.-K. punch
    S.-K. rongeur
    S.-K. rongeur forceps
Spurling-Love-Gruenwald-Cushing rongeur
squamosal suture
squamosomastoid suture
squamosoparietal suture
squamososphenoid suture
squamous suture
squares of dressing
square specimen forceps
square-tipped arterial dissector
squeeze-handle forceps
Squibb urostomy pouch
squint hook
Squire catheter
SR-Isosit
    S.-I. dental restorative material
    S.-I. teeth
SR-Ivocap denture material
SR-Ivolen impression material
SR-Ivoseal impression material
S-ROM
    S-ROM acetabular cup
    S-ROM prosthesis
SS
    stainless steel
    SS suture
    SS white mercury
Ssabanejeu-Frank gastrostomy

S-shaped
    S.-s. brain retractor
    S.-s. brain spatula
    S.-s. peripheral vascular clamp
    S.-s. retractor
SSI
    shoulder subluxation inhibitor
    SSI brace
SSW forceps
stab
    s. drain
    s. needle
stabilizer
    Claussen fragment s.
stabilizing bar
stabilocondylar knee prosthesis
Stabilor alloy
stable access cannula (SAC)
stab-wound drain
Stack
    S. perfusion catheter
    S. perfusion coronary dilatation catheter
    S. retractor
    S. splint
Stacke
    S. gouge
    S. probe
Stader
    S. connecting rod
    S. extraoral apparatus
    S. pin
    S. pin guide
    S. splint
    S. wrench
staff
    fiberglass s.
    piano-wire s.
    Sippy esophageal dilator piano-wire s.
    Turner-Warwick urethral s.
    urethral s.
Sta-Fix tape
Stahl
    S. calipers
    S. calipers block
    S. calipers plate
    S. lens gauge
stainless
    s. spatula
    s. steel (SS)
    s. steel blade

s. steel clamp
s. steel cup
s. steel flexible ruler
s. steel guide wire
s. steel implant
s. steel mesh
s. steel suture
s. steel suture wire
s. steel wire
s. steel wire suture
s. steel with molybdenum
(SMo)
Stalite root canal post
Stallard
S. blunt dissector
S. dissector
S. head clamp
S. scleral hook
S. stricturotome
S. suture
Stallard-Liegard suture
stall bar
Stalzner rectal scissors
STA-MCA
superior temporal artery-middle
cerebral artery
Stamey
S. catheter
S. needle
S. ureteral catheter
Stamm
S. bone-cutting forceps
S. gastrostomy
Stammberger antral punch
stamp
Sklar medical breast s.
stand
Mayo s.
standard
s. arterial forceps
s. arthroscope
s. forceps
s. full-lumen esophagoscope
s. head halter
s. Jackson laryngoscope
s. laryngoscope
s. 6-lumen perfused catheter
s. pattern mallet
standby pacemaker
standing frame orthosis
Stanford end-hole pigtail catheter
Stangel
S. fallopian tube cannula

S. fallopian tube miniclip
S. modified Barraquer
microsurgical needle holder
Stange laryngoscope
Stanicor
S. Gamma pacemaker
S. Lambda demand
pacemaker
S. pacemaker
**Stankiewicz iris clip intraocular
lens**
Stanmore
S. shoulder prosthesis
S. total knee
Stanton
S. cautery clamp
S. clamp
Stanzel needle holder
stapedectomy
s. footplate pick
s. forceps
s. knife
s. prosthesis
stapedial footplate auger
stapes
s. chisel
s. curette
s. dilator
s. elevator
s. excavator
s. forceps
s. hoe
s. hook
s. needle
s. pick
s. speculum
staphylorrhaphy
s. elevator
s. needle
staple
ASP clip s.
barbed s.
barbed Richards s.
Bio-Absorbable s.
Blount epiphyseal s.
Blount fracture s.
Bostick s.
DePalma s.
duToit shoulder s.
Ellison fixation s.
Fastlok implantable s.
s. forceps
GIA s.

staple *(continued)*
    Krackow HTO blade s.
    Nakayama s.
    Richards fixation s.
    skin s.
    s. suture
    TA metallic s.
    TA Premium 30 s.
    TA Premium 55 s.
    TA Premium 90 s.
    Wiberg fracture s.
    Zimaloy epiphyseal s.

stapler
    American vascular s.
    Appose disposable skin s.
    Appose skin s.
    arcuate skin s.
    Auto Suture s.
    Auto Suture GIA s.
    Auto Suture surgical s.
    barbed s.
    bullet-shaped tip s.
    circular s.
    circular intraluminal s.
    circular mechanical s.
    Concorde disposable skin s.
    copolymer s.
    Coventry s.
    Cricket disposable skin s.
    Day s.
    disposable intraluminal s.
    Downing s.
    duToit s.
    Dwyer spinal mechanical s.
    EEA s.
    EEA Auto Suture s.
    Endopath ES endoscopic s.
    gastroplasty s.
    GIA s.
    Hall double-hole spinal s.
    Inokucki vascular s.
    intraluminal s. (ILS)
    Lactomer copolymer
      absorbable s.
    linear s.
    Multifire GIA 50 s.
    Multifire GIA 60 s.
    Multifire TA s.
    Multifire TA 30 s.
    Multifire TA 50 s.
    Multifire TA 60 s.
    Nakayama microvascular s.

    Ni-Ti Shape Memory alloy
      compression s.
    One-Time disposable skin s.
    Oswestry-O'Brien spinal s.
    PC EEA s.
    PKS-25 apparatus s.
    Polysorb 55 s.
    Premium CEEA s.
    Premium Poly CS-57 s.
    Proximate s.
    Proximate disposable skin s.
    Proximate-ILS circular s.
    Proximate ILS curved
      intraluminal s.
    PSS Powered disposable
      skin s.
    Reflex skin s.
    Roticulator s.
    Roticulator 30 s.
    Roticulator 55 s.
    Roticulator 55 Poly s.
    Royal disposable skin s.
    SGIA 50 disposable s.
    Signet disposable skin s.
    sliding s.
    Soviet s.
    Soviet mechanical
      bronchial s.
    SPTU Soviet s.
    STI-1 needle-shaped
      tissue s.
    Surgiport s.
    TA s.
    TA-30 s.
    TA-55 s.
    TA-90 s.
    UG-70 s.
    UPO-16 s.
    Vital skin s.
    Vogelfanger-Beattie s.
    Vogelfanger blood vessel s.
    Wiberg fracture s.
    Yamagishi s.

Staples osteotomy nail
stapling device
starch bandage
Starck dilator
Stark vulsellum forceps
Starlinger
    S. dilator
    S. uterine dilator

Starlite
S. endodontic implant
starter kit
S. point
Star Optica hearing aid
Starr
S. fixation forceps
S. forceps
S. prosthesis
S. Surgical polyimide loop
intraocular lens
Starr-Edwards
S.-E. ball valve
S.-E. cloth-covered metallic
ball heart valve
S.-E. heart valve
S.-E. heart valve prosthesis
S.-E. hermetically sealed
pacemaker
S.-E. pacemaker
S.-E. prosthesis
Starrett pin vise
starter
s. awl
s. broach
Ritchey nail s.
Statak soft tissue attachment
device
Statham
S. cautery
S. flowmeter
static topical occlusive hemostatic
pressure device
Sta-Tite gauze dressing
Stat 2 Pumpette
Staude
S. forceps
S. tenaculum
S. tenaculum forceps
S. uterine tenaculum
S. uterine tenaculum forceps
Staude-Jackson
S.-J. tenaculum
S.-J. tenaculum forceps
S.-J. uterine tenaculum
Staude-Moore
S.-M. forceps
S.-M. tenaculum
S.-M. tenaculum forceps
S.-M. uterine forceps
S.-M. uterine tenaculum
S.-M. uterine tenaculum
forceps

Stavis fixation forceps
Stax
S. fingertip splint
S. splint
stay
s. suture
s. suture retractor
Stayce adjustable clamp
Stay-Rite clamp
Staze denture adhesive
St. Bartholomew barium catheter
St. Clair forceps
St. Clair-Thompson abscess
forceps
St. Clair-Thompson adenoidal
curette
St. Clair-Thompson adenoidal
forceps
St. Clair-Thompson adenotome
St. Clair-Thompson curette
St. Clair-Thompson forceps
St. Clair-Thompson peritonsillar
abscess forceps
STD+ Titanium total hip
prosthesis
Stearnes speculum
Stecher
S. arachnoid knife
S. microruler
Stedman
S. aspirator
S. continuous suction tube
S. suction pump aspirator
steel
s. mesh suture
s. rule
s. suture
Steele
S. articulator
S. bronchial dilator
S. dilator
S. fiberoptics system
S. filling instrument
S. periosteal elevator
S. scaler
steerable catheter
Steiner-Auvard
S.-A. speculum
S.-A. vaginal retractor
Steinhauser-Castroviejo
electromucotome
Steinhauser orotome

Steinmann
- S. extension bow
- S. fixation pin
- S. holder
- S. intestinal forceps
- S. intestinal-grasping forceps
- S. nail
- S. pin
- S. traction tractor

Stein membrane perforator
Steldent alloy
Stellbrink synovectomy rongeur
Stellite
- S. ball heart valve
- S. cage heart valve

stem
- APF Moore-type femoral s.
- Bio-Groove s.
- calcar replacement s.
- collarless s.
- s. extractor
- femoral s.
- fenestrated s.
- fenestrated Moore-type femoral s.
- Frankfeldt rectal snare bushing for s.
- Frankfeldt rectal snare insulated s.
- KMP fenestrated femoral s.
- MAPF (textured surface) femoral s.
- modular calcar replacement s.
- Morse taper s.
- nonfenestrated Moore-type femoral s.
- Omnifit HA s.
- PCA total hip s.
- s. pessary
- rectal snare insulated s.
- TC femoral s.
- VS femoral s.

Stemp clamp
stencil
- electro-etching kit s.
- Etch-Master electronic s.

stenopaic goggle
stenosis clamp
Stenstrom
- S. nerve holder
- S. raspatory

stent
- activated balloon expandable intravascular s.
- adjustable vaginal s.
- American Heyer-Schulte s.
- Amsterdam s.
- Amsterdam biliary s.
- AMS urethral s.
- antegrade internal s.
- balloon expandable intravascular s.
- Bard coil s.
- Bardex s.
- Bard soft double-pigtail s.
- biliary s.
- Carey-Coons soft s.
- Carpentier s.
- coil vascular s.
- Conley tracheal s.
- Cook ureteral s.
- Cook Urosoft s.
- core mold s.
- s. creep of porcine heart valve
- s. cutter
- Dacron s.
- diversion s.
- Dobbhoff biliary s.
- double-J indwelling catheter s.
- double-J silicone internal ureteral catheter s.
- double-J ureteral s.
- double-J urinary s.
- double-pigtail s.
- s. dressing
- endoluminal s.
- esophageal s.
- foam rubber s.
- foam rubber vaginal s.
- French s.
- gauze s.
- Geenen pancreatic s.
- Gianturco s.
- Gianturco-Rosch bilary Z s.
- Gibbon indwelling ureteral s.
- Gibbon ureteral s.
- indwelling s.
- indwelling ureteral s.
- intraoral s.
- iridium-192 loaded s.
- J-s.

Kaminsky s.
keel s.
lacrimal s.
Medinvent vascular s.
Mentor biliary s.
Montgomery laryngeal s.
Ossoff-Sisson surgical s.
Palmaz s.
Palmaz arterial s.
Palmaz-Schatz coronary s.
Palmaz vascular s.
pancreatic duct s.
Percuflex biliary s.
percutaneous s.
pigtail s.
pigtail biliary s.
polyethylene s.
ring biliary s.
Schnieder wall s.
Silastic s.
Silitek ureteral s.
single-J urinary diversion s.
spring-loaded vascular s.
straight s.
Surgitek double-J ureteral s.
Surgitek Tractfinder
  ureteral s.
Surgitek Uropass s.
ties-over-s.
transhepatic biliary s.
Trimble suture s.
T-tube s.
ureteral s.
Urosoft s.
U-tube s.
vaginal s.
Vantec urinary s.
Wall arterial s.
Wilson-Cook French s.
stented homografts heart valve
Stenzel
  S. fracture rod
  S. rod prosthesis
step-down drill
Stephenson holder
Stepita
  S. clamp
  S. meatal clamp
stepped-down cautery
stepwise suture
stereoencephalotome
  Spiegel-Wycis s.
stereoscope

stereotaxic, stereotactic
  s. device
  s. instrument
  s. laser
Steri-Band
Steri-Drape drape
sterile
  s. compression dressing
  s. drape
  s. dressing
  s. electrodermatome blade
  s. field barrier
  s. forceps holder
  s. stockinette
sterilizer
  Anprolene s.
  autoclave s.
  Bard s.
  s. box
  Buffalo dental s.
  Dry-Therm s.
  Esquire dental s.
  glass bead s.
  Stermatic s.
  Wallach Bio-Tool s.
sterilizing
  s. basket
  s. forceps
  s. instrument tray
  s. and storage container
Steri-Pad
  S.-P. gauze pad
Steri-Probe explorer
steriscope
  Krumeich s.
Steri-Sleeve
Steri-Strips dressing
Steritapes
Sterivac drain
Sterling iris spatula
Sterling-Spring orthodontic wire
Sterling-Sylva irrigator
Stermatic sterilizer
sternal
  s. approximator
  s. blade
  s. knife
  s. needle
  s. needle holder
  s. notch stethoscope
  s. perforating awl
  s. punch forceps
  s. puncture needle

693

sternal *(continued)*
    s. retractor
    s. retractor blade
    s. saw
    s. shears
    s. spreader
    s. wire suture
sternal occipital mandibular immobilization (SOMI)
Stern-Castroviejo
    S.-C. forceps
    S.-C. locking forceps
    S.-C. suturing forceps
Stern dental attachment
Stern-McCarthy
    S.-M. electrode
    S.-M. electrotome
    S.-M. electrotome resectoscope
    S.-M. resectoscope
sternotome
sternotomy retractor
sternum-perforating awl
Stertzer
    S. brachial guiding catheter
    S. catheter
stethoscope
    Andries s.
    Argyle esophageal s.
    Boston s.
    DeLee s.
    DeLee fetal s.
    DeLee-Hillis s.
    DeLee-Hillis fetal s.
    Doppler s.
    electronic s.
    electronic-amplified s.
    fetal s.
    Hillis s.
    Hillis fetal s.
    Leff s.
    Pinard fetal s.
    Rusch esophageal s.
    sternal notch s.
Stetten
    S. intestinal clamp
    S. spur crusher
Stevens
    S. eye scissors
    S. fixation forceps
    S. forceps
    S. iris forceps
    S. lacrimal retractor

    S. muscle hook
    S. needle holder
    S. scissors
    S. stitch scissors
    S. tenotomy hook
    S. tenotomy scissors
Stevenson
    S. alligator scissors
    S. capsular punch
    S. clamp
    S. cupped-jaw forceps
    S. forceps
    S. grasping forceps
    S. lacrimal retractor
    S. lacrimal sac retractor
    S. microsurgical forceps
    S. needle holder
    S. retractor
Stevenson-LaForce adenotome
Stevens-Street
    S.-S. elbow prosthesis
    S.-S. elbow prosthesis template
Stewart
    S. cartilage knife
    S. cruciate ligament guide
    S. crypt hook
    S. lenticular nuclear snare
    S. ligament guide
    S. rectal hook
    S. suture
St. George prosthesis
STI-1 needle-shaped tissue stapler
Stichs wound clip
Stick
    Instrument Makar Switching S.
    Lollipop S.
stick
    bite s.
    Grafco seizure s.
    sponge s.
    switching s.
"stick-and-carrot" appliance
stick-on electrode
stick-tie suture
Stiegler unipolar nasal snare
Stieglitz splinter forceps
Stierlen lens loupe
Stik-Temp thermometer
stiletto knife
Stilith implantable cardiac pulse generator

Stille
- S. bone chisel
- S. bone drill
- S. bone drill set
- S. bone gouge
- S. bone rongeur
- S. brace
- S. cast cutter
- S. cheek retractor
- S. chisel
- S. clamp
- S. coarctation hook
- S. conchotome
- S. cranial drill
- S. dissecting scissors
- S. drill
- S. flat pliers
- S. forceps
- S. gallstone forceps
- S. Gigli-saw guide
- S. gouge
- S. hand drill
- S. heart retractor
- S. insufflator
- S. kidney clamp
- S. kidney forceps
- S. kidney pedicle forceps
- S. laryngeal applicator
- S. mallet
- S. osteotome
- S.-pattern bone chisel
- S.-pattern bone gouge
- S.-pattern trephine and bone drill set
- S. periosteal elevator
- S. plaster shears
- S. plaster spreader
- S. rongeur forceps
- S. scissors
- S. Super Cut scissors
- S. tissue forceps
- S. trephine
- S. uterine dilator
- S. vessel clamp
- S. wrench

Stille-Adson forceps
Stille-Aesculap plaster shears
Stille-Babcock forceps
Stille-Bailey-Senning rib contractor
Stille-Barraya
- S.-B. intestinal forceps
- S.-B. intestinal-grasping forceps
- S.-B. vascular forceps

Stille-Beyer rongeur
Stille-Björk forceps
Stille-Broback knee retractor
Stille-Crafoord
- S.-C. forceps
- S.-C. raspatory

Stille-Crawford coarctation clamp
Stille-Crile forceps
Stille-Doyen raspatory
Stille-Edwards raspatory
Stille-Ericksson rib shears
Stille-French cardiovascular needle holder
Stille-Giertz shears
Stille-Gigli wire saw
Stille-Halsted forceps
Stille-Horsley
- S.-H. bone-cutting forceps
- S.-H. forceps
- S.-H. rib forceps
- S.-H. rongeur
- S.-H. shears

Stille-Langenbeck elevator
Stille-Leksell rongeur
Stille-Liston
- S.-L. bone-cutting forceps
- S.-L. bone forceps
- S.-L. forceps
- S.-L. rib-cutting forceps
- S.-L. rongeur

Stille-Luer
- S.-L. angled rongeur
- S.-L. angular duckbill rongeur
- S.-L. bone rongeur
- S.-L. forceps
- S.-L. rongeur
- S.-L. rongeur forceps

Stille-Luer-Echlin rongeur
Stille-Mayo
- S.-M. dissecting scissors
- S.-M. scissors

Stille-Mayo-Hegar needle
Stillenberg raspatory
Stille-pattern osteotome
Stille-Quervain spreader
Stille-Ruskin rongeur
Stille-Russian forceps
Stille-Seldinger needle

Stille-Sherman
  S.-S. bone drill
  S.-S. drill
Stille-Stiwer
  S.-S. gouge
  S.-S. osteotome
  S.-S. plaster shears
Stille-Waugh forceps
Stille-Zaufal-Jansen rongeur
Stimoceiver implant material
Stimson pedicle clamp
stimulating
  s. catheter
  s. electrode
stimulation
  dorsal column s. (DCS)
stimulator
  ACUTENS transcutaneous nerve s.
  Anustim electronic neuromuscular s.
  Bionicare s.
  Bipulse micro s.
  Butler s.
  Concept nerve s.
  Digitimer pattern reversal s.
  direct current bone growth s. (DCBGS)
  Dormed cranial electrotherapy s.
  electronic muscle s.
  external functional neuromuscular s.
  facial nerve s.
  Ganzfeld s.
  Gatron s.
  Gatron nerve s.
  Hilger facial nerve s.
  implantable neural s.
  Myopulse muscle s.
  Myosynchron muscle s.
  oculogyric s.
  Optokinetic s.
  Orthofuse implantable growth s.
  OrthoGen bone growth s.
  OrthoPak II bone growth s.
  personal portable s. (PPS)
  photic-evoked response s.
  Smoke Control Porta-Pack aversive s.
  surgical nerve s.
  transcutaneous electrical nerve s. (TENS)
  transcutaneous nerve s. (TNS)
  Ultratone electrical transcutaneous neuromuscular s.
  Waters muscle s.
  Whistle-Stop wireless aversive s.
  WR surgical nerve s.
stirrup brace
stirrup-loop curette
stitch scissors
Stitt catheter
Stiwer
  S. biopsy forceps
  S. bone-holding forceps
  S. curette
  S. dissector
  S. dressing forceps
  S. finger ring saw
  S. furuncle knife
  S. grooved director
  S. hand drill
  S. laryngeal mirror
  S. retractor
  S. scalpel handle
  S. scissors
  S. sponge forceps
  S. tendon dissector
  S. tissue forceps
  S. towel clamp
  S. trocar
St. Jude annuloplasty ring
St. Jude composite valve graft
St. Jude heart valve prosthesis
St. Jude medical heart valve
St. Jude Medical prosthesis
St. Luke's double-action rongeur
St. Luke's retractor
St. Mark clamp
St. Mark's Hospital retractor
St. Mark's lipped retractor
St. Mark's pelvis retractor
St. Martin eye forceps
St. Martin forceps
St. Martin-Franceschetti cataract hook
St. Martin suturing forceps

Stocker
    S. cyclodiathermy puncture
        needle
    S. needle
Stockert cardiac pacing electrode
Stock finger splint splint
Stockfisch appliance
stockinette
    s. amputation bandage
    s. bandage
    s. dressing
    orthopaedic s.
    sterile s.
stockings
    antiembolism s.
    Atkins-Tucker
        antiembolism s.
    Bellavar medical support s.
    Carolon life support
        antiembolism s.
    Comtesse medical support s.
    Florex medical
        compression s.
    sequential compression s.
    Sigvaris medical s.
    TED antiembolism s.
    Venofit medical
        compression s.
    Venoflex medical
        compression s.
    Zimmer antiembolism s.
Stockman
    S. clamp
    S. meatal clamp
    S. penile clamp
Stoesser stripper
Stolte
    S. dissector
    S. tonsillar dissector
Stolte-Stille elevator
Stoltz laparoscope
stoma button
stoma-centering guide
stomach
    s. brush
    s. clamp
Stomahesive
    S. paste
    S. powder
    S. sterile wafer
stomal bag
stoma-measuring device

Stone
    S. clamp
    S. clamp-applying forceps
    S. clamp-locking device
    S. eye implant
    S. forceps
    S. implant
    S. intestinal anastomosis
        clamp
    S. intestinal clamp
    S. intestinal forceps
    S. lens nucleus prolapser
    S. stomach clamp
    S. tissue forceps
stone
    s. basket
    s. basket outer catheter
    s. basket screw mounted
        handle
    s. dislodger
    s. forceps
    s. retrieval balloon
    s. retrieval basket
    s. retriever
stone-crushing forceps
stone-extraction forceps
stone-grasping forceps
Stone-Holcombe
    S.-H. anastomosis clamp
    S.-H. clamp
    S.-H. intestinal clamp
stone-holding basket
stone-locking device
Stoneman forceps
Stony splenorenal shunt clamp
Stookey
    S. cranial rongeur
    S. retractor
    S. rongeur
stool
    s. collector
    foot s.
    Fuchs surgical s.
stop
    Bowman needle s.
    s. cock
    s. collar telescope
    Devonshire-Mack s.
    s. needle
stopcock
    Ayer s.
    Morse s.
Stop eye speculum

Storer
- S. retractor
- S. thoracoabdominal retractor

Storey
- S. clamp
- S. forceps
- S. gall duct forceps
- S. thoracic forceps
- S. thoracic hemostatic forceps

Storey-Hillar dissecting forceps
Story orbital elevator
Storz
- S. adjustable headrest
- S. anterior commissure laryngoscope
- S. antral punch
- S. applicator
- S. arthroscope
- S. aspiration biopsy needle
- S. band
- S. biopsy forceps
- S. blade
- S. bougie-urethrotome
- S. bronchial catheter
- S. bronchoscopic forceps
- S. bronchoscopic telescope
- Calcutript by Karl S.
- S. calipers
- S. camera
- S. catheter
- S. catheter adapter
- S. ceiling-mounted microscope system
- S. chalazion trephine
- S. choledochoscope-nephroscope
- S. ciliary forceps
- S. cleaning brush
- S. coagulator
- S. continuous flow rectoscope
- S. corneal bur
- S. cotton carrier
- S. curved forceps
- S. cystoscopic electrode
- S. cystoscopic forceps
- S. diagnostic laparoscope
- S. diagnostic microscope system
- S. direct-view resectoscope
- S. disposable blade
- S. disposable fiberoptic light pipe
- S. double-fixation hook
- S. duckbill rongeur
- S. ear knife handle
- S. ear knife set
- S. ear, nose and throat (ENT) camera system
- S. Easy shield
- S. endo camera
- S. esophagoscope
- S. esophagoscopic forceps
- S. examining arthroscope
- S. face shield headband
- S. fiberoptic cable adapter
- S. flexible injection needle
- S. folding-handle ear knife
- S. forceps
- S. grasping biopsy forceps
- S. hair transplant trephine
- S. head holder
- S. hysteroscope
- S. infection ventilation laryngoscope
- S. insertor
- S. intranasal antral punch
- S. intraocular scissors
- S. iris hook
- S. iris scissors
- S. keratometer
- S. kidney stone forceps
- S. knife
- S. Laparocam
- S. laparoscope
- S. laser
- S. laser resectoscope
- S. meatal clamp
- S. microcalipers
- S. microserrefine
- S. microsurgical bipolar coagulator
- S. miniature forceps
- S. nasal speculum
- S. nasopharyngeal biopsy forceps
- S. needle cannula
- S. needle holder
- S. operating esophagoscope
- S. operating laparoscope
- S. optical biopsy forceps
- S. optical esophagoscope
- S. orbital elevator-retractor
- S. pediatric esophagoscope

S. pigtail probe
S. resectoscope
S. resectoscope curette
S. resectoscope electrode
S. retractor
S. scleral buckling balloon catheter
S. septal speculum
S. sheath
S. sheath-handle ear knife
S. shield
S. sinus biopsy forceps
S. stitch scissors
S. stone-crushing forceps
S. stone dislodger
S. stone-extraction forceps
S. suction tube
S. Teflon forceps guard
S. telescope
S. tonographer
S. tonometer
S. twisted snare wire
S. twist hook
S. Universal lens loupe
S. urethrotome
S. vent tube introducer
S. Vienna nasal speculum
S. wire-cutting scissors
Storz-Atlas eye magnet
Storz-Beck tonsillar snare
Storz-Bell erysiphake
Storz-Bonn
    S.-B. forceps
    S.-B. suturing forceps
Storz-Bowman lacrimal probe
Storz-Bruening
    S.-B. anastigmatic aural magnifier
    S.-B. diagnostic head
    S.-B. magnifier
Storz-DeKock two-way bronchial catheter
Storz-Duredge
    S.-D. cataract knife
    S.-D. keratome
Storz-Hopkins
    S.-H. laryngoscope
    S.-H. telescope
Storz-Kirkheim urethrotome
Storz-LaForce adenotome
Storz-LaForce-Stevenson adenotome
Storz-Moltz tonsillectome

Storz-Riecker laryngoscope
Storz-Schitz tonometer
Storz-Vienna nasal speculum
Storz-Westcott scissors
strabismus
    s. forceps
    s. hook
    s. needle
    s. scissors
Strach spring
straight
    s. bistoury
    s. blade
    s. catheter
    s. catheter guide
    s. clamp
    s. clip
    s. coagulating forceps
    s. Crile clamp
    s. flush percutaneous catheter
    s. forceps
    s. guide wire
    s. hemostat
    s. hex screwdriver
    s. knife
    s. lacrimal cannula
    s. needle
    s. osteotome
    s. rasp
    s. reamer
    s. retractor
    s. scissors
    s. shank bur
    s. single tenaculum forceps
    s. stent
    s. suturing needle
    s. tenaculum
    s. tube
    s. tube stylet
straight-blade
    s.-b. electrode
    s.-b. laryngoscope
straight-end cup forceps
straightener
    Asch septal s.
    Cottle-Walsham septal s.
    septal s.
    Walsham septal s.
straight-point
    s.-p. electrode
    s.-p. needle

straight-tip
>   s.-t. electrode
>   s.-t. jeweler's bipolar forceps

straight-wire electrode

Straith
>   S. chin implant
>   S. nasal implant
>   S. nasal splint kit
>   S. profilometer

Strampelli
>   S. eye splint
>   S. implant
>   S. lens

Strandell retractor

Strandell-Stille
>   S.-S. retractor
>   S.-S. tendon hook

strap
>   Circumpress chin s.
>   s. clavicle splint
>   Dermicel Montgomery s.
>   latex rubber tourniquet s.
>   Meek-style clavicular s.
>   Rotalok wrist s.
>   Rusch head s.
>   tourniquet s.

Strassburger tissue forceps

Strassmann
>   S. uterine-elevating forceps
>   S. uterine forceps

Stratte
>   S. clamp
>   S. forceps
>   S. kidney clamp
>   S. needle holder

Strauss
>   S. cannula
>   S. clamp
>   S. dental attachment
>   S. meatal clamp
>   S. needle
>   S. penile clamp
>   S. sigmoidoscope

Strauss-Valentine penis clamp

Strayer meniscal knife

Streak resectoscope

streak retinoscope

Street pin

Streli forceps

Strelinger
>   S. catheter-introducing
>   forceps
>   S. colon clamp

>   S. right-angle clamp
>   S. right-angle colon clamp

Strempel dermatome

Stress Cath catheter

stretcher
>   Kuttner wound s.

Stretzer bent-tip USCI catheter

Stribs strut

stricturotome
>   Stallard s.
>   Werb angled s.

Stringer
>   S. catheter-introducing
>   forceps
>   S. forceps
>   S. newborn throat forceps
>   S. tracheal catheter

stringer
>   instrument s.

strip
>   Codman surgical s.
>   G-C polishing s.
>   GHM polishing s.
>   Mosher s.
>   PD polishing s.
>   s. and point sponge
>   Urihesive moldable
>   adhesive s.

Stripper

stripper
>   Babcock jointed vein s.
>   Bartlett fascial s.
>   Brand tendon s.
>   Bunnell tendon s.
>   Bunt tendon s.
>   Cannon-type s.
>   Carroll forearm tendon s.
>   chest tube s.
>   Clark vein s.
>   Codman disposable vein s.
>   Codman vein s.
>   Cole polyethylene vein s.
>   Crawford fascial s.
>   Crile vagotomy s.
>   DeBakey intraluminal s.
>   Doyen rib s.
>   Doyle vein s.
>   Dunlop s.
>   Emerson vein s.
>   Endostat fiber s.
>   external vein s.
>   fascial s.
>   Friedman olive-tip vein s.

Friedman vein s.
Furlong tendon s.
Grierson s.
Hall-Chevalier s.
hydraulic vein s.
IM tendon s.
interchangeable vein s.
Joplin tendon s.
Keeley vein s.
Kurtin vein s.
LaVeen helical s.
Lempka vein s.
Levy-Okun s.
Linton vein s.
Martin endarterectomy s.
Masson fascial s.
Matson-Alexander rib s.
Matson-Mead periosteum s.
Matson rib s.
Mayo external vein s.
Mayo-Myers s.
Mayo-Myers external vein s.
Mayo vein s.
Meyer olive-tipped vein s.
Meyer spiral vein s.
Meyer vein s.
Myers interchangeable
  vein s.
Myers spiral vein s.
Myers vein s.
Nabatoff vein s.
Nelson rib s.
Nelson-Roberts s.
New Orleans s.
orthopaedic surgical s.
Phelan vein s.
Price-Thomas rib s.
reusable vein s.
rib s.
rib edge s.
ring s.
Roberts-Nelson rib s.
Samuels vein s.
Shaw carotid artery clot s.
Smith posterior cartilage s.
spiral vein s.
Stoesser s.
Stukey s.
surgical s.
tendon s.
Trace hydraulic vein s.
vagotomy s.
vein s.

Verner s.
Webb interchangable vein s.
Webb vein s.
Wilson vein s.
Wurth vein s.
Wylie endarterectomy s.
Zollinger-Gilmore vein s.
stripping
Stripseal catheter
**Strobex Mark II electrosurgical
  unit**
stroboscope
  rhinolarynx s.
Stromeyer splint
**strontium-90 ophthalmic beta ray
  applicator**
Stroud-Baron ear suction tube
Strubel lid everter
Struck
  S. laminectomy retractor
  S. spreader
Struempel, Strümpel
  S. ear alligator forceps
  S. ear forceps
  S. ear punch forceps
  S. forceps
  S. rongeur
Struempel-Voss
  S.-V. ethmoidal forceps
  S.-V. nasal forceps
Strully
  S. cardiovascular scissors
  S. curette
  S. dissecting scissors
  S. dressing forceps
  S. dural scissors
  S. dural twist hook
  S. Gigli-saw handle
  S. hook scissors
  S. nerve root retractor
  S. neurosurgical scissors
  S. retractor
  S. ruptured disk curette
  S. scissors
  S. tissue forceps
Strully-Kerrison rongeur
Strümpel (*var. of* Struempel)
strut
  Adkins s.
  Anderson nasal s.
  s. bar
  s. bar hook
  s. calipers

strut *(continued)*
    s. forceps
    Harrington s.
    s. hook
    House calipers s.
    Judet s.
    Magneson s.
    s. measuring instrument
    Nalebuff-Goldman s.
    s. pick
    polyethylene s.
    Rehbein internal steel s.
    Robinson s.
    Stribs s.
    Teflon s.
    TORP s.
    tricuspid valve s.
    valve outflow s.
    wire-loop s.
strut-type pin
Struyken
    S. angular punch tip
    S. conchotome
    S. ear forceps
    S. forceps
    S. nasal-cutting forceps
    S. nasal forceps
    S. punch
    S. turbinate forceps
Stryker
    S. autopsy saw
    S. blade
    S. bur
    S. camera
    S. cast cutter
    S. chip camera
    S. chondrotome
    S. CircOlectric fracture
      frame
    S. Constavac closed wound
      suction apparatus
    S. dermatome
    S. drill
    S. lag screw
    S. micro-irrigator
    S. resector
    S. Rolo-dermatome
    S. saw
    S. screw
    S. screwdriver
    S. SE3 drive system
    S. shaver
    S. turning fracture frame

Stryker-School meniscal knife
Stuart Gordon hand splint
Stubbs
    S. adenoidal curette
    S. curette
Stucker
    S. bile duct dilator
    S. gall duct dilator
Stuck laminectomy self-retaining
  retractor
Stuckrad magnifying
  laryngopharyngoscope
study
    rectosphincteromanometric s.
Stuhler-Heise fixator
Stukey stripper
Stumer perforating bur
Sturmdorf
    S. cervical needle
    S. cervical reamer
    S. needle
    S. obstetrical suture
    S. pedicle needle
    S. suture
Stutsman nasal snare
St. Vincent forceps
St. Vincent tube clamp
St. Vincent tube-clamping forceps
St. Vincent tube-occluding forceps
Styles forceps
stylet, stylette
    bipolar irrigating s.
    Bruening forceps s.
    cardiovascular s.
    Cooper endotracheal s.
    curved tube s.
    Frigitronics disposable
      cryosurgical s.
    Jelco intravenous s.
    Malis irrigating forceps s.
    malleable s.
    Rumel ratchet tourniquet
      eyed s.
    straight tube s.
    surgical s.
    tourniquet-eyed ratchet s.
    transmyocardial pacing s.
    transthoracic pacing s.
    Universal curved-tube s.
    Universal straight-tube s.
    ureteral s.

styletted
>s. catheter
>s. tracheobronchial catheter

stylus
>IM/EM tibial resection s.
>tibial s.

S-type dental implant
styptics
Styrofoam dressing
Suarez spreader
subclavian
>s. cannula
>s. catheter
>s. dialysis catheter
>s. Tegaderm dressing

subcostal trocar
subcutaneous port
subcuticular suture
subdermal implant
subglottic forceps
subglottiscope
>Healy-Jako pediatric s.

subimplant
>Spencer silicone s.

sublaminar wire
submammary dissector
submucosal implant
submucous
>s. chisel
>s. curette
>s. dissector
>s. resection (SMR)
>s. retractor

Subortholen sheet
subperiosteal
>s. glass bead insertor
>s. implant

Subramanian
>S. aortic clamp
>S. clamp
>S. classic miniature aortic
> clamp
>S. miniature aortic clamp
>S. sidewinder aortic clamp

subretinal fluid cannula
substitute
>Accu-Flo dural s.
>dural s.
>U-channel stripping dural s.

sucker
>Churchill s.
>intercardiac s.

>intracardiac s.
>s. tip

suction
>s. adapter
>s. apparatus
>s. aspirator
>Barton s.
>s. biopsy needle
>s. biter
>s. cannula
>s. catheter
>s. cautery
>s. cup
>s. curette
>s. device
>s. dissector
>s. drain
>ear forceps with s.
>s. elevator
>s. forceps
>Frazier s.
>s. irrigator
>s. magnet
>s. pistol
>Pleur-Evac s.
>s. probe
>s. pump aspirator
>s. punch
>Rosen s.
>s. tip
>s. tip curette
>s. tonsillar dissector
>s. tube
>s. tube-cleaning wire
>s. tube clip
>s. tube-holding forceps
>s. tube obturator

suction-coagulation tube
suction-irrigator
>Jako s.-i.
>Kurze s.-i.
>William-House s.-i.

Sudarsky cryoprobe
SUE
>single-use electrode

Sugar
>S. aneurysm clip
>S. clip

Sugarbaker retrocolic clamp
sugar-tong splint
Suggs catheter
Sugita
>S. aneurysm clip

Sugita *(continued)*
  S. catheter
  S. clip
  S. jaws clip applier
Suker
  S. cyclodialysis spatula
  S. iris forceps
  S. spatula knife
Sullival gum scissors
Sullivan
  S. sinus rasp
  S. variable stiffness cable
SULP II catheter
Sulze diamond-point needle
Summar alloy
Summit alloy
Sumner clamp
sump
  s. catheter
  Cooley vertricular s.
  s. drain
  s. Penrose drain
  s. pump catheter
  s. suction tube
  s. tube
  ventricular s.
Sumpter clasp spring-lock
Sunday staphylorrhaphy elevator
Sundt
  S. aneurysm clip-applier
  S. carotid endarterectomy
    shunt
  S. clip
  S. encircling clip
  S. shunt
Sundt-Kees
  S.-K. aneurysm clip
  S.-K. booster clip
  S.-K. clip
  S.-K. Slim-Line aneurysm
    clip
Superblade
Supercath intravenous catheter
Super-Dent orthodontic cement
**Super Epitron high-frequency
  epilator**
superficial
  s. implant
  s. suture
Superflex elastic dressing
superior
  s. rectus bridle suture

  s. rectus forceps
  s. rectus traction suture
**superior temporal artery-middle
  cerebral artery (STA-MCA)**
Super-Soft denture reliner
**Super-Trac adhesive traction
  dressing**
Supolene suture
Support
  Well Leg S.
support
  cock-up wrist s.
  Dr. Gibaud thermal
    health s.
  flat brain spatula s.
  Grotena abdominal s.
  IMP-Capello arm s.
  s. kit
  Schillinger suture s.
  Surgi-Bra breast s.
  s. suture
supporter
  Malis vessel s.
  vessel s.
supracondylar
  s. barrel/plate component
  s. nail
suprahepatic caval cuff
Supramead nose splint
Supramid
  S. Extra suture
  S. eye muscle sleeve
  S. graft
  S. implant
  S. lens
  S. mesh
  S. prosthesis
  S. quarter globe caps
  S. snare
  S. suture
suprapubic
  s. bag
  s. cannula
  s. catheter
  s. drain
  s. hemostatic bag
  s. retractor
  s. self-retaining retractor
  s. suction drain
  s. trocar
Suraci
  S. elevator hook

S. hook elevator
S. zygoma hook elevator
Surcan
S. knee holder
S. leg holder
Sure-Cut needle
Surefit
S. intraocular lens
S. lens
Sureflow catheter
surface
s. electrode
s. eye implant
Surfasoft dressing
Sur-Fit
S.-F. colostomy bag
S.-F. colostomy irrigation
sleeve
S.-F. loop
S.-F. urinary drainage bag
S.-F. urostomy pouch
Surgair bur
Surgairtome air drill
Surgaloy
S. metallic suture
S. suture
Surgibone implant
Surgi-Bra breast support
surgical
s. blade
s. cannula
s. chromic suture
s. clamp
s. clip applier
s. contractor
s. curette
s. cutter
s. dissector
s. drape
s. dressing
s. electrode
s. exhaust apparatus
s. file
s. general rasp
s. gouge
s. gut suture
s. hammer
s. handle
s. hood
s. instrument guide
s. instrument post
s. keratometer
s. laser

s. linen suture
s. loupe
s. mallet
s. marking pen
s. mask
s. metallic mesh
s. microscope
s. nerve stimulator
s. otoscope
s. pin driver
s. power magnet
s. retractor
s. saw
s. saw blade
s. scissors
s. silk suture
s. skin graft expander
s. snare
s. spatula
s. staple applier
s. stapling gun
s. steel gauze
s. steel suture
s. stripper
s. stylet
s. suction pump
s. suture
s. telescope
surgical-orthopaedic
s.-o. drill
Surgical Simplex P bone cement
Surgicel
S. absorbable hemostat
S. dressing
S. gauze
S. gauze dressing
S. implant
S. implantation
S. Nu-Knit absorbable
hemostat
Surgiclip
S. clip
McDermott S.
McFadden S.
Poly S.
Surgicraft
S. electrode
S. pacemaker electrode
S. suture
S. suture needle
Surgidev
S. intraocular lens
S. iris clip

Surgidev *(continued)*
    S. Leiske anterior chamber
      intraocular lens
Surgifix dressing
Surgiflex
    S. bandage
    S. dressing
Surgi-Flo leg bag
Surgigrip sleeve
Surgikit Velcro tourniquet
Surgikos cleaner
Surgilar suture
Surgilav drain
Surgilene
    S. blue monofilament
      polypropylene suture
    S. suture
Surgiloid suture
Surgilon
    S. braided nylon suture
    S. suture
Surgilone
    S. monofilament
      polypropylene suture
    S. suture
Surgilope suture
Surgi-Med
    S.-M. clamp
    S.-M. umbiliclamp
Surgineedle pneumoperitoneum
  needle
Surgin hemorrhage occluder pin
Surgi-Pad combined dressing
Surgiport
    S. disposable trocar
    S. stapler
Surgi-Prep
Surgiscribe
Surgiset suture
Surgi-Site Incise drape
Surgitable hand surgery table
Surgitek
    S. catheter
    S. double-J ureteral catheter
    S. double-J ureteral stent
    S. Flexi-Flate II penile
      implant
    S. graduated cystoscope
    S. implant
    S. mammary implant
    S. prosthesis
    S. Tractfinder ureteral stent
    S. Uropass stent

Surgitie ligating loops
Surgitome bur
Surgitube dressing
suspended operating illuminator
suspension
    s. apparatus
    s. laryngoscope
suspensory
    s. bandage
    s. dressing
Sustagen nasogastric tube
Sutherland
    S. eye scissors
    S. scissors
    S. vitreous forceps
Sutter MCP finger joint prosthesis
Sutter-Smeloff heart valve
  prosthesis
Sutton
    S. biopsy needle
    S. needle
Sutupak suture
suture
    absorbable s.
    absorbable surgical s.
    Acutrol s.
    Albert s.
    Alcon s.
    Allgower s.
    Allison s.
    already-threaded s.
    alternating s.
    aluminum-bronze wire s.
    aluminum wire s.
    Ancap braided silk s.
    Ancap silk s.
    anchor s.
    anchoring s.
    angle s.
    anterior palatine s.
    Appolito s.
    apposition s.
    approximation s.
    arcuate s.
    Argyll Robertson s.
    Arlt s.
    Arruga encircling s.
    arterial silk s.
    atraumatic s.
    atraumatic braided silk s.
    atraumatic chromic s.
    Aureomycin s.
    Auto Suture s.

Axenfeld s.
Babcock wire s.
back-and-forth s.
Barraquer s.
Barraquer silk s.
barrel knot s.
baseball s.
basilar s.
bastard s.
Bauer-Black s.
Béclard s.
Bell s.
Bertrandi s.
Bigelow s.
biparietal s.
16-bite nylon s.
black s.
black braided s.
black silk s.
black twisted s.
Blalock s.
blanket s.
blue-black monofilament s.
blue cotton s.
blue twisted cotton s.
bolster s.
bone wax s.
Bonney s.
bony s.
Bozeman s.
braided s.
braided Ethibond s.
braided Mersilene s.
braided Nurolone s.
braided nylon s.
braided polyamide s.
braided silk s.
braided wire s.
bregmatomastoid s.
bridle s.
bronchial s.
bronze s.
bronze wire s.
Brown-Sharp gauge s.
B&S gauge s.
Buckston s.
bulb s.
bunching s.
Bunnell s.
buried s.
button s.
s. button
cable wire s.

Callaghan s.
capitonnage s.
cardinal s.
cardiovascular s.
cardiovascular Prolene s.
Cargile s.
Carrel s.
s. carrier
catgut s. (CGS, CS)
celluloid s.
celluloid linen s.
cervical s.
chain s.
Champion s.
Cherney s.
Chinese twisted silk s.
chloramine catgut s.
chromated catgut s.
chromic s.
chromic blue dyed s.
chromic catgut s.
chromic catgut mattress s.
chromic collagen s.
chromic gut s.
chromicized catgut s.
circular s.
circumcisional s.
clavate s.
clavate clove-hitch s.
s. clip
s. clip-applying forceps
s. clip forceps
s. clip-removing forceps
clove-hitch s.
clovehitch s.
Cloward stitch s.
Coakley s.
coaptation s.
coated s.
coated polyester s.
coated Vicryl s.
cobbler's s.
cocoon thread s.
collagen s.
comeoscleral s.
compound s.
Connell s.
Connell inverting s.
continuous s.
continuous catgut s.
continuous circular
  inverting s.
continuous cuticular s.

suture *(continued)*
    continuous interlocking s.
    continuous inverting s.
    continuous key-pattern s.
    continuous Lembert s.
    continuous locked s.
    continuous mattress s.
    continuous over-and-over s.
    continuous running s.
    continuous running
      locked s.
    continuous silk s.
    continuous U-shaped s.
    contiunous hemostatic s.
    Cooley U-s.
    corneal s.
    corneoscleroconjunctival s.
    cotton s.
    cotton Duknatel s.
    cotton nonabsorbable s.
    Cottony Dacron s.
    cranial s.
    crown s.
    Cushing s.
    s. cushion
    cushioning s.
    Custodis s.
    cutaneous s.
    cuticular s.
    s. cutter
    Czerny s.
    Czerny-Lembert s.
    Dacron s.
    Dacron bolstered s.
    Dacron traction s.
    Daily s.
    Davis-Geck s.
    Davis-Geck eye s.
    40-day chromic catgut s.
    20-day gut s.
    Degnon s.
    dekalon s.
    Deklene s.
    Deklene polypropylene s.
    Deknatel s.
    Deknatel silk s.
    delayed s.
    DeMartel s.
    dentate s.
    dermal s.
    Dermalene s.
    Dermalene polyethylene s.
    Dermalon s.

    Dermalon cuticular s.
    dermal tension
      nonabsorbing s.
    Dexon s.
    Dexon absorbable synthetic
      polyglycolic acid s.
    Dexon II s.
    Dexon Plus s.
    Dexon subcuticular s.
    D&G s.
    DG Softgut s.
    direct radial s.
    Docktor s.
    Donnati s.
    double-armed s.
    double-armed mattress s.
    double-armed retention s.
    double-button s.
    doubled s.
    doubled black silk s.
    doubled chromic catgut s.
    doubled pursestring s.
    double-stop s.
    doubly-ligated s.
    Douglas s.
    Drews s.
    s. drill
    Dulox s.
    Dupuytren s.
    dural-tenting s.
    Duvergier s.
    echelon s.
    edge-to-edge s.
    Edinburgh s.
    EEA Auto s.
    elastic s.
    Emmet s.
    end-on mattress s.
    end-over-end running s.
    EPTFE s.
    EPTFE vascular s.
    Equisetene s.
    erthmoidomaxillary s.
    Ethibond s.
    Ethibond polyester s.
    Ethicon s.
    Ethicon-Atraloc s.
    Ethicon silk s.
    Ethiflex s.
    Ethiflex retention s.
    Ethilon s.
    Ethilon nylon s.
    Ethi-pack s.

everting s.
everting interrupted s.
expanded
  polytetrafluoroethylene s.'s
extrachromic s.
eye s.
Faden s.
false s.
far s.
far-and-near s.
far-near s.
figure-of-eight s.
filament s.
fine s.
fine chromic s.
fine silk s.
Finsterer s.
fish-mouth s.
fixation s.
flat s.
Flaxedil s.
Flexitone s.
Flexon s.
Flexon steel s.
s. forceps
formaldehyde catgut s.
forty-day chromic catgut s.
Fothergill s.
free ligature s.
free-tie s.
French s.
frontal s.
frontal zygomatic s.
frontoethmoidal s.
frontolacrimal s.
frontomalar s.
frontonasal s.
frontoparietal s.
frontosphenoid s.
frontozygomatic s.
Frost s.
funicular s.
Furness s.
furrier's s.
Gaillart-Arlt s.
Gambee s.
Gamophen s.
gastrointestinal surgical
  gut s.
gastrointestinal surgical
  linen s.
gastrointestinal surgical
  silk s.

Gely s.
general closure s.
general eye surgery s.
Gianturco s.
Gibson s.
Gillies horizontal dermal s.
GI pop-off silk s.
GI silk s.
Glover's s.
glue-in s.
Goethe s.
Gore-Tex s.
gossamer silk s.
Gould s.
granny knot s.
green braided s.
green monofilament
  polyglyconate s.
Gregory stay s.
groove s.
Gudebrod s.
guide s.
Gussenbauer s.
gut s.
gut chromic s.
gut plain s.
guy s.
guy steading s.
Guyton s.
Guyton-Friedenwald s.
half-hitch s.
Halsted interrupted
  mattress s.
Halsted mattress s.
Hamis s.
harelip s.
harmonic s.
Harrington s.
Harris s.
Heaney s.
heavy gauge s.
heavy retention s.
heavy silk s.
heavy silk retention s.
heavy wire s.
helical s.
hemostatic s.
Herculon s.
Hill s.
s. holder
s. hole drill
horizontal s.
horizontal mattress s.

suture *(continued)*
    horseshoe s.
    Horsley s.
    IKI catgut s.
    imbricating s.
    implanted s.
    incisive s.
    India rubber s.
    infraorbital s.
    insert mattress s.
    interdermal buried s.
    interlocking s.
    intermaxillary s.
    intermittent s.
    internasal s.
    interpalpebral s.
    interrupted s.
    interrupted black silk s.
    interrupted chromic s.
    interrupted chromic
     catgut s.
    interrupted cotton s.
    interrupted far-near s.
    interrupted fine silk s.
    interrupted Lembert s.
    interrupted mattress s.
    interrupted near-far s.
    interrupted nylon s.
    interrupted plain catgut s.
    interrupted silk s.
    interrupted vertical
     mattress s.
    intestinal s.
    intracuticular s.
    intracuticular nylon s.
    intradermal s.
    intradermal mattress s.
    inverted s.
    inverted knot s.
    inverting s.
    iodine catgut s.
    iodized surgical gut s.
    iodochromic catgut s.
    Ivalon s.
    Jobert s.
    Jobert de Lamballe s.
    Jones s.
    jugal s.
    Kal-Dermic s.
    Kalt s.
    kangaroo tendon s.
    Keisley s.
    Kelly s.

Kelly-Kennedy s.
Kelly plication s.
Kessler s.
Kirby s.
Kirschner s.
Kleinert s.
Krause transverse s.
Küstner s.
Kypher s.
lace s.
lacidem s.
lacrimoconchal s.
lacrimoethmoidal s.
lacrimomaxillary s.
lacrimoturbinal s.
Lahey s.
lambdoid s.
Lang s.
LaRoque s.
lead s.
lead-shot tie s.
LeDentu s.
LeDran s.
LeFort s.
Lembert s.
Lespinasse s.
Ligapak s.
ligation s.
ligature s.
limbal s.
limbic s.
Lindner comeoscleral s.
linear polyethylene s.
linen s.
linen thread s.
lip s.
Littre s.
living s.
lock s.
locked s.
locking s.
locking running s.
lock-stitch s.
Loeffler s.
longitudinal s.
loop s.
Lukens catgut s.
lumbar s.
Lytle s.
malomaxillary s.
mamillary s.
Marlex s.
Marshall V-s.

mastoid s.
mattress s.
Maunsell s.
Maxam s.
Maxon s.
Maxon absorbable s.
Mayo s.
Mayo linen s.
McCannel s.
McGraw s.
McKissock s.
McLean corneoscleral s.
Measuroll s.
median palatine s.
medium chromic s.
Medrafil s.
Medrafil wire s.
Meigs s.
Mers s.
Mersilene s.
mesh s.
metal band s.
metopic s.
middle palatine s.
Millipore s.
monofilament s.
monofilament clear s.
monofilament green s.
monofilament nylon s.
monofilament steel s.
monofilament wire s.
multifilament s.
multifilament steel s.
multistrand s.
Mustarde s.
nasal s.
nasofrontal s.
nasomaxillary s.
natural s.
near-and-far s.
near-far s.
nerve s.
Nesta stitch s.
neurosurgical s.
Nissen s.
nonabsorbable s.
nonabsorbable surgical s.
noneverting s.
noose s.
Novofil s.
Nurulon s.
nylon s.
nylon monofilament s.

nylon retention s.
obstetrical double-armed s.
occipital s.
occipitomastoid s.
occipitoparietal s.
occipitosphenoidal s.
O'Connell s.
Oertli s.
oiled silk s.
on-edge mattress s.
Ophthalon s.
outer interrupted silk s.
over-and-over whip s.
overlapping s.
Owen s.
Oyloidin s.
Pagenstecher s.
Pagenstecher linen thread s.
palatine s.
palatoethmoidal s.
palatomaxillary s.
Palfyn s.
Pancoast s.
pants-over-vest s.
Paré s.
parietal s.
parietomastoid s.
parieto-occipital s.
Parker-Kerr s.
s. passer
patch-reinforced mattress s.
PDS s.
PDS Vicryl s.
Pearsall Chinese twisted s.
Pearsall silk s.
pericostal s.
perineal support s.
Perlon s.
Perma-Hand s.
Perma-Hand braided silk s.
Perma-Hand silk s.
Petit s.
petrobasilar s.
petrosphenobasilar s.
petrosquamous s.
Pilling s.
pin s.
pink twisted cotton s.
plain s.
plain catgut s.
plain gut s.
plain interrupted s.
plastic s.

suture *(continued)*
pledget s.
pledgeted s.
pledgeted Ethibond s.
plicating s.
plication s.
polyamide s.
Polydek s.
polydioxanone s.
polyester s.
polyester fiber s.
polyethylene s.
polyfilament s.
polyglycolic s.
polypropylene s.
polypropylene button s.
pop-off s.
posterior palatine s.
postplaced s.
Potts tie s.
precut s.
preplaced s.
presection s.
primary s.
Prolene s.
Prolene polypropylene s.
Proxi-Strip s.
pulley s.
pull-out s.
pull-out wire s.
Pulvertaft s.
Purlon s.
pursestring s.
PVB s.
pyoktanin s.
pyoktanin catgut s.
Quickert s.
quilt s.
quilted s.
radial s.
Ramdohr s.
Ramsey County pyoktanin
  catgut s.
Rankin s.
reconstructive s.
rectus traction s.
reef knot s.
reinforcing s.
relaxation s.
Reo Macrodex s.
retained s.
retention s.
reverse-cutting s.

rhabdoid s.
ribbon gut s.
Richardson s.
Richardson angle s.
Richter s.
Rigal s.
right-angle mattress s.
s. ring
Ritisch s.
rubber s.
running s.
running chromic s.
running continuous s.
running imbricating s.
running-locked s.
running nylon s.
running subcuticular s.
Sabreloc s.
Saenger s.
safety-bolt s.
sagittal s.
scalp s.
s. scissors
secondary s.
seminal s.
seromuscular s.
seromuscular-to-edge s.
seroserosal s.
seroserosal silk s.
seroserous s.
serrated s.
seton s.
sewing-machine stitch s.
Shirodkar s.
shorthand vertical mattress
  stitch s.
shotted s.
Siemens PTCA open-
  heart s.
silicone-treated s.
silicone-treated surgical
  silk s.
silk s.
silk braided s.
silk interrupted mattress s.
silk nonabsorbable s.
silk pop-off s.
silk stay s.
silk traction s.
silkworm gut s.
Silky Polydek s.
silver s.
silverized catgut s.

Simon s.
simple s.
Sims s.
single-armed s.
single-handed knot s.
skin s.
sleeper s.
sling s.
slotted s.
Smead-Jones s.
Snellen s.
Softgut s.
Softgut chromic s.
Softgut surgical chromic
  catgut s.
solid-state silk s.
Spanish blue virgin silk s.
spatula needle s.
sphenoethmoidal s.
sphenofrontal s.
sphenomalar s.
sphenomaxillary s.
spheno-occipital s.
spheno-orbital s.
sphenoparietal s.
sphenopetrosal s.
sphenosquamous s.
sphenotemporal s.
sphenozygomatic s.
spiral s.
Sprong s.
squamosal s.
squamosomastoid s.
squamosoparietal s.
squamososphenoid s.
squamous s.
SS s.
stainless steel s.
stainless steel wire s.
Stallard s.
Stallard-Liegard s.
staple s.
stay s.
steel s.
steel mesh s.
stepwise s.
sternal wire s.
Stewart s.
stick-tie s.
Sturmdorf s.
Sturmdorf obstetrical s.
subcuticular s.
superficial s.

superior rectus bridle s.
superior rectus traction s.
Supolene s.
support s.
Supramid s.
Supramid Extra s.
Surgaloy s.
Surgaloy metallic s.
surgical s.
surgical chromic s.
surgical gut s.
surgical linen s.
surgical silk s.
surgical steel s.
Surgicraft s.
Surgilar s.
Surgilene s.
Surgilene blue monofilament
  polypropylene s.
Surgiloid s.
Surgilon s.
Surgilon braided nylon s.
Surgilone s.
Surgilone monofilament
  polypropylene s.
Surgilope s.
Surgiset s.
Sutupak s.
swaged s.
swaged-on s.
Swedgeon s.
Swiss blue virgin silk s.
synthetic s.
synthetic absorbable s.
tacking s.
s. tag forceps
Tagima s.
tantalum wire s.
tantalum wire
  monofilament s.
Tapercut s.
Taylor s.
Teflon-coated Dacron s.
Teflon-pledgeted s.
temporal s.
temporomalar s.
temporozygomatic s.
tendon s.
tension s.
tenting s.
Tevdek s.
Tevdek pledgeted s.
thermo-flex s.

suture *(continued)*
    Thiersch s.
    thoracic s.
    thread s.
    through-and-through s.
    through-and-through
      continuous s.
    Ti-Cron s.
    tie s.
    tiger gut s.
    Tinel s.
    Tom Jones s.
    tongue s.
    tongue-and-groove s.
    tongue-in-groove s.
    tonsillar s.
    track s.
    traction s.
    transfixing s.
    transfixion s.
    transition s.
    transverse s.
    traumatic s.
    true s.
    Trumbull s.
    twenty-day gut s.
    twisted s.
    twisted cotton s.
    twisted dermal s.
    twisted linen s.
    twisted silk s.
    Tycron s.
    s. and tying forceps
    Tyrrell-Gray s.
    U-s.
    U-double-barrel s.
    umbilical tape s.
    unabsorbable s.
    undyed s.
    uninterrupted s.
    U-shaped continuous s.
    uteroparietal s.
    Van Hillman s.
    vascular silk s.
    Verhoeff s.
    vertical s.
    vertical mattress s.
    VEST traction s.
    Vicryl s.
    Vicryl pop-off s.
    Vicryl SH s.
    Vienna wire s.
    virgin silk s.

    Viro-Tec s.
    visceroparietal s.
    von Pirquet s.
    Werner s.
    whipstitch s.
    white s.
    white braided s.
    white nylon s.
    white silk s.
    white twisted s.
    wing s.
    s. wire
    wire s.
    s. wire-cutting scissors
    s. wire scissors
    wire Zytor s.
    Wölfler s.
    Woodbridge s.
    Worst medallion s.
    Wysler s.
    Y-s.
    Z-s.
    zygomatic s.
    zygomaticofrontal s.
    zygomaticomaxillary s.
    zygomaticotemporal s.
    Zytor s.
suture-carrying
    s.-c. forceps
    s.-c. scissors
suture-holding forceps
sutureless pacemaker electrode
suture-pulling forceps
suture-release needle
suture-removing
    s.-r. forceps
    s.-r. scissors
suture-spreading forceps
suture-tying
    s.-t. forceps
    s.-t. platform forceps
Suture VesiBand organizer
suturing
    s. forceps
    s. instrument
    s. needle
Suxion denture adhesive
Sven Johansson hip nail
swab
    Chamois s.
    Janet bladder s.
    KBM gauze s.

Koenig tonsillar s.
Merthiolate s.
swaged
  s. needle
  s. suture
swaged-on
  s.-o. needle
  s.-o. suture
Swan
  S. aortic clamp
  S. clamp
  S. corneoscleral punch
  S. knife
  S. knife-needle
  S. needle eye holder
  S. spade-type needle knife
Swan-Brown arterial forceps
Swan-Ganz
  S.-G. balloon type catheter
  S.-G. catheter
  S.-G. guide-wire TD
    catheter
  S.-G. pulmonary artery
    catheter
  S.-G. thermodilution
    catheter
  S.-G. tube
Swan-Jacob
  S.-J. gonioprism
  S.-J. gonioscopic prism
  S.-J. goniotomy pliers
Swank high-flow arterial blood
  filter
swan-neck
  s.-n. clamp
  s.-n. gouge
Swann-Morton
  S.-M. blade
  S.-M. surgical blade
Swanson
  S. carpal lunate implant
  S. carpal scaphoid implant
  S. dynamic toe splint splint
  S. finger joint implant
  S. finger joint prosthesis
  S. flexible hallux valgus
    prosthesis
  S. great toe implant
  S. hand splint
  S. hemi-implant
  S. implant
  S. intramedullary broach
  S. radial head implant

S. radiocarpal implant
S. reamer
S. Silastic elbow prosthesis
S. trapezium implant
S. ulnar head implant
S. wrist joint implant
Sweaper curette
Swede-O brace
Swedgeon
  S. already-threaded needle
  S. suture
Swedish-pattern chisel
Sweeney
  S. posterior vaginal
    retractor
  S. posterior vaginal
    speculum
  S. retractor
sweeper
  Cottle spicule s.
  periosteal spicule s.
Sweet
  S. amputation retractor
  S. antral trocar
  S. clip-applying forceps
  S. delicate pituitary scissors
  S. dissecting forceps
  S. esophageal scissors
  S. eye magnet
  S. forceps
  S. ligature forceps
  S. modified sternal punch
  S. retractor
  S. rib spreader
  S. scissors
  S. sternal punch
  S. two-point discriminator
Sweet-Burford rib spreader
sweetheart retractor
Swenko
  S. bag
  S. gastric-cooling apparatus
Swenson
  S. cholangiography tube
  S. ring-jawed clamp
  S. ring-jawed holding clamp
  S. wire-guided
    papillotome/sphincterotome
Swiderski nasal chisel
Swiss
  S. blade
  S. bladebreaker
  S. blade holder

Swiss *(continued)*
    S. blue virgin silk suture
    S. bulldog clamp
    S. MP joint implant
Swissedent wax
Swiss-pattern speculum
switch box
    Elecath s.b.
switching stick
Switzerland dilatation catheter
swivel
    Erich s.
    facial fracture appliance s.
    s. joint suture holder
    s. knife
    Universal s.
Swolin self-retaining vaginal
  speculum
Sword knife
Syark vulsellum forceps
Sydenham mouth gag
Syed-Neblett implant
Syed template implant
Sylva
    S. anterior chamber
      irrigator
    S. irrigating cannula
Sylver-Wax dental wax
Symbion
    S. pneumatic assist device
    S. total artificial heart
Symbios pacemaker
symblepharon ring
Syme prosthesis
Symmonds hysterectomy retractor
Symonds needle
sympathectomy
    s. hook
    s. retractor
sympathetic raspatory
Syms tractor
Synapse electrocardiographic cream
Synatomic total knee prosthesis
SynchroMed pump
synchronous
    s. burst pacemaker
    s. mode pacemaker
    s. pacemaker
Synchrony
    S. II pacemaker
    S. pacemaker
Synevac vacuum curettage system
Syn-optics camera

synoptophore
synovectomy rongeur
synovium biopsy forceps
Synthaderm dressing
Synthes
    S. drill
    S. facial curette
    S. screw
synthetic
    s. absorbable suture
    s. suture
Syrex syringe
syringe
    Aeroflow s.
    Alcock bladder s.
    Alexander-Reiner ear s.
    Asepto bulb s.
    aspirating s.
    Boehm drop s.
    Bruening pressure s.
    bulb s.
    bulbous-tip ear s.
    Carti-Loid s.
    Cilacalcin double-
      chambered s.
    C-R resin s.
    Cuchica s.
    DeVilbiss s.
    Dynacor ear s.
    Dynacor ulcer s.
    ear s.
    E-Z s.
    Fink-Weinstein s.
    Fluorescite s.
    Fuchs two-way s.
    Gabriel s.
    G-C s.
    Gemini s.
    glycerine s.
    Green-Armytage s.
    Higginson s.
    Ilopan disposable s.
    impression material s.
    intraligamentary s.
    IPAS s.
    Irrigo s.
    Isosal s.
    Lewy Teflon glycerine-
      mixture s.
    MPL aspirating s.
    Multi-Fit Luer-Lok control
      tonsillar s.
    Namic angiographic s.

Nourse bladder s.
Pallin spring-assisted s.
PDL intraligamentary s.
Politzer air s.
Pomeroy ear s.
Pritchard s.
Proetz s.
Reiner-Alexander s.
Reiner-Alexander ear s.
Reiner ear s.
Rochester s.
Rudolph calibrated super s.
Sana-Lok s.
Schein s.
SEMI bulb irrigation s.
spring-assisted s.
Syrex s.
tapered-tip ear s.
Teflon glycerine-mixture s.
Tobald s.
tonsillar s.
Toomey s.
Tubex metal s.
Visitec s.

Syrrat scoop

system

Accuflo ultrafiltration s.
Ace intramedullary femoral
  nail s.
Advanced Medical Systems
  fetal monitoring s.
AGC Biomet total knee s.
AIM femoral nail s.
Alta modular s.
AMBI compression hip
  screw s.
Amplatz anchor s.
Anatomic hip s.
Anchor IIa osseointegrated
  titanium implant s.
Anspach s.
Arthro-Flo powered
  irrigation s.
Arthroscan video s.
Artus power s.
Asnis guided screw s.
Bateman UPF II bipolar s.
BIAS total hip s.
Bio-Fit total hip s.
Biofix absorbable fixation s.
Bioport collection and
  transportation s.
biotelemetry s.

Brown-Roberts-Wells
  stereotactic s.
BTM hip s.
CAPIS bone plate s.
capsule applier s.
Castle Daystar surgical
  television s.
C-2 hip s.
Clark hemoperfusion s.
CMI vacuum delivery s.
Codman external
  drainage s.
Cofield total shoulder s.
Coltene direct inlay s.
Compass CT stereotaxic
  adaptation s.
Concept arthroscopy
  power s.
Concept beachchair shoulder
  positioning s.
Concept Precise ACL
  guide s.
Concept rotator cuff
  repair s.
Concept self-compressing
  cannulated screw s.
Concept Sterling arthroscopy
  blade s.
Concept video imaging s.
Concept zone-specific
  cannula s.
Coombs bone biopsy s.
Corometrics Medical
  Systems Inc. fetal
  monitoring s.
coronary angiography
  analysis s.
CPT hip s.
curved Küntscher nail s.
cutaneous pO2
  monitoring s.
CVP s.
Cygnet Laboratories fetal
  monitoring s.
Dall-Miles cable grip s.
Denver hydrocephalus
  shunt s.
Dimension hip s.
Dupont distal humeral
  plate s.
Dyonics PS3500 drive s.
Ectra s.
Endocam video camera s.

system *(continued)*
Ergo irrigation s.
Estilux ultraviolet s.
Evoport auditory evoked
potential s.
extracorporeal membrane
oxygenation s.
Fenlin total shoulder s.
Fetasonde fetal
monitoring s.
Flexiflo gastrostomy tube
enteral delivery s.
Gambro s.
Gambro hemofiltration s.
Gastroscan motility s.
Genesis total knee s.
gravity assist s.
HA-biointegrated dental
implant s.
Hakim valve s.
Hall mandibular implant s.
Hall modular acetabular
reamer s.
Halo CO_2 laser s.
HJD total hip s.
Holter external drainage s.
Holter hydrocephalus
shunt s.
Hopkins II optical s.
Howmedica pediatric
osteotomy s.
Howmedica total ankle s.
HybridFit total hip s.
HybridFit total knee s.
Ilizarov limb-lengthening s.
Integral hip s.
IntraArc 9963 arthroscopic
power s.
irrigation-aspiration s.
Jimmy John colonic
irrigation s.
J-Vac closed wound
drainage s.
Kinematic II condylar and
stabilizer total knee s.
Kinematic II rotating-hinge
knee s.
Kinemax modular condylar
and stabilizer total knee s.
Kinemetric guide s.
Kirschner II-C shoulder s.
KMC hip s.
KMW hip s.

KTP/532 surgical laser s.
KTP/YAG surgical laser s.
Lamis infusion s.
Laparomed cholangiogram
vacuum s.
Laparo Vac irrigation and
aspiration s.
Leukotrap red cell
storage s.
Luhr fixation s.
Luhr MRS s.
Marion oxygen
resuscitation s.
Mark III halo s.
Maxi-Myst nebulizer s.
McIntire aspiration-
irrigation s.
McIntyre coaxial irrigating-
aspirating s.
McIntyre irrigation-
aspiration s.
Medelec-Van Gogh
electroencephalographic
recording s.
Medi-Tech catheter s.
Medwatch telemetry s.
Meniscus Mender II s.
MG II total knee s.
Micro-Aire pulse lavage s.
Micro-Aire surgical
instrument s.
Microloc knee s.
Microstar dialysis s.
Miller-Galante revision
knee s.
Miller-Galante total knee s.
Mitek anchor s.
Mityvac vacuum delivery s.
Mityvac vacuum
extraction s.
modular Lenbach hip s.
MOD unicompartmental
knee s.
Moore hip endoprosthesis s.
Mouradian humeral
fixation s.
Neer II shoulder s.
Neff femorotibial nail s.
Neuroguide interoperative
viewing s.
Neuroprobe pain control s.
Ogden plate s.

Omega Plus compression
hip s.
Omnifit HA hip s.
Opti-Fix total hip s.
OR-340 imaging s.
Orth-evac autotransfusion s.
Osteobond vacuum
mixing s.
Panoview arthroscopic s.
Parr closed irrigation s.
P.A.S. Port Fluoro-Free
peripheral access s.
Patil stereotaxic s.
PCA total knee s.
PerFixation s.
Performance total knee s.
Performance
unicompartmental knee s.
peripheral atherectomy s.
peritoneal dialysis s. (PDS)
Peritronics Medical Inc.
fetal monitoring s.
PGP flexible nail s.
Pie Medical ultrasound s.
Pleur-Evac autotransfusion s.
Precision Osteolock femoral
component s.
Press-Fit total condylar
knee s.
Pump Vac Plus s.
punch myringotomy s.
Redy 2000 dialysis s.
Redy Sorbent dialysis s.
Renatron II dialyzer
reprocessing s.
Richards fixator s.
Richards hip
endoprosthesis s.
Richards Solcotrans
orthopaedic drainage-
reinfusion s.
Richards Solcotrans Plus
drainage s.
Rogozinski screw s.
Rogozinski spinal rod s.
Rudolph breathing s.
Russell-Taylor femoral
interlocking nail s.
Safestretch incontinence s.
Sandhill esophageal
motility s.
self-injurious-behavior
inhibiting s. (SIBIS)

Seraton dialysis control s.
Shimadzu ultrasound s.
Simcoe irrigation-
aspiration s.
Simmons plating s.
Simpson-Robert vascular
dilation s.
Simpulse lavage s.
SITE TXR
phacoemulsification s.
Soehendra endoscopic biliary
stent s.
Solcotrans Plus drainage
reinfusion s.
Souter Strathclyde total
elbow s.
Spectron EF total hip s.
Sperm Select s.
Steele fiberoptic s.
Storz ceiling-mounted
microscope s.
Storz diagnostic
microscope s.
Storz ear, nose and throat
(ENT) camera s.
Stryker SE3 drive s.
Synevac vacuum
curettage s.
Systems Flow colonic
irrigation s.
TAB tibial augmentation
block s.
TAG s.
TCIV knee s.
telemetry s.
Thompson hip
endoprosthesis s.
Thora-Klex chest drainage s.
Ti-Fit total hip s.
tissue anchor guide s.
TPL-6 hip s.
Tri-Wedge total hip s.
Ultra-Drive bone cement
removal s.
Ultra-X external fixation s.
Uniflex nailing s.
Uni-Shunt hydrocephalus
shunt s.
Vacupac portable vacuum s.
Vector II guide s.
vessel occlusion s.
Visio-Gem color s.
VTCB biliary s.

system *(continued)*
    White s. for pediatric percutaneous catheterization
    Wit portable TENS s.
    Zimmer Anatomic hip prosthesis s.
    Zimmer-Hall drive s.
    ZMS intramedullary fixation s.
Systems Flow colonic irrigation system
Syticon 5950 bipolar demand pacemaker

Sztehlo
    S. clamp
    S. umbilical clamp
Szulc
    S. bone cutter
    S. eye magnet
    S. grommet
    S. orbital implant material
    S. vascular dilator
Szuler
    S. eustachian bougie
    S. forceps
    S. vascular forceps
Szultz corneal forceps

T-28 hip prosthesis
TA
>TA II loading unit
>TA metallic staple
>TA Premium 30 staple
>TA Premium 55 staple
>TA Premium 90 staple
>TA stapler

TA-30 stapler
TA-55 stapler
TA-90 stapler
TAB
>tibial augmentation block
>TAB acrylic
>TAB tibial augmentation block system

Tabb
>T. crural nipper
>T. curette
>T. double-ended flap knife
>T. ear curette
>T. ear elevator
>T. ear knife
>T. elevator
>T. flap knife
>T. knife pick
>T. knife-pick
>T. 3-millimeter ruler
>T. myringoplasty knife
>T. pick knife
>T. ruler

table
>Albee orthopaedic t.
>arthroscopic surgical t.
>t. band
>chemonucleolysis t.
>Chick surgical t.
>Heidelberg-R t.
>IMSI-Metripond operating room t.
>Jackson spinal surgery t.
>Maquet operating t.
>Maquet velox t.
>Mayfield instrument t.
>Mayo t.
>Mayo instrument t.
>Surgitable hand surgery t.
>Telos fracture t.
>tilt t.

table-fixed retractor

TAC atherectomy catheter
Tach-EZ dental attachment
tachycardia-terminating pacemaker
Tachylog pacemaker
tack
>Cody t.
>Cody sacculotomy t.
>titanium retinal t.

tack-and-pin forceps
tacking suture
Tactaid I vibrotactile aid
tactile probe
Tactylon surgical gloves
TAG
>tissue anchor guide
>TAG anchor
>TAG instrumentation
>TAG system

Tager lever
Tagima suture
Takagi arthroscope
Takahashi
>T. cutting forceps
>T. ethmoidal forceps
>T. ethmoidal punch
>T. forceps
>T. nasal forceps
>T. nasal punch
>T. neurosurgical forceps
>T. punch
>T. rongeur

Takaro clip
Take-Me-Along Personal Shocker pocket shocker
TALC
>transairway laryngeal control

Tallerman apparatus
Talley pump
Tamai clamp approximator
tamp
>CPT revision t.
>interbody graft t.
>Kiene bone t.
>Robinson-Smith t.
>tension band wire t.

tamper
>McIntyre suture t.

tampon
>t. forceps
>nasal t.

Tamsco
T. curette
T. forceps
T. periodontic scaler
T. wire-cutting scissors
tandem and ovoid
tangential
t. clamp
t. forceps
t. occlusion clamp
t. pediatric clamp
tangent screen
Tanne corneal cutting block
Tanner mesh graft dermacarrier
Tanner-Vandeput
T.-V. mesh dermatome
T.-V. mesh graft dermatome
Tan spatula
tantalum
t. clip
t. eye implant
t. gauze
t. hemostasis clip
t. implant
t. mesh eye implant
t. "O" ring
t. ring
t. wire monofilament suture
t. wire suture
tap
t. drill
Richards bone t.
screw t.
tape
t. board
brow t.
Dacron retraction t.
Dermicare hypoallergenic
paper t.
Dermicel hypoallergenic
cloth t.
Dermicel hypoallergenic
knitted t.
Dermiclear t.
Elastikon elastic t.
instrument coding t.
Mefix adhesive t.
Microfoam surgical t.
3M matrix t.
polyethylene retractor t.
Scanpor surgical t.
Sta-Fix t.
umbilical t.

Vascor sterile retraction t.
Zonas porous t.
taper
laser t.
Morse t.
t. needle
t. tip catheter
t. with Zimmer shank
Tapercut
T. needle
T. suture
tapered
t. catheter
t. needle
t. reamer
tapered-spring
t.-s. holder
t.-s. needle holder
tapered-tip ear syringe
taper-jaw
t.-j. rongeur
t.-j. rongeur forceps
Taperloc femoral prosthesis
taper-point suture needle
tapper
rectangular t.
round t.
tapping hammer
TARA
total articular replacement
arthroplasty
TARA total hip prosthesis
Tara retropubic retractor
Tarlov nerve elevator
Tarnier
T. axis-traction forceps
T. basiotribe
T. cephalotribe
T. cranioclast
T. forceps
T. obstetrical forceps
tarsal bar
Tassett vaginal cup bag
tattoo
Derma-Tattoo surgical t.
tattooing needle
Tatum
T. clamp
T. meatal clamp
T. Tee intrauterine device
T. ureteral transilluminator
Tauber
T. catheter

T. ligature carrier
T. ligature hook
T. male urethrographic catheter
T. needle
T. speculum
T. vaginal spatula
Taufic cholangiography clamp
T-auger
Taylor
T. apparatus
T. aspirator
T. back brace
T. blade
T. brace
T. brain scissors
T. Britetrac retractor
T. catheter holder
T. curette
T. dissecting forceps
T. dural scissors
T. fiberoptic retractor
T. forceps
T. gastric balloon
T. gastroscope
T. knife
T. laminectomy blade
T. percussion hammer
T. pulmonary dilator
T. reflex hammer
T. retractor
T. retractor blade
T. spinal retractor
T. spinal retractor blade
T. spinal support apparatus
T. spine brace
T. splint
T. suture
T. tissue forceps
T. vaginal speculum
Taylor-Cushing dressing forceps
Taylor-Knight brace
T-band
T-bandage dressing
t-bar
T-binder pressure dressing
^{99m}Tc
^{99m}Tc Cardiolyte contrast material
^{99m}Tc Cardiotech contrast material
^{99m}Tc disofenin contrast material

^{99m}Tc DTPA contrast material
^{99m}Tc MDP contrast material
^{99m}Tc sulfur colloid contrast material
TC femoral stem
TCIV knee system
T clamp
T-clamp
Pratt T.-c.
TD
thermodilution
TDC
thermal dilution catheter
TDM
thermodeltameter
TDMAC heparin shunt
teacher
Resnick speech t.
Teale
T. forceps
T. gorget
T. gorget lithotrite
T. tenaculum
T. tenaculum forceps
T. uterine forceps
T. uterine vulsellum forceps
T. uterine vulsellum tenaculum
T. vulsellum
T. vulsellum forceps
tear
t. away introducer sheath
t. duct tube
Teare
T. arm splint
T. snare
TEC
transluminal extraction-endarterectomy catheter
technetium-99m
TED
thromboembolic disease
TED antiembolism stockings
teeth
Astron t.
Logan bow with t.
Logan traction bow with t.
Planustar t.
SR-Isosit t.
Vita t.
Vitapan t.

723

Teflon
- T. button
- T. cannula
- T. catheter
- T. clip
- T. coating
- T. collar button
- T. ERCP cannula
- T. glycerine-mixture injection needle
- T. glycerine-mixture syringe
- T. implant
- T. injection needle
- T. intracardiac patch
- T. mesh implant
- T. nasobiliary drain
- T. needle
- T. needle catheter
- T. orbital floor implant
- T. pledget
- T. pledget suture buttress
- T. plug
- T. probe
- T. strut
- T. tri-leaflet prosthesis

Teflon-coated
- T.-c. Dacron suture
- T.-c. guide wire

Teflon-covered needle
Teflon-pledgeted suture
Teflon-tipped catheter
Tef-wire prosthesis
Tegaderm
- T. dressing
- T. occlusive dressing
- T. transparent dressing

Tegagel nonocclusive dressing
Tegasorb occlusive dressing
Tehl clamp
Teknamed drape sheet
Tekno
- T. coagulator
- T. forceps

Tek-Pro needle
Tel-A-Fever forehead thermometer
Telectronics pacemaker
telemetry
- Bio-sentry t.
- t. receiver
- t. system

telephone probe
telescope
- ACMI t.
- ACMI microlens t.
- ACMI microlens Foroblique t.
- Atkins esophagoscopic t.
- Best t.
- Best direct forward-vision t.
- biopsy t.
- bioptic t.
- Bridge t.
- bronchoscopic t.
- Broyles t.
- Burns t.
- Burns bridge t.
- catheterizing Foroblique t.
- clamp-on t.
- convertible t.
- direct forward-vision t.
- direct-vision t.
- double-catheterizing t.
- endoscopic t.
- examining t.
- fiberoptic t.
- fiberoptic right-angle t.
- Foroblique t.
- Holinger t.
- Holinger bronchoscopic t.
- Hopkins t.
- Hopkins direct-vision t.
- Hopkins endoscopy t.
- Hopkins fiber-shaft t.
- Hopkins forward-oblique t.
- Hopkins lateral t.
- Hopkins nasal endoscopy t.
- Hopkins pediatric t.
- Hopkins retrospective t.
- Hopkins rigid t.
- Hopkins rod-lens t.
- infant t.
- Keeler panoramic surgical t.
- Kramer t.
- Kramer direct-vision t.
- laryngeal-bronchial t.
- lateral microlens t.
- LUMINA operating t.
- LUMINA-SL t.
- McCarthy t.
- McCarthy fiberoptic Foroblique t.
- McCarthy Foroblique operating t.
- McCarthy miniature t.
- microlens direct-vision t.
- microlens Foroblique t.

Mueller t.
nasal endoscopic t.
Negus t.
pediatric t.
retrospective t.
right-angle t.
right-angle examining t.
Selsi sport t.
stop collar t.
Storz t.
Storz bronchoscopic t.
Storz-Hopkins t.
surgical t.
transilluminating t.
Tucker t.
Tucker direct-vision t.
Vest t.
Vest direct forward-vision t.
Walden t.
telescoping
t. guide
t. rod
Telfa
T. dressing
T. gauze dressing
T. pad
T. plastic film dressing
T. 4 x 4 bandage
Telos fracture table
Temens curette
Tempbond dental cement
temperature
t. and galvanic skin
response biofeedback
device
t. probe
template
Mallory-Head modular
acetabular t.
McKissock keyhole
areolar t.
rod t.
Stevens-Street elbow
prosthesis t.
total toe t.
Temple
T. University nail
T. University plate
Temple-Fay
T.-F. laminectomy retractor
T.-F. retractor
Tempo denture liner

temporal
t. bone holder
t. electrode
t. suture
temporalis transfer clamp
temporary
t. clip
t. clip-applying forceps
t. pacemaker
t. pacing catheter
t. pervenous lead
t. transvenous pacemaker
t. vascular clip
t. vessel clamp-applying
forceps
t. vessel clip
temporomalar suture
temporomandibular joint (TMJ)
temporozygomatic suture
Temrex dental cement
tenaculum
Abel-Aesculap-Pratt t.
Adair breast t.
Aesculap-Pratt t.
Barrett t.
Barrett uterine t.
Braun t.
Braun-Schroeder single-
tooth t.
Braun uterine t.
breast t.
Brophy t.
Collen-Pozzi t.
Corey t.
Cottle t.
Cottle single-prong t.
double-tooth t.
Duplay t.
Duplay uterine t.
Emmet t.
t. forceps
t. holder
t. hook
Hulka t.
Hulka uterine t.
Jackson t.
Jackson tracheal t.
Jacob t.
Jacobs t.
Jacob uterine t.
Jacob vulsellum uterine t.
Jarcho t.
Jarcho uterine t.

tenaculum *(continued)*
    Kahn traction t.
    Küstner t.
    Lahey goiter t.
    Martin t.
    Museux t.
    nasal t.
    New t.
    Newman t.
    Potts t.
    Pozzi t.
    Pratt t.
    Revots vulsellum t.
    Ritchie cleft palate t.
    Sargis uterine t.
    Schroeder t.
    Schroeder uterine t.
    Schroeder vulsellum
      uterine t.
    single t.
    single-tooth t.
    Skene t.
    Skene uterine t.
    Staude t.
    Staude-Jackson t.
    Staude-Jackson uterine t.
    Staude-Moore t.
    Staude-Moore uterine t.
    Staude uterine t.
    straight t.
    Teale t.
    Teale uterine vulsellum t.
    Thoms t.
    toothed t.
    tracheal t.
    traction t.
    uterine t.
    Watts t.
    Weisman t.
    Wylie t.
    Wylie uterine t.
Tenckhoff
    T. catheter
    T. peritoneal catheter
    T. renal dialysis catheter
Tenderfoot incision-making device
tendinosuture
tendon
    t. carrier
    t. forceps
    t. hook
    t. implant
    t. knife

    t. needle
    t. passer
    t. prosthesis
    t. stripper
    t. suture
    t. tucker
tendon-holding forceps
tendon-passing forceps
tendon-pulling forceps
tendon-tunneling forceps
Tennant
    T. Anchorflex intraocular
      lens
    T. Anchorflex lens implant
    T. anchor lens-insertion
      hook
    T. eye needle holder
    T. forceps
    T. hook
    T. intraocular lens forceps
    T. iris hook
    T. lens forceps
    T. lens-inserting forceps
    T. lens-manipulating hook
    T. spatula
    T. thumb-ring needle holder
    T. tying forceps
Tennant-Colibri corneal forceps
Tennant-Maumenee forceps
**Tennant-Troutman superior rectus
  forceps**
Tenner
    T. cannula
    T. eye cannula
    T. lacrimal cannula
Tennessee capsular polisher
Tennis
    T. Racquet angiographic
      catheter
    T. Racquet catheter
tennis elbow splint
Ten-O-Matic TENS unit
tenometer
    Schivitz t.
Tenoplast elastic adhesive dressing
tenosuture
tenotome
    Dieffenbach t.
    Ljunggren-Stille t.
    Ryerson t.
tenotomy
    t. hook
    t. scissors

TENS
transcutaneous electrical nerve
stimulator
Tensilon implant
tension
t. band wire tamp
t. clamp
t. suture
tensioner
Tensmax TENS unit
Tensor elastic dressing
TENS unit (*See also* unit)
Accucare TENS u.
Accu-o-Matic TENS u.
Dybex TENS u.
Electrorelaxor TENS u.
EMPI Neuropacer TENS u.
Meda 2500 TENS u.
Micro-Pulsar TENS u.
Ministem TENS u.
Mr. PainAway Health-
Up TENS u.
Neuromod TENS u.
Neuro-Pulse TENS u.
Pulsar TENS u.
Pulsar obstetrical two-
channel TENS u.
Skylark TENS u.
Ten-O-Matic TENS u.
Tensmax TENS u.
tent
KTK laminaria t.
laminaria t.
laminaria cervical t.
Mizutani laminaria t.
tenting suture
Tenzel
T. bipolar forceps
T. double-end periosteal
elevator
T. elevator
T. forceps
T. periosteal elevator
Tepas retractor
Terino anatomical chin implant
terminal
t. adapter electrode
t. electrode
t. electrode adapter
**Ter-Pogossian cervical radium
applicator**
terres knife
Terry keratometer

Terry-Mayo needle
Terson
T. capsular forceps
T. extracapsular forceps
T. forceps
T. speculum
Terumo
T. AV fistula needle
T. dental needle
T. Doppler fetal heart rate
monitor
T. guide wire
T. hypodermic needle
T. Surflo intravenous
catheter
T. transducer protector
T. tube sealer
Terumo-Clirans dialyzer
Tesberg esophagoscope
Tessier
T. disimpaction device
forceps
T. dislodger
T. osteotome
test
Catford visual acuity t.
Clearview hCG one-step
pregnancy t.
color vision t.
duochrome t.
Farnsworth t.
HemoCue blood
hemoglobin t.
Ishihara color t.
Schirmer tear t.
Snellen t.
thallium-102 stress t.
Titmus vision t.
t. tube holder
Tes Tape dressing
tester
finger muscle t.
House-Urban taste t.
Phoropter vision t.
testicular implant
testing drum knife
Teufel
T. brace
T. cervical brace
Tevdek
T. implant
T. pledgeted suture

Tevdek *(continued)*
    T. prosthesis
    T. suture
Texal-Muller chest binder
Texas
    T. catheter
    T. Scottish Rite Hospital (TSRH)
    T. Scottish Rite Hospital instrumentation
Textor vasectomy clamp
T-finger splint
TF needle
TG140 needle
T-grommet ventilation tube
Thackray
    T. dental forceps
    T. mouth gag
Thackston
    T. retropubic bag
    T. retropublic hemostatic bag
thallium-102 stress test
Thal-Mantel obturator
T-handle
    T.-h. reamer
    T.-h. Zimmer chuck
T-handled cup curette
Tharies prosthesis
Thatcher
    T. nail
    T. screw
Theden bandage
Theis
    T. infant rib spreader
    T. retractor
    T. self-retaining retractor
    T. vein retractor
Theobald
    T. lacrimal dilator
    T. probe
    T. sinus probe
TheraBand
therapeutic splint
Thermaderm epilator
thermal
    t. dilution catheter (TDC)
    t. knife
thermistor
    t. catheter
    nostril t.
    t. probe

thermocautery
thermodeltameter (TDM)
thermodilution (TD)
    t. balloon catheter
    t. cardiac output computer
    t. catheter
    t. catheter introducer kit
    t. pacing catheter
    t. Swan-Ganz catheter
thermo-flex suture
Thermograph temperature monitor
thermometer
    ATI forehead t.
    EZ Temp t.
    Farenheit and centigrade flat bath t.
    Instant Fever Tester t.
    Quik-Temp t.
    Stik-Temp t.
    Tel-A-Fever forehead t.
Thermophore bandage
thermopore
    Shahan t.
Thermos pacemaker
Theurig sterilizer forceps
Thiersch
    T. graft
    T. implant
    T. prosthesis
    T. skin graft knife
    T. suture
Thillaye
    T. bandage
    T. dressing
THI needle
Thinlith II pacemaker
thin-walled needle
Thole
    T. goniometer
    T. pelvimeter
Thoma
    T. clamp
    T. tissue retractor
Thomas
    T. brace
    T. bur
    T. cervical collar brace
    T. cryoptor
    T. curette
    T. femoral shunt
    T. forceps
    T. fracture frame
    T. full-ring splint

T. hinged splint
T. irrigating-aspirating cannula
T. keratome
T. knee splint
T. Kodel sling
T. leg splint
T. magnet
T. pelvimeter
T. pessary
T. posterior splint
T. shot compression forceps
T. spatula
T. splint with Pearson attachment
T. suspension splint
T. uterine curette
T. uterine tissue-grasping forceps
T. walking brace
T. wrench

Thommy lid clamp

Thompson
T. adenoid curette
T. bronchial catheter
T. carotid artery clamp
T. carotid clamp
T. carotid vascular clamp
T. catheter
T. cervical transilluminator
T. clamp
T. curette
T. direct full-vision resectoscope
T. drape
T. endoprosthesis
T. evacuator
T. frontal sinus rasp
T. hemiarthroplasty hip prosthesis
T. hip endoprosthesis system
T. hip prosthesis
T. hip prosthesis forceps
T. hyperextention fracture frame
T. modification of Denis Browne splint
T. punch
T. rasp
T. rasp forceps
T. retractor

T. rib shears
T. stem rasp

Thoms
T. forceps
T. pelvimeter
T. tenaculum
T. tissue forceps
T. tissue-grasping forceps

Thoms-Allis
T.-A. forceps
T.-A. intestinal forceps
T.-A. tissue forceps
T.-A. vulsellum

Thomsen rib shears

Thoms-Gaylor
T.-G. biopsy forceps
T.-G. biopsy punch
T.-G. forceps
T.-G. forceps
T.-G. uterine biopsy forceps
T.-G. uterine biopsy punch
T.-G. uterine forceps

Thomson
T. adenoidal punch
T. lung clamp

Thomson-Walker
T.-W. scissors
T.-W. urethrotome

thoracic
t. artery forceps
t. catheter
t. clamp
t. drain
t. forceps
t. hemostatic forceps
Lahey t.
t. scissors
t. suture
t. tissue forceps
t. trocar

thoracolumbar standing orthosis brace (TLSO brace)

thoracoscope
Coryllos t.
Cutler forceps t.
Jacobaeus t.
Jacobaeus-Unverricht t.
Moore t.
Sarot t.

thoracotome
Bettman-Forvash t.

Thora-Klex chest drainage system

Thoratec
- T. biventricular assist device
- T. right ventricular assist device
- T. ventricular assist device

Thorek
- T. aspirator
- T. gallbladder aspirator
- T. gallbladder forceps
- T. gallbladder scissors
- T. scissors
- T. thoracic scissors

Thorek-Feldman gallbladder scissors

Thorek-Mixter
- T.-M. forceps
- T.-M. gallbladder forceps
- T.-M. gall duct forceps

Thorlakson
- T. deep abdominal retractor
- T. lower occlusive clamp
- T. multipurpose retractor
- T. retractor
- T. upper occlusive clamp

Thornton
- T. corneal marker
- T. corneal press-on ruler
- T. episcleral forceps
- T. fixating ring
- T. fixation forceps
- T. incision-spreading forceps
- T. intraocular forceps
- T. iris retractor
- T. low-profile marker
- T. nail
- T. open-wire lid speculum
- T. optical center marker
- T. plate
- T. ruler
- T. speculum
- T. T-incision diamond knife

Thornwald
- T. antral drill
- T. antral irrigator
- T. antral perforator
- T. antral trephine
- T. drill
- T. irrigator

Thorpe
- T. calipers
- T. conjunctival fixation forceps
- T. conjunctival forceps
- T. corneal forceps
- T. corneoscleral forceps
- T. cup-jaw forceps
- T. curette
- T. forceps
- T. foreign body forceps
- T. gonioprism lens
- T. 4-mirror goniolaser
- T. 4-mirror goniolaser lens
- T. 4-mirror goniolens
- T. 4-mirror vitreous fundus laser lens
- T. pupillary membrane scissors
- T. slit lamp
- T. surgical gonioscope
- T. suture-spreading forceps

Thorpe-Castroviejo cataract scissors
Thorpe-Westcott cataract scissors
Thrasher intraocular forceps
thread
- SMIC nylon t.
- t. suture
- Wi-Last-Ic t.

threaded
- t. eye needle
- t. guide pin
- t. pin
- t. rod

threader
- Allen wire t.
- Borchard wire t.
- cannulated wire t.
- Frackelton wire t.
- Hamby wire t.
- t. rod holder pliers
- wire t.

three-armed basket forceps
three-bladed clamp
three-bottle tidal suction tube
three-footed lens intraocular lens
three-hole aspiration cannula
three-legged cage heart valve
three-mirror intraocular lens
three-piece modified J-loop intraocular lens
three-point fixation intraocular lens
three-prong
- t.-p. grasping forceps
- t.-p. retractor
- t.-p. sterilizer forceps

three-way
    t.-w. bridge
    t.-w. catheter
    t.-w. Foley catheter
    t.-w. irrigating catheter
Thriftcast alloy
Throat-E-Vac suction device
throat forceps
thrombectomy catheter
thromboembolic disease (TED)
Thrombogen absorbable hemostat
through-and-through
    t.-a.-t. continuous suture
    t.-a.-t. suture
through-cutting forceps tip
through-the-scope (TTS)
    t.-t.-s. dilator
throw-away manual dermatome
   blade
Thruflex PTCA balloon catheter
Thrust femoral prosthesis
Thudichum nasal speculum
thulium holmium:YAG laser
thumb
    t. forceps
    t. retractor
    t. tissue forceps
thumb-dressing forceps
Thurmond
    T. iris retractor
    T. nucleus-irrigating cannula
    T. retractor
    T. two-way air bubble
      removal cannula
Thurston-Holland fragment forceps
thymus retractor
thyroid
    t. drain
    t. forceps
    t. retractor
    t. traction forceps
Ti-BAC
    T.-B. acetabular cup
    T.-B. II acetabular cup
Tibbs
    T. arterial cannula
    T. semi-automatic suturing
      device
tibial
    t. augmentation block
     (TAB)
    t. bolt
    t. broach

    t. calipers
    t. collet
    t. cutting block
    t. driver
    t. guide pin
    t. pin
    t. plate
    t. plateau prosthesis
    t. retractor
    t. stylus
Tickner
    T. forceps
    T. tissue forceps
Ti/CoCr hip prosthesis
Ticonium splint
Ti-Cron suture (*See also* Tycron
   suture)
Ticsay transpubic needle
Tieck-Halle
    T.-H. infant nasal speculum
    T.-H. nasal speculum
Tieck nasal speculum
Tiemann
    T. bullet forceps
    T. catheter
    T. coudé catheter
    T. Foley catheter
    T. nail
    T. Neoflex catheter
tie-over
    t.-o. bolster
    t.-o. dressing
tier
    Adson knot t.
    knot t.
tie suture
Ti-Fit total hip system
tiger gut suture
tightener
    Harris wire t.
    Loute wire t.
    Shiffrin bone wire t.
    Verner-Joseph wire t.
    wire t.
Tiko rake retractor
Tiley dressing forceps
Tillary
    T. double-ended retractor
    T. retractor
Tilley-Henckel forceps
Tilley-Lichwitz trocar
tilting disk heart valve
tilt table

Timberlake
   T. catheter
   T. electrode
   T. evacuator
   T. irrigating tip
   T. obturator
   T. obturator electrotome
   T. obturator resectoscope
timer
   Medela Apgar t.
TiMesh
tin-bullet probe
T-incision marker
Tindall scissors
tined lead pacemaker
Tinel
   T. suture
   T. tapered reamer
Ti-Nidium surface hardening process
Tinnant gauge
Tiny-Tef ventilation tube
Tiny Tytan ventilation tube
tip
   ACMI cystoscopic t.
   Acufex femoral guide t.
   Air-Shield-Vickers syringe t.
   Bard t.
   Berkeley Medevices, Inc. syringe t.
   Boies cutting forceps t.
   Bruening biting t.
   Cloward cervical drill t.
   conical t.
   conical inserter t.
   Cordes punch forceps t.
   Cordes square punch t.
   coronary perfusion t.
   cutting forceps t.
   t. deflecting
   double-articulated forceps t.
   double-articulated grasping forceps t.
   esophageal dilating flexible metal spiral t.
   Fell sucker t.
   femoral guide t.
   Flateau oval t.
   Frazier suction t.
   grasping forceps t.
   t. guard
   Henke punch forceps t.
   irrigating t.

Jackson square punch t.
Kahler double-action t.
Kahn uterine trigger cannula extension t.
Killian cutting forceps t.
Killian double-articulated forceps t.
Krause oval punch t.
Krause punch forceps t.
Krause square-basket t.
Krause through-cutting forceps t.
Kurze micro-instrument with scissors t.
Leasure round punch t.
Mayo coronary perfusion t.
Myerson biting t.
Patterson double-action biting t.
Patterson oval biting t.
plastic cone t.
punch forceps t.
pyramidal t.
Radovan tissue expander t.
rubber acorn t.
Scheinmann biting t.
Schuknecht suction t.
screw t.
Seiffert double-articulated grasping forceps t.
Seiffert grasping t.
serrated grasping t.
Spencer oval t.
Spencer triangular t.
Spencer Universal adenoid punch t.
Struyken angular punch t.
sucker t.
suction t.
through-cutting forceps t.
Timberlake irrigating t.
Universal t.
Universal adenoid punch t.
uterine trigger cannula extension t.
venous cannula t.
vessel t.
V. Mueller cystoscopy t.
Welsh flat-olive t.
tip-deflecting
   t.-d. catheter
   t.-d. wire
Tip-Trol handle

tire eye implant
tire-grooved silicone
Tischer biopsy forceps
Tischler
    T. cervical biopsy forceps
    T. cervical biopsy punch
    T. cervical biopsy punch
      forceps
    T. cervical forceps
    T. forceps
Tischler-Morgan biopsy forceps
tissue
    Adson-Callison t. forceps
    t. anchor guide (TAG)
    t. anchor guide system
    t. band
    t. bed
    Callison-Adson t.
    t. desiccation needle
    t. dessication needle
      electrode
    t. dissector
    t. drain
    t. forceps
    t. graft press
    t. lifter
    t. mandrel implant material
    t. occlusion clamp
    t. press
    t. protector
    t. retractor
tissue-dressing forceps
tissue-grasping forceps
tissue-holding forceps
tissue-protective, end-cutting (TPE)
Titan
    T. hip cup
    T. scaler
titanium
    t. ball heart valve
    t. bipolar forceps
    t. cage heart valve
    t. implant material
    t. mesh
    t. needle
    t. prosthesis
    t. retinal tack
    t. screw
Titmus vision test
Titus
    T. forearm splint
    T. needle

    T. tongue depressor
    T. venoclysis needle
    T. wrist splint
Tivanium
    T. hip prosthesis
    T. Ti-6A1-4V alloy
Tivnen
    T. forceps
    T. tonsillar forceps
    T. tonsil-seizing forceps
TJF endoscope
TLC Baxter balloon catheter
TLS
    TLS drain
    TLS suction drain
    TLS surgical marker
TLSO brace
    thoracolumbar standing orthosis
    brace
T-malleable retractor
TMJ
    temporomandibular joint
    TMJ acrylic
    TMJ head positioner
T-model endaural retractor
TNS
    transcutaneous nerve stimulator
Toad finger splint
Tobald syringe
Tobey
    T. ear forceps
    T. ear rongeur
    T. forceps
Tobold
    T. apparatus
    T. forceps
    T. laryngeal forceps
    T. laryngeal knife
    T. laryngoscopic apparatus
    T. tongue depressor
Tobold-Fauvel grasping forceps
Tobolsky elevator
Tobruk splint
Tocantins bone marrow needle
tocotonometer
Todd
    T. bur hole button
    T. button
    T. eye cautery needle
    T. foreign body gouge
    T. needle
    T. stereotaxic guide

Todd-Wells
T.-W. human stereotaxic instrument
T.-W. stereotaxic apparatus
Todt-Heyer cannula guide
toedrop brace
Toennis
T. director
T. dissecting scissors
T. dissector
T. dural hook
T. dural knife
T. needle holder
T. retractor
T. tumor-grasping forceps
Toennis-Adson
T.-A. dural scissors
T.-A. forceps
T.-A. scissors
Toennis-Adson dissector
toe prosthesis
Tofflemire
T. matrix band
T. retainer
Tokodynamometer
Tolantins bone marrow infusion catheter
Tolentino
T. cutter
T. vitrectomy lens
T. vitreoretinal cutter
Tolman
T. micrometer
T. tonometer
Tomac
T. catheter
T. clip
T. foam rubber traction dressing
T. forceps
T. goniometer
T. knitted rubber elastic dressing
T. Nélaton catheter
T. vest-style holder
Tomasini brace
Tomasino cryostylet
Tomas iris hook
Tomenius gastroscope
Tomey trabeculectomy punch
Tom Jones suture

Tommy
T. bar
T. hip bar
Tomomatic brain scanner
Tompkins aspirator
tongs
adjustable skull traction t.
Barton-Cone t.
Barton skull traction t.
Böhler t.
Cherry traction t.
Crutchfield t.
Crutchfield adjustable skull traction t.
Crutchfield-Raney skull traction t.
Crutchfield skull t.
Crutchfield skull traction t.
Crutchfield traction t.
Gardner-Wells skull t.
Gardner-Wells traction t.
Hinz t.
Raney-Crutchfield skull t.
Reynolds skull traction t.
skull traction t.
traction t.
University of Virginia skull t.
Vinke t.
tongue
t. blade
t. depressor
t. forceps
t. plate
t. plate electrode
t. retractor blade
t. suture
tongue-and-groove suture
tongue-holding forceps
tongue-in-groove suture
tongue-seizing forceps
tonograph
tonographer
Storz t.
Tonomat applanation tonometer
tonometer
Allen-Schiotz plunger retractor t.
applamatic t.
applanation t.
Bailliart t.
Barraquer t.
CT-10 computerized t.

Gartner t.
Goldmann applanation t.
Jena-Schiotz t.
Keeler Pulsair noncontact t.
Mack t.
Mackay-Marg t.
Maklakoff t.
McLean t.
Meding tonsil enucleator t.
Mueller electronic t.
Musken t.
Non-Contact t. (NCT)
Non-Contact II t.
Nuvistor electronic t.
Pach-Pen t.
Perkins t.
pneumatic t.
Recklinghausen t.
Reichert t.
Roush t.
Sauer t.
Sauer-Storz t.
Schiøtz t.
Sklar t.
Sklar-Schitz jewel t.
Sluder t.
Sluder-Demarest t.
Storz t.
Storz-Schitz t.
Tolman t.
Tonomat applanation t.
Tonotips
tonsil
tonsil-holding forceps
tonsillar
    t. abscess forceps
    t. artery forceps
    t. calipers
    t. clamp
    t. compressor
    t. curette
    t. dissector
    t. electrode
    t. expressor
    t. forceps
    t. guillotine
    t. hemostatic forceps
    t. hook
    t. knife
    t. loop
    t. needle
    t. needle holder forceps
    t. pillar grasping forceps

    t. pillar retractor
    t. punch
    t. punch forceps
    t. retractor
    t. scissors
    t. screw
    t. snare
    t. snare wire
    t. sponge
    t. suction tube
    t. suture
    t. suture needle
    t. syringe
tonsillar
tonsillectome
    Ballenger-Sluder t.
    Beck-Mueller t.
    Beck-Schenck t.
    Brown t.
    Daniels hemostatic t.
    hemostatic t.
    LaForce hemostatic t.
    t. loop
    Mack lingual tonsillar t.
    Meding tonsil enucleator t.
    Moltz-Storz t.
    Myles guillotine t.
    Sauer t.
    Sauer hemostatic t.
    Sauer-Sluder t.
    Sauer-Storz t.
    Searcy t.
    Seiffert t.
    Sluder-Ballenger t.
    Sluder-Demarest t.
    Sluder-Sauer t.
    Sluder tonsillar t.
    Storz-Moltz t.
    tonsillectome t.
    Tydings t.
    Van Osdel tonsil
      enucleator t.
    Whiting t.
tonsil-ligating forceps
tonsillotome
    Sluder-Ballenger t.
tonsil-seizing forceps
tonsil-suction dissector
tonsil-suturing
    t.-s. forceps
    t.-s. hook
Tooke
    T. angled knife

Tooke *(continued)*
    T. angled splitter
    T. blade
    T. corneal forceps
    T. corneal knife
    T. cornea-splitting knife
    T. iris knife
    T. knife
tool
    Lillie-Koffler t.
Toomey
    T. bladder evacuator
    T. forceps
    T. syringe
tooth
    t. band
    t. guard
toothbrush
    Water Pik t.
toothed
    t. forceps
    t. retractor
    t. tenaculum
    t. thumb forceps
    t. tissue forceps
tooth-extracting forceps
toothless forceps
Topax gel
Topcon
    T. camera
    T. microscope
    T. SL-45 camera
    T. slit lamp
toposcopic catheter
Topper
    T. cannula
    T. dressing sponge
    T. sponge
Torchia
    T. aspirating cannula
    T. calipers
    T. cannula
    T. capsular forceps
    T. capsular polisher
    T. conjunctival scissors
    T. corneal knife
    T. eye speculum
    T. lens hook
    T. lens implantation forceps
    T. microbipolar forceps
    T. microcorneal scissors
    T. nucleus cannula
    T. tissue forceps

    T. tying forceps
    T. vectis loop
Torchia-Colibri forceps
Torchia-Kuglen hook
Torchia-Vannas micro-iris scissors
Torcon
    T. angiographic catheter
    T. catheter
toric
    crimped t.
    Durasoft t.
    t. lens
    2-optifit t.
Torkildsen shunt
Torktherm torque control catheter
Toronto splint
TORP
    total ossicular replacement
    prosthesis
        TORP ossicular prosthesis
        Proplast TORP
        TORP strut
Torpedo eye patch
Torpin
    T. automatic uterine gauze
    packer
    T. obstetrical lever
    T. vectis
    T. vectis blade
    T. vectis extractor
torque
    t. eliminator
    t. wrench
torque-control balloon catheter
torque-type prosthesis
Torre cryojet
Torres
    T. cross-action forceps
    T. needle holder
Torrington French spring needle
torsion
    t. bar splint
    t. forceps
Toshiba
    T. brain scanner
    T. video endoscope
total
    t. articular replacement
    arthroplasty (TARA)
    t. ossicular replacement
    t. ossicular replacement
    prosthesis (TORP)

t. parenteral nutrition
(TPN)
t. toe template
t. top implant

Totco

T. Autoclip
T. clip

Toti trephine
Tott ring remover
Touchless catheter
Touchup acrylic coating liquid
Touma

T. dissector
T. T-type grommet
ventilation tube

tourniquet

Adams modification of
Bethune t.
automatic t.
Bethune lung t.
Campbell-Boyd t.
Carr lobectomy t.
Conn pneumatic t.
Conn Universal t.
t. cuff
Disposiquet disposable t.
Dupuytren t.
Esmarch t.
Field t.
Fouli t.
Grafco t.
Holcombe gastric t.
horseshoe t.
Ideal t.
Johnson & Johnson t.
Kidde t.
Kidde-Robbins t.
Linton t.
Momberg t.
nonpneumatic t.
Pac-Kit Army-type t.
Petit t.
pneumatic t.
Quicket t.
ratchet t.
Robbins automatic t.
Roberts-Nelson lobectomy t.
Roper-Rumel t.
Rumel t.
Rumel-Belmont t.
Rumel cardiovascular t.
Rumel ratchet t.
Samway t.

Sebra arm t.
Signorini t.
SMIC auricular t.
t. strap
Surgikit Velcro t.
Tourniquick t.
Trussdale t.
Universal t.
U.S. Army t.
Velcro t.
Velket Velcro t.
Weiner t.
Wright pneumatic t.

tourniquet-eyed

t.-e. obturator
t.-e. ratchet stylet

Tourniquick tourniquet
towel

t. clamp
t. clip
t. clip forceps
t. drape
t. forceps

Tower

Concept Traction T.
T. forceps
T. interchangeable retractor
T. muscle forceps
T. retractor
T. rib retractor
T. spinal retractor

Townley

T. bone graft screw
T. calipers
T. femur calipers
T. forceps
T. implant
T. inside-outside femur
calipers
T. tissue forceps
T. total knee prosthesis

Townsend biopsy punch
Townsend-Gilfillan

T.-G. plate
T.-G. screw

toxemia curette
Toynbee

T. curette
T. diagnostic tube
T. ear speculum
T. otoscope
T. speculum

TPE
    tissue-protective, end-cutting
T-pin handle
TPL-6 hip system
TPN
    total parenteral nutrition
        TPN catheter
trabeculotome
    Allen-Burian t.
    Harms t.
    McPherson t.
trabeculotomy probe
Trace hydraulic vein stripper
Tracer wire guide
tracheal
    t. bistoury
    t. cannula
    t. catheter
    t. dilator
    t. forceps
    t. hemostatic forceps
    t. hook
    t. retractor
    t. scalpel
    t. tenaculum
    t. tube
    t. tube brush
    t. tube cuff
trachelotome
    Spencer t.
tracheobronchoesophagoscope
    Haslinger t.
tracheoscope
    Fearon t.
    Haslinger t.
    Jackson t.
    Tucker t.
tracheostomy
    t. button
    t. cannula
    t. hook
    t. tube
tracheotome
    Salvatore-Maloney t.
    Sierra-Sheldon t.
tracheotomic bistoury
tracheotomy
    t. cannula
    t. hook
    t. sponge
trachoma forceps
Tracker knee brace
track suture

Tracoe tracheostomy tube
traction
    t. apparatus
    t. bar
    t. belt
    t. bow (*See* bow)
    Buck t.
    t. device
    t. forceps
    t. handle
    leg and ankle t.
    t. legging
    lumbosacral support
        pelvic t.
    t. suture
    t. tenaculum
    t. tongs
    t. tongs screw
    transfer t.
Tracto-Halter
tractor
    Anderson t.
    axial t.
    banjo t.
    Barton-Cone traction t.
    Blackburn skull traction t.
    Böhler t.
    Bryant t.
    Buck extension t.
    Cherry traction t.
    Dunlop t.
    Exo-bed t.
    Exo-static overhead t.
    Fisk t.
    Freiberg traction t.
    halo t.
    Hamilton pelvic traction
        screw t.
    Handy-Buck extension t.
    Hoke-Martin t.
    Kestler ambulatory head t.
    Kirschner wire t.
    Lowsley prostatic t.
    Lyman-Smith t.
    Muirhead-Little pelvic
        rest t.
    Naugh os calcis
        apparatus t.
    Neufeld t.
    Orr-Buck extension t.
    Perkins split-weight t.
    prostatic t.
    Pugh t.

Rankin prostatic t.
Russell-Beck extension t.
Steinmann traction t.
Syms t.
Trimline mobile t.
Vinke skull t.
Watson-Jones t.
Wells t.
Young prostatic t.
Zim-Trac traction splint t.
tragus House hook
trainer
auditory t.
transairway laryngeal control (TALC)
transcatheter
t. umbrella implant material
transcricothyroid selective bronchography set
transcutaneous
t. electrical nerve stimulator (TENS)
t. nerve stimulator (TNS)
t. pacemaker
transducer
Array ultrasound t.
Mikro-tip t.
Millar t.
Millar Mikro-Tip catheter pressure t.
transducer-tipped catheter
Transelast surgical drape
transesophageal probe
transfer
t. forceps
t. traction
transfixing suture
transfixion
t. bolt
t. screw
t. suture
transhepatic biliary stent
transilluminating telescope
transilluminator
all-purpose t.
Briggs t.
Coldite t.
Finnoff t.
Finnoff sinus t.
Hildreth t.
hooded t.
Jako t.
Lancaster ocular t.

National all-metric t.
National opal-glass t.
O'Malley-Skia t.
rotating t.
speculum illuminator t.
Tatum ureteral t.
Thompson cervical t.
Welch Allyn t.
Widner t.
transition suture
transluminal
t. angioplasty catheter
t. balloon
t. extraction catheter
t. extraction-endarterectomy catheter (TEC)
transmyocardial pacing stylet
transnasal drain
transoral retractor
transosteal pin implant
transpapillary drain
transparent
t. drape
t. dressing
transpericardial pacemaker
transphenoidal forceps
transplant-grafting forceps
transplant trephine
Transpore surgical tape dressing
transpubic needle
transseptal
t. cannula
t. catheter
transsphenoidal
t. bipolar forceps
t. curette
t. enucleator
t. forceps
t. speculum
transthoracic
t. catheter
t. pacemaker
t. pacing stylet
transurethral
t. resection (TUR)
t. resection of prostate (TURP)
transvenous
t. electrode
t. pacemaker
t. pacemaker catheter
t. ventricular demand pacemaker

transventricular dilator
transverse suture
trap
    Concept digit t.
    Rusch mucous t.
trapeze bar
trapeziometacarpal joint
  replacement prosthesis
trapezium implant
Traquair
    T. elevator
    T. periosteal elevator
Trattner
    T. catheter
    T. urethrographic catheter
Traube neurological hammer
traumatic suture
Travenol
    T. bag
    T. biopsy needle
    T. heart bag
    T. infusor device
    T. needle
Travert needle
tray
    Alcon Instrument Delivery
      System t. (AIDS tray)
    Budde halo patty t.
    cannula holder t.
    CAPIS screw assortment t.
    CAPIS sterilizing t.
    Codman-Shurtleff surgical
      instrument t.
    curette sterilizing t.
    Curity irrigation t.
    eye instrument rack t.
    flash t.
    glenoid metal t.
    t. handle
    Henry t.
    Henry instrument t.
    HSG t.
    t. insert
    instrument t.
    t. instrument
    I-tech cannula t.
    Kormed peritoneal lavage t.
    large t.
    Mayo t.
    Mayo instrument t.
    micro-instrument t.
    Monoject laceration
      irrigation t.

    Papanicolaou smear t.
    percutaneous aspiration
      biopsy t.
    perforated Mayo t.
    Russell gastrostomy t.
    safety handles t.
    small t.
    sterilizing instrument t.
    urological system instrument
      soaking/storage t.
    Weck microsurgical t.
Treace
    T. drill
    T. stapes drill
Trefoil balloon for percutaneous
  valvuloplasty
Trelat
    T. palate raspatory
    T. vaginal speculum
Tremble sphenoid cannula
Trendelenburg cannula
Trendelenburg-Crafoord
    T.-C. clamp
    T.-C. coarctation clamp
Trent
    T. eye retractor
    T. pick
trephine
    Arruga t.
    Arruga eye t.
    Arruga lacrimal t.
    Barraquer corneal t.
    Becker skull t.
    Blackburn t.
    t. blade
    Blakesley lacrimal t.
    Boiler septal t.
    Brown-Pusey corneal t.
    Cam guided t.
    Cardona corneal t.
    Castroviejo t.
    Castroviejo corneal t.
    Castroviejo improved t.
    Castroviejo transplant t.
    corneal t.
    Cross scleral t.
    Damshek sternal t.
    DeMartel t.
    D'Errico t.
    D'Errico skull t.
    DeVilbiss skull t.
    Dimitry chalazion t.

Dimitry
   dacryocystorhinostomy t.
disposable t.
t. drill
Elliot t.
Elliot corneal t.
Franceschetti corneal t.
Galt t.
Galt skull t.
Gradle corneal t.
Green automatic corneal t.
Greenwood spinal t.
Grieshaber t.
Grieshaber corneal t.
GTS t.
Guyton corneal t.
hand t.
Hanna t.
Harris t.
Hessburg t.
Hessburg-Barron t.
Hessburg vacuum t.
Hippel t.
Horsley t.
Iliff t.
Iliff lacrimal t.
Jentzer t.
Keyes cutaneous t.
King corneal t.
Lahey Clinic skull t.
Leksell t.
Lichtenberg corneal t.
Lorie antral t.
t. marker
Martinez corneal t.
Martinez disposable t.
Michele t.
Mueller electric corneal t.
Paton t.
Paton corneal t.
Paton see-through t.
pattern t.
Paufique corneal t.
Polley-Bickel t.
Robertson corneal t.
Schuknecht temporal t.
Scoville skull t.
Searcy chalazion t.
Sidney Stephenson
   corneal t.
sinus t.
Sisler lacrimal t.
skull t.

Stille t.
Storz chalazion t.
Storz hair transplant t.
Thornwald antral t.
Toti t.
transplant t.
Turkel t.
Von Hippel mechanical t.
Walker corneal t.
Wilder t.
Wilkins t.
Triad prosthesis
trial
   t. acetabular cup
   t. component
   t. cup
   t. driver
   t. fracture frame
   t. implant
   t. prosthesis
   radius t.
   ulnar t.
triangle Secto dissector
triangular
   t. arm sling
   t. bandage
   t. dressing
   t. encompassing clip
   t. punch forceps
Trichodemolus epilator
tricuspid valve strut
trifacet knife
tri-fin chisel
trigeminal
   t. knife
   t. retractor
   t. scissors
   t. self-retaining retractor
trigeminus cannula
trigger cannula
trileaflet prosthesis
Trilicon external breast prosthesis
Triloc acetabular cup
Tri-lock total hip prosthesis with
   Porocoat
Trimble suture stent
Trimline mobile tractor
trimmer
   calcar t.
   Mallory-Head Interlok
     calcar t.
   Nordent margin t.

Trinkle
- T. bone drill
- T. brace
- T. chuck
- T. power drill
- T. screwdriver
- T. socket wrench
- T. Super-Cut twist drill

Trios M pacemaker
Trio-Temp X biofil
triple
- t. hook
- t. thermistor coronary sinus catheter

triple-edge diamond-blade knife
triple-lumen
- t.-l. biliary manometry catheter
- t.-l. catheter
- t.-l. central catheter
- t.-l. manometric catheter
- t.-l. needle
- t.-l. sump drain

triple-syringe
- NTS-4 t.-s.

tripod
- t. intraocular lens

tri-point
- t.-p. bullet
- t.-p. K-Wire sleeve

tripolar
- t. catheter
- t. W/Damato curve catheter

tri-pronged loop
Tri-Wedge total hip system
trocar, trochar
- abdominal t.
- Abelson cricothyrotomy t.
- Allen cecostomy t.
- American Heyer-Schulte-Robertson suprapubic t.
- antral t.
- Arbuckle-Shea t.
- Argyle t.
- Babcock empyema t.
- Barnes internal decompression t.
- Barnes intestinal decompression t.
- Beardsley cecostomy t.
- Birch t.
- blunt t.
- Boettcher antral t.

- Boettcher-Schmidt antral t.
- Buelan empyema t.
- Bülau t.
- Campbell suprapubic t.
- Castens ascites t.
- Castens hydrocele t.
- Charlton antral t.
- Coakley antral t.
- Cross needle t.
- Curschmann t.
- Davidson t.
- Dean antral t.
- Denker t.
- Diederich empyema t.
- Douglas antral t.
- Douglas nasal t.
- Dr. White t.
- Duchenne's t.
- Duke t.
- Durham tracheotomy t.
- Emmet t.
- Emmet ovarian t.
- Endopath disposable surgical t.
- Faulkner t.
- Fein antral t.
- Fleurant bladder t.
- Frazier brain-exploring t.
- Gallagher t.
- Haeggstrom antral t.
- Hargin antral t.
- Havlicek t.
- Hunt angiographic t.
- Hurwitz t.
- Hurwitz thoracic t.
- Ingram t.
- intercostal t.
- intestinal decompression t.
- Jako laser t.
- Johanson-Stille cystotomy t.
- Judd t.
- Kidd t.
- Kido suprapubic t.
- Kolb t.
- Krause antral t.
- Kreutzmann t.
- Landau t.
- laryngeal t.
- Lichtwicz abdominal t.
- Lichtwicz antral t.
- Lillie antral t.
- Livermore t.
- Mayo-Ochsner t.

Morson t.
Myerson antral t.
Nagashima antroscope t.
Neal catheter t.
t. needle
Nelson t.
Nelson empyema t.
Nelson-Patterson
 empyema t.
Nelson thoracic t.
nested t.
Ochsner t.
Ochsner gallbladder t.
Ochsner thoracic t.
Patterson t.
Patterson empyema t.
Patterson-Nelson
 empyema t.
Peterson t.
Pierce antral t.
Pierce-Kyle t.
plain vesical t.
t. point Kirschner wire
Pool t.
Potain aspirating t.
rectal t.
Rica Universal t.
Roberts abdominal t.
Ruskin antral t.
Schwartz t.
t. set
Sewall antral t.
sharp t.
Singleton empyema t.
sinoscopy t.
Snyder Urevac t.
Southey anasarca t.
Southey-Leech t.
Stiwer t.
subcostal t.
suprapubic t.
Surgiport disposable t.
Sweet antral t.
thoracic t.
Tilley-Lichwitz t.
Ueckermann-Denker t.
Uni-Shunt split t.
Universal abdominal t.
Van Alyea antral t.
Veirs t.
Viers t.
Walther aspirating
 bladder t.

Wangensteen internal
 decompression t.
Wiener-Pierce antral t.
Wilson amniotic t.
Wilson-Baylor amniotic t.
Wolf-Cottle t.
Wolf needle t.
Wright-Harloe empyema t.
Yankauer antral t.
Trocath peritoneal dialysis catheter
trochanter-holding clamp
trochanteric
 t. awl
 t. pin
 t. plate
 t. router
trochar (*var. of* trocar)
Troeltsch, Tröltsch
 T. ear-dressing forceps
 T. ear forceps
 T. ear speculum
 T. eustachian catheter
 T. forceps
 T. nasal-dressing forceps
Tromner percussion hammer
Troncoso
 T. implant
 T. tubular lens
Tronzo elevator
Trotter forceps
Trough gouge
Trousseau
 T. dilating forceps
 T. dilator
 T. esophageal bougie
 T. forceps
 T. mouth gag
 T. tracheal dilator
Trousseau-Jackson
 T.-J. dilator
 T.-J. esophageal dilator
 T.-J. tracheal dilator
Troutman
 T. alpha-chymotrypsin
 cannula
 T. blade
 T. bladebreaker
 T. cannula
 T. cataract extractor
 T. chisel
 T. conjunctival scissors
 T. corneal dissector
 T. corneal forceps

Troutman *(continued)*
- T. corneal knife
- T. corneal scissors
- T. corneal splitter
- T. eye dissector
- T. eye implant
- T. forceps
- T. implant
- T. lens loop
- T. lens loupe
- T. lens spatula
- T. magnetic implant
- T. mastoid chisel
- T. microsurgery forceps
- T. needle
- T. needle holder
- T. punch
- T. rectal forceps
- T. superior rectus forceps
- T. wave edge corneal dissector

Troutman-Barraquer
- T.-B. Colibri forceps
- T.-B. corneal forceps
- T.-B. corneal utility forceps
- T.-B. forceps
- T.-B. iris forceps
- T.-B. iris spatula
- T.-B. minibladebreaker
- T.-B. needle holder

Troutman-Castroviejo
- T.-C. corneal section scissors
- T.-C. scissors

Troutman-Katzin
- T.-K. corneal transplant scissors
- T.-K. scissors

Troutman-Llobera
- T.-L. fixation forceps
- T.-L. Flieringa forceps
- T.-L. forceps

Troutman-Tooke corneal knife
Trowbirdge-Campau bone drill
Trowbridge-Campau eye magnet
Trowbridge triple-speed drill
Tru-Arc blood vessel ring
Tru-Arch preformed archwire
Tru-Chrome band material
Tru-clip
Tru-Cut
- T.-C. biopsy needle
- T.-C. biopsy needle holder

- T.-C. liver biopsy needle
- T.-C. needle

true suture
Truflex
Trulife silicone breast form
Trumbull suture
trummion bearing hip prosthesis
trumpet
- Iowa t.
- t. needle guide

truncus clamp
Trupp ventricular needle
Trush grasping forceps
Trusler
- T. clamp
- T. infant vascular clamp

Trusler-Dean scissors
truss
- Hood t.
- inguinal t.
- Kansas City band t.
- Nu-Form t.
- scrotal t.

Trussdale tourniquet
Tru-Stain acrylic powder
Truszkowski dural dissector
Truvision Omni lens
Trylon hemostatic forceps
T-shaped
- T.-s. angled forceps
- T.-s. forceps

"T" spatula
TSRH
- Texas Scottish Rite Hospital
- TSRH instrumentation
- TSRH plate

T-stack
- Hagie T.-s.

TTS
- through-the-scope
- TTS dilator

T-tube
- bar T.-t.
- T.-t. catheter
- Deaver T.-t.
- T.-t. drain
- T.-t. drain for hysterectomy procedures
- Goode T.-t.
- Kehr T.-t.
- Kelly inflatable T.-t.
- Montgomery tracheal T.-t.
- T.-t. round suction tube

silicone T.-t.
T.-t. stent
T-type
   T.-t. dental implant
   T.-t. matrix band
tubal
   t. hook
   t. insufflation cannula
   t. scissors
Tubbs
   T. aortic dilator
   T. dilator
   T. mitral valve dilator
   T. two-bladed dilator
   T. valvulotome
Tubby tenotomy knife
tube
   Abbott t.
   Abbott-Rawson t.
   abdominal suction t.
   Adson aspirating t.
   Adson brain suction t.
   Adson neurosurgical
     suction t.
   Adson suction t.
   AF t.
   Air-Lon laryngectomy t.
   Air-Lon tracheal t.
   Alesen t.
   American circle
     nephrostomy t.
   American Heyer-Schulte
     suction t.
   American Heyer-Schulte T-t.
   Andersen mercury-
     weighted t.
   Anderson flexible suction t.
   Andrews-Pynchon
     aspirating t.
   Andrews-Pynchon suction t.
   Anthony aspirating t.
   Anthony mastoid suction t.
   Anthony suction t.
   antifog t.
   antral wash t.
   aortic sump t.
   Argyle-Dennis t.
   Argyle endotracheal t.
   Armstrong grommet
     ventilation t.
   Armstrong ventilation t.
   Armstrong V-Vent t.
   Arrow t.

Asepto suction t.
aspirating t.
Atkins-Cannard
   tracheotomy t.
Ayre t.
Baker jejunostomy t.
Baldwin butterfly
   ventilation t.
Bardic t.
Barnes suction t.
Baron ear t.
Baron ear suction t.
Baron-Frazier suction t.
Baron suction t.
Baylor intracardiac sump t.
Baylor sump t.
Beall-Feldman-Cooley
   sump t.
Beardsley empyema t.
Bellocq t.
Bellucci t.
Bellucci suction t.
Bel-O-Pak suction t.
Bettman empyema t.
Billroth t.
Biolite ventilation t.
Bivona tracheostomy t.
Blakemore esophageal t.
Blakemore nasogastric t.
Blakemore-Sengstaken t.
Bonney uterine t.
Bouchut laryngeal t.
Brawley nasal suction t.
bronchial t.
bronchoscopy disposable
   suction t.
Broyles esophagoscope t.
Bruecke t.
Bucy-Frazier suction t.
Bucy suction t.
Buie t.
Buie rectal suction t.
Buie suction t.
Butler tonsillar suction t.
Buyes air-vent suction t.
calibrated grasping t.
Cantor t.
Cantor intestinal t.
Carabelli endobronchial t.
Carlens t.
Carl Zeiss myringotomy t.
Carman rectal t.
Carrel t.

tube *(continued)*
  t. carrier
  Casselberry sphenoid t.
  Castelli-Paparella colar
    button t.
  Cattell forked-type T- t.
  Cattell gallbladder t.
  Celestin t.
  Celestin endoesophageal t.
  Chaffin-Pratt bedside
    suction t.
  Charnley drain t.
  Chauffen-Pratt t.
  Chaussier t.
  Clerf laryngectomy t.
  closed suction t.
  closed water-seal suction t.
  coagulation-aspirator t.
  coagulation suction t.
  Coakley wash t.
  collar button t.
  Colton empyema t.
  Cone-Bucy suction t.
  Cone suction t.
  continuous suction t.
  Cook County tracheal
    suction t.
  Cooley-Anthony suction t.
  Cooley aortic sump t.
  Cooley graft suction t.
  Cooley intracardiac
    suction t.
  Cooley suction t.
  Cooley sump suction t.
  Cooley vascular suction t.
  Coolidge t.
  Costen suction t.
  Cottle suction t.
  Coupland nasal suction t.
  Crawford t.
  cricothyrotomy trocar t.
  cuffed t.
  CUI myringotomy t.
  curved t.
  Dandy suction t.
  David
    pharyngolaryngectomy t.
  Davol t.
  Dawson-Yuhl suction t.
  Dean wash t.
  Deaver t.
  DeBakey-Adson suction t.
  DeBakey suction t.

Debove t.
Denker t.
DePaul t.
Devers gall bladder t.
DeVilbiss suction t.
Devine-Millard-Frazier
  fiberoptic suction t.
diagnostic t.
disposable Yankauer
  aspirating t.
disposable Yankauer
  suction t.
Donaldson eustachian t.
Donaldson ventilation t.
drain-to-wall suction t.
Dr. Bruecke aspirating t.
t. dressing
Dr. Twiss duodenal t.
Duke t.
Dundas-Grant t.
Duralite t.
Durham tracheostomy t.
Eastman suction t.
E. Benson Hood
  Laboratories esophageal t.
E. Benson Hood
  Laboratories salivary
  bypass t.
Einhorn t.
endoesophageal t.
endotracheal t.
Ethox rectal t.
Ewald t.
extension t.
Fay suction elevator
  suction t.
Ferguson-Frazier suction t.
Feuerstein drainage t.
Feuerstein split
  ventilation t.
fiberoptic suction t.
Finsterer myringotomy
  split t.
Finsterer suction t.
Fitzpatrick suction t.
flanged Teflon t.
Flexiflo t.
Flexiflo enteral feeding t.
Flexiflo gastrostomy t.
Flexiflo Sachs-Veni t.
Flexiflo Stomate
  gastrostomy t.
Flexiflo suction feeding t.

Flexiflo tap-fill enteral t.
Flexiflo Taptainer t.
t. forceps
Franco triflange
ventilation t.
Fraser suction t.
Frazier aspirating t.
Frazier brain suction t.
Frazier Britetrac nasal
suction t.
Frazier disposable suction t.
Frazier-Ferguson
aspirating t.
Frazier-Ferguson ear
suction t.
Frazier-Ferguson suction t.
Frazier fiberoptic suction t.
Frazier modified suction t.
Frazier nasal suction t.
Frazier obturator aspirating
suction t.
Frazier-Paparella mastoid t.
Frazier-Paparella mastoid
suction t.
Frazier-Paparella suction t.
Frazier suction t.
frontal sinus wash t.
Gavriliu gastric t.
GBH bypass t.
Gillquist-Stille arthroplasty
suction t.
Gillquist suction t.
Glover suction t.
Gomco suction t.
Goode t.
Goodhill-Pynchon tonsillar
suction t.
Gott t.
Grafco Martin
laryngectomy t.
t. graft
graft suction t.
Great Ormand Street
tracheostomy t.
Great Ormond Street
pediatric tracheostomy t.
Greiling gastroduodenal t.
Guibor t.
Guilford-Wright suction t.
Gwathmey suction t.
Haering t.
Hagan surface suction t.
Hardy suction t.

Heimlich-Gavrilu gastric t.
Helsper tracheostomy
vent t.
Hemovac t.
Hemovac suction t.
heparin-bonded t.
heparin-bonded Bott-type t.
Hi-Lo Jet tracheal t.
Holinger open-end
aspirating t.
Hossli suction t.
Hotchkiss ear suction t.
Hough-Cadogan suction t.
House-Baron t.
House-Baron suction t.
House endolymphatic
shunt t.
Houser t.
House-Radpour suction t.
Houser silicone T-tube t.
House-Stevenson suction t.
House suction t.
House-Urban t.
Hubbard airplane vent t.
Hugly aspirating t.
Humphrey coronary sinus-
sucker suction t.
Immergut suction t.
Immergut suction-
coagulation t.
infusion t.
intracardiac suction t.
intracardiac sump t.
Israel suction suction t.
Jackson aspirating t.
Jackson cone-shaped
tracheal t.
Jackson laryngectomy t.
Jackson open-end
aspirating t.
Jackson-Pratt suction t.
Jackson-Rees endotracheal t.
Jackson silver
tracheostomy t.
Jackson tracheal t.
Jackson velvet-eye t.
Jackson velvet-eye
aspirating t.
Jackson warning stop t.
Jacques gastric t.
Jako laryngeal suction t.
Jako laser aspirating t.
Jako suction t.

tube *(continued)*
Jarit-Poole abdominal suction t.
Jarit-Yankauer suction t.
Javid bypass t.
Jesberg aspirating t.
Johnson coagulation suction t.
Johnson intestinal t.
Jones tear duct t.
Jutte t.
Kaslow t.
Kaslow gastrointestinal t.
Kay-Cross suction tip suction t.
Kehr gallbladder t.
Kelly t.
Keymed esophageal t.
Kidd U-t.
Killian t.
Kistner plastic tracheostomy t.
Klein ventilation t.
Knoche t.
Kos ear suction t.
Kozlowski t.
Kuhn endotracheal t.
Kurze suction t.
Lacor t.
Lahey Y-tube t.
Lar-A-Jext laryngectomy t.
LaRocca nasolacrimal t.
laryngeal suction t.
laryngectomy t.
laser laryngeal suction t.
Leiter t.
Lell tracheal t.
Lepley-Ernst t.
Levin-Davol t.
Levin duodenal t.
Lewis laryngectomy t.
Lezius suction t.
life-saving t.
Lindeman-Silverstein Arrow t.
Lindeman-Silverstein ventilation t.
Linton esophageal t.
Linton-Nachlas t.
Lonnecken t.
Lord-Blakemore t.
Lore-Lawrence tracheotomy t.
Lore suction t.
Luer t.
Luer speaking t.
Luer tracheal t.
Lyon t.
MacKenty laryngectomy t.
Mackler intraluminal t.
Madoff suction t.
Magill t.
Maingot gallbladder t.
Malis-Frazier suction t.
Mallinckrodt Laser-Flex t.
Martin laryngectomy t.
Martin tracheostomy t.
Mason suction t.
Massie sliding nail t.
mastoid suction t.
McGowan-Keeley t.
McMurtry-Schlesinger shunt t.
mesh myringotomy t.
Methodist vascular suction t.
MIC gastrostomy t.
micro "penny" sucker suction t.
Miller t.
Miller-Abbott double-lumen intestinal t.
Miller-Abbott intestinal t.
Miller endotracheal t.
Millin suction t.
Mill-Rose t.
Milroy-Piper suction t.
Minnesota t.
Mixter t.
modified suction t.
Momberg t.
Montefiore tracheal t.
Montgomery esophageal t.
Montgomery tracheal t.
Morch swivel tracheostomy t.
Moretz Tiny Tytan ventilation t.
Moretz Tytan ventilation t.
Morse-Andrews suction t.
Morse-Ferguson suction t.
Morse suction t.
Mosher intubation t.
Mosher life-saving t.
Mosher life-saving suction t.

Moss gastric
  decompression t.
Moulton lacrimal t.
Mousseau-Barbin
  esophageal t.
Mueller-Frazier suction t.
Mueller-Pool suction t.
Mueller-Pynchon suction t.
Mueller suction t.
Mueller-Yankauer suction t.
Muldoon t.
Myerson wash t.
myringotomy drain t.
Nachlas gastrointestinal t.
Nachlas-Linton t.
nasal suction t.
nephrostomy t.
Neuber bone t.
New Luer-type speaking t.
New speaking t.
New York glass suction t.
Nilsson-Stille abortion
  suction t.
Nilsson suction t.
Norton endotracheal t.
Nunez ventricular
  ventilation t.
Nyhus-Nelson gastric
  decompression t.
Nyhus-Nelson jejunal
  feeding t.
Nystroem abdominal
  suction t.
O'Beirne sphincter t.
Ochsner gallbladder t.
O'Dwyer t.
O'Hanlon-Pool suction t.
Ommaya ventricular t.
open-end aspirating t.
Ossoff-Karlan laser
  suction t.
Oxford nonkinking cuffed t.
Panje t.
Paparella-Frazier suction t.
Paparella myringotomy t.
Paparella ventilation t.
Parker t.
Paul intestinal drainage t.
Paul-Mixter t.
PEG t.
PEJ t.
Per-Lee equalizing t.
Per-Lee myringotomy t.

Per-Lee ventilation t.
Pertrach percutaneous
  tracheostomy t.
Pierce antrum wash t.
Pilling duralite t.
plastic-cuffed
  tracheostomy t.
Pleur-Evac suction t.
Polisar-Lyons adapted
  tracheal t.
polyethylene t.
polyvinyl t.
Pool abdominal suction t.
Poole abdominal-
  aspirating t.
Poole abdominal suction t.
Poole suction t.
Poppen suction t.
Portex t.
Porto-vac suction t.
Pribram suction t.
Proctor suction t.
proctosigmoid disposable
  suction t.
Puestow-Olander
  gastrointestinal t.
Pynchon suction t.
Radpour-House suction t.
RAE endotracheal t.
Rand-House suction t.
Rand-Radpour suction t.
rectal t.
Redivac t.
Redivac suction t.
Rehfuss duodenal t.
Reinecke-Carroll lacrimal t.
Reuter bobbin ventilation t.
Rhoton-Merz suction t.
Rica mastoid suction t.
Ritter suprapubic suction t.
Robinson equalizing t.
Rochester suction t.
Rochester tracheal t.
Roller pump suction t.
Rosen suction t.
Rusch t.
Rusch laryngectomy t.
Russell suction t.
Ryle duodenal t.
Sachs t.
Sachs suction t.
Sacks-Vine PEG t.

tube *(continued)*

Salem sump action
nasogastric t.
salivary bypass t.
Samson-Davis infant t.
Samson-Davis infant
suction t.
Schall laryngectomy t.
Schmiedt t.
Schuknecht suction t.
Schuler
aspiration/irrigation t.
Scott-Harden t.
Scott nasal suction t.
Securat suction t.
Sengstaken-Blakemore t.
Sengstaken nasogastric t.
Senstaken esophageal t.
Seroma-cath feeding t.
Shah ventilation t.
Sheehy collar button t.
Sheehy Tytan ventilation t.
Shepard drain t.
Shepard grommet
ventilation t.
Sherman suction t.
Shiley French sump t.
Shiley sump t.
Silastic eustachian t.
Silastic intestinal t.
Silastic sucker suction t.
Silastic tracheostomy t.
silicone t.
Silverstein permanent
aeration t. (SPAT)
Singer-Bloom t.
siphon suction t.
SMIC mastoid suction t.
Smith t.
Snyder Hemovac t.
Snyder Hemovac suction t.
Snyder Surgivac suction t.
Snyder Urevac t.
Snyder Urevac suction t.
Soileau Tytan ventilation t.
Southey capillary drainage t.
Souttar t.
speaking t.
Stedman continuous
suction t.
Storz suction t.
straight t.
Stroud-Baron ear suction t.

suction t.
suction-coagulation t.
sump t.
sump suction t.
Sustagen nasogastric t.
Swan-Ganz t.
Swenson cholangiography t.
tear duct t.
T-grommet ventilation t.
three-bottle tidal suction t.
Tiny-Tef ventilation t.
Tiny Tytan ventilation t.
tonsillar suction t.
Touma T-type grommet
ventilation t.
Toynbee diagnostic t.
tracheal t.
tracheostomy t.
Tracoe tracheostomy t.
T-tube round suction t.
Tucker aspirating t.
Tucker flexible tip t.
Tucker tracheal t.
Turkel t.
Turner-Warwick fiberoptic
suction t.
Turner-Warwick illuminating
suction t.
Turner-Warwick suction t.
Tytan grommet
ventilation t.
Tytan ventilation t.
U-t.
underwater-seal suction t.
urinary drainage t.
Valentine irrigation t.
Van Alyea t.
Van Alyea antral wash t.
vascular suction t.
velvet-eye t.
velvet-eye aspirating t.
Venturi t.
Vernon antral wash t.
Vinyon-N cloth t.
Vivonex gastrostomy t.
V. Mueller Frazier
suction t.
V. Mueller Pool suction t.
Voltolini ear t.
Von Eichen antral wash t.
Vortex tracheotomy t.
Wangensteen t.
Wannagat suction t.

wash t.
Watske t.
Webster infusion t.
Weck coagulating suction t.
Weck suction t.
Welch Allyn t.
Welch Allyn suction t.
Wendl t.
Wepsic suction t.
Williams esophageal t.
Winsburg-White bladder t.
Woodbridge t.
Wullstein microsuction t.
Xomed endotracheal t.
Xomed straight-shank t.
Xomed-Treace ventilation t.
Yankauer t.
Yankauer aspirating t.
Yankauer suction t.
Yasargil microsuction t.
Yasargil suction t.
Yeder suction t.
Zollner suction t.
Zyler t.
Tube-Lok tracheotomy dressing
tube-occluding
t.-o. clamp
t.-o. forceps
Tube-Tainer
Clemons T.-T. suction tube
Tubex metal syringe
Tubigrip elastic support bandage
tubing
t. adapter
angiographic t.
Argyle Penrose t.
t. clamp
t. clamp forceps
t. compressor
connecting t.
dialysate t.
evacuator t.
t. hand roller
Hi Vac t.
Lifemed blood t.
Ott insufflator filter t.
Perry latex Penrose
drainage t.
polyvinyl t.
PVC t.
Simcoe connecting t.
wound t.

Tubinger
T. gall stone forceps
T. self-retaining retractor
Tubiton tubular bandage
tuboplasty surgical kit
tubular
t. dressing
t. forceps
t. plate
Tubulitec cavity liner
Tucker
T. anterior commissure
laryngoscope
T. appendix clamp
T. aspirating tube
T. aspirating valve
T. bead forceps
T. bronchoscope
T. cardiospasm dilator
T. dilator
T. direct-vision telescope
T. esophagoscope
T. flexible tip tube
T. forceps
T. hallux forceps
T. hemorrhoidal ligator
T. laryngoscope
T. mid-lighted optic slide
laryngoscope
T. reach-and-pin forceps
T. retrograde bougie
T. slotted laryngoscope
T. tack-and-pin forceps
T. telescope
T. tracheal tube
T. tracheoscope
T. vertebrated guide
T. vertebrated lumen finder
tucker
Bishop-Black tendon t.
Bishop-DeWitt tendon t.
Bishop-Peter tendon t.
Bishop tendon t.
Burch-Greenwood tendon t.
Burch tendon t.
Fink tendon t.
Green stabismus t.
Harrison t.
ligature t.
McGuire tendon t.
Ruedemann-Todd tendon t.
Smuckler t.
tendon t.

tucker *(continued)*
    Twirlon ligature t.
    Wayne t.
Tucker-Holinger laryngoscope
Tucker-Jako laryngoscope
Tucker-Levine vocal cord retractor
Tucker-Luikart blade
Tucker-McLane
    T.-M. axis-traction forceps
    T.-M. forceps
    T.-M. obstetrical forceps
Tucker-McLane-Luikart forceps
Tudor-Edwards
    T.-E. costotome
    T.-E. forceps
    T.-E. rib shears
    T.-E. rib spreader
    T.-E. spreader
Tufcote epilation probe
Tuffier
    T. abdominal retractor
    T. abdominal spatula
    T. artery traction forceps
    T. forceps
    T. retractor
    T. rib retractor
    T. rib spreader
Tuffier-Raney
    T.-R. laminectomy retractor
    T.-R. retractor
Tuffnell bandage
Tuke bone saw
Tulevech lacrimal cannula
tulip probe
tulle gras dressing
Tum-E-Vac gastric lavage
tumor
    t. forceps
    t. probe
    t. screw
tunable dye laser
tungsten microdissection needle
tuning fork
tunneled eye implant
tunneler
    Cooley cardiac t.
    Crawford-Cooley t.
    Davol t.
    DeBakey t.
    DeBakey femoral bypass t.
    DeBakey vascular t.
    Diethrich-Jackson femoral graft t.

    Dosick t.
    Hallman t.
    Jackson t.
    Kelly-Wick vascular t.
    Noon AV fistular t.
    Noon modified vascular access t.
    Scanlan vascular t.
    vascular t.
    vascular access t.
tunnel graft
tunnel-type implant material
Tuohy
    T. aortography needle
    T. catheter
    T. lumbar aortography needle
    T. needle
Tuohy-Borst side-arm introducer
Tupman osteotomy plate
TUR
    transurethral resection
    TUR drape
turbinate
    t. electrode
    t. forceps
    t. scissors
turbine
    air t.
    Allen-Powell air t.
    BT 77 t.
Turbo-Inhaler
    Spinhaler T.-I.
Turbo-Jet dental bur
Turchik instrument holder
Turek spinous process spreader
Turkel
    T. bone biopsy trephine set
    T. liver biopsy needle
    T. needle
    T. prostatic punch
    T. sternal needle
    T. trephine
    T. tube
turkey-claw clamp
turnbuckle
    Giannestras t.
Turnbull
    T. adhesions forceps
    T. applicator
    T. cannula
    T. forceps
    T. nail nipper

Turner
- T. biopsy needle
- T. cord elevator
- T. cystoscopic fulgurating electrode
- T. dilator
- T. periosteal elevator
- T. pin
- T. prosthesis
- T. spinal gouge

Turner-Babcock tissue forceps
Turner-Doyen retractor
Turner-Waru ring
Turner-Warwick
- T.-W. adult retractor ring
- T.-W. bladder neck spreader
- T.-W. blade
- T.-W. diathermy scissors
- T.-W. fiberoptic suction tube
- T.-W. illuminating suction tube
- T.-W. malleable spoon
- T.-W. needle
- T.-W. needle holder
- T.-W. pediatric perineal retractor ring
- T.-W. posterior urethral retractor
- T.-W. post-urethroplasty review speculum
- T.-W. prostate retractor
- T.-W. retractor
- T.-W. speculum
- T.-W. stone forceps
- T.-W. suction tube
- T.-W. urethral staff
- T.-W. urethroplasty needle

Turner-Warwick-Adson forceps
TURP
- transurethral resection of prostate

Turrell
- T. biopsy forceps
- T. forceps
- T. rectal biopsy forceps
- T. sigmoidoscope
- T. specimen forceps

Turrell-Wittner
- T.-W. rectal biopsy forceps
- T.-W. rectal forceps

Tuttle
- T. dressing forceps
- T. forceps
- T. obstetrical forceps
- T. proctoscope
- T. sigmoidoscope
- T. thoracic forceps
- T. thumb forceps
- T. tissue forceps

Tuttle-Singley thoracic forceps
Twardon grommet
Tweedy canaliculus knife
tweezers
- Arti-holder t.
- Dumont t.
- soldering t.

twenty-day gut suture
twill dressing
twin
- t. coil dialyzer
- t. knife

Twin Cities Lo-Profile halo
twin-pattern chisel
Twirlon ligature tucker
Twisk forceps
twist
- t. drill
- t. drill catheter
- Hamby t.

twisted
- t. cotton nonabsorbable surgical suture material
- t. cotton suture
- t. dermal suture
- t. linen suture
- t. silk suture
- t. sister
- t. suture
- t. wire snare loop

twister
- Baumgarten wire t.
- Corwin wire t.
- Ochsner wire t.
- Richards wire t.
- Vital Cooley-Baumgarten wire t.
- Vital Cooley wire t.
- Vital wire t.
- wire t.

twist-in drain tube inserter
Twist-Mate ligator
two-bladed dilator
two-by-two strung sponge
two-point discriminator

two-pronged
> t.-p. dural hook
> t.-p. stem finger prosthesis

two-prong rake retractor

Tworek
> T. bone marrow-aspirating needle
> T. screw guide
> T. transorbital leukotome
> T. Universal gouge

two-stage Sarns cannula

two-stream irrigating forceps

two-toothed forceps

two-way
> t.-w. bag
> t.-w. cataract aspirating cannula
> t.-w. catheter
> t.-w. hemostatic bag

two-wing
> t.-w. drain
> t.-w. Malecot drain

Tycron suture (*See also* Ti-Cron suture)

Tydings
> T. automatic ratchet snare
> T. forceps
> T. tonsillar clamp
> T. tonsillar forceps
> T. tonsillar knife
> T. tonsillar snare
> T. tonsillectome
> T. tonsil-seizing forceps

Tydings-Lakeside
> T.-L. forceps

T.-L. tonsillar forceps
T.-L. tonsil-seizing forceps

Tygon
> T. catheter
> T. esophageal prosthesis
> T. tubing circuit

tying forceps

Tyler
> T. Gigli saw
> T. spiral Gigli saw

tympanometer
> diagnostic t.

tympanoplasty forceps

tympanoscope
> Hopkins t.
> ulcer marker Quinton t.

tympanum
> t. perforator
> t. perforator handle

Tyrer nerve root retractor

Tyrrell
> T. clamp
> T. foreign body forceps
> T. hook
> T. hook retractor
> T. iris hook
> T. skin hook

Tyrrell-Gray suture

Tytan
> T. grommet ventilation tube
> T. tube inserter
> T. ventilation tube

UAC
  umbilical artery catheter
UBC brace
U-channel stripping dural
  substitute
UCI prosthesis
Uckermann cotton applicator
UCLA functional long-leg brace
U-double-barrel suture
Uebe applicator
Ueckermann-Denker trocar
Uffenorde bone curette
UG-70 stapler
Ulbrich wart curette
ulcer
  u. bed
  u. marker Quinton
    tympanoscope
Uldall subclavian hemodialysis
  cannula
Ullrich
  U. bone-holding forceps
  U. dressing forceps
  U. drill guard
  U. drill guard drill
  U. fistular knife
  U. forceps
  U. laminectomy retractor
  U. retractor
  U. self-retaining retractor
  U. small bone-holding
    forceps
  U. tubing clamp
  U. uterine knife
  U. vaginal speculum
Ullrich-Aesculap forceps
Ullrich-St. Gallen forceps
Ullrich-St. Gallen self-retaining
  retractor
ulnar
  u. bearing
  u. rasp
  u. ruler
  u. trial
Ultec dressing
Ultex
  U. implant
  U. lens
Ultracast alloy

Ultra-Cut
  U.-C. Cobb curette
  U.-C. Cobb spinal gouge
  U.-C. Cobb spinal
    instrument
  U.-C. Hibbs gouge
  U.-C. Hoke osteotome
  U.-C. Smith-Petersen
    osteotome
Ultra-Drive bone cement removal
  system
Ultramatic Rx master phoroptor
  refractor
Ultramer catheter
Ultra pacemaker
Ultra-Select Nitinol PTCA guide
  wire
ultrasonic
  u. bone-cutting instrument
  u. cleaner basket
  u. cleaner with folding
    handles instrument basket
  u. cleaner with rigid
    handles instrument basket
  u. denture cleaner
  u. diathermy electrosurgical
    unit
  u. dissector
  u. electrode
  u. harmonic scalpel
  u. nebulizer
  u. scaler
  u. stone crusher
ultrasonoscope
  Bronson u.
ultrasound
  u. inhaler
  intravascular u. (IVUS)
  u. monitor
  OR 340 Intraoperative u.
Ultratome sphincterotome
Ultratone electrical transcutaneous
  neuromuscular stimulator
ultraviolet-blocking intraocular lens
ultraviolet light
ultraviolet radiation (UVR)
Ultra-X external fixation system
Ultrex
  U. penile prosthesis
  U. Plus penile prosthesis

Ultroid coagulator
Ultrox implant
umbilical
  u. artery catheter (UAC)
  u. catheter
  u. clamp
  u. clip
  u. cord clamp
  u. scissors
  u. tape
  u. tape drain
  u. tape suture
  u. vein catheter
umbiliclamp
  u. clamp
  Surgi-Med u.
umbiliclip
  Hesseltine u.
umbrella-type prosthesis
UMI
  UMI amniocentesis kit
  UMI Cath-Seal sheath
  UMI transseptal Cath-Seal
    catheter introducer
unabsorbable suture
unconstrained prosthesis
underwater
  u. Bovie
  u. diathermy
  u. electrode
underwater-seal suction tube
undyed suture
UNI
  UNI reservoir
  UNI shunt
  UNI shunt catheter
Unicare breast pump
Unicath all-purpose catheter
unicompartmental knee implant
unicondylar prosthesis
Unifile
Uniflex
  U. calibrated step drill
  U. distal targeting awl
  U. dressing
  U. drill bushing
  U. guide bushing
  U. nailing system
Unilab Surgibone surgical implant
unilateral bar
Unilink system for hand surgery
Unilith pacemaker
Unimar Cervex-Brush

uninterrupted suture
union
  u. broach retention drill
  u. broach retention pin
uniplanar intraocular lens
unipolar
  u. atrial pacemaker
  u. atrioventricular
    pacemaker
  u. cautery
  u. electrode
  u. pacemaker
  u. sequential pacemaker
Uni-Shunt
  U.-S. abdominal slip clip
  U.-S. anchoring clip
  U.-S. catheter passer
  U.-S. cranial anchoring clip
  U.-S. hydrocephalus shunt
    system
  U.-S. right-angle clip
  U.-S. split trocar
  U.-S. with elliptical
    reservoir
  U.-S. with reservoir
  U.-S. with reservoir
    introducer
unisplint
Uni-sump drain
Unis Universal guide
unit (*See also* TENS unit)
  AG Bovie electrosurgical u.
  Amoils-Keeler cryo u.
  Atmolit suction u.
  AVIT u.
  BiLAP bipolar cautery u.
  Birtcher hyfrecator
    electrosurgical u.
  Bovie electrosurgical u.
  Buck convoluted traction u.
  Buck Universal convoluted
    traction u.
  Burdick microwave
    diathermy electrosurgical u.
  Burdick short-wave
    diathermy electrosurgical u.
  Cal-20 central dialysate
    preparation u.
  Centry 2 cps dialysis u.
  Centry 2 dialysis control u.
  combilan electrosurgical u.
  complete traction u.
  CSV Bovie electrosurgical u.

diathermy u.
EEA disposable loading u.
Elan electrosurgical u.
electricator electrosurgical u.
electrosurgical u.
forearm reduction u.
Frac-Sur u.
Freedom dental u.
GIA II loading u.
Hampton electrosurgical u.
Heliodent dental x-ray u.
LDS disposable u.
L-F Uniflex diathermy
  electrosurgical u.
Lithostar lithotripsy u.
Lumix dental x-ray u.
McKesson suction bottle u.
Mettler Dia-Sonic
  electrosurgical u.
microcautery u.
Osada beaver-XL
  handpiece u.
Oti Vac lighted suction u.
Portaray dental x-ray u.
Premier irrigation-
  aspiration u.
Resuscitaire neonatal
  resuscitation u.
Ritter-Bantam Bovie
  electrosurgical u.
Ritter coagulator
  electrosurgical u.
Sensimatic electrosurgical u.
SITE irrigating-aspirating u.
SM disposable loading u.
Strobex Mark II
  electrosurgical u.
TA II loading u.
ultrasonic diathermy
  electrosurgical u.
Visitec vitrectomy u.
Wangensteen suction u.
Windmill suction
  evacuation u.
X-Cel dental x-ray u.
Yoshida dental x-ray u.
unitome knife
Unitron hearing aid
Universal
U. abdominal trocar
U. adenoid punch tip
U. appliance
U. aspirator

U. cannula
U. chuck handle
U. clip remover
U. connector
U. curved-tube stylet
U. drainage catheter
U. drill
U. drill point
U. esophagoscope
U. eye shield
U. forceps
U. gastroscope
U. goniometer
U. handle
U. head holder
U. hex screwdriver
U. joint device
U. Kerrison rongeur
U. laminectomy set
U. lamp
U. Mack lamp
U. malleable valvulotome
U. nasal instrument handle
U. nasal saw
U. nasal saw blade
U. pelvic traction belt
U. prosthesis
U. radial component
U. retractor
U. screwdriver
U. speculum
U. speculum holder
U. straight-tube stylet
U. support splint
U. swivel
U. T-adapter
U. tip
U. tourniquet
U. two-speed hand drill
U. wire clamp
U. wire scissors
Universal-Endoscope
Uni-Versatil sling
University
U. of British Columbia
  brace
U. forceps
U. of Illinois biopsy needle
U. of Illinois marrow
  needle
U. of Illinois needle
U. of Illinois sternal needle

University *(continued)*
U. of Illinois sternal
puncture needle
U. of Iowa cotton
applicator
U. of Kansas corneal
forceps
U. of Kansas forceps
U. of Kansas hook
U. of Kansas spatula
U. of Michigan gonioscope
U. of Michigan Mixter
forceps
U. of Michigan Mixter
thoracic forceps
U. of Virginia skull tongs
Unna comedo extractor
unsegmented bar
unstented pulmonary homograft
heart valve
up-angle hook
upbiting
u. biopsy forceps
u. cup forceps
u. forceps
upcurved basket forceps
Updegraff
U. cleft palate needle
U. needle
U. staphylorrhaphy needle
UPF prosthesis
UPO-16 stapler
upper
u. body dressing
u. esophagoscope
u. lateral scissors
u. occlusive clamp
upper-hand retractor
upper-lateral exposing retractor
Upper 7 model head halter
Uppsala gall duct forceps
Urban
U. microsurgery closed-
circuit color TV camera
U. retractor
Urbanski strut guide
Urbantschitsch
U. eustachian bougie
U. forceps
U. nasal forceps
Uresil
U. biliary catheter
U. carotid shunt

U. embolectomy-
thrombectomy catheter
U. irrigation catheter
U. occlusion balloon
catheter
U. radiopaque silicone-band
vessel loops
U. Vascu-Flo carotid shunt
ureteral
u. basket stone dislodger
u. brush biopsy kit
u. catheter
u. catheter forceps
u. catheter obturator
u. clamp
u. dilatation catheter
u. dilator
u. forceps
u. implant
u. isolation forceps
u. meatotomy electrode
u. occlusion catheter
u. pigtail stent set
u. stent
u. stone basket
u. stone dilator
u. stone dislodger
u. stone extractor
u. stone forceps
u. stone isolation forceps
u. stone retriever
u. stylet
u. visualization instrument
ureteropyeloscope
Karl Storz flexible u.
ureterotome
Campbell u.
Korth u.
Optic u.
Otis u.
ureterscope
urethral
u. catheter
u. dilator
u. female dilator
u. instillation cannula
u. male dilator
u. male follower dilator
u. meatus dilator
u. sound
u. staff
urethrographic
u. cannula

u. cannula clamp
u. catheter
u. clamp
urethroplasty needle
urethro-profilometer
urethroscope
Judd u.
microlens u.
urethrotome
u. blade
bougie u.
Hertel bougie u.
infant u.
Keitzer infant u.
Kirkheim-Storz u.
Maisonneuve u.
Otis u.
Riba u.
Sachs u.
Storz u.
Storz bougie-u.
Storz-Kirkheim u.
Thomson-Walker u.
Urias pressure splint
Uribe
U. implant
U. orbital implant
Uridome catheter
Uridrop catheter
Urihesive moldable adhesive strip
urinary
u. catheter
u. drainage tube
u. incontinence clamp
u. incontinence prosthesis
Urocare Foley catheter
Urocath external catheter
Uroflo cystometer
uroflowmeter
urological
u. catheter
u. soaking basin
u. system instrument
soaking/storage tray
UroLume Endourethral Wallstent prosthesis
Uro-San Plus external catheter
Uroseal valve
Urosheath incontinence device
Urosoft stent
Urquhart periosteal elevator
Urrets-Zavalia
U.-Z. depressor

U.-Z. localizer
U.-Z. probe
Urschel-Leksell rongeur
Urschel rongeur
U.S.
U.S. Army bone chisel
U.S. Army chisel
U.S. Army double-ended retractor
U.S. Army gauze scissors
U.S. Army gouge
U.S. Army osteotome
U.S. Army-pattern retractor
U.S. Army-pattern umbilical scissors
U.S. Army retractor
U.S. Army tourniquet
USA
USA plaster spreader
USA retractor
USCI
USCI Bard catheter
USCI bifurcated Vasculour II prosthesis
USCI catheter
USCI Finesse guiding catheter
USCI guiding catheter
USCI introducer
USCI Mini-Profile balloon dilatation catheter
USCI pacing electrode
USCI Positrol coronary catheter
USCI Vario permanent pacemaker
USCI-DeBakey vascular prosthesis
U-shaped
U-s. cannula
U-s. continuous suture
U-s. forceps
U-s. retractor
Usher
U. Marlex mesh dressing
U. Marlex mesh implant
U. Marlex mesh implant material
U. Marlex mesh prosthesis
Uslenghi drill guide
U-splint
uterine
u. artery forceps
u. aspirator

uterine *(continued)*
- u. biopsy curette
- u. biopsy forceps
- u. biopsy punch
- u. biopsy punch forceps
- u. clamp
- u. cuff
- u. curette
- u. dilator
- u. elevator
- u. forceps
- u. injector
- u. irrigating curette
- u. manipulator
- u. needle
- u. polyp forceps
- u. probe
- u. punch
- u. scissors
- u. scoop
- u. self-retaining cannula
- u. sound
- u. specimen forceps
- u. suction curette
- u. tenaculum
- u. tenaculum forceps
- u. trigger cannula
- u. trigger cannula extension tip
- u. vacuum aspirating curette (UVAC)
- u. vacuum cannula
- u. vertebrated probe
- u. vulsellum forceps

uterine-dressing forceps
uterine-elevating forceps
uterine-holding forceps
uterine-manipulating forceps
uterine-packing forceps
uteroparietal suture
utility
- u. bandage scissors
- u. forceps
- u. scissors
- u. shears

UTK alloy
Utrata
- U. capsulorrhexis forceps
- U. forceps

U-tube
- U.-t. drain
- U.-t. stent

U-type dental implant
UVAC
- uterine vacuum aspirating curette

uvea-fixated intraocular lens
uvea-supported
- u.-s. intraocular lens
- u.-s. lens

Uviolite lamp
UVR
- ultraviolet radiation

UVR-absorbing
- UVR-a. intraocular lens
- UVR-a. lens

uvular retractor

VA
   visual acuity
      VA implant
      VA magnetic implant
      VA magnetic orbital
         implant
Vabra
      V. aspirator
      V. cannula
      V. catheter
      V. cervical aspirator
Vacher
      V. retractor
      V. self-retaining retractor
Vac-Pac positioner
Vacuconstrictor erection device
Vacupac portable vacuum system
Vacurette
      V. catheter
      V. suction curette
Vacutainer
      V. drain
      V. holder
      V. needle
Vacu-tome
      Barker V.-t.
      V.-t. knife
vacuum
      v. apparatus
      v. aspiration catheter
      v. aspirator
      v. curette
      v. drain
      v. erection device (VED)
      v. fixation ring
      v. intrauterine cannula
      v. intrauterine probe
      v. retractor
      Semm v.
      v. tumescence-constrictor
         device
      v. uterine cannula (VUC)
vacuuming needle
vacuum-operated viscous restraint
VAD
   vascular/venous access device
   ventricular assist device
vaginal
      v. aluminum electrode
      v. bag

      v. cuff
      v. cuff clamp
      v. dilating set
      v. dilator
      v. forceps
      v. hysterectomy forceps
      v. laser measuring rod
      v. retractor
      v. spatula
      v. speculum
      v. stent
Vaginard metal speculum
vaginoscope
      Huffman-Huber v.
      Huffman-Huber infant v.
      Huffman infant v.
      infant v.
vagotometer
      Burge v.
vagotomy
      v. retractor
      v. stripper
Vail
      V. lid everter
      V. lid retractor
Vaiser-Dibis muscle retractor
Vakutage curette
Valdoni clamp
Valentine
      V. irrigation tube
      V. splint
valgus bar
Valin
      V. hemilaminectomy
         retractor
      V. hemilaminectomy self-
         retaining retractor
Valleylab
      V. electrocautery
      V. laparoscopic instrument
Valliex uterine probe
Valls prosthesis
Valtrac anastomosis ring
valve
      Abrams-Lucas flap heart v.
      Accu-Flo pressure v.
      4-A Magovern heart v.
      Ambu-E v.
      Angell-Shiley heart v.
      apicoaortic conduit heart v.

valve *(continued)*
apicoaortic shunt heart v.
Beall disk heart v.
Beall heart v.
Bicer-val mitral heart v.
Bioprosthesis heart v.
Björk-Shiley heart v.
Braunwald v.
Braunwald heart v.
Carpentier-Edwards heart v.
Carpentier ring heart v.
convexoconcave heart v.
Cutter-Smeloff heart v.
DeBakey heart v.
Delrin disk heart v.
v. dilator
dual-chamber flushing v.
Duostat rotating
  hemostatic v.
Duraflow heart v.
Duromedics bileaflet
  heart v.
Edwards seamless heart v.
Emiks heart v.
fascia lata heart v.
floating disk heart v.
flushing v.
four-legged cage heart v.
Hall-Kaster heart v.
Hammersmith heart v.
Hancock bioprosthetic
  heart v.
Hancock heterograft
  heart v.
Hancock modified orifice
  heart v.
Harken ball v.
Harken ball heart v.
Harken-Starr v.
Hasner v.
heart v.
Heidbrink expiratory spill v.
Heimlich chest drain v.
Heimlich heart v.
Heimlich Vygon
  pneumothorax v.
Heyer-Schulte v.
v. holder
hollow Silastic disk heart v.
Holter v.
Holter elliptical v.
Holter mini-elliptical v.
Holter straight v.

Hufnagel-Kay v.
Hufnagel-Kay heart v.
Intact xenograft v.
Ionescu-Shiley heart v.
Kay-Shiley heart v.
Kay-Suzuki heart v.
v. leaflet excision scissors
lens mitral heart v.
Lewis-Leigh positive-pressure
  nonrebreathing v.
Lifemed heterologous
  heart v.
Liks Russian disk rotation
  heart v.
Lillehei-Kaster heart v.
low-profile v.
low-profile mitral heart v.
low-profile with
  antisiphon v.
Magovern-Cromie heart v.
Magovern heart v.
Medtronic Hall prosthetic
  heart v.
Mishler dual-chamber v.
Mishler flushing v.
Mitamura fine ceramic
  heart v.
monostrut heart v.
multipurpose v.
Omniscience heart v.
v. outflow strut
polyethylene seat heart v.
porcine heart v.
Pudenz flushing v.
pyrolyte ball heart v.
pyrolyte cage heart v.
v. redo forceps
Rudolph one-way
  respiratory v.
Sanders v.
SCDK heart v.
SCDT heart v.
Shiley convexoconcave
  heart v.
Shiley monostrut heart v.
silicone ball heart v.
silicone disk heart v.
sixty-degree valve heart v.
Smeloff-Cutter heart v.
Smeloff heart v.
Spitz-Holter v.
Starr-Edwards ball v.

Starr-Edwards cloth-covered
metallic ball heart v.
Starr-Edwards heart v.
Stellite ball heart v.
Stellite cage heart v.
stent creep of porcine
heart v.
stented homografts heart v.
St. Jude medical heart v.
three-legged cage heart v.
tilting disk heart v.
titanium ball heart v.
titanium cage heart v.
Tucker aspirating v.
unstented pulmonary
homograft heart v.
Uroseal v.
Wada-Cutter heart v.
valvuloplasty balloon catheter
valvulotome
antegrade v.
Bakst v.
break knife v.
Brock v.
Chalnot v.
Derra v.
Dogliotti v.
Dubost v.
Gerbode v.
Gohrbrand v.
Harken v.
Himmelstein pulmonary v.
Leather antegrade v.
Leather retrograde v.
Longmire v.
Longmire-Mueller curved v.
Malm-Himmelstein
pulmonary v.
Mills v.
Neider v.
Potts expansile v.
Potts-Riker v.
retrograde v.
Sellor v.
Tubbs v.
Universal malleable v.
Van Alyea antral cannula
Van Alyea antral trocar
Van Alyea antral wash tube
Van Alyea cannula
Van Alyea frontal sinus cannula
Van Alyea sphenoid cannula
Van Alyea tube

Van Aman pigtail catheter
Van Buren bone-holding forceps
Van Buren canvas roll sound
Van Buren catheter guide
Van Buren curve catheter guide
Van Buren dilating sound
Van Buren dilator
Van Buren forceps
Van Buren sequestrum forceps
Van Buren urethral sound
Vance
V. percutaneous Malecot
nephrostomy catheter
V. prostatic aspiration
cannula
**Vance-Kish urethral illuminated
catheter**
Vanderbilt
V. arterial forceps
V. clamp
V. deep-vessel forceps
V. forceps
V. hemostatic forceps
V. University hemostatic
forceps
V. University vessel clamp
V. University vessel forceps
V. vessel clamp
Van Der Pas hysteroscope
Vander Pool sterilizer forceps
Van Doren forceps
**Van Doren uterine biopsy punch
forceps**
Van Doren uterine forceps
Vanghetti limb prosthesis
Van Hillman suture
Van Hove bag
**Van Mandach capsule fragment
and clot forceps**
Vannas
V. abscess knife
V. capsulotomy scissors
V. corneal scissors
V. fixation forceps
V. iridocapsulotomy scissors
V. scissors
Van Osdel guillotine
Van Osdel irrigating cannula
**Van Osdel tonsil enucleator
tonsillectome**
Van Rosen splint
Van Ruben forceps
van Sonnenberg catheter

van Sonnenberg sump catheter
van Sonnenberg sump drain
Van Struyken forceps
Van Struyken nasal-cutting forceps
Van Struyken nasal forceps
Van Struyken nasal punch
Vantage tube-occluding forceps
Van Tassel angled pigtail catheter
Van Tassel pigtail catheter
Vantec
    V. dilator
    V. grasping forceps
    V. loop retriever
    V. occlusion balloon
      catheter
    V. stone basket
    V. ureteral balloon
      dilatation catheter
    V. urinary stent
vaporizing rust inhibitor
Varco
    V. dissecting clamp
    V. forceps
    V. gallbladder clamp
    V. gallbladder forceps
    V. thoracic forceps
variable
    v. axis knee
    v. flow insufflator
    v. rate pacemaker
variable-focus scope
Variable Spot Dermastat
vari-angle
    v.-a. clip
    v.-a. McFadden clip applier
    v.-a. temporary clip-applying
      forceps
    v.-a. temporary clip
      approximator
    v.-a. temporary vessel clip
Varick elastic dressing
Variflex catheter
Varigray lens
Varilux
    V. implant
    V. infinity lens
    V. Plus lens
Vari-Mix II amalgamator
VariMoist dressing
Varivas R vein graft
varnish
    Copal cavity v.
    Copalite cavity v.

    Fuji cavity v.
    Opotow cavity v.
vas
    v. clamp
    v. hook
    v. isolation forceps
Vas-Cath
    V.-C. Opti-Plast peripheral
      angioplasty catheter
    V.-C. peritoneal dialysis
      catheter
Vasconcelos-Barretto clamp
Vasco-Posada orbital retractor
Vascor sterile retraction tape
Vascuclamp
    V. minibulldog vessel clamp
    V. vascular clamp
vascular
    v. access catheter
    v. access set
    v. access tunneler
    v. bed
    v. catheter
    v. clamp
    v. clip
    v. dilator
    v. dissector
    v. forceps
    v. graft clamp
    v. graft prosthesis
    v. loop
    v. needle holder
    v. and needle-pulling
      forceps
    v. retractor
    v. scissors
    v. silk suture
    v. spring retractor
    v. suction tube
    v. tissue forceps
    v. tunneler
vascular/venous access device
  (VAD)
Vascushunt carotid balloon shunt
Vascutech circular blade
Vascutek vascular prosthesis
vasectomy forceps
Vaseline
    V. dressing
    V. gauze dressing
    V. petroleum gauze dressing
    V. wick dressing

Vasocillator
    V. fracture appliance
    V. fracture frame
vasodilator
vasovasostomy clamp
Vastrip
VAT pacemaker
Vauban speculum
Vaughan
    V. abscess knife
    V. periosteotome
Vaughn sterilizer forceps
V-blade plate plate
VCU
    videocystourethrography
VDD pacemaker
VDS plate
vectis
    v. blade
    v. cesarean forceps
    v. cesarean section forceps
    Drews-Knolle reverse
      irrigating v.
    v. forceps
    irrigating v.
    Knolle-Pearce v.
    v. loop
    Sheets irrigating v.
    Torpin v.
Vector II guide system
VED
    vacuum erection device
Vedder loop
Veeder tip snare
Veenema
    V. retractor
    V. retropubic retractor
    V. retropubic self-retaining
      retractor
Veenema-Gusberg
    V.-G. needle
    V.-G. prostatic biopsy cup
    V.-G. prostatic biopsy
      needle
    V.-G. prostatic punch
Vehmehren costotome
Veidenheimer
    V. clamp
    V. resection clamp
vein
    v. dilator
    v. graft cannula
    v. graft ring marker

    v. retractor
    v. stripper
Veirs
    V. canaliculus rod
    V. cannula
    V. dacryocystorhinostomy
      set
    V. needle
    V. trocar
Velcro
    V. dressing
    V. extenders splint
    V. fastener dressing
    V. tourniquet
Velex woven Dacron vascular graft
Veley headrest
Velket Velcro tourniquet
velocimeter
Velpeau
    V. bandage
    V. dressing
    V. sling-dressing
    V. snare
Velpeau-style shoulder immobilizer
Velroc dressing
velvet-eye
    v.-e. aspirating tube
    v.-e. tube
vena
    v. caval cannula
    v. caval clamp
    v. caval clip
    v. caval forceps
Venable
    V. bone plate
    V. screw
Venable-Stuck
    V.-S. fracture pin
    V.-S. nail
Venaflo needle
Vena-Tech dual vena caval filter
veneer retention wire
venesuture
Venflon cannula
venipuncture needle
Vennes pancreatic dilation set
venoclysis cannula
**Venodyne pneumatic inflation
    device**
**Venofit medical compression
    stockings**
**Venoflex medical compression
    stockings**

venous
    v. cannula
    v. cannula tip
    v. catheter
    v. irrigation catheter
    v. needle
    v. sheath
    v. thrombectomy catheter
    v. Y-adapter
    v. Y connector
venouscapacitance bed
Ventak AICD pacemaker
Ventifoam traction dressing
ventilation adapter
ventilator
    Bear v.
    Bear adult-volume v.
    Bear Cub infant v.
    Bennett v.
    Bennett pressure-cycled v.
    Bio-Med MVP-10
      pediatric v.
    Bird pressure-cycled v.
    blow-by v.
    Bourns-Bear v.
    Bourns infant v.
    Carass v.
    Emerson postoperative v.
    IVAC v.
    mechanical v.
    Monaghan v.
    Morch v.
    Ohio critical care v.
    pneuPAC v.
    Puritan-Bennett v.
    Sechrist infant v.
    Sechrist neonatal v.
    Servo v.
    Siemens Servo v.
    Venturi v.
    Vix infant v.
venting
    v. aortic Bengash needle
    v. catheter
Vent-O-Vac aspirator
Ventricor pacemaker
ventricular
    v. assist device (VAD)
    v. bands
    v. cannula
    v. catheter
    v. catheter introducer
    v. demand pacemaker
    v. demand pulse generator
    v. needle
    v. pacemaker
    v. sump
ventricular-suppressed pacemaker
ventricular-triggered pacemaker
ventriculogram retractor
ventriculography catheter
Ventura spreader
Venturi
    V. apparatus
    V. tube
    V. ventilation adapter
    V. ventilator
Vera bond alloy
Veratex cotton roll
Verbrugge
    V. bone clamp
    V. bone-holding forceps
    V. clamp
    V. forceps
    V. retractor
Verbrugge-Müller bone lever
Verbrugge-Souttar craniotome
Veress
    V. cannula
    V. laparoscopic cannula
    V. needle
    V. peritoneum cannula
    V. pneumoperitoneum
      needle
    V. spring-loaded
      laparoscopic needle
Veress-Frangenheim needle
Verhoeff
    V. capsular forceps
    V. cataract forceps
    V. dissecting scissors
    V. expressor
    V. forceps
    V. lens expressor
    V. suture
Veri-Flex guide wire
Verlow brace
Verner
    V. speculum
    V. stripper
Verner-Joel cutter
Verner-Joseph
    V.-J. scissors
    V.-J. wire tightener
Verner-Kalinowski speculum
Verner-Smith monitor

Vernier calipers
Vernon
 V. antral wash tube
 V. David sigmoidoscope
 V. scissors
 V. wire cutter
 V. wire-cutting scissors
Vernon-David
 V.-D. proctoscope
 V.-D. rectal speculum
Versadopp Doppler probe
Versafix external fracture fixation device
Versaflex steerable catheter
Versa-lite
 Lubke-Berci V.-l.
Versatrax
 V. cardiac pacemaker
 V. II pacemaker
 V. pacemaker
Verse-Webster clamp
vertebral body biopsy instrument
vertebrated
 v. catheter
 v. probe
vertical
 v. bone self-retaining retractor
 v. mattress suture
 v. retractor
 v. ring curette
 v. suture
Vesely nail
Vesely-Street nail
vesical retractor
vessel
 v. band
 v. clamp
 v. clip
 v. clip-applying forceps
 v. dilator
 v. forceps
 v. knife
 v. loop
 v. occlusion system
 v. pediatric forceps
 v. peripheral clamp
 v. peripheral forceps
 v. punch
 v. retractor
 v. supporter
 v. tip
vessel-occluding clamp

Vest
 V. direct forward-vision telescope
 V. telescope
vest
 Circumpress gynecomastia v.
vestibular clamp
VEST traction suture
Vezien abdominal scissors
Viasorb dressing
Viboch
 V. graft retractor
 V. iliac graft retractor
Vibrasonic hearing instrument
Vibrodilator probe
Vibro-Graver
 Burgess V.-G.
vibrometer
Vic
 V. hair transplant knife
 V. Vallis running hair knife
Vicat needle
Vick-Blanchard
 V.-B. forceps
 V.-B. hemorrhoidal forceps
Vickers
 V. isolator
 V. Treonic hemoheater
Vicor pacemaker
Vicryl
 V. pop-off suture
 V. SH suture
 V. suture
Victor-Bonney forceps
Victorian collar dressing
Victory alloy
Vidal-Ardrey modified Hoffman device
Vidal device
Vidal-Hoffman fixator frame
video
 v. camera
 v. endoscope
 v. otoscope
 Wallach Zoomscope with v.
videocystourethrography (VCU)
videoscope
 Cabot Medical Corporation v.
Vi-Drape
 V.-D. drape
 V.-D. dressing

Vienna
    V. nasal speculum
    V. original nasal speculum
    V. speculum
    V. wire suture
Vienns Britetrac nasal speculum
Viers
    V. erysiphake
    V. trocar
Vigger-5 eye forceps
Vigilon
    V. drain
    V. dressing
Viking
    V. cannula
    V. needle
Villard button
Vimedic articulating paper
Vim needle
Vim-Silverman
    V.-S. biopsy needle
    V.-S. needle
Vimule pessary
Vinke
    V. retractor
    V. skull tractor
    V. tongs
Vinyon-N cloth tube
Vioform
    V. dressing
    V. gauze dressing
Viomedex surgical marking pen
Virchow
    V. brain knife
    V. cartilage knife
    V. chisel
    V. skin graft knife
Virden
    V. catheter
    V. rectal catheter
Virgin hip screw
virgin silk suture
Viro-Tec suture
Virtus
    V. forceps
    V. splinter clamp
    V. splinter forceps
Visalens contact lens cleaning and soaking solution
VISC
    vitreous infusion suction cutter
viscera-holding forceps
visceral forceps

viscera retainer
visceroparietal suture
Viscoadherent Occucoat viscoelastic
Viscoat
    V. viscoelastic
viscoelastic
    Cilco v.
    CooperVision v.
    sodium hyaluronate v.
    Viscoadherent Occucoat v.
    Viscoat v.
Viscoflow angled cannula
vise
    Benda finger v.
    v. forceps
    Gam-Mer v.
    pin v.
    Starrett pin v.
vise-grip pliers
Visi-Black
    V.-B. needle
    V.-B. surgical needle
Visicath viewing catheter
Visiline disposable sigmoidoscope
Visio-Gem color system
Visitec
    V. anterior chamber cannula
    V. cannula
    V. cystitome
    V. needle
    V. retrobulbar needle
    V. syringe
    V. vitrectomy unit
Vismark surgical skin marker
Vista pacemaker
Vistec x-ray detectable sponge
Vistnes
    V. applier bar
    V. rubber band applier band
visual acuity (VA)
visual hemostatic forceps
Visulas Nd:YAG laser
Vitacrilic
Vitacuff
Vitadur-N porcelain powder
Vita-Gel acrylic
Vitagraft vascular graft
Vital
    V. Adson tissue forceps
    V. Babcock tissue forceps

V. Baumgartner needle
holder
V. Castroviejo eye needle
holder
V. Castroviejo needle holder
V. Cooley-Baumgarten wire
twister
V. Cooley French eye
needle holder
V. Cooley general tissue
holder
V. Cooley intracardiac
needle holder
V. Cooley microsurgery
needle holder
V. Cooley microvascular
needle holder
V. Cooley needle holder
V. Cooley neurosurgical
needle holder
V. Cooley operating scissors
V. Cooley wire-cutting
scissors
V. Cooley wire twister
V. Cottle dorsal angled
scissors
V. Crile-Wood needle
holder
V. Cushing tissue forceps
V. DeBakey cardiovascular
needle holder
V. Derf eye needle holder
V. Duval intestinal forceps
V. Evans pelvic tissue
forceps
V. Finochietto needle
holder
V. Fomon angular scissors
V. forceps
V. French-eye needle holder
V. general tissue forceps
V. Halsey eye-needle holder
V. Heaney needle holder
V. intestinal forceps
V. Jacobson needle holder
V. Jacobson spring-handled
needle holder
V. Julian needle holder
V. Kalt eye needle holder
V. Knapp iris scissors
V. Knapp strabismus
scissors
V. lung-grasping forceps

V. Masson needle holder
V. Mayo dissecting scissors
V. Mayo-Hegar needle
holder
V. Metzenbaum dissecting
scissors
V. Metzenbaum scissors
V. microsurgery needle
holder
V. microvascular needle
holder
V. Mills vascular needle
holder
V. needle holder forceps
V. Neivert needle holder
V. Nelson dissecting scissors
V. neurosurgical needle
holder
V. New Orleans needle
holder
V. Olsen-Hegar needle
holder
V. operating scissors
V. Potts-Smith forceps
V. Rochester needle holder
V. Ryder needle holder
V. Sarot needle holder
V. skin stapler
V. Stratte needle holder
V. tissue forceps
V. Wangensteen needle
holder
V. Wangensteen tissue
forceps
V. Webster needle holder
V. wire-cutting scissors
V. wire twister
Vitalcor
V. cardioplegia infusion
cannula
V. catheter
V. venous catheter
V. venous return catheter
Vitallium
V. clip
V. cup
V. drill
V. Elliott knee plate
V. eye implant
V. Hicks radius plate
V. implant
V. implant material
V. mesh component

Vitallium *(continued)*
>V. Moore self-locking prosthesis
>V. nail
>V. plate
>V. screw
>V. Wainwright blade plate
>V. Walldius mechanical knee plate

Vitapan teeth
Vita teeth
Vitatrax II pacemaker
Vitatron pacemaker
Vitax female catheter
vitrectomy instrument
vitrector
>Kaufman eye v.
>Kaufman II v.
>Machemer VISC v.
>ocutome v.
>O'Malley v.
>Peeler-Cutter v.
>Peyman v.

vitreous
>v. cutter
>v. infusion suction cutter (VISC)
>v. scissors

vitreous-grasping forceps
Vivalith-10 pacemaker
Vivalith II pulse generator
Vivant ultrasonic scaler
Vivatron pacemaker
Vivonex
>V. gastrostomy tube
>V. jejunostomy catheter

Vivosil
>V. implant
>V. prosthesis

Vix infant ventilator
V-lance eye knife
VLC compression screw
V. M. & Co. *(See* V. Mueller)
V-medullary nail
V. Mueller *(See also* Mueller, Müller)
>V. M. amputating saw
>V. M. aortic clamp
>V. M. auricular appendage clamp
>V. M. biopsy forceps
>V. M. blade
>V. M. blunt hook

V. M. bone-cutting forceps
V. M. bulldog clamp
V. M. catheter
V. M. cross-action bulldog clamp
V. M. curved operating scissors
V. M. cystoscopy tip
V. M. diamond rasp
V. M. ear blade
V. M. embolectomy catheter
V. M. fiberoptic retractor
V. M. Frazier suction tube
V. M. Gigli saw
V. M. laser Adson tissue forceps
V. M. laser Backhaus towel forceps
V. M. laser Crile micro-arterial forceps
V. M. laser micro-Allis forceps
V. M. laser Rhoton microforceps
V. M. laser Rhoton microneedle holder
V. M. laser Rhoton microscissors
V. M. laser Rhoton microtying forceps
V. M. laser Singley tissue forceps
V. M. laser tubal scissors
V. M. mastoid curette
V. M. mini blade
V. M. myringotomy ear blade
V. M. nonperforating towel forceps
V. M. operating scissors
V. M. paracervical nerve block needle
V. M. Pool suction tube
V. M. pudendal nerve block needle
V. M. ruler
V. M. ruler calipers
V. M. screwdriver
V. M. Tip-Trol handle
V. M. TUR drape
V. M. tying forceps
V. M. Universal handle

V. M. vascular loop
V. M. vena caval clamp
V. Mueller-Balfour abdominal
retractor
V. Mueller-LaForce adenotome
V. Mueller-Vital laser Babcock
forceps
V. Mueller-Vital laser Heaney
needle holder
V. Mueller-Vital laser Julian
needle holder
V. Mueller-Vital laser Mayo
dissecting scissors
V. Mueller-Vital laser Potts-Smith
forceps
Vogel
V. adenoid curette
V. curette
V. infant adenoid curette
Vogelfanger-Beattie stapler
Vogelfanger blood vessel stapler
Vogler hysterectomy forceps
Vogt
V. forceps
V. toothed capsular forceps
Vogt-Barraquer
V.-B. corneal needle
V.-B. eye needle
voice button
Volk
V. conoid implant
V. conoid lens
Volkmann
V. bone curette
V. curette
V. finger retractor
V. hand retractor
V. oval curette
V. pocket retractor
V. rake retractor
V. retractor
V. scoop
V. splint
V. spoon
V. vas hook
Voller curette
voltage clamp
Voltolini
V. ear tube
V. nasal speculum
V. speculum
Voltz wrist joint prosthesis
Volutrol apparatus

vomer
v. forceps
v. septal forceps
Von Andel biliary dilation catheter
Von Andel catheter
Von Eichen antral cannula
Von Eichen antral wash tube
Von Eichen cannula
von Graefe (See Graefe)
Von Hippel mechanical trephine
Von Lackum transection shift
jacket
Von Lackum transection shift
jacket brace
von Langenbeck periosteal elevator
von Mandach forceps
von Petz
von Petz apparatus
von Petz clamp
von Petz clip
von Petz forceps
von Petz intestinal clamp
von Petz stomach clamp
von Petz suturing apparatus
von Pirquet suture
von Saal medullary pin
von Seemen rongeur
von Szulec hook
Voorhees
V. bag
V. needle
Voris intervertebral disk rongeur
Voris-Oldberg intervertebral disk
forceps
Voris-Wester forceps
Vorse
V. occluding clamp
V. tube-occluding clamp
V. tube-occluding forceps
Vorse-Webster
V.-W. clamp
V.-W. tube-occluding clamp
Vorse-Wester forceps
Vortex tracheotomy tube
VPI
VPI stone basket
VPI urethral meatal dilator
VPI-Ambrose resectoscope forceps
VPI-Jacobellis microhematuria
catheter set
VPL
VPL electrode
VPL thalamic electrode

VS femoral stem
VSP
>VSP bone plate
>VSP plate

VTCB biliary system
V-type intertrochanteric plate
VUC
>vacuum uterine cannula

vulcanite
>v. bur
>v. chisel

vulsellum
>Bland v.
>cervical v.
>Donald v.
>Fenton bulldog v.
>v. forceps
>Henrotin v.
>Jacob v.
>Jacobs v.

>Kelly v.
>MGH v.
>Schroeder v.
>Seyand v.
>Skene v.
>Teale v.
>Thoms-Allis v.

VVI
>VVI bipolar Programalith
> pacemaker
>VVI pacemaker
>VVI single-chamber
> pacemaker

VVI/AAI pacemaker
VVIR single-chamber rate-adaptive
pacemaker
VVT pacemaker
Vygon Nutricath S catheter
Vynacron resin
Vynagel dental resin

Wachsberger bur
Wachtenfeldt
    W. butterfly clip
    W. clip
    W. clip-applying forceps
    W. clip-removing forceps
    W. forceps
    W. suture clip
    W. wound clip
Wachtenfeldt-Stille retractor
Wada-Cutter heart valve
Wada hingeless heart valve prosthesis
Wadsworth
    W. lid clamp
    W. lid forceps
    W. scissors
Wadsworth-Todd
    W.-T. cautery
    W.-T. eye cautery
wafer
    Stomahesive sterile w.
Wagener hook
Wagensteen tissue forceps
Wagner
    W. antral punch
    W. apparatus
    W. bone lever
    W. knife
    W. laryngeal brush
    W. leg-lengthening device
    W. punch
    W. resurface prosthesis
    W. rongeur
Wainstock eye forceps
WAK
    wearable artificial kidney
Wakeling fetal heart monitor
Walb knife
Waldeau
    W. fixation forceps
    W. forceps
Waldenberg apparatus
Waldenstrom laryngeal forceps
Walden telescope
Waldeyer forceps
Waldon wrench
Waldron forceps
Wales
    W. dilator

    W. rectal bougie
    W. rectal dilator
Walker
    W. aspirator
    W. cautery
    W. coagulating electrode
    W. corneal scissors
    W. corneal trephine
    W. curette
    W. dissector
    W. electrode
    W. forceps
    W. gallbladder retractor
    W. hollow quill pin
    W. lid everter
    W. lid retractor
    W. needle
    W. retractor
    W. ring curette
    W. ruptured disk curette
    W. scleral ruler
    W. submucous elevator
    W. suction tonsillar dissector
    W. tonsillar dissector
    W. tonsillar needle
    W. tonsil-suction dissector
    W. ureteral meatotomy electrode
Walker-Apple scissors
Walker-Atkinson scissors
Walker-Lee sclerotome
walking brace
Wallace cesarean forceps
Wallach
    W. Bio-Tool sterilizer
    W. cryosurgical pain blocker
    W. freezer cryosurgical device
    W. mini-freezer cryosurgical instrument
    W. pencil cryosurgical device
    W. Zoomscope with video
Wall arterial stent
Walldius Vitallium mechanical knee prosthesis
Wallich
    W. abortion scoop

Wallich *(continued)*
- W. curette
- W. placental scoop

Walser matrix

Walsh
- W. chisel
- W. cortex extractor
- W. curette
- W. dermal curette
- W. footplate chisel
- W. forceps
- W. hook
- W. hook-type dermal curette
- W. pressure ring
- W. tissue forceps

Walsham
- W. forceps
- W. nasal forceps
- W. septal forceps
- W. septal straightener
- W. septum-straightening forceps

Walter
- W. corneal spud
- W. forceps
- W. Reed implant
- W. splinter forceps

Walter-Deaver retractor

Waltham-Street bougie

Walther
- W. aspirating bladder trocar
- W. catheter
- W. clamp
- W. dilator
- W. dilator-catheter
- W. female catheter
- W. female dilator catheter
- W. forceps
- W. kidney pedicle clamp
- W. pedicle clamp
- W. tissue forceps
- W. urethral dilator
- W. urethral sound

Walther-Crenshaw
- W.-C. clamp
- W.-C. meatal clamp

Walton
- W. clamp
- W. comedo extractor
- W. corneoscleral punch
- W. curette
- W. ear knife

- W. forceps
- W. foreign body gouge
- W. gouge
- W. meniscal clamp
- W. meniscal forceps
- W. rib shears
- W. rongeur
- W. round gauge spud
- W. scissors

Walton-Allis tissue forceps

Walton-Liston forceps

Walton-Ruskin rongeur

Walton-Schubert
- W.-S. forceps
- W.-S. punch
- W.-S. uterine biopsy forceps

waltzing areolar lifter

Walzl hysterectomy forceps

wandering
- w. atrial pacemaker
- w. pacemaker

Wang
- W. lens
- W. needle

Wangensteen
- W. anastomosis clamp
- W. apparatus
- W. awl
- W. carrier
- W. clamp
- W. deep ligature carrier
- W. dissector
- W. drain
- W. dressing
- W. forceps
- W. gastric-crushing anastomotic clamp
- W. internal decompression trocar
- W. intestinal forceps
- W. intestinal needle
- W. ligature carrier
- W. needle
- W. needle holder
- W. patent ductus clamp
- W. retractor
- W. suction unit
- W. tissue forceps
- W. tissue inverter
- W. tube
- W. Vital needle holder

Wannagat
- W. injection needle

W. sponger
W. suction tube
Wappler
W. bridge
W. cautery
W. cold cautery
W. cystoscope with
microlens optics
W. cystourethroscope
W. electrode
W. microlens
cystourethroscope
W. pneumotome
W. polypectomy snare
W. resectoscope with
microlens optics
Ward
W. French-eye needle
W. French needle
W. nasal chisel
W. nasal osteotome
W. needle
W. periosteal elevator
Ward-Lempert lens loupe
Ware cancer cell collector
warmer
hypothermia oxygen w.
(HOW)
Warm Springs brace
Warne penile sheath
Warren-Mack
W.-M. drill
W.-M. rotating drill
Warren-Wilder retriever
Wartenberg
W. neurological hammer
W. pinwheel
Warthen
W. clamp
W. forceps
W. spur crusher
W. spur-crushing clamp
Warwick James elevator
wash
w. catheter
w. tube
washer
barbed plastic w.
connector with lock w.
contoured w.
w. crimper
w. holder
male/female w.

narrow w.
rotation-stop w.
spiked w.
wide w.
washing catheter
washout cannula
Wasko
W. common duct probe
W. probe
wasp-waist laryngoscope
Watanabe
W. apparatus for
cystolithotripsy
W. arthroscope
W. catheter
W. pin
W. pin holder
watchmaker forceps
water
w. bed
w. dressing
w. probe
w. scalpel
water-infusion esophageal
manometry catheter
Waterman
W. folding bronchoscope
W. rib contractor
W. sump drain
Water Pik
W. P. irrigator
W. P. toothbrush
water-seal drain
Waters muscle stimulator
water-trap drain
Watske tube
Watson
W. angular forceps
W. forceps
W. heart value holder
W. intestinal biopsy capsule
W. skin graft knife
W. speculum
W. tonsil-seizing forceps
Watson-Cheyne
W.-C. dissector
W.-C. dry dissector
Watson-Jones
W.-J. dressing
W.-J. elevator
W.-J. gouge
W.-J. guide pin

Watson-Jones *(continued)*
  W.-J. nail
  W.-J. tractor
Watson-Williams
  W.-W. conchotome
  W.-W. ethmoidal punch
  W.-W. ethmoid-biting
    forceps
  W.-W. forceps
  W.-W. intervertebral disk
    rongeur
  W.-W. nasal forceps
  W.-W. needle
  W.-W. polyp forceps
  W.-W. sinus rasp
Watts
  W. clamp
  W. locking clamp
  W. tenaculum
Watzke
  W. forceps
  W. sleeve
  W. sleeve-spreading forceps
Waugh
  W. dissection forceps
  W. dressing forceps
  W. prosthesis
  W. tissue forceps
Waugh-Brophy forceps
wave
  w. guide catheter
  Parama pulse w.
wave-tooth forceps
wax
  Aluwax impression w.
  Astron dental w.
  Bite wafer denture bite w.
  bone w.
  w. bougie
  Carver dental w.
  dental w.
  Flex-E-Z w.
  Flexo w.
  Godiva w.
  Kwik w.
  Parafil w.
  PD dental w.
  Peck inlay w.
  Plastodent w.
  w.-removing spatula
  Swissedent w.
  Sylver-Wax dental w.
  w. up coping

3-way
  3-w. catheter
  3-w. Foley catheter
  3-w. irrigating catheter
Wayne
  W. tucker
  W. U. crimper
W. Dean McDonald gastric clamp
weapon
  Sheehy w.
wearable artificial kidney (WAK)
Weary
  W. brain spatula
  W. nerve hook
  W. nerve root retractor
Weavenit
  W. implant
  W. prosthesis
  W. vascular prosthesis
Weaver
  W. chalazion clamp
  W. chalazion curette
  W. chalazion forceps
  W. clamp
  W. forceps
  W. sinus probe
Webb
  W. bolt
  W. bolt nail
  W. cannula
  W. interchangable vein
    stripper
  W. pin
  W. retractor
  W. stove bolt
  W. vein stripper
Webb-Balfour
  W.-B. abdominal retractor
  W.-B. retractor
  W.-B. self-retaining retractor
Weber
  W. aortic clamp
  W. canaliculus knife
  W. catheter
  W. colonic insufflator
  W. hip implant
  W. implant
  W. iris knife
  W. knife
  W. lens scoop
  W. rectal catheter
  W. retractor

W. tissue scissors
W. winged catheter
Weber-Elschnig
W.-E. lens loupe
W.-E. loop
Web needle holder
Webril
W. bandage
W. dressing
Webster
W. abdominal retractor
W. coronary sinus catheter
W. infusion cannula
W. infusion tube
W. needle holder
W. retractor
W. ruler
W. skin graft knife
W. Vital needle holder
Webster-Halsey needle holder
Webster-Kleinert needle holder
Weck
W. astigmatism ruler
W. clamp
W. clip
W. clip applier
W. coagulating suction tube
W. dermatome
W. electrosurgery pencil
W. eye speculum
W. forceps
W. hemoclip
W. hysterectomy forceps
W. instrument cleaner
W. instrument holder
W. iris scissors
W. knife
W. liquid detergent
W. microsurgical tray
W. rectal biopsy forceps
W. shears
W. sponge
W. suction tube
W. suture-removal scissors
W. suture scissors
W. towel forceps
W. uterine biopsy forceps
W. wire-cutting scissors
Weck-cel
W.-c. dressing
W.-c. implant
W.-c. microsponge sponge
W.-c. prosthesis

W.-c. sponge
W.-c. surgical spear sponge
Weck-Edna nonperforating towel clamp
Wecker iris spatula
Weck-Harms forceps
Weck-Kare
W.-K. instrument lubricant
W.-K. kit instrument cleaner
Weck-Kleen instrument cleaner
Weck-Lube instrument lubricant
Weck-Prep
W.-P. blade
W.-P. infant soap
W.-P. orderly razor
Weck-Rack instrument holder
Wec-Kreem instrument lubricant
Weck-Spencer suture scissors
Weck-Wash detergent
Wec-Wash instrument cleaner
Weder
W. dissector
W. retractor
W. tongue depressor
Weder-Solenberger
W.-S. pillar retractor
W.-S. retractor
W.-S. tonsillar pillar retractor
W.-S. tonsillar retractor
wedge
w. balloon catheter
w. catheter
w. pressure balloon catheter
w. resection clamp
Wedge Cook catheter
wedge-line needle
Weeks
W. eye forceps
W. eye speculum
W. needle
Weerda laryngoscope
Wehmer TMJ radiographer
Wehrs incus prosthesis
Weider depressor
Weiger-Zollner forceps
weightbearing brace
weighted
w. posterior retractor
w. retractor
w. speculum

weighted *(continued)*
  w. speculum-retractor
  w. vaginal speculum
Weil
  W. cannula
  W. ear forceps
  W. ethmoidal forceps
  W. forceps
  W. lacrimal cannula
  W. pelvic sling
  W. pelvic snare
  W. pituitary rongeur
Weil-Blakesley
  W.-B. conchotome
  W.-B. ethmoidal forceps
  W.-B. rongeur
Weinberg
  W. blade
  W. "Joe's hoe" double-
  ended retractor
  W. retractor
  W. rib spreader
  W. vagotomy retractor
Weiner
  W. cannula
  W. speculum
  W. tourniquet
  W. uterine biopsy forceps
Weingartner
  W. ear forceps
  W. forceps
  W. rongeur
Weinstein
  W. horizontal retractor
  W. intestinal retractor
Weis chalazion forceps
Weise jack screw
Weisenbach
  W. forceps
  W. sterile forceps holder
Weisman
  W. cannula
  W. curette
  W. ear curette
  W. forceps
  W. infant ear curette
  W. tenaculum
  W. uterine tenaculum
  forceps
Weisman-Graves vaginal speculum
Weiss
  W. needle

  W. speculum
  W. spring
Weissbarth vaginal speculum
Weiss-pattern knife
Weitlaner
  W. brain retractor
  W. hinged retractor
  W. microsurgery retractor
  W. retractor
  W. self-retaining retractor
Welch
  W. Allyn anal biopsy
  forceps
  W. Allyn anoscope
  W. Allyn disposable
  laryngoscope
  W. Allyn dual-purpose
  otoscope
  W. Allyn fiberoptic
  sigmoidoscope
  W. Allyn flexible
  sigmoidoscope
  W. Allyn forceps
  W. Allyn hook
  W. Allyn illuminated
  speculum
  W. Allyn KleenSpec
  disposable laryngoscope
  W. Allyn KleenSpec
  fiberoptic disposable
  sigmoidoscope
  W. Allyn KleenSpec vaginal
  speculum
  W. Allyn laryngoscope
  W. Allyn laryngoscope blade
  W. Allyn operating otoscope
  W. Allyn ophthalmoscope
  W. Allyn probe
  W. Allyn proctoscope
  W. Allyn rectal probe
  W. Allyn scope
  W. Allyn sigmoidoscope
  W. Allyn standard
  retinoscope
  W. Allyn streak retinoscope
  W. Allyn suction tube
  W. Allyn transilluminator
  W. Allyn tube
  W. Allyn video endoscope
Weldon miniature bulldog clamp
Wellaminski antral perforator
Weller
  W. cartilage forceps

W. cartilage scissors
W. meniscal forceps
W. total hip joint
  prosthesis
Wellington
W. Hospital vaginal
  retractor
W. Hospital vaginal
  speculum
well-leg holder
Well Leg Support
Wells
W. cannula
W. clamp
W. enucleation scoop
W. enucleation spoon
W. forceps
W. irrigator
W. Johnson cannula
W. pedicle clamp
W. scleral suture pick
W. tractor
Wellwood-Ferguson introducer
Welsh
W. cannula
W. cortex extractor
W. erysiphake
W. flat-olive tip
W. forceps
W. olive-tipped needle
W. ophthalmological forceps
W. pupil spreader-retractor
  forceps
W. rubber bulb erysiphake
W. Silastic erysiphake
Wendl tube
Wenger slotted plate
Wepsic
W. fiberoptic cautery
W. suction tube
Werb
W. angled stricturotome
W. scissors
Werner suture
Wertheim
W. clamp
W. forceps
W. hysterectomy forceps
W. kidney pedicle clamp
W. needle holder
W. pedicle clamp
W. splint

W. uterine forceps
W. vaginal forceps
Wertheim-Cullen
W.-C. clamp
W.-C. compression forceps
W.-C. forceps
W.-C. hysterectomy forceps
W.-C. kidney pedicle clamp
W.-C. kidney pedicle
  forceps
W.-C. pedicle clamp
W.-C. pedicle forceps
Wertheim-Navratil
W.-N. forceps
W.-N. needle
Wertheim-Reverdin
W.-R. clamp
W.-R. pedicle clamp
Weser dental hinge
Wesolowski
W. bypass graft
W. prosthesis
W. Teflon graft
Wesson
W. mouth gag
W. perineal retractor
W. perineal self-retaining
  retractor
W. retractor
W. vaginal retractor
West
W. blunt dissector
W. blunt elevator
W. bone chisel
W. bone gouge
W. cannula
W. chisel
W. and elevator
W. hand dissector
W. lacrimal cannula
W. lacrimal chisel
W. lacrimal sac chisel
W. nasal chisel
W. nasal-dressing forceps
W. nasal gouge
W. plastic dissector
W. Shur cartilage clamp
West-Beck
W.-B. periosteotome
W.-B. spoon curette
Westcott
W. biopsy needle
W. conjunctival scissors

Westcott *(continued)*
  W. double-end scissors
  W. scissors
  W. spring-action scissors
  W. stitch scissors
  W. tenotomy scissors
  W. utility scissors
Westcott-Scheie scissors
Westcott-type stitch scissors
Wester
  W. clamp
  W. meniscal clamp
  W. meniscectomy scissors
Westerman-Jansen needle
Westermark
  W. forceps
  W. uterine dressing forceps
Westermark-Stille forceps
Western external urinary catheter
Westfield-style
  W.-s. acromioclavicular immobilizer
  W.-s. envelope sling
Westmacott
  W. dressing forceps
  W. forceps
Weston rectal snare
Westphal
  W. forceps
  W. gall duct forceps
  W. hemostatic forceps
wet
  w. bandage
  w. cup
  w. dressing
wet-field
  w.-f. cautery
  w.-f. coagulator
  w.-f. device
wet-to-dry dressing
Weve electrode
Wexler
  W. abdominal retractor
  W. deep-spreader blade abdominal retractor
  W. expandable-blade abdominal retractor
  W. large-frame abdominal retractor
  W. lateral side-blade abdominal retractor
  W. malleable-blade abdominal retractor

  W. retractor
  W. self-retaining retractor
  W. standard abdominal retractor
  W. standard-frame abdominal retractor
  W. Universal-joint abdominal retractor
  W. vaginal retractor
  W. X-P large abdominal retractor
Wexler-Balfour retractor
Wexler-Bantam retractor
Wexler-Deaver blade abdominal retractor
Wextran sponge
whalebone
  w. eustachian probe
  w. filiform bougie
  w. filiform catheter
wheel
  Excell polishing w.
Wheeler
  W. blade
  W. cyclodialysis spatula
  W. cystitome
  W. discission knife
  W. eye implant
  W. implant
  W. iris knife
  W. iris spatula
  W. knife
  W. plaque forceps
  W. sphere eye implant
  W. vessel forceps
Whip appliance
whip bougie
whipstitch suture
whirlybird
  w. excavator
  Hough w.
  w. needle
  w. probe
  w. stapes excavator
whisker, wisker
  slotted w.
whisk-packets dressing
whistle
  Bárány noise apparatus w.
  Galton ear w.
Whistler bougie
Whistle-Stop wireless aversive stimulator

(handwritten: locking device)

whistle-tip
> w.-t. catheter
> w.-t. drain
> w.-t. Foley catheter
> w.-t. ureteral catheter

Whitacre needle
Whitcomb-Kerrison
> W.-K. laminectomy punch
> W.-K. rongeur

White
> W. bone chisel
> W. chisel
> W. foam pessary
> W. forceps
> W. mallet
> W. Plume absorbent gauze
> W. scissors
> W. screwdriver
> W. system for pediatric percutaneous catheterization
> W. tonsillar forceps
> W. tonsillar hemostatic forceps
> W. tonsil-seizing forceps

white
> w. braided suture
> w. nylon suture
> w. silk suture
> w. suture
> w. twisted suture

Whitehead-Jennings mouth gag
Whitehead mouth gag
White-Lillie
> W.-L. forceps
> W.-L. tonsillar forceps
> W.-L. tonsil-seizing forceps

White-Oslay
> W.-O. forceps
> W.-O. prostatic forceps
> W.-O. prostatic lobe-holding forceps

White-Proud
> W.-P. retractor
> W.-P. uvular retractor

Whiteside prosthesis
White-Smith forceps
Whiting
> W. mastoid curette
> W. mastoid rongeur
> W. tonsillectome

Whitman
> W. fracture appliance
> W. fracture frame

Whitmore bag
Whittle spud
Whitver
> W. clamp
> W. penile clamp

Wholey-Edwards catheter
Wholey Hi-Torque modified J-guide wire
Whylie uterine dilator
Wiberg
> W. fracture staple
> W. fracture stapler
> W. raspatory

wick
> Bone-Dri femoral surgical w.
> w. dressing

Wick catheter
Wickman uterine forceps
wide
> w. seal diaphragm
> w. washer

Widex hearing aid
Widner transilluminator
Wiechel scissors
Wiechel-Stille bile duct scissors
Wieder
> W. dental retractor
> W. pillar retractor
> W. tonsillar dissector

Wieder-Solenberger pillar retractor
Wiegerinck culdocentesis puncture set
Wiener
> W. antral rasp
> W. corneal hook
> W. eye needle
> W. eye speculum
> W. hook
> W. hysterectomy forceps
> W. keratome
> W. nasal rasp
> W. scleral hook
> W. suture hook
> W. Universal frontal sinus rasp

Wiener-Pierce
> W.-P. antral rasp
> W.-P. antral trocar

Wies
- W. chalazion forceps
- W. forceps

Wiet
- W. graft-measuring instrument
- W. otologic cup forceps
- W. otologic scissors
- W. retractor

Wigand endoscopic instrument
Wigderson ribbon retractor
Wigmore
- W. plaster saw
- W. plaster saw with lift

Wikstroem
- W. arterial forceps
- W. forceps

Wikstrom gallbladder clamp
Wikstrom-Stilgust clamp
Wi-Last-Ic thread
Wilauer-Deaver retractor
Wilde
- W. ear forceps
- W. ear polyp snare
- W. ethmoidal exenteration forceps
- W. ethmoidal forceps
- W. ethmoidal punch
- W. forceps
- W. intervertebral disk forceps
- W. intervertebral disk rongeur
- W. laminectomy forceps
- W. nasal-cutting forceps
- W. nasal-dressing forceps
- W. nasal punch
- W. nasal snare
- W. rongeur
- W. septal forceps

Wilde-Blakesley
- W.-B. ethmoidal forceps
- W.-B. forceps

Wilde-Bruening
- W.-B. ear snare
- W.-B. nasal snare

Wilder
- W. cystitome
- W. cystitome knife
- W. dilating forceps
- W. dilator
- W. foreign body hook
- W. lacrimal dilator
- W. lens loop
- W. lens loupe
- W. lens scoop
- W. pick
- W. retractor
- W. scleral depressor
- W. scleral retractor
- W. scleral self-retaining retractor
- W. scleral wound retractor
- W. trephine

Wilde-Troeltsch forceps
Wildgen-Reck metal locator magnet
Wildhirt laparoscope
Wild laser
Wiles prosthesis
Wilgnath alloy
Wilkadium alloy
Wilke
- W. boot brace
- W. boot prosthesis
- W. brace

Wilkerson
- W. bur
- W. choanal bur

Wilkes self-retaining retractor
Wilkinson
- W. abdominal retractor
- W. abdominal self-retaining retractor
- W. retractor
- W. ring-frame abdominal retractor

Wilkinson-Deaver blade abdominal retractor
Wilkins trephine
Wilkoro alloy
Willauer
- W. intrathoracic forceps
- W. raspatory
- W. scissors

Willauer-Allis
- W.-A. forceps
- W.-A. thoracic forceps
- W.-A. thoracic tissue forceps
- W.-A. tissue forceps

Willauer-Deaver retractor
Willauer-Gibbon
- W.-G. elevator
- W.-G. periosteal elevator

Willett
- W. clamp
- W. forceps
- W. placental forceps
- W. placenta previa forceps
- W. scalp flap forceps

William
- W. Dixon collar scissors
- W. Dixon Cratex point
- W. Harvey arterial blood filter
- W. Harvey cardiotomy reservoir

William-House suction-irrigator
Williams
- W. brace
- W. cartilage knife
- W. catheter
- W. clamp
- W. craniotome
- W. cystoscopic needle
- W. dilator
- W. diskectomy forceps
- W. esophageal tube
- W. eye speculum
- W. forceps
- W. gastrointestinal forceps
- W. internal pelvimeter
- W. intestinal forceps
- W. lacrimal dilator
- W. lacrimal probe
- W. L-R guiding catheter
- W. microclip
- W. microlumbar diskectomy retractor
- W. microlumbar diskectomy suction retractor
- W. microlumbar retractor
- W. needle
- W. pediatric eye speculum
- W. perforator
- W. probe
- W. screwdriver
- W. splinter forceps
- W. tissue forceps
- W. tonsillar electrode
- W. uterine forceps
- W. vessel-holding forceps

Williamsburg forceps
Williamson biopsy needle
Williams-Watson ethmoidal punch
Williger
- W. bone curette

- W. ear curette
- W. elevator
- W. hammer
- W. raspatory

Willock
- W. jacket
- W. respiratory jacket

Wills
- W. eye lacrimal retractor
- W. Hospital eye cautery
- W. Hospital forceps
- W. Hospital ophthalmology forceps
- W. Hospital utility forceps
- W. spatula
- W. spoon with spatula
- W. utility eye forceps
- W. utility forceps

Wilman clamp
Wilmer
- W. chisel
- W. cryosurigal iris retractor
- W. iris forceps
- W. iris retractor
- W. iris scissors
- W. retractor
- W. scissors
- W. wedge chisel

Wilmer-Bagley
- W.-B. expressor
- W.-B. iris expressor
- W.-B. lens expressor
- W.-B. retractor

Wilmer-Converse conjunctival scissors
Wilmington jacket
Wilson
- W. amniotic trocar
- W. awl
- W. bolt
- W. clamp
- W. fracture appliance
- W. frame
- W. hand retractor
- W. intraocular scissors
- W. retractor
- W. rib spreader
- W. right-angled awl
- W. spinal frame
- W. spinal fusion plate
- W. vein stripper
- W. vitreous foreign body forceps

Wilson-Baylor amniotic trocar
Wilson-Cook
  W.-C. biopsy forceps
  W.-C. bronchoscope biopsy
    forceps
  W.-C. Carey capsule set
  W.-C. catheter
  W.-C. coagulation electrode
  W.-C. colonoscope biopsy
    forceps
  W.-C. cytology brush
  W.-C. eight-wire basket
    stone extractor
  W.-C. electrode needle
  W.-C. endoprosthesis
  W.-C. esophageal balloon
    prosthesis
  W.-C. esophageal prosthesis
  W.-C. French stent
  W.-C. gastric balloon
  W.-C. gastroscope biopsy
    forceps
  W.-C. grasping forceps
  W.-C. hot biopsy forceps
  W.-C. low-profile esophageal
    prosthesis set
  W.-C. minibasket
  W.-C. ministent retriever
  W.-C. papillotome
  W.-C. polypectomy snare
  W.-C. prosthesis repositioner
  W.-C. retrieval forceps
  W.-C. standard wire guide
  W.-C. stone basket
  W.-C. tripod retrieval
    forceps
  W.-C. wire-guided
    sphincterotome
Wilson-Kirbe speculum
Wiltberger spinous process
  spreader
Wil-Tex alloy
Wilton-Webster coronary sinus
  catheter
Wiltse-Bankart retractor
Wiltse-Gelpi
  W.-G. retractor
  W.-G. self-retaining retractor
Wiltse iliac retractor
Wincor enucleation scissors
Windmill suction evacuation unit

window
  Buie sigmoidoscope
    dilating w.
  w. clip
  w. rasp
  w. rasp marker
Winer catheter
wing
  w. clip
  w. suture
winged
  w. catheter
  w. retractor blade
Wingfield fracture frame
Winkelmann circumcision clamp
Winsburg-White
  W.-W. bladder tube
  W.-W. retractor
Winston SD catheter
Winter
  W. arch bar
  W. elevator
  W. facial fracture appliance
  W. ovum forceps
  W. splint
Winter-Nassauer placental forceps
Winternitz sound
wipes
  Microclens w.
wire
  AES Amplatz guide w.
  Amplatz guide w.
  Ancrofil clasp w.
  angled guide w.
  angle-tipped guide w.
  anterior chamber
    retaining w.
  w. appliance
  argon guide w.
  Australian orthodontic w.
  Babcock w.
  Babcock stainless steel
    suture w.
  Babcock suture w.
  Baron suction tube-
    cleaning w.
  beaded cerclage w.
  beaded guide w.
  Becton-Dickinson guide w.
  w. bending die
  Benson w.
  Bentson exchange straight
    guide w.

Bentson guide w.
w. bivalve vaginal speculum
bone fixation w.
Cannu-Flex guide w.
catheter guide w.
cerclage w.
Charnley trochanter w.
coiled spiral pusher w.
Compere fixation w.
Cook straight guide w.
Cope mandril guide w.
w. crimper
Crozat orthodontic w.
cut snare w.
w. cutter
Dentaflex w.
w. drill
w. and drill guide
w. driver
ear snare w.
Elastorc catheter guide w.
Eve-Neivert tonsillar w.
E wildcat orthodontic w.
exchange w.
w. fixation bolt
flexible-tip J-guide w.
floppy guide w.
Frankfeldt rectal snare
  hinged-loop w.
Geenen Endotorque
  guide w.
Gigli spiral saw w.
glide w.
Glidewire guide w.
w. guide
guide w.
Hahnenkratt orthodontic w.
Hancock temporary cardiac
  pacing w.
heparin-coated guide w.
Hi-Per Flex w.
Hi-Per Flex exchange w.
Hi-Torque floppy exchange
  guide w.
Hi-Torque floppy guide w.
Hi-Torque intermediate
  guide w.
House piston w.
Hyperflex flexible guide w.
intermaxillary w.
interosseous w.
Isotac pilot w.
J-guide w.

Johnson canaliculus w.
Kadir Hi-Torque guide w.
Katzen w.
Kirchner w.
Kirschner w., K-wire
Kirschner boring w.
w. lid speculum
Linx extension w.
w. loop
w. loop dilator
w. loop stapes dilator
Lunderquist guide w.
w. mandrin
Markley orthodontic w.
Medi-Tech guide w.
w. mesh eye implant
nasal snare w.
Neivert-Eves tonsillar w.
Newton guide w.
Newton LLT guide w.
New Yorker guide w.
olive w.
w. pass bur
w. passer
PD orthodontic w.
PDT guide w.
phantom w.
phantom guide w.
piston w.
w. probe
w. prosthesis
w. prosthesis-crimping
  forceps
prosthesis smooth w.
Radiofocus catheter
  guide w.
rectal cautery w.
rectal snare hinged-loop w.
rectal snare replacement w.
Reflex SuperSoft steerable
  guide w.
Remaloy w.
Remanium w.
Rosen guide w.
Rosen J-guide w.
round chuck-end
  Kirschner w.
Saf-T J guide w.
Sage w.
w. saw
w. scissors
w. side blade
silk guide w.

wire *(continued)*
>>Simcoe anterior chamber-retaining w.
>>Sippy esophageal dilator coiled spiral pusher w.
>>smooth transfixion w.
>>w. snare
>>snare w.
>>w. speculum
>>w. speculum wire guide
>>w. splint
>>stainless steel w.
>>stainless steel guide w.
>>stainless steel suture w.
>>w. stapes prosthesis
>>Sterling-Spring orthodontic w.
>>Storz twisted snare w.
>>straight guide w.
>>w. stylet catheter
>>sublaminar w.
>>suction tube-cleaning w.
>>w. suture
>>suture w.
>>w. suture scissors
>>Teflon-coated guide w.
>>Terumo guide w.
>>w. threader
>>w. tightener
>>tip-deflecting w.
>>tonsillar snare w.
>>trocar point Kirschner w.
>>w. twister
>>Ultra-Select Nitinol PTCA guide w.
>>veneer retention w.
>>Veri-Flex guide w.
>>Wholey Hi-Torque modified J-guide w.
>>Wironit clasp w.
>>Wirotom clasp w.
>>Zimaloy beaded suture w.
>>Zimaloy suture w.
>>w. Zytor suture

wire-closure forceps
wire-crimping forceps
wire-cutting scissors
wire-fat ear prosthesis
wire-guided
>>w.-g. biliary manometry catheter set
>>w.-g. papillotome
>>w.-g. sphincterotome

wire-loop strut
wire-pulling forceps
wire-tightening clamp
wire-twisting forceps
wire-wound cannula
wiring retractor
Wironit clasp wire
Wirosol investment material
Wirotom clasp wire
Wirovest investment material
Wirthlin
>>W. splenorenal clamp
>>W. splenorenal shunt clamp
Wisap/USA
>>W. diagnostic laparoscope
>>W. operating laparoscope
Wisconsin
>>W. laryngoscope
>>W. laryngoscope blade
>>W. stainless steel laryngoscope blade
Wise
>>W. dilator
>>W. orbital retractor
>>W. retractor
Wis-Foregger laryngoscope
Wishard
>>W. catheter
>>W. tip catheter
>>W. tip ureteral catheter
Wis-Hipple laryngoscope
wisker *(var. of* whisker)
Wissinger
>>W. rod
>>W. set
Wister
>>W. clamp
>>W. forceps holder
>>W. nipper
>>W. vascular clamp
Withers tendon passer
Wit portable TENS system
Witt
>>W. dental light
>>W. fiberoptic hand piece
Wittmoser optical arm
Wittner
>>W. cervical biopsy punch
>>W. forceps
>>W. uterine biopsy forceps
Witzel enterostomy catheter
Witzel gastrostomy
Wizard disposable inflation device

Woakes nasal saw
Wolf
- W. antral needle
- W. biopsy forceps
- W. biting-basket forceps
- W. cannula
- W. catheter
- W. curved-basket forceps
- W. drainage cannula
- W. endoscope
- W. hemostatic bag
- W. insufflation laparoscope
- W. laparoscope
- W. Loktite mouth gag
- W. meniscal retractor
- W. mouth gag
- W. needle trocar
- W. nephrostomy bag catheter
- W. nephrostomy catheter
- W. photolaparoscope
- W. return-flow cannula

Wolf-Cottle trocar
Wolfe
- W. cataract delivery forceps
- W. eye forceps
- W. graft
- W. implant
- W. prosthesis
- W. uterine cuff forceps

Wölfe-Böhler, Wolfe-Boehler
- W.-B. cast breaker
- W.-B. cast remover
- W.-B. plaster cast spreader

Wölfe-Krause
- W.-K. graft
- W.-K. implant

Wolferman drill
Wolff
- W. dermal curette
- W. drain

wolffian drain
Wolf-Henning gastroscope
Wolf-Knittlingen gastroscope
Wölfler suture
Wolf-Post rhinoscope
Wolf-Schindler gastroscope
Wolfson
- W. clamp
- W. forceps
- W. gallbladder retractor
- W. intestinal clamp
- W. retractor

- W. spur crusher
- W. spur-crushing clamp

Wolf Veress needle
Wolf-Yoon
- W.-Y. applicator
- W.-Y. ring

Wolvek
- W. approximator
- W. fixation device
- W. sternal approximator

Wood
- W. aortography needle
- W. bulldog clamp
- W. colonic kit
- W. needle
- W. screw

wood
- w. roll dressing
- w. tongue blade
- w. tongue depressor

Woodbridge
- W. suture
- W. tube

Woodruff
- W. catheter
- W. screw
- W. screwdriver
- W. spatula knife
- W. ureteropyelographic catheter

Woodson
- W. dental periosteal elevator
- W. double-ended dissector
- W. dural separator
- W. elevator
- W. elevator spatula
- W. obstetrical spoon
- W. packer
- W. plug
- W. spatula

Woods Surgitek bra
Woodward
- W. antral rasp
- W. forceps
- W. hemostatic forceps
- W. retractor
- W. sound
- W. thoracic artery forceps
- W. thoracic hemostatic forceps

Woodward-Potts intestinal forceps
Wooten eye needle

Worcester
W. City Hospital speculum
W. instrument holder
Word catheter
Work-Bruening diagnostic head
work station
Coritaxic multimodal
stereotaxic w.s.
Worrall
W. deep retractor
W. headband
W. retractor
Worst
W. corneal contact glass
W. double-ended pigtail
probe
W. lens
W. lobster-claw lens
W. Medallion lens
W. medallion suture
W. pigtail probe
W. probe
Wort antral retractor
Worth
W. advancement forceps
W. chisel
W. cystitome
W. forceps
W. muscle forceps
W. strabismus forceps
wound
w. clip
w. drain
w. drainage reservoir
w. dressing
w. forceps
w. tubing
wound-clip forceps
Wound-Evac kit
woven
w. catheter
w. elastic bandage
w. loop stone dislodger
woven-loop
w.-l. dislodger
w.-l. stone dislodger
woven-silk catheter
woven-tube vascular graft
prosthesis
Wozniak Sur-Lok chuck
wrap
Ace w.

wraparound
w. dressing
w. inactive electrode
wrench
Barton w.
beaded pin w.
Budde halo w.
Canakis w.
Cloward spanner w.
Hagie w.
Halifax w.
hex w.
hexagonal w.
hex socket w.
Kurlander orthopaedic w.
Richmond subarachnoid w.
Santa Casa w.
slotted w.
socket w.
spanner w.
spinal slip w.
Stader w.
Stille w.
Thomas w.
torque w.
Trinkle socket w.
Waldon w.
Wright
W. Care-TENS device
W. fascial needle
W. knee plate
W. knee prosthesis
W. nasal snare
W. needle
W. ophthalmic needle
W. peak-flow meter
W. pneumatic tourniquet
W. prosthesis
W. ptosis needle
W. tonsillar snare
W. Universal brace
Wright-Crawford needle
Wright-Guilford
W.-G. curette
W.-G. cutting block
W.-G. double-edged knife
W.-G. drum elevator
W.-G. elevator-flap knife
W.-G. elevator knife
W.-G. fenestrometer
W.-G. flap knife
W.-G. footplate pick
W.-G. incudostapedial knife

W.-G. microbone curette
W.-G. middle ear
instrument
W.-G. roller knife
W.-G. stapes pick
W.-G. wire cutter
Wright-Harloe empyema trocar
Wright-Rubin
W.-R. forceps
W.-R. forceps guard
Wrigley forceps
wrist
WR surgical nerve stimulator
W-shape forceps
Wullen
W. dislodger
W. stone dislodger
Wullstein
W. bur
W. chuck adapter
W. contra-angle handpiece
W. curette
W. diamond bur
W. double-edged knife
W. drill
W. ear forceps
W. ear scissors
W. ear self-retaining
retractor
W. forceps
W. handpiece
W. high-speed bur
W. microsuction tube
W. ototympanoscope
otoscope
W. retractor
W. ring curette
W. scissors
W. transplant spatula
W. tympanoplasty forceps
Wullstein-House forceps
Wullstein-Paparella forceps

Wullstein-Weitlaner
W.-W. retractor
W.-W. self-retaining
retractor
Wunderer modification activator
Wurd catheter
Wurmuth spatula
Wurth
W. spur crusher
W. vein stripper
Wurzelheber dental elevator
Wutzler scissors
W. W. Walker appliance
Wyler
W. electrode
W. subdural strip electrode
Wylie
W. carotid artery clamp
W. clamp
W. dilator
W. drain
W. endarterectomy set
W. endarterectomy stripper
W. forceps
W. hypogastric clamp
W. "J" clamp
W. lumbar bulldog clamp
W. renal vein retractor
W. retractor
W. spatula
W. splanchnic retractor
W. stem pessary
W. tenaculum
W. tenaculum forceps
W. uterine dilator
W. uterine forceps
W. uterine tenaculum
W. uterine tenaculum
forceps
Wylie-Post rhinoscope
Wynne-Evans tonsillar dissector
Wysler suture

X-Acto utility knife
Xanar
  X. 20 Amulase CO2 laser
  X. laser adapter
Xaner laser bronchoscope
X-Cel dental x-ray unit
xenograft
  Carpentier-Edwards x.
  Ionescu-Shiley pericardial x.
xenon
  x. arc coagulator
  x. arc photocoagulator
  x. coagulator
  x. cold light fountain
  x. lamp
  x. light source
  x. photocoagulator
Xenophor femoral prosthesis
Xeroflo dressing
Xeroform dressing
XGT ultrasonic scaler
XL-11 Ranfac percutaneous
  cholangiographic catheter

X-long cement forceps
Xomed
  X. Audiant bone conductor
  X. Doyle nasal airway
    splint
  X. endotracheal tube
  X. intraoral artificial larynx
  X. micro-oscillating saw
  X. rectal probe
  X. Silastic splint
  X. sinus irrigation kit
  X. straight-shank tube
Xomed-Treace ventilation tube
Xpanderm
x-ray
  x.-r. calipers
  x.-r. detectable laparotomy
    sponge
  x.-r. overlay
X-ray translucent retractor
Xyrel pacemaker

YAG
  yttrium-aluminum-garnet
  YAG laser
Yalon intraocular lens
Yamagishi stapler
Yamanda knife
Yankauer
  Y. antral punch
  Y. antral trocar
  Y. aspirating tube
  Y. bronchoscope
  Y. catheter
  Y. curette
  Y. ear curette
  Y. esophagoscope
  Y. ethmoidal forceps
  Y. ethmoid-cutting forceps
  Y. eustachian catheter
  Y. forceps
  Y. hook
  Y. laryngoscope
  Y. ligature passer
  Y. middle meatus cannula
  Y. nasopharyngeal speculum
  Y. needle
  Y. probe
  Y. punch
  Y. salpingeal curette
  Y. salpingeal probe
  Y. scissors
  Y. septal needle
  Y. suction tube
  Y. suture needle
  Y. tube
Yankauer-Little
  Y.-L. forceps
  Y.-L. tube forceps
Yarmo morcellizer
Yasargil
  Y. alligator-type forceps
  Y. aneurysm clip-applier
  Y. angled forceps
  Y. applying forceps
  Y. arachnoid knife
  Y. arterial forceps
  Y. bayonet needle holder
  Y. bayonet scissors
  Y. bayonet-shaped forceps
  Y. bipolar forceps
  Y. carotid clamp

  Y. clamp
  Y. clip
  Y. clip applier
  Y. clip-applying forceps
  Y. curette
  Y. dissector
  Y. forceps
  Y. ligature carrier
  Y. microclip
  Y. microdissector
  Y. microforceps
  Y. microneedle holder
  Y. microraspatory
  Y. microscissors
  Y. microsuction tube
  Y. microvascular bayonet
    scissors
  Y. microvessel clip applying
    forceps
  Y. needle holder
  Y. neurosurgical bipolar
    forceps
  Y. raspatory
  Y. retractor
  Y. scissors
  Y. scoop
  Y. spring hook
  Y. straight forceps
  Y. suction tube
  Y. tissue lifter
Yazujian
  Y. bur
  Y. cataract bur
Y-bandage dressing
Y-bone plate
Yeates drain
Yeder suction tube
Yellen
  Y. circumcision clamp
  Y. clamp
yellow-eyed dilating bougie
Yellow Springs probe
yellow-tip aspirator
Yeoman
  Y. biopsy forceps
  Y. biopsy punch
  Y. forceps
  Y. probe
  Y. proctoscope
  Y. rectal biopsy forceps

Yeoman *(continued)*
  Y. sigmoidoscope
  Y. uterine forceps
Yeoman-Wittner
  Y.-W. rectal biopsy forceps
  Y.-W. rectal forceps
Yoon
  Y. applicator
  Y. ring
  Y.-ring applicator
  Y. tubal sterilization ring
Yoshida
  Y. aspirating tonsillar
    dissector
  Y. dental x-ray unit
  Y. dissector
  Y. tonsillar dissector
Young
  Y. anterior prostatic
    retractor
  Y. anterior retractor
  Y. bifid retractor
  Y. bladder retractor
  Y. boomerang needle holder
  Y. bulb retractor
  Y. clamp
  Y. cystoscope
  Y. cystoscopic rongeur
  Y. dilator
  Y. dissector
  Y. forceps
  Y. intestinal forceps
  Y. lateral prostatic retractor
  Y. lateral retractor
  Y. ligature carrier
  Y. lobe forceps
  Y. needle holder
  Y. pediatric rectal dilator
  Y. prostatectomy forceps
  Y. prostatic enucleator
  Y. prostatic forceps
  Y. prostatic retractor
  Y. prostatic tractor

  Y. rectal dilator
  Y. renal pedicle clamp
  Y. retractor
  Y. rongeur
  Y. rubber dam fracture
    frame
  Y. rubber-jaws forceps
  Y. tongue forceps
  Y. tongue-holding forceps
  Y. tongue-seizing forceps
  Y. urological dissector
  Y. uterine forceps
  Y. vaginal dilator
  Y. vaginal dilator set
Younge
  Y. endometrial curette
  Y. forceps
  Y. irrigator
  Y. modified endometrial
    biopsy curette
  Y. uterine biopsy curette
  Y. uterine biopsy forceps
  Y. uterine curette
  Y. uterine forceps
Younge-Kevorkian forceps
**Young-Hryntschak boomerang
  needle holder**
Young-Millin
  Y.-M. boomerang needle
    holder
  Y.-M. holder
Younken double-lumen drain
**Yours Truly asymmetrical external
  breast form**
Y-trough catheter
yttrium-aluminum-garnet (YAG)
Yuan screw
Yucca wood splint
Yund
  Y. acetabular skid
  Y. knife
  Y. ligamentum teres knife
  Y. skid

Zachary-Cope clamp
Zachary-Cope-DeMartel
    Z.-C.-D. clamp
    Z.-C.-D. colon clamp
    Z.-C.-D. triple-colon clamp
Zalkind-Balfour
    Z.-B. blade
    Z.-B. center-blade retractor
    Z.-B. self-retaining retractor
Zalkind lung retractor
Zander apparatus
Zarski gallstone scoop
Zaufel-Jansen
    Z.-J. bone rongeur
    Z.-J. ear hook
    Z.-J. rongeur
Zavod
    Z. aneroid pneumothorax
      apparatus
    Z. bronchospirometry
      catheter
    Z. catheter
Zawadzki cystitome
Zeeifel angiotribe forceps
Zein loupe
Zeiss
    Z. aspheric lens
    Z. camera
    Z. coagulator
    Z. colposcope
    Z. H laser
    Z. laser
    Z. lens loupe
    Z. MD laser
    Z. operating camera
    Z. operating microscope
    Z. ophthalmoscope
    Z. photocoagulator
    Z. small beam splitter
    Z. stone dislodger
    Z. ureteral stone dislodger
    Z. xenon arc
      photocoagulator
Zeiss-Scheimpflug camera
Zenker
    Z. dissecting and ligature
      forceps
    Z. forceps
    Z. raspatory
    Z. retractor

Zephyr rubber elastic dressing
Zeppelin obstetrical forceps
zero-degree laparoscope
Zest subperiosteal implant
Z-fixation nail
Zickel
    Z. II subtrochanteric rod
    Z. nail
    Z. supracondylar rod
Ziegler
    Z. blade
    Z. cautery
    Z. cautery electrode
    Z. ciliary forceps
    Z. dilator
    Z. double-ended lacrimal
      dilator
    Z. eye speculum
    Z. forceps
    Z. iris knife
    Z. iris knife-needle
    Z. knife-needle
    Z. lacrimal dilator
    Z. lacrimal probe
    Z. needle
    Z. needle-knife
    Z. needle probe
    Z. probe
Ziegler-Furness clamp
Zielke
    Z. instrumentation
    Z. scoliosis gouge
Zilkie device
Zimalate
    Z. drill
    Z. twist drill
Zimaloy
    Z. beaded suture wire
    Z. cobalt-chromium-
      molybdenum alloy
    Z. epiphyseal staple
    Z. femoral head prosthesis
    Z. suture wire
Zimberg esophageal hiatal
  retractor
Zimcode traction frame
Zim-Flux dressing
Zimfoam
    Z. head halter

Zimfoam *(continued)*
- Z. pin
- Z. splint

Zimmer
- Z. airplane splint
- Z. Anatomic hip prosthesis system
- Z. antiembolism stockings
- Z. bolt
- Z. bone cement
- Z. bur
- Z. cartilage clamp
- Z. clamp
- Z. clavicular cross splint
- Z. drill
- Z. driver
- Z. extractor
- Z. fracture frame
- Z. Gigli-saw blades
- Z. goniometer
- Z. hand drill
- Z. head halter
- Z. Orthair ream driver
- Z. pin
- Z. protractor
- Z. screw
- Z. screwdriver
- Z. shoulder prosthesis
- Z. skin graft mesher
- Z. snare
- Z. splint
- Z. telescoping nail
- Z. tibial bolt
- Z. tibial nail cap
- Z. tibial prosthesis
- Z. Total Shoulder II
- Z. Universal drill

Zimmer-Hall drive system
Zimmer-Hoen forceps
Zimmer-Hudson shank
Zimmer-Kirschner hand drill
Zimmer-Schlesinger forceps
Zimmon
- Z. catheter
- Z. endoscopic biliary stent set
- Z. endoscopic pancreatic stent set
- Z. papillotome/sphincterotome

Zimocel dressing

Zim-Trac
- Z.-T. traction splint
- Z.-T. traction splint tractor

Zim-Zip rib belt splint
zinc ball electrode
Zinn endoilluminiation infusion cannula
Zipser
- Z. clamp
- Z. meatal clamp
- Z. meatal dilator
- Z. penile clamp

Zipster rib guillotine
Zirconia orthopaedic prosthetic head
Ziskie operating laparoscope
Ziski iris clip intraocular lens
Zitron pacemaker
ZIV laryngeal depressor
ZMS intramedullary fixation system
Zmurkiewicz
- Z. brain clip
- Z. clip applier

Zobec sponge dressing
Zoeffle soft intraocular lens
Zoellner
- Z. hook
- Z. needle
- Z. raspatory
- Z. scissors

Zoll
- Z. NTP pacemaker
- Z. pacemaker

Zollinger
- Z. forceps
- Z. multipurpose tissue forceps
- Z. splint

Zollinger-Gilmore vein stripper
Zollner suction tube
Zonas
- Z. porous adhesive tape dressing
- Z. porous tape

zonule separator
Zoroc resin plaster dressing
Zower speculum
Z-plate plate
Z retractor
Zucker
- Z. cardiac catheter
- Z. catheter

Z. multipurpose bipolar
catheter
Z. splint
Zuelzer
Z. awl
Z. hook plate
Zuker bipolar pacing electrode
Zund-Burguet apparatus
Zurich dilatation catheter
Zutt clamp
Zwanck radium pessary
Zweifel
Z. angiotribe
Z. appendectomy clamp
Z. needle holder
Z. pressure clamp
Zweifel-DeLee cranioclast
Zweymuller hip prosthesis
Zyderm
Z. collagen implant
Z. implant
zygoma
z. elevator
z. hook

zygomaticofrontal suture
zygomaticomaxillary suture
zygomaticotemporal suture
zygomatic suture
Zyler
Z. head halter
Z. tube
Zylik
Z. cannula
Z. microclip
Z. ophthalmoendoscope
Zylik-Joseph hook
Zylik-Michaels
Z.-M. retractor
Z.-M. scissors
Z.-M. speculum
Zyplast implant
Zytor suture
Zywiec electrode

GOT A GOOD WORD FOR THE NEXT EDITION OF

THIS **STEDMAN'S WORD BOOK?**

Help us keep future editions of this **Stedman's Word Book** fresh and up-to-date with new words and new ideas!

What's going on in your field? Are there new terms being used in this specialty? Are there better, easier ways for organizing the book's content?

Be specific! We want to know how we can make this **Stedman's Word Book** the very best specialty medical word reference possible for you. So go ahead and fill-in the lines below with your best thoughts and recommendations. Attach a separate sheet of paper if you have to—*you* are our most important contributor and we want to know what's on *your* mind!

Thanks!

(PLEASE TYPE OR PRINT CLEARLY)

OK, here's what I think: _____

_____

_____

_____

_____

_____

_____

_____

_____

_____

All done? Great, just detach this card and mail today. No postage necessary, and thanks again!

Name _____ Title _____

Facility _____

Address _____

_____

City _____ State _____ Zip _____-____

Day Telephone No. ( ) _____

Williams & Wilkins
428 East Preston Street • Baltimore, MD 21202-6564

7954-9 MEDEQUIP

BUSINESS REPLY MAIL

FIRST CLASS   PERMIT NO. 724   BALTIMORE, MD

POSTAGE WILL BE PAID BY ADDRESSEE

Williams & Wilkins
ATTN: REFERENCE DIVISION/Gail Russell
P.O.Box Box 1496
Baltimore, Maryland 21298-9724

Appendix 1
Cesarean Delivery

Adson forceps
Adson pickup
Allis clamp
Army-Navy retractor
Babcock clamp
Balfour retractor
bandage scissors
Billroth tumor forceps
bladder retractor
Bookwalter retractor
Crile-Wood needle holder
curved hemostat
DeLee Universal retractor
Heaney needle holder
Kelly clamp
Kocher clamp
Lister scissors
malleable retractor
Mayo curved scissors

Mayo-Hegar needle holder
Mayo straight scissors
Metzenbaum long scissors
Metzenbaum scissors
Murless head retractor
Ochsner forceps
O'Sullivan-O'Connor retractor
Pennington clamp
Phaneuf uterine artery forceps
rat-tooth pickup
Richardson retractor
Rochester-Péan forceps
Schroeder tenaculum forceps
Schroeder uterine vulsellum forceps
Singley forceps
sponge forceps
thumb retractor
tissue forceps

Appendix 2
Cholecystectomy

Balfour retractor with fenestrated
  blade
bayonet forceps
Crile forceps
Cushing dressing forceps
Cushing forceps
cystic duct catheter clamp
Doyen intestinal forceps
Frazier suction tip
French-eye Vital needle holder
gallbladder ring clamp
hemostatic clamp
Jarit forceps
Jarit mosquito forceps

Kelly forceps
Lahey thoracic
Mayo scissors
Mayo scoop
Metzenbaum scissors
Mixter ligature-carrier clamp
mosquito forceps
Ochsner forceps
Péan forceps
Rochester-Ochsner forceps
Rochester-Péan forceps
Stille Super Cut scissors
subcostal trocar
towel clip

Appendix 3
Dilatation and Curettage (D & C)

Auvard speculum
Backhaus clamp
Bozeman uterine-dressing forceps
Braun-Schroeder single-tooth
  tenaculum
Crile forceps
Crile hemostat
Deaver retractor
dressing forceps
Duncan curette
Graves bivalve speculum
Green uterine curette
Heaney curette
Hegar dilator
Jackson right-angle retractor
Jacobs tenaculum
Kelly clamp
Kelly-Gray curette
Kevorkian-Younge biopsy forceps

Kevorkian-Younge curette
Laufe polyp forceps
Mayo-Hegar needle holder
Mayo scissors
Pratt dilator
progressive dilators
Randall stone forceps
Rochester-Péan forceps
Schroeder uterine tenaculum
Schubert uterine biopsy forceps
Sims curette
sponge forceps
sponge stick
Thomas curette
Thoms-Gaylor biopsy forceps
tissue forceps
towel clip
uterine sound
weighted speculum

Appendix 4
Cardiac Catheterization

Activase
angiogram
angled pigtail catheter
bicycle ergometry
cineangiogram
flash-lamp excited pulsed dye
flexible-tip J-guide wire
floppy guide wire
guide wire
Hartzler ACS coronary dilation
   catheter
HDL — high-density lipoprotein
Hemashield collagen-enhanced graft
high-density lipoprotein (HDL)

Inoue balloon catheter
Judkins catheter
laser taper
LDL — low-density lipoprotein
low-density lipoprotein (LDL)
Reflex pacemaker
Relay pacemaker
scattergram
Seldinger catheter
side port
thallium-102 stress test
USCI catheter
venous sheath

Appendix 5
Cataract Lens Extraction

Allergan Medical Optics (AMO)
AMO — Allergan Medical Optics
AMO intraocular lens implant
anchor suture
Anis forceps
argon laser
balanced salt solution (BSS)
#15 Bard-Parker blade
Beaver blade
16-bite nylon suture
biting rongeur
bridle suture
brow tape
BSS — balanced salt solution
BV100 needle
capsulorrhexis forceps
cardiac monitor
cardinal suture
Cavitron I&A handpiece
Charles irrigating lens
Cilco intraocular lens
clovehitch suture
Coburn intraocular lens
collagen shield
collar button
CooperVision I&A machine
corneoscleral scissors
cortex-aspirating cannula
cryopexy
cryotherapy probe
cutter
cystitome
Dacron suture
Descemet punch
diathermy electrode
Diode endolaser
disposable trephine
1021 drape
endodiathermy
endo-illuminator
endolaser
eraser cautery
eraser-tip cautery
exoplant
explant
Flieringa ring
flute needle

Fox eye shield
gentian violet marking pen
Geuder implanter
girth hitch
Graefe forceps
Graefe strabismus hook
Grieshaber blade
Grieshaber endo-illuminator
Guibor tube
Honan balloon
Hyde astigmatism ruler
I&A — irrigation and aspiration
I&A machine
Iliff trephine
indirect ophthalmoscope
interrupted nylon suture
IOLAB intraocular lens
Ioptex intraocular lens
irrigating cystitome
irrigation and aspiration (I&A)
Jaffe lid speculum
Jarit bladebreaker
Kaufman eye vitrector
Kelman-McPherson corneal forceps
keratome
Kratz polisher
Kratz scratcher
Kuglen hook
lens loop
lid speculum
light pipe
loupe magnification
Maumenee forceps
Mayo stand
McPherson forceps
microvitrector
microvitreoretinal (MVR)
mosquito clamp
muscle hook
MVR — microvitreoretinal
MVR blade
nasal-tip dressing
Novus 2000 ophthalmoscope
ocutome vitrector
ophthalmoscope
Ophthalon suture
ORC intraocular lens

Cataract Lens Extraction

oximeter
pencil cautery
pencil-tip cautery
Peyman vitrector
Pharmacia intraocular lens
Pierse Colibri utility forceps
Prolene suture
pulse oximeter
radial keratotomy (RK)
radial keratotomy marker
RK — radial keratotomy
RK marker
running nylon suture
scarifier knife
Schiøtz tonometer
scleral band
scleral shell
Sheets glide
Shepard forceps
sickle-shaped blade
silicone explant
silicone tube
silk traction suture
Simcoe loop
Sinskey hook
SITE I&A instrument

SITE irrigating-aspirating unit
SITE needle
SITE TXR phacoemulsification system
Steri-Strips dressing
Storz band
Superblade
Sutherland scissors
Telfa pad
TG140 needle
Troutman punch
Utrata forceps
Vicryl suture
vitrector
vitreous cutter
Weck astigmatism ruler
Weck-cel
Weck sponge
Weiner speculum
Westcott scissors
wet-field cautery
Wheeler blade
Wheeler knife
wire lid speculum
Y-hook
Zeiss operating microscope

Appendix 6
Total Abdominal Hysterectomy

Adson ganglion scissors
Allis clamp
Allis forceps
Army-Navy retractor
Babcock clamp
Balfour bladder blade
Balfour retractor
Ballantine clamp
Billroth tumor forceps
bladder blade
Bookwalter retractor
Deaver retractor
DeBakey clamp
DeBakey tissue forceps
double-tooth tenaculum
Goulet retractor
Harrington retractor
Heaney clamp
Heaney hysterectomy forceps
Heaney needle holder
Jacobs tenaculum
Jorgenson scissors

Kelly clamp
Kocher clamp
Mayo scissors
Ochsner forceps
O'Sullivan-O'Connor retractor
Péan forceps
pedicle clamp
right-angle scissors
Roberts thumb retractor
Rochester-Ochsner forceps
Russian tissue forceps
Schroeder tenaculum
Schroeder tenaculum forceps
Schroeder vulsellar forceps
self-retaining retractor
single-tooth tenaculum
sponge forceps
sponge-holding forceps
thoracic clamp
tissue forceps
uterine clamp

Appendix 7
Vaginal Delivery

Allis clamp
Auvard speculum
Backhaus clamp
Barton forceps
Baumberger forceps
Billroth tumor forceps
Bill traction handle forceps
Bird vacuum extractor
Braun episiotomy scissors
Crile forceps
DeLee forceps
DeWeese axis traction obstetrical
  forceps
Dewey forceps
dressing forceps
Elliott obstetrical forceps
English lock
French lock
Gelpi perineal retractor
German lock
Haig Ferguson obstetrical forceps
Halsted mosquito hemostatic
  forceps
Hawk-Dennen forceps
Hodge forceps
Kelly clamp
Kelly retractor
Kjelland-Barton forceps
Kjelland forceps

Kjelland-Luikart forceps
Kobayashi vacuum extractor
Luikart forceps
Malström vacuum extractor
Mayo-Hegar needle holder
Mayo scissors
McLane obstetrical forceps
Mityvac extractor
Mityvac vacuum delivery system
Mityvac vacuum extractor
Murless head extractor
Naegele forceps
Ochsner forceps
Piper forceps
pivot lock
Russian tissue forceps
Schroeder tenaculum
Shute forceps
Silastic cup extractor
Simpson forceps
sliding lock
sponge stick
straight scissors
Tarnier axis-traction forceps
tissue forceps
towel clip
Tucker-McLane axis-traction
  forceps
Tucker-McLane-Luikart forceps

Appendix 8
Transurethral Prostatectomy

Adson clamp
Adson forceps
Alexander elevator
Allis clamp
Army-Navy retractor
Babcock clamp
Bovie electrocautery
Bovie holder
bulldog clamp
Crile angle retractor
curved hemostat
Cushing forceps
Deaver retractor
Ellik evacuator
Foroblique resectoscope
Frazier suction tube
Gerald forceps
Gil-Vernet retractor
hemostat
Herrick clamp
Herrick kidney clamp
Iglesias fiberoptic resectoscope
kidney pedicle clamp
Kocher clamp
long scalpel
long tissue forceps

malleable retractor
Mayo-Hegar needle holder
Mayo scissors
McBurney retractor
Metzenbaum scissors
Millin bladder retractor
Millin forceps
Moynihan clamp
Poole suction tube
Potts forceps
Randall stone forceps
resectoscope
resectoscope sheath
ribbon retractor
Richardson retractor
right-angle clamp
sponge forceps
straight hemostat
suture scissors
Timberlake obturator
towel clip
tubing clamp
urethrotome
wire scissors
Young needle holder
Young prostatic retractor

Appendix 9
Appendectomy

Adson clamp
Allis tissue clamp
Babcock clamp
Balfour center-blade retractor
Balfour retractor with fenestrated
  blade
bladder blade
Bookwalter retractor
Bovie cautery holder
Crile-Wood Vital needle holder
Harrington deep surgical scissors
Long forceps with teeth
Masson-Mayo-Hegar needle holder
Mayo-Hegar curved-jaw needle
  holder
Mayo needle holder

multitoothed cartilage forceps
needle holder
Ochsner scissors
probe with eye
regular forceps with teeth
Rochester-Ochsner scissors
Rochester scissors
self-retaining retractor
single-tooth forceps
smooth dressing forceps
sponge stick
Stille scissors
Stille Super Cut scissors
U.S. Army double-ended retractor
Weck clip applier
wire suture scissors

Appendix 10
Myringotomy

Armstrong grommet ventilation tube
Armstrong ventilation tube
Baldwin butterfly ventilation tube
Barton suction
Biolite ventilation tube
cotton ball
Donaldson ventilation tube
ear knife handle
ear speculum
Feuerstein split ventilation tube
Franco triflange ventilation tube
Frazier suction
Gelfoam pledget
Goode T-tube
Hubbard airplane vent tube
Klein ventilation tube
Lindeman-Silverstein ventilation tube
Moretz Tiny Tytan ventilation tube
Moretz Tytan ventilation tube
myringotomy drain tube
Paparella ventilation tube
Per-Lee ventilation tube

pledget
punch myringotomy system
Reuter bobbin collar button
Reuter bobbin ventilation tube
Rosen suction
Shah ventilation tube
Shea speculum
Sheehy collar button
Sheehy Tytan ventilation tube
Shepard grommet ventilation tube
Silverstein permanent aeration tube (SPAT)
Soileau Tytan ventilation tube
SPAT — Silverstein permanent aeration tube
Teflon collar button
T-grommet ventilation tube
Tiny-Tef ventilation tube
Tiny Tytan ventilation tube
Touma T-type grommet ventilation tube
T-tube
Tytan ventilation tube
Xomed-Treace ventilation tube

Appendix 11
Percutaneous Transluminal Coronary Angioplasty (PTCA)

angioplasty
arterial sheath
ASC Alpha balloon
ASC RX perfusion balloon catheter
atheroblation laser
balloon angioplasty
balloon-centered argon laser
balloon pump
Baxter Intrepid balloon
ELCA — Excimer laser coronary angioplasty
Eppendorfer catheter
exchange wire
Excimer laser
Excimer laser coronary angioplasty (ELCA)
fluorescence-guided "smart" laser
French JR4 Schneider catheter
French SAL catheter
French sheath
Goodale-Lubin catheter
guider
guide wire
guiding catheter with side hole
Hartzler dilatation catheter
helium-cadmium diagnostic laser
Hemashield collagen-enhanced graft
high-flow catheter
Hi-Per Flex wire
Hi-Torque floppy guide wire
Hi-Torque floppy with Propel
holmium laser
hot-tipped laser probe
Inoue balloon catheter
intra-aortic balloon
intravascular ultrasound (IVUS)
IVUS — intravascular ultrasound

J-guide wire
Kay balloon
Linx extension wire
Lo-Profile balloon
manifold
Medi-Tech balloon catheter
Mylar catheter
Nd:YAG laser
Nestor-3
Nestor guiding catheter
NL3 guider
Olbert balloon
percutaneous transluminal coronary angioplasty (PTCA)
phantom guide wire
phantom wire
Propel
PTCA — percutaneous transluminal coronary angioplasty
radiocontrast dye
rotational ablation laser
sapphire lens
scattergram
Seldinger arterial needle
Seldinger cardiac catheter
silk guide wire
Skinny balloon catheter
Slinky balloon
spectroscopy-directed laser
spirometer
TEC — transluminal extraction-endarterectomy catheter
Teflon coating
tip-deflecting wire
transluminal extraction-endarterectomy catheter (TEC)
ultrasound
USCI introducer